OXFORD CLINICAL GUIDELINES

Newly Qualified Doctor

OXFORD CLINICAL GUIDELINES

Newly Qualified Doctor

EDITED BY

David Fisher
Specialist in Internal Medicine, Clalit Healthcare Services, Israel

Liora Wittner
Resident in Family Medicine, Clalit Healthcare Services, Israel

WITH CONSULTANT EDITOR

Deborah Gill
Vice-President (Education & Student Experience), University of Southampton, Southampton, UK

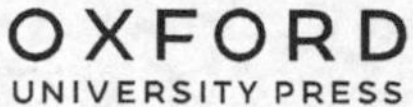

OXFORD
UNIVERSITY PRESS

OXFORD
UNIVERSITY PRESS

Great Clarendon Street, Oxford, OX2 6DP,
United Kingdom

Oxford University Press is a department of the University of Oxford. It furthers the University's objective of excellence in research, scholarship, and education by publishing worldwide. Oxford is a registered trade mark of Oxford University Press in the UK and in certain other countries

First Edition published in 2023

Published in the United States of America by Oxford University Press
198 Madison Avenue, New York, NY 10016, United States of America

British Library Cataloguing in Publication Data
Data available

Library of Congress Control Number: 2021947301

ISBN 978–0–19–883450–2

DOI: 10.1093/med/9780198834502.001.0001

Printed in the UK by
Ashford Colour Press Ltd, Gosport, Hampshire

Preface

Evidence-based guidelines have played an increasing role in medical practice in recent years. Healthcare professionals use guidelines to contend with the overwhelming wealth of available information and to translate scientific advances and new knowledge into safe clinical care.

The popularity of clinical guidelines has led to an exponential rise in guidelines being created since the 1980s and modern healthcare professionals are expected to be familiar with them. The General Medical Council's (GMC) *Good Medical Practice* guidance, which records what is expected of every GMC-registered doctor, states: 'You must be familiar with guidelines ... that affect your work'. Such a directive is challenging to uphold. First, the range of available guidelines in every speciality is vast and constantly expanding. Furthermore, individual guidelines can be dense and lengthy, and are therefore impractical to comb through for a professional wishing to acquaint themselves quickly with current clinical approaches.

This publication seeks to address that challenge. Written by junior doctors, each chapter summarizes the key clinical evidence-based guidelines which shape UK practice and presents the information in an accessible and concise format. Where relevant, chapters provide brief additional contextual points in order to explain the guideline for those less familiar with the field. Junior doctors, in particular foundation doctors, will find this resource useful to rapidly familiarize themselves with the latest clinical guidelines for the commonest conditions that they encounter in both primary and secondary care. Students will find this book useful as a quick reference guide to better understand the patient journey. They can also use it as a revision aid, as knowledge of guidelines is increasingly tested in medical school examinations.

Reading and learning every clinical guideline that is relevant to junior doctors is an arduous and almost impossible task. We hope that this book helps to bridge the gap and makes clinical guidelines more accessible to junior doctors, both for their benefit and also for the benefit of the patients that they treat.

Introduction: how to use this book

This book contains 123 chapters, covering a wide range of topics within internal medicine, surgery, emergency medicine, paediatrics, obstetrics and gynaecology, and psychiatry. The book is designed to cover the breadth of knowledge expected of a foundation doctor and it is pitched at this level. However, we would expect it to also be useful for medical students, specialist nurses, and junior specialist trainees (ST/CT 1–3 level).

This book is intended to be concise. Content which is relevant to multiple chapters will usually be noted once and other chapters will signpost to the primary mention.

Multiple guidelines exist for some topics and occasionally they conflict with each other in terms of their conclusions. It can be challenging for non-specialists to know which guideline they should follow. Each specialty section in this book has been overseen by at least one senior specialist consultant who has provided direction in identifying the most relevant and widely used guideline (or guidelines) to base each chapter upon. Readers should be aware that institutions often have their own local protocols which supersede the guidelines used in this publication.

The information in each chapter refers to adult patients only, except for chapters in the Resuscitation section (Part 17) where paediatric content is highlighted and chapters in the Paediatric section (Part 10). Where a drug is suggested as a treatment option, any dosages mentioned assume an otherwise healthy, non-pregnant adult with normal hepatic and renal function, and of average height and weight. Exceptions include chapters dealing with obstetrics, paediatrics, elderly medicine, hepatology, and nephrology. In all cases, the most recent *British National Formulary* or local protocols should be consulted to verify the drug choice, dosage, and any contraindications.

This book includes some investigation and management options that should only be considered under the guidance of a senior or specialist clinician, and they are highlighted as such. It is vital that junior professionals should be aware of their own limitations and not do anything that they are not competent to do.

Finally, please note that the information contained within these pages is for educational purposes only and should not be solely relied upon to direct the management of patients. The full guidelines are referenced at the start of each chapter and can be accessed online.

Acknowledgements

First and foremost, this book would not have been possible without the hard work of each chapter contributor. We are also grateful for the dedication of the Senior Editorial Board and for all of the reviews and advice that they provided.

We are appreciative of Professor Deborah Gill for her thoughtful oversight and helpful suggestions over the course of writing this book.

We are of course indebted to the wonderful team at Oxford University Press. We are grateful to each of the project managers that we have been fortunate to work with including Sam Callard, Mark Knowles, Fiona Sutherland, and most recently Sylvia Warren.

Most of all we would like to thank our commissioning editors Elizabeth Reeve and Geraldine Jeffers, who have provided us with their wealth of expert experience and have guided every step of this project to fruition. They have been a pleasure to work with and we are grateful for their support. As a brand-new concept which took time to perfect, this book has been a long time in the making, so finally, we would like to acknowledge all the 'OCG babies' born to the team since the start of this process, Tessa, Aurora, and Gidon!

Contents

Part 16 **Professional guidelines**

Part 17 **Resuscitation**

A-Z of all conditions

Index of emergency topics

Section editors

Rachel Ayers
2. Care of the elderly
Consultant in Geriatric Medicine, John Radcliffe Hospital, Oxford, UK

Andrew Baldwin
15. Cancer guidelines
GP Partner, East Sussex, UK

Robin Basu Roy
10. Paediatrics
Clinical Lecturer in Paediatric Infectious Disease, London School of Hygiene & Tropical Medicine, London, UK

Oliver Brain
4. Gastrointestinal
Consultant Gastroenterologist, Oxford University Hospitals NHS Trust, Oxford, UK

Laura Brown
2. Care of the elderly
Consultant in Geriatric Medicine, John Radcliffe Hospital, Oxford, UK

Chris Carson
Emergency editor
Accident and Emergency Registrar, University of Sheffield, Sheffield, UK

Jeremy Cobbold
5. Hepatobiliary
Consultant Hepatologist and Gastroenterologist, John Radcliffe Hospital, Oxford, UK

Ryan Devlin
6. Mental health
ST5 Doctor in General Adult Psychiatry, NHS Greater Glasgow and Clyde, Glasgow, UK

Andrew Greer
Emergency editor
Specialist in Intensive Care, Barnsley District General Hospital, UK

James Harrison
1. Cardiology
Consultant Cardiologist and Honorary Senior Lecturer, King's College Hospital NHS Foundation Trust, London, UK

Abdullah Jibawi
13. Surgery
Consultant Vascular, Endovascular, and General Surgeon; Academic Instructor to the Royal College of Surgeons of England, Ashford, and St Peter's Hospitals NHS Foundation Trust, UK

Nigel Lane
14. Miscellaneous
Consultant Physician, North Bristol NHS Trust, Bristol, UK

Suzanne Mason
Emergency editor
Professor of Emergency Medicine, University of Sheffield, Sheffield, UK

Kerry Munro
9. Obstetrics and gynaecology
Consultant Obstetrician, Queen Charlotte's and Chelsea Hospital, London, UK

Eleana Ntatsaki
12. Rheumatology and musculoskeletal
Consultant Rheumatologist, Ipswich Hospital NHS Trust, Ipswich, and Honorary Senior Lecturer, University College London, London, UK

William Petchey
7. Nephrology
Consultant Nephrologist, West Sussex NHS Foundation Trust, Bury St Edmonds, and Cambridge University Hospitals NHS Foundation Trust, Cambridge, UK

Bernard Prendergast
1. Cardiology
Professor of Interventional Cardiology and Valvular Heart Disease, Department of Cardiology, St Thomas' Hospital, London, UK

Rustam Rea
3. Endocrinology
Consultant in Diabetes and Acute Medicine, Oxford Centre for Diabetes, Endocrinology and Metabolism, Oxford University Hospitals NHS Foundation Trust, Oxford, UK

David Semple
6. Mental health
Consultant Psychiatrist, University Hospital Hairmyres, East Kilbride, and Honorary Fellow, Division of Psychiatry, University of Edinburgh, UK

Manjeet Shehmar
9. Obstetrics and gynaecology
Consultant in Gynaecology and Deputy Medical Director, Walsall Healthcare NHS Trust, Birmingham, UK

Helen Turner
3. Endocrinology and 16. Professional guidelines
Consultant in Endocrinology, Oxford Centre for Diabetes, Endocrinology and Metabolism, Radcliffe Department of Medicine, University of Oxford, Oxford, UK

Richard A. Watts
12. Rheumatology and musculoskeletal
Consultant Rheumatologist and Honorary Professor, Norwich Medical School, University of East Anglia, UK

Alastair Webb
8. Neurology
Consultant Neurologist and Wellcome Trust CRCD Fellow, Nuffield Department of Clinical Neurosciences, University of Oxford, Oxford, UK

Stephanie Wittmann
10. Paediatrics
Paediatrician, St Mary's Hospital, London, UK

Andrew Zurek
11. Respiratory
Consultant Respiratory Physician, Royal Berkshire Hospital, Reading, UK

Contributors

Sabrina Ahmed
GP Trainee
General Practice, Barking, Havering Redbridge University Hospitals NHS Trust
London, UK

Anna Maria Albert
Salaried GP
Manor Surgery
Oxford, UK

Mohammed Al-Talib
NIHR Academic Clinical Fellow in Renal Medicine
North Bristol NHS Trust
UK

James Andren
Anaesthetic Registrar
University Hospitals Sussex
Brighton, UK

Gabriella Bathgate
GP
North Central London CCG
London, UK

Darryl Ethan Bernstein
Core Surgical Trainee in Urology
East & North Hertfordshire NHS Trust
UK

George Blanchard
Specialist Registrar in Adult and Old Age Psychiatry
Mental Health Services for Older People Barnet
Enfield and Haringey Mental Health NHS Trust
UK

Harriet Blundell
General Medicine Registrar
St Bernard's Hospital
Gibraltar

Laura Brodie
Registered Medical Practitioner
Centre for Health and Disability Assessments
Maximus, Newcastle Upon Tyne
UK

Benjamin Bussmann
Cardiology Registrar
Royal Berkshire Hospital
Reading, UK

Stephanie Mei Yann Choo
Specialist Registrar in Renal Medicine
Hull Royal Infirmary
West Yorkshire, UK

Georgina Clark
Registrar
Obstetrics and Gynaecology
West Suffolk Hospital
Suffolk, UK

Ben Coombs
Specialty registrar in anaesthetics & intensive care medicine
Royal Air Force
Oxford, UK

John Creamer
Gastroenterology Registrar
Southmead Hospital
Bristol, UK

Angharad Everden
ST3 Haematology Registrar
Royal Cornwall Hospital
NHS Trust

David Fisher
Specialist in Internal Medicine
Clalit Healthcare Services
Israel

Harriet Gardner
ST3 in Obstetrics and Gynaecology
James Cook University Hospital
Middlesbrough, UK

Alison Hare
Core Trainee
Anaesthetics, Aneurin Bevan University Health Board
Wales

Vanessa Jessop
Adam Maxwell Internal Medicine Trainee Year 3
University Hospitals Bristol and Weston NHS Foundation Trust
UK

Georgios Karagiannis
Consultant Cardiologist
Department of Transplant
Harefield Hospital
London, UK

Thomas McCabe
NHS Ayrshire and Arran
Kilmarnock, UK
School of Medicine, Dentistry & Nursing
University of Glasgow
Glasgow, UK

Clemency Nye
Registrar in Infectious Diseases and Microbiology
University Hospital Wales
Cardiff, UK

Sarah Orr
Psychiatric Higher Trainee
South West Yorkshire Partnership

Tom Owens
ST4 in Emergency Medicine
Barts Health NHS Trust
London, UK

Bina Patel
Academic Clinical Fellow in Neurology
Addenbrookes Hospital
Cambridge, UK

Catharine Pearce
Speciality Training Registrar in Respiratory and General Internal Medicine
University Hospitals Plymouth NHS Trust
Devon, UK

Shervin Poladi
Royal Brompton and Harefield NHS
UK

Emma Shephard
Specialist Registrar in Obstetrics and Gynaecology
Torbay Hospital
Devon, UK

Prabhsimran Singh
Specialist Registrar in Gastroenterology
Hull University Teaching Hospitals
Hull, UK

Yasmin Smith
Obstetrics & Gynaecology Registrar
South West Deanery

Matthew Sutton
Anaesthetic Registrar
James Cook University Hospital
Middlesbrough, UK

Elizabeth Tan
ST3 in Geriatric Medicine
North West London Deanery
London, UK

Dinta Thakkar
General Practitioner and Health Tech Clinical Lead
Leicester, UK

Ashwini Virgincar
Anaesthetic Registrar
Chelsea and Westminster Hospital
London, UK

Rebecca Webb-Mitchell
Cardiology Registrar
South Tyneside and Sunderland NHS Foundation Trust
Newcastle upon Tyne, UK

Nicola West
GP ST3
West Midlands Deanery
UK

Samantha Williamson
Paediatric ST5 Doctor
North West Deanery
England

Liora Wittner
Resident in Family Medicine
Clalit Healthcare Services
Israel

Emily Yeung
Gateshead Health NHS Foundation Trust
QE Hospital
UK

Symbols and abbreviations

>	greater than
≥	greater than or equal to
<	less than
≤	less than or equal to
↓	decreased
↑	increased
↔	normal
⚑	red flag
±	with or without
2WW	2-week wait
4AT	4 'A's Test
5-ASA	5-aminosalicyclic acid
ABCDE	Airway, Breathing, Circulation, Disability, and Exposure
ABG	arterial blood gas
ABPM	ambulatory blood pressure monitoring
ACE	angiotensin-converting enzyme
ACR	albumin:creatinine ratio
ACS	acute coronary syndrome
ACTH	adrenocorticotropic hormone
AED	antiepileptic drug
AF	atrial fibrillation
AHT	antihypertensive treatment
AKI	acute kidney injury
ALF	acute liver failure
ALP	alkaline phosphatase
ALS	advanced life support
ALT	alanine aminotransferase
AMTS	Abbreviated Mental Test Score
ANA	antinuclear antibody
ANCA	antineutrophil cytoplasmic antibody
AP	anteroposterior
APH	antepartum haemorrhage
APTT	activated partial thromboplastin time
ARB	angiotensin receptor blocker
ArLD	alcohol-related liver disease
AS	aortic stenosis
ASA	American Society of Anesthesiologists
AST	aspartate aminotransferase
AUDIT	Alcohol Use Disorders Identification Test
AV	atrioventricular
AVPU	Alert, Voice, Pain, Unresponsive
BD	twice daily (*bis die*)
βHCG	beta-human chorionic gonadotropin
BMD	bone mineral density
BMI	body mass index
BNF	*British National Formulary*
BNP	B-type natriuretic peptide
BPE	benign prostatic enlargement
BPPV	benign paroxysmal positional vertigo
BSG	British Society of Gastroenterology
CABG	coronary artery bypass grafting
CAD	coronary artery disease
CAM	Confusion Assessment Method
CAMHS	child and adolescent mental health services
CBG	capillary blood glucose
CBT	cognitive behavioural therapy
CCP	cyclic citrullinated peptide
CD	Crohn's disease
CHF	chronic heart failure
CJD	Creutzfeldt–Jakob disease
CLD	chronic liver disease
COPD	chronic obstructive pulmonary disease
COX	cyclooxygenase
CPAP	continuous positive airway pressure
CPR	cardiopulmonary resuscitation
CRP	C-reactive protein
CRT	cardiac resynchronization therapy
CSF	cerebrospinal fluid
CT	computed tomography
CTG	cardiotocograph
CTPA	computed tomography pulmonary angiogram
DIC	disseminated intravascular coagulation

DKA	diabetic ketoacidosis
DMARD	disease-modifying antirheumatic drug
DNACPR	do not attempt cardiopulmonary resuscitation
DOAC	direct oral anticoagulant
DRE	digital rectal examination
DSM-5	*Diagnostic and Statistical Manual of Mental Disorders*, fifth edition
DVLA	Driver and Vehicle Licensing Agency
DVT	deep vein thrombosis
DXA	dual-energy X-ray absorptiometry
EACTS	European Association for Cardio-Thoracic Surgery
EASL	European Association for the Study of the Liver
ECG	electrocardiogram
EEG	electroencephalogram
eGFR	estimated glomerular filtration rate
ENT	ear, nose, and throat
EPU	early pregnancy unit
ESC	European Society of Cardiology
ESR	erythrocyte sedimentation rate
FFP	fresh frozen plasma
FiO_2	fraction of inspired oxygen
FMH	fetomaternal haemorrhage
FRII	fixed rate insulin infusion
FT3	free triiodothyronine
FT4	free thyroxine
GAD	generalized anxiety disorder
GBS	group B *Streptococcus*
GCA	giant cell arteritis
GCS	Glasgow Coma Scale
GDM	gestational diabetes mellitus
GFR	glomerular filtration rate
GI	gastrointestinal
GMC	General Medical Council
GORD	gastro-oesophageal reflux disease
GP	general practitioner
GTN	glyceryl trinitrate
Hb	haemoglobin
HbA1c	glycated haemoglobin
HBc	hepatitis B core antigen
HBPM	home blood pressure monitoring
HBsAg	hepatitis B surface antigen
HCC	hepatocellular carcinoma
HE	hepatic encephalopathy
HFpEF	heart failure with preserved ejection fraction
HFrEF	heart failure with reduced ejection fraction
HHS	hyperglycaemic hyperosmolar syndrome
HIV	human immunodeficiency virus
HLA	human leucocyte antigen
HRT	hormone replacement therapy
HSV	herpes simplex virus
IBD	inflammatory bowel disease
IBS	irritable bowel syndrome
ICD	implantable cardioverter defibrillator
ICS	inhaled corticosteroid
IL	interleukin
IM	intramuscular
INR	international normalized ratio
IPSS	International Prostate Scoring System
ITU	intensive therapy unit
IV	intravenous
JBDS	Joint British Diabetes Societies
JVP	jugular venous pressure
KDIGO	Kidney Disease: Improving Global Outcomes
LABA	long-acting beta-2 agonist
LBBB	left bundle branch block
LDH	lactate dehydrogenase
LFT	liver function tests
LKMA	liver kidney microsomal antibody
LMWH	low-molecular-weight heparin
LP	lumbar puncture
MC&S	microscopy, culture, and sensitivity
MDT	multidisciplinary team
MELD	Model for End-Stage Liver disease
MI	myocardial infarction
MPS	myocardial perfusion scintigraphy
MR	mitral regurgitation
MRI	magnetic resonance imaging
MSCC	metastatic spinal cord compression
NICE	National Institute for Health and Care Excellence

NSAID	non-steroidal anti-inflammatory drug
NSTEMI	non-ST-segment elevation myocardial infarction
NT-proBNP	N-terminal pro-B-type natriuretic peptide
NVP	nausea and vomiting in pregnancy
NYHA	New York Heart Association
OD	once daily (*omnie die*)
OGD	oesophagogastroduodenoscopy
$PaCO_2$	partial pressure of carbon dioxide in arterial blood
PaO_2	partial pressure of oxygen in arterial blood
PCI	percutaneous coronary intervention
PCR	polymerase chain reaction
PD	Parkinson's disease
PE	pulmonary embolism
PEF	peak expiratory flow
PET	positron emission tomography
PMR	polymyalgia rheumatica
PO	orally (*per os*)
PPH	postpartum haemorrhage
PPI	proton pump inhibitor
PRN	as required (*pro re nata*)
PSA	prostate-specific antigen
PSC	primary sclerosing cholangitis
PT	prothrombin time
PTH	parathyroid hormone
PTSD	post-traumatic stress disorder
QDS	four times daily (*quater die sumendus*)
RAS	renin–angiotensin system
RBBB	right bundle branch block
RCOG	Royal College of Obstetricians and Gynaecologists
RF	rheumatoid factor
S2	second heart sound
S3	third heart sound
S4	fourth heart sound
SABA	short-acting beta-2 agonist
SAVR	surgical aortic valve replacement
SC	subcutaneous
SGLT2	sodium–glucose cotransporter-2
SIGN	Scottish Intercollegiate Guidelines Network
SMA	smooth muscle antibody
SNRI	serotonin–noradrenaline reuptake inhibitor
SPECT	single-photon emission computed tomography
SpO_2	oxygen saturation
SSRI	selective serotonin reuptake inhibitor
STEMI	ST-segment elevation myocardial infarction
T1DM	type 1 diabetes mellitus
T2DM	type 2 diabetes mellitus
T3	triiodothyronine
T4	thyroxine
TAVI	transcatheter aortic valve implantation
TB	tuberculosis
TCA	Tricyclic antidepressants
TDS	three times daily (*ter die sumendus*)
TED	thyroid eye disease
TENS	transcutaneous electrical nerve stimulation
TFT	thyroid function tests
TIA	transient ischaemic attack
TIPSS	transjugular intrahepatic portosystemic shunt
TLoC	transient loss of consciousness
TNF	tumour necrosis factor
TSH	thyroid-stimulating hormone
TTE	transthoracic echocardiography
U&E	urea and electrolytes
UA	unstable angina
UC	ulcerative colitis
UGIB	upper gastrointestinal bleed
UKELD	United Kingdom Model of End-Stage Liver Disease
UPT	urine pregnancy test
USS	ultrasound scan
VBG	venous blood gas
VRII	variable rate insulin infusion
VT	ventricular tachycardia
VTE	venous thromboembolism
VZV	varicella zoster virus
WHO	World Health Organization

A note on terminology

It should be noted that where the term 'child' has been used, this refers to a 'child or young person'. The term 'parent' refers to 'parent, carer, or legal guardian'. Where guidelines apply to pregnancy, childbirth and other aspects of reproductive healthcare, the terms 'woman' or 'women' should be assumed to cover all people who can become pregnant and would need access to healthcare services in this capacity. Their gender identity should be respected at the point of care.

Part 1

Cardiology

Chapter 1

Acute coronary syndromes

Guidelines:
National Institute for Health and Care Excellence (NICE) CG95 (Recent-onset chest pain of suspected cardiac origin: assessment and diagnosis): https://www.nice.org.uk/guidance/cg95

NICE NG185 (Acute coronary syndromes): https://www.nice.org.uk/guidance/ng185

OUP disclaimer: Oxford University Press makes no representation, express or implied, that the drug dosages are correct and that the recommendations are an exclusive or mandatory course of care. All health professionals reading this text have a responsibility to evaluate its appropriateness and take the individual needs of the patient into account.

Local trust guidelines: please refer to your local guidelines as necessary.

Overview

Acute coronary syndrome (ACS) covers a spectrum of myocardial ischaemia (from least to most severe):

- Unstable angina (UA)—chest pain due to myocardial ischaemia at rest or minimal exertion, without myocardial necrosis
- Myocardial infarction (MI)—myocardial ischaemia resulting in myocardial necrosis. There are two types of MI:
    - Non-ST-segment elevation myocardial infarction (NSTEMI)
    - ST-segment elevation myocardial infarction (STEMI).

Diagnosis

The diagnosis of MI requires a rise and/or fall of cardiac biomarker values (preferably troponin), with at least one value above the 99th percentile of the upper reference limit and at least one of the following:

1. Symptoms of myocardial ischaemia (see 'History')
2. New (or presumed new) significant ST-segment/T wave changes or new left bundle branch block (LBBB) (Fig. 1.1)
3. Development of pathological Q waves (Fig. 1.2)
4. Imaging evidence of new myocardial loss or regional wall motion abnormality
5. Identification of an intracoronary thrombus by angiography.

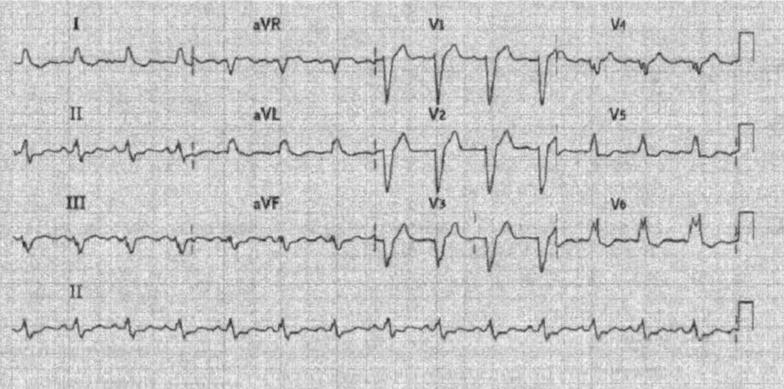

Fig. 1.1 Left bundle branch block.

Reproduced from Wilkinson I B et al (2017) 'Oxford Handbook of Clinical Medicine 10e' Oxford University Press: Oxford, with permission from Oxford University Press.

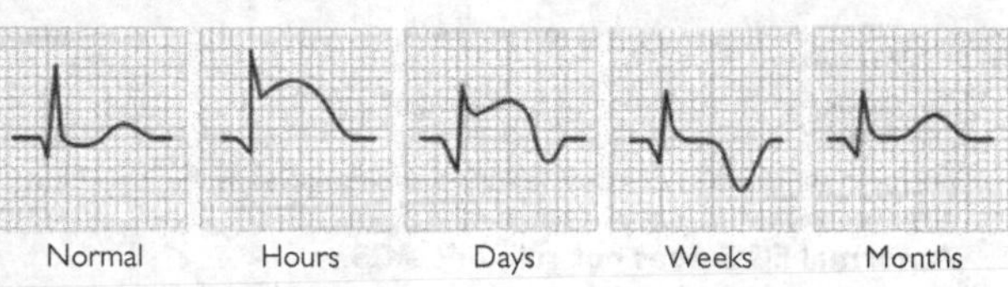

Fig. 1.2 Sequential electrocardiogram (ECG) changes following acute MI.

Reproduced from Wilkinson I B et al (2017) 'Oxford Handbook of Clinical Medicine 10e' Oxford University Press: Oxford, with permission from Oxford University Press.

History

- Characteristics of pain (site, whether pain is ongoing, time of onset, duration (>15 minutes), character, provoking and relieving factors, radiation)
- Associated symptoms, such as sweating, breathlessness, palpitations, and nausea or vomiting
- Presence of cardiovascular risk factors, e.g. type 2 diabetes mellitus, obesity, or hypercholesterolaemia

- Pre-existing diagnosis of ischaemic heart disease
- Previous investigations and interventions for ischaemic heart disease, e.g. percutaneous coronary intervention (PCI) or coronary artery bypass grafting (CABG)
- Bleeding risk factors which may be a contraindication for antithrombin therapy.

Examination

Assess haemodynamic status, the presence of ACS complications, and signs pointing to a non-ACS cause of chest pain.

Some examination findings may indicate heart failure (Table 1.1). This may be pre-existing, due to an unrelated cause such as decompensated aortic stenosis, or have developed as a result of a previous infarction.

Table 1.1 Possible ACS examination findings

B	Hypoxia Orthopnoea Bilateral crepitations
C	Blood pressure and heart rate changes (hypotension/hypertension ± bradycardia/tachycardia) Cool and clammy peripheries Arrhythmias Murmurs Raised jugular venous pressure (JVP)
E	Peripheral oedema Midline sternotomy scar

Investigations

- ECG—look for the presence of ST-segment and T wave changes, pathological Q waves, and new LBBB:
  - Perform serial ECGs or consider using additional leads if initial ECGs are non-diagnostic, e.g. posterior MI.
  - **A normal ECG does not rule out ACS.**
- Bloods—cardiac troponins, urea and electrolytes (U&E), full blood count (FBC), glycated haemoglobin (HbA1c), and lipid profile (Table 1.2)
- Chest X-ray—look for pulmonary oedema (see Chapter 2) or non-ACS causes of chest pain
- Echocardiogram:
  - Bedside echocardiography can detect new regional wall motion abnormalities or non-ACS causes of chest pain.

Table 1.2 Bloods in ACS

Cardiac troponins	Be aware that multiple troponin assays exist with different sensitivities and normal ranges. Interpret any results in line with local guidelines
U&E	Renal disease is a risk factor for ischaemic heart disease Knowledge of renal function is required when prescribing ACS treatments
FBC	Anaemia may exacerbate chest pain and is a relative contraindication for antithrombotic therapy
HbA1c	Diabetes is a risk factor for ischaemic heart disease
Lipid profile	Hyperlipidaemia is a risk factor for ischaemic heart disease

Management

Acute management

- Pain management:
  - Use intravenous (IV) opioids, e.g. diamorphine 1–5mg IV or morphine sulphate 5–10mg IV, titrated to effect. Also offer an antiemetic, e.g. metoclopramide 10mg IV
  - Give sublingual glyceryl trinitrate (GTN) if blood pressure allows (systolic blood pressure >100mmHg) or a GTN infusion if pain continues
- Antiplatelet therapy:
  - Aspirin 300mg loading dose unless known allergy
- Oxygen:
  - Do not give oxygen unless oxygen saturations <94% on room air
- Hyperglycaemia:
  - Keep glucose levels <11mmol/L. Use a variable rate insulin infusion if required
- Monitoring:
  - All patients with ACS should have regular pulse, blood pressure, heart rhythm, oxygen saturation, and pain monitoring.

STEMI

All patients with STEMI should be discussed with cardiology **immediately** as they may require emergency primary PCI or fibrinolysis—see Box 1.1.

Box 1.1 ACS reperfusion strategy

- Patients with STEMI should be considered for angiography with follow-on PCI if:
  - Presentation is within 12 hours of symptom onset and PCI can be delivered within 120 minutes
  - Presentation was >12 hours ago, but there is ongoing evidence of ischaemia or cardiogenic shock
- If angiography cannot be delivered within 120 minutes, offer fibrinolysis instead
- If an ECG shows residual ST elevation 60–90 minutes following fibrinolysis, offer immediate coronary angiography
- If there is recurrent myocardial ischaemia following successful fibrinolysis, consider angiography and PCI.

Source: data from NICE NG185.

STEMI with primary PCI

- Add prasugrel (or ticagrelor) alongside aspirin unless:
  - Age >75 years with a high bleeding risk (consider clopidogrel instead)
  - Patient already taking an oral anticoagulant (give clopidogrel instead)
- Drug-eluting stents are recommended
- If multivessel disease is found, it may be elected to perform PCI for all the diseased vessels and not just the vessel that is thought to have caused the STEMI.

STEMI without primary PCI

- Add ticagrelor (or prasugrel) alongside aspirin unless:
  - Bleeding risk is high (add clopidogrel or use aspirin alone).

NSTEMI

- Antithrombin therapy:
  - Fondaparinux 2.5mg subcutaneously (SC) to those without a high bleeding risk unless immediate coronary angiography is planned
  - Unfractionated heparin is preferred if significant renal impairment
- Perform Global Registry of Acute Coronary Events (GRACE) score (predicts 6-month mortality):
  - Offer coronary angiography as soon as possible if clinically unstable
  - Offer coronary angiography within 72 hours to patients with a predicted 6-month mortality >3%
  - Consider coronary angiography for patients with a predicted 6-month mortality ≤3% and subsequent ischaemia
  - Consider conservative management for patients with a predicted 6-month mortality ≤3% without ischaemia
- Antiplatelet therapy:
  - In patients undergoing angiography:
    - Add either ticagrelor (or prasugrel) alongside aspirin if not already taking an oral anticoagulant
    - Add clopidogrel alongside aspirin if already taking an oral anticoagulant
  - In patients not undergoing angiography:
    - Add ticagrelor (or prasugrel) alongside aspirin unless high bleeding risk
    - If bleeding risk is high, add clopidogrel alongside aspirin or use aspirin alone
- Drug-eluting stents are preferred.

Treatment after stabilization

Patient education

See Chapter 115 for driving restrictions following ACS

Lifestyle advice

- All patients should be offered a cardiac rehabilitation programme
- Offer smoking cessation support
- Provide lifestyle advice:
  - Encourage a Mediterranean-style diet
  - 20–30 minutes/day of exercise
  - Weight management
  - Moderation of alcohol intake.

Pharmacological therapy

- **Angiotensin-converting enzyme inhibitor** (ACE; e.g. ramipril 5mg) or **angiotensin receptor blocker** (ARB; e.g. valsartan 20mg BD) if intolerant:
  - Titrate to the maximum tolerated dose and continue long-term
  - Check renal function, electrolytes, and blood pressure prior to starting, after 1–2 weeks and then annually if stable
- **Dual antiplatelet therapy** (lifelong aspirin 75mg plus a second antiplatelet agent as previously specified for 12 months)

- **Beta-blocker** (e.g. bisoprolol 2.5mg), once haemodynamically stable:
  - Continue long-term if reduced left ventricular ejection fraction
  - Consider stopping after 12 months in patients with preserved left ventricular ejection fraction
  - **Calcium channel blockers** (e.g. diltiazem or verapamil) may be used if beta-blockers are contraindicated
- **Statin** (e.g. atorvastatin 80mg)
- For patients who have symptoms and/or signs of heart failure with reduced left ventricular ejection fraction, initiate treatment with an **aldosterone antagonist** (e.g. spironolactone 25mg).

Testing prior to discharge

- Perform an echocardiogram (to assess left ventricular function) for all patients who have had an MI. Consider performing for patients with UA
- Consider ischaemia testing in NSTEMI patients who have been managed conservatively
- Patients with reduced left ventricular ejection fraction should be considered for an implantable cardioverter defibrillator prior to discharge
- Check HbA1c levels and fasting glucose (≥4 days after onset of ACS) for any patients who were hyperglycaemic but without known diabetes:
  - Patients with hyperglycaemia are at ↑ risk for developing type 2 diabetes and should be monitored annually.

Further reading

1. European Society of Cardiology (2020). 2020 ESC Guidelines for the management of acute coronary syndromes in patients presenting without persistent ST-segment elevation. Available at: https://www.escardio.org/Guidelines/Clinical-Practice-Guidelines/Acute-Coronary-Syndromes-ACS-in-patients-presenting-without-persistent-ST-segm
2. European Society of Cardiology (2017). 2017 ESC/EACTS Guidelines for the management of valvular heart disease. Available at: https://www.escardio.org/Guidelines/Clinical-Practice-Guidelines/Acute-Myocardial-Infarction-in-patients-presenting-with-ST-segment-elevation-Ma

Chapter 2

Acute heart failure

Guideline:
NICE CG187 (Acute heart failure: diagnosis and management):https://www.nice.org.uk/guidance/cg187

OUP disclaimer: Oxford University Press makes no representation, express or implied, that the drug dosages are correct and that the recommendations are an exclusive or mandatory course of care. All health professionals reading this text have a responsibility to evaluate its appropriateness and take the individual needs of the patient into account.

Local trust guidelines: please refer to your local guidelines as necessary.

Overview

Acute heart failure is a medical emergency and arises when cardiac output cannot meet the requirements of the body. In adults, it is usually a consequence of myocardial damage, valvular dysfunction, and/or arrhythmias. For chronic heart failure, see Chapter 5.

Diagnosis

History

Patients with acute heart failure may present with:

- Shortness of breath on exertion or at rest
- Paroxysmal nocturnal dyspnoea
- Productive cough
- Orthopnoea
- Worsening peripheral oedema
- Generalized lethargy.

Examination

Systematically examine the patient using an ABCDE approach. On examination, you may find the following (Table 2.1):

Table 2.1 Acute heart failure examination findings

B	Cyanosis Bibasal coarse crepitations
C	Raised JVP (Box 2.1) Cool peripheries Prolonged capillary refill time Added S3 heart sound—'gallop' rhythm Irregularly irregular pulse (atrial fibrillation (AF)) Conjunctival pallor (anaemia)
E	Pitting oedema

Box 2.1 JVP

If you can't find the JVP, sit the patient up at a 45° angle and check below the earlobe.

Investigations

Investigations aim to demonstrate acute heart failure, and rule out common causes for decompensation, e.g. infection, acute cardiac events, arrhythmias, and malignant hypertension.

Bedside

ECG to indicate possible cause of heart failure e.g. ST/T wave changes (ACS; see Chapter 1), left ventricular hypertrophy (aortic stenosis or hypertension; see Chapter 3 or 6, respectively), or arrhythmias (e.g. AF; see Chapter 4)

Bloods

See Table 2.2.

Imaging

- **Chest X-ray**—posteroanterior film (Fig. 2.1)
- **Transthoracic echocardiogram**—perform within 48 hours to:
  - Measure severity of systolic/diastolic dysfunction
  - Identify structural abnormalities, e.g. valvular defects.

Table 2.2 Bloods for acute heart failure

Test	Indication
FBC	Anaemia may exacerbate heart failure
U&E	Renal disease is both a risk factor for heart failure and a potential consequence
HbA1c and lipid profile	Diabetes mellitus and hyperlipidaemia are risk factors for heart failure
Thyroid function tests (TFT)	Thyroid disease may cause heart failure
Liver function tests (LFT)	Liver damage can result from heart failure and alcohol can cause cardiomyopathy
B-type natriuretic peptide (BNP) or N-terminal pro-B-type natriuretic peptide (NT-proBNP)	These peptides are secreted in response to ventricular wall stress. AF, age, and renal failure may cause elevated levels. Obesity may be associated with lower levels **BNP <100ng/L** or **NT-proBNP <300ng/L suggests that heart failure is unlikely**

Source: data from NICE CG187.

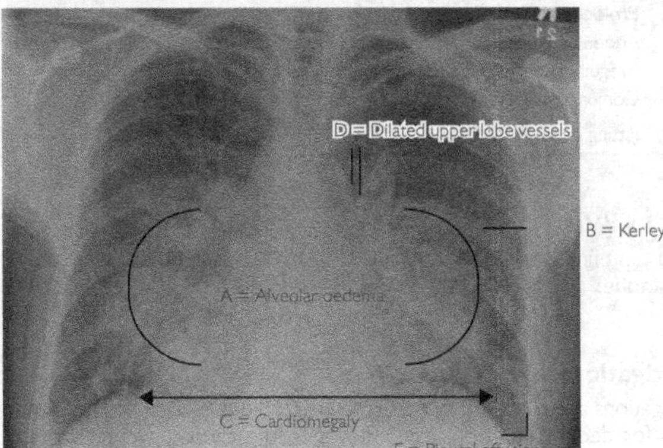

Fig. 2.1 Chest X-ray showing ABCDE findings suggestive of acute heart failure. A, alveolar oedema (batwing perihilar shadowing); B, Kerley B lines; C, cardiomegaly (cardiothoracic ratio of >0.5); D, dilated upper lobe vessels; E, pleural effusions.

Adapted from Wilkinson I B et al (2017) 'Oxford Handbook of Clinical Medicine 10e' Oxford University Press: Oxford, with permission from Oxford University Press.

Management

Acute management

- Oxygen if required to target saturations >94%. Sitting the patient up may improve oxygenation
- IV diuretics, unless hypoperfused, e.g. IV furosemide 40mg twice daily (BD). If already prescribed diuretics, consider a higher dosage
- Monitor U&E, weight, and urine output daily. Consider urinary catheterization.

Second-line options—discuss with a senior

- Nitrates are not routinely indicated and are contraindicated if the patient is hypotensive; however, they may be useful if the patient is extremely unwell, has coexisting myocardial ischaemia, or is hypertensive
- Inotropes or vasopressors should be considered in cardiogenic shock. Consider whether escalation to higher dependency care is appropriate
- Non-invasive ventilation is an option if the patient has cardiogenic pulmonary oedema, dyspnoea, or acidaemia. Invasive ventilation should be used if worsening respiratory failure, reduced consciousness, or exhaustion despite the above-mentioned treatments
- Consider renal replacement therapy if diuretic therapy is inadequate
- Opiates are not routinely indicated but may be used under specialist guidance.

Treatment after stabilization

All of the following apply to patients with reduced left ventricular ejection fraction.

Beta-blockers (first line)

- Decrease mortality
- Continue unless heart rate <50bpm, shock, or second/third-degree heart block
- Start or restart when patient is stable and monitor for 48 hours, e.g. bisoprolol 2.5mg once daily (OD) (uptitrate as tolerated)
- Side effects: bradycardia, hypotension.

ACE inhibitors (first line)

- Decrease mortality, e.g. ramipril 2.5mg OD (uptitrate as tolerated)
- Side effects: dry cough, hypotension
- Second line if ACE inhibitor not tolerated: ARB, e.g. losartan 12.5mg OD (uptitrate as tolerated).

Aldosterone receptor antagonists (first line)

- Decrease mortality, e.g. spironolactone 25mg OD or eplerenone 25mg OD.

Monitor clinical observations, serum creatinine, and electrolyte levels closely after any changes in treatment regimen.

Surgical management

- **Valve surgery:** surgical repair or replacement or percutaneous valve intervention (e.g. transcatheter aortic valve implantation (TAVI)) may be required for those with acute heart failure secondary to valve disease
- **Mechanical circulatory support:** for patients with potentially reversible severe acute heart failure or those who are candidates for transplantation. Specialist input ± transfer to tertiary centre required.

Further reading

1. Ramrakha P, Hill J (eds) (2012). Heart failure. In: *Oxford Handbook of Cardiology*, 2nd ed (pp. 367–416). Oxford: Oxford University Press. Available at: https://doi.org/10.1093/med/9780199643219.003.0007

Chapter 3

Aortic stenosis and mitral regurgitation

Guideline:
European Society of Cardiology (ESC)/ European Association for Cardio-Thoracic Surgery (EACTS) (2017 ESC/EACTS Guidelines for the management of valvular heart disease): https:// academic.oup.com/eurheartj/article/38/36/2739/4095039

OUP disclaimer: Oxford University Press makes no representation, express or implied, that the drug dosages are correct and that the recommendations are an exclusive or mandatory course of care. All health professionals reading this text have a responsibility to evaluate its appropriateness and take the individual needs of the patient into account.

Local trust guidelines: please refer to your local guidelines as necessary.

Overview

Aortic stenosis (AS) and mitral regurgitation (MR) are the two most common valvular pathologies in high-income countries. Patients often remain asymptomatic for an extended period before cardiovascular decompensation which leads to the onset of symptoms. In the asymptomatic phase, management involves optimization of cardiovascular risk factors and regular surveillance. The onset of symptoms is associated with a significant increase in adverse events and sudden cardiac death. Boxes 3.1 and 3.2 describe the aetiology of AS and MR, respectively.

Box 3.1 Aetiology of aortic stenosis

- Calcific degeneration of the aortic valve
- Bicuspid aortic valve
- Rheumatic heart disease
- Congenital.

Box 3.2 Aetiology of mitral regurgitation

- Primary—abnormality of mitral valve apparatus:
  - Degenerative
  - Connective tissue disease
  - Rheumatic fever
  - Infective endocarditis
  - Papillary muscle rupture
- Secondary—functional regurgitation due to distortion of the subvalvular apparatus with a structurally normal valve and chordae:
  - Left ventricular dilatation (ischaemic and non-ischaemic).

Diagnosis

History

Ask about:

- Presence of symptoms such as fatigue, exertional dyspnoea, angina, syncope, light headedness, and palpitations
- Presence of cardiovascular risk factors and comorbidities
- Functional status
- History of rheumatic fever.

Examination

Focus on detecting signs and complications of valvular heart disease (Table 3.1 and Fig. 3.1).

Table 3.1 Possible examination findings in patients with valvular pathology

	Aortic stenosis	Mitral regurgitation
B	Basal crepitations due to pulmonary oedema Hypoxia Orthopnoea	
C	Heaving apex beat Slow-rising central pulse Crescendo–decrescendo mid-systolic murmur radiating to the carotid arteries Soft second heart sound	Displaced apex beat Pansystolic murmur radiating to the axilla Third heart sound Soft first heart sound AF is common
E	Evidence of infective endocarditis (splinter haemorrhages, Osler nodes, Janeway lesions) Ankle oedema	

Investigations

Bedside

- **ECG:** look for evidence of left ventricular hypertrophy, left atrial dilatation, left axis deviation, LBBB, AF, or Q waves due to a previous infarct.

Bloods

See Table 3.2.

Imaging

- **Chest X-ray:** look for evidence of heart failure or valve calcification. In MR, cardiomegaly may be present due to left ventricular and atrial dilatation.

Other

- **Transthoracic echocardiography (TTE):** confirms diagnosis, severity, and aetiology.
- **Transoesophageal echocardiography:** sometimes used in MR or AS to further assess for concomitant valve pathology.

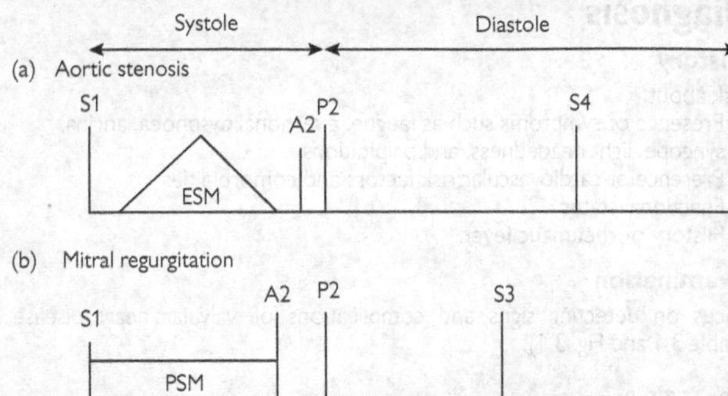

Fig. 3.1 Auscultation findings in aortic stenosis and mitral regurgitation. (a) There is a mid-systolic crescendo–decrescendo ejection systolic murmur that radiates to the carotid arteries. There may be reverse splitting or only a single audible second heart sound, due to delayed and softer aortic valve closure (A2). A fourth heart sound may be present due to forceful atrial contraction. (b) There is a pan-systolic murmur that radiates to the axilla. There is a soft first heart sound (S1) due to incomplete mitral valve closure, and there is splitting of the second heart sound due to early closure of the aortic valve (A2). A fourth heart sound may be present due to rapid ventricular filling. A2, aortic second heart sound; ESM, ejection systolic murmur; PSM, pansystolic murmur; P2, pulmonary second heart sound; S1, first heart sound; S3, third heart sound; S4, fourth heart sound.

Table 3.2 Blood

U&E	Kidney disease is a risk factor for atherosclerotic disease Knowledge of renal function is required when prescribing diuretics
FBC	Anaemia may exacerbate symptoms
HbA1c	Diabetes is a risk factor for atherosclerotic disease
Lipid profile	Hyperlipidaemia is a risk factor for atherosclerotic disease
BNP	Elevated BNP is a predictor of poorer outcomes

- **Exercise echocardiography:** sometimes used when there is evidence of severe AS or MR on echocardiography but the patient is asymptomatic. This test provides prognostic information and the presence of symptoms may justify early surgical management.
- **Cardiac magnetic resonance imaging (MRI), cardiac computed tomography (CT), and cardiac angiography:** these can provide additional information for surgical planning and prognostication.

Diagnostic criteria

See Table 3.3.

Table 3.3 Criteria for severe valvular disease

	Aortic stenosis	Mitral regurgitation
Clinical	Presence of symptoms (angina, dyspnoea, syncope)	
Qualitative	Left ventricular hypertrophy Valve morphology	
Quantitative	Peak trans-valvular pressure gradient >40mmHg Peak trans-valvular velocity >4m/s Valve area <1cm^2	Effective regurgitant orifice area >40mm^2 Regurgitant volume >60mL/beat Left atrial or left ventricular enlargement

Source: data from 2017 ESC/EACTS Guidelines for the management of valvular heart disease.

Management

Patient education

- Educate patients about the importance of follow-up and reporting symptoms as soon as they occur.

Lifestyle and simple interventions

- Support patients with weight loss, smoking cessation, diet modification, and exercise.
- Vigorous or anaerobic exercise is **contraindicated** in symptomatic AS patients.

Psychological interventions

- Palliative care input should be considered for symptomatic patients not eligible for interventional management.

Pharmacological management

There is no evidence that medical therapy improves the natural progression of AS or MR. The focus of medical management is:

1. To treat any modifiable cardiovascular risk factors (hypertension (see Chapter 6), Type 2 diabetes mellitus (see Chapter 26), hyperlipidaemia)
2. To manage underlying/concurrent heart failure (see Chapter 5)
3. To reduce preload in acute MR using nitrates and diuretics ± to use inotropes if there is haemodynamic instability
4. To attempt to maintain sinus rhythm in patients with AF (see Chapter 4).

Surgical management

The strongest indication for intervention is the onset of symptoms. Intervention can be surgical or percutaneous depending on the surgical risk of the patient. Decisions about timing and mode of intervention need to be made by a multidisciplinary heart team after considering individual risks and benefits of intervention.

Mitral regurgitation

- **Primary MR:** surgical repair is the preferred method of intervention, with percutaneous edge-to-edge repair reserved for patients with a high surgical risk. Surgery is indicated in severe disease, which is determined by the presence of symptoms, left ventricular ejection fraction (<60mmHg), pulmonary artery pressure (>50mmHg), and presence of AF
- **Acute MR:** if there is haemodynamic instability, an intra-aortic balloon pump may be used prior to intervention.

Aortic stenosis

- **Surgical aortic valve replacement (SAVR):** preferred mode of intervention in younger patients with severe symptomatic AS and low surgical risk
- **Transcatheter aortic valve implantation (TAVI):** intervention of choice in patients aged >75 years
- **Balloon valvuloplasty:** can be considered in haemodynamically unstable patients as a bridge to surgery or TAVI.

Valvular pathology and coronary heart disease

- In the presence of moderate AS, if CABG surgery is also required, patients should have an SAVR
- In the presence of moderate symptomatic MR, if CABG surgery is also required, patients should have a mitral valve repair at the same time.

Complications

Left ventricular remodelling (hypertrophy and/or dilatation), pulmonary hypertension, heart failure, AF (see Chapter 4), LBBB, and sudden cardiac death may occur as complications of the conditions. Infective endocarditis may occur as a complication of an intervention.

Monitoring and follow-up

In asymptomatic patients with severe MR or AS, 6-monthly follow-up is advised with careful screening for onset of symptoms and progression of echocardiographic parameters.

Further reading

1. EuroSCORE II surgical risk calculator. Available at: http://www.euroscore.org/calc.html

Chapter 4

Atrial fibrillation

Guideline:
NICE NG196 (Atrial fibrillation: diagnosis and management): https://www.nice.org.uk/guidance/ng196

OUP disclaimer: Oxford University Press makes no representation, express or implied, that the drug dosages are correct and that the recommendations are an exclusive or mandatory course of care. All health professionals reading this text have a responsibility to evaluate its appropriateness and take the individual needs of the patient into account.

Local trust guidelines: please refer to your local guidelines as necessary.

Overview

Atrial fibrillation (AF) is a common arrhythmia that results in dyssynchronous contraction of the atria relative to the ventricles. Patients with this condition have an increased risk of thromboembolism that may lead to stroke.

Diagnosis

History

About 25–30% of AF patients are asymptomatic (incidental finding). Others may present with:

- Shortness of breath
- Palpitations
- Chest discomfort
- Syncope or light-headedness
- Fatigue
- An embolic event (stroke, transient ischaemic attack (TIA); see Chapter 56).

Aim to identify any possible predisposing causes:

- Underlying infection
- Heavy alcohol intake
- Cocaine or marijuana use
- High caffeine intake
- Hypertension (see Chapter 6)
- Heart failure
- Structural heart disease:
  - Valvular (mitral stenosis or MR; see Chapter 3)
  - Congenital (atrial septal defect)
- Coronary artery disease
- Hyperthyroidism (see Chapter 19)
- Pulmonary conditions, e.g. chronic obstructive pulmonary disease (COPD; see Chapter 81), obstructive sleep apnoea.

Examination

- Perform a full cardiac examination including blood pressure
- Palpate for an irregularly irregular ± tachycardic pulse
- Auscultate for irregularly irregular tachycardia (if in AF with rapid ventricular rate) ± murmurs.

Investigations

Bedside

A 12-lead ECG (Fig. 4.1 and Box 4.1).

Box 4.1 Diagnosing atrial fibrillation

A diagnosis of AF requires ECG evidence of the following:

- Irregular RR intervals

AND

- Absence of visible P waves.

Bloods

Use blood tests to screen for possible underlying factors which might cause or exacerbate AF:

- FBC (anaemia)
- U&E and bone profile (electrolyte abnormalities, e.g. hyperkalaemia)

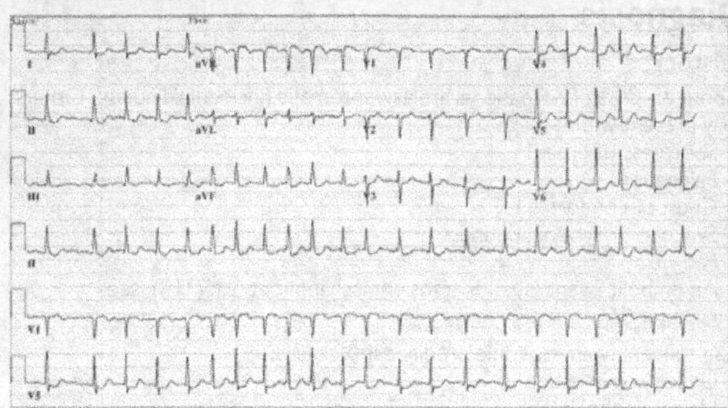

Fig. 4.1 Electrocardiogram rhythm strip demonstrating atrial fibrillation.

Reproduced from Wijdicks EFM et al (2016) 'Neurocritical Care 2e' Oxford University Press: Oxford, with permission from Oxford University Press.

- Thyroid screen (hyperthyroidism)
- Venous blood gas (lactate for infection)
- Coagulation profile (anticoagulation may be required)

Imaging

Transthoracic echocardiography

May reveal structural heart disease and/or presence of thrombus. It should be offered to all patients with AF.

Other

Ambulatory ECG monitoring

If suspected paroxysmal AF with multiple episodes in 24 hours, consider an ambulatory ECG monitor ('Holter'). If episodes are >24 hours apart, consider using a longer ambulatory ECG or other ECG technology (including an implantable loop recorder).

Management

Acute management

Aim to correct any reversible causes of recent-onset AF, such as infection and hypovolaemia, and consider the need for anticoagulation (Box 4.2). An overview of acute management is covered in Fig. 4.2.

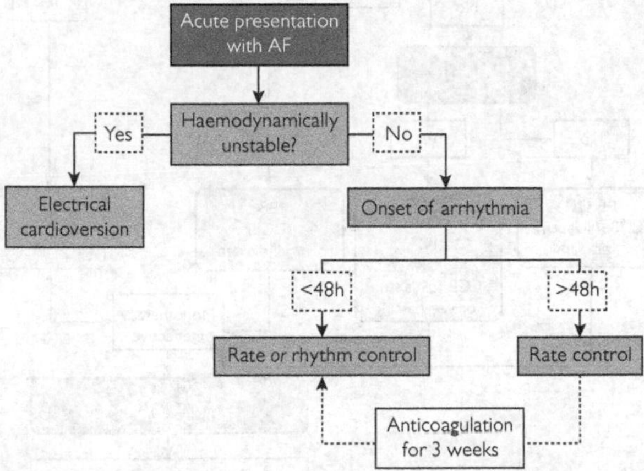

Fig. 4.2 The acute management of atrial fibrillation.

Box 4.2 Anticoagulation in the acute phase

- Do not delay emergency electrical cardioversion solely for achieving anticoagulation if haemodynamically unstable
- Give low-molecular-weight heparin (LMWH) until full risk assessment can be carried out.

Haemodynamically unstable

Urgent cardioversion is required (see Chapter 123).

Haemodynamically stable

Acute rate control

There is no clear evidence of an optimal target ventricular rate. A resting heart rate of <110bpm is acceptable. See Fig. 4.3, Box 4.3, and Table 4.1.

Acute rhythm control

If a rate control strategy has not worked, or if symptoms persist despite the heart rate being brought down, rhythm control should be considered.

This may be achieved using electrical or pharmacological cardioversion.

A rhythm control strategy is also more preferable than rate control for the following patient groups:

- AF with reversible cause
- Heart failure caused by AF
- New-onset AF (within 48 hours).

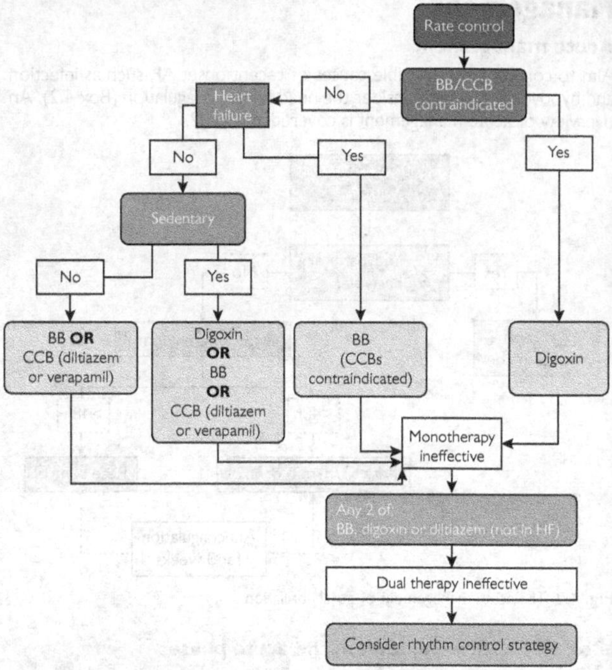

Rate control

BB/CCB contraindicated

No

Heart failure

No

Yes

Yes

Sedentary

No

Yes

BB **OR** CCB (diltiazem or verapamil)

Digoxin **OR** BB **OR** CCB (diltiazem or verapamil)

BB (CCBs contraindicated)

Digoxin

Monotherapy ineffective

Any 2 of: BB, digoxin or diltiazem (not in HF)

Dual therapy ineffective

Consider rhythm control strategy

Fig. 4.3 Choice of rate control therapy. BB, beta-blocker; CCB, calcium channel blocker; HF, heart failure.

Box 4.3 Which rate control therapy to choose?

- Beta-blockers or calcium channel blockers are first line
- Calcium channel blockers are contraindicated in pulmonary oedema or when left ventricular ejection fraction is <40%
- Digoxin may also be used first line if the patient is sedentary and/or a beta-blocker or calcium channel blocker cannot be given
- Any two of beta-blocker, diltiazem, and digoxin may be used in combination if rate control is inadequate with a single agent. Specialist advice is needed as this may cause bradycardia.
- Drug doses are listed in Table 4.1.

Source: data from NICE CG180.

Table 4.1 Drug doses for rate control in atrial fibrillation

Drug	Oral dose	IV dose (boluses)
Bisoprolol	1.25–10mg daily	
Metoprolol		2.5–10mg
Diltiazem (standard release)	120mg daily (unlicensed)	
Verapamil (standard release)	Up to 120 mg TDS	2.5–10mg
Digoxin	62.5–250mcg	500mcg (max. 1.5mg/24 hours)

Electrical cardioversion

This requires short-acting general anaesthesia or conscious sedation with anaesthetic support.

It may be used in conjunction with antiarrhythmic therapy (e.g. amiodarone) to increase the chance of success and lower the energy requirement.

If elective cardioversion is planned for AF which has been present for >48 hours, anticoagulation should be given for 3 weeks until cardioversion takes place, and then the need for long-term anticoagulation should be assessed (see 'Long-term anticoagulation'). Anticoagulation may not be necessary in this setting if a transoesophageal echocardiogram has excluded the possibility of a clot in the left atrium or left atrial appendage.

Pharmacological cardioversion

Flecainide can be given in an acute setting or may be self-administered by the patient ('pill in the pocket') as a single bolus (oral, 100 150mg) in an outpatient setting.

This is contraindicated in patients with structural, valvular, or ischaemic heart disease. Amiodarone is an alternative choice in these patients (IV, 5mg/kg over 20–120 minutes, maximum 1.2g/24 hours).

Treatment after stabilization

Long-term rhythm control

If onset of AF was >48 hours ago, electrical cardioversion can be considered after a period of at least 3 weeks of anticoagulation. To increase the success rate of electrical cardioversion, the use of amiodarone for **4 weeks before** and up to **12 months after** can be considered.

Long-term rate control

Drug choices are similar to those used in acute rate control (Table 4.1). Combination therapy is often required to achieve adequate control. Amiodarone is not normally offered as long-term rate control.

Long-term anticoagulation

The decision should be guided by clinical risk scores (Table 4.2) and reviewed at least annually.

Table 4.2 Stroke versus bleeding risks

CHA_2DS_2-VASc stroke risk score	ORBIT bleeding risk score
Congestive heart failure = 1 **H**ypertension (treated or untreated) = 1 **A**ge ≥75 = 2 **D**iabetes mellitus = 1 **S**troke or TIA = 2 **V**ascular (myocardial infarction, peripheral arterial disease, aortic plaque) = 1 **A**ge 65–74 = 1 **S**ex, female = 1	Anaemia (<13mg/dL in men, <12mg/dL in women) = 2 Age >74 = 1 Bleeding history = 2 GFR <60mL/min/1.73m² = 1 Treatment with antiplatelet agents = 1

CHA_2DS_2-VASc score: *consider* anticoagulation if score ≥1 in men and *offer* to men and women if ≥2

ORBIT score: ≤2 = low bleeding risk; 3 = medium bleeding risk; 4–7 = high bleeding risk

Adapted from Lip GYH, Nieuwlaat R, Pisters R, Lane DA, Crijns HJGM. Refining clinical risk stratification for predicting stroke and thromboembolism in atrial fibrillation using a novel risk factor-based approach: the Euro Heart Survey on atrial fibrillation. Chest. 2010 Feb;137(2):263–72 and O'Brien EC, Simon DN, Thomas LE, Hylek EM, Gersh BJ, Ansell JE, Kowey PR, Mahaffey KW, Chang P, Fonarow GC, Pencina MJ, Piccini JP, Peterson ED. The ORBIT bleeding score: a simple bedside score to assess bleeding risk in atrial fibrillation. Eur Heart J. 2015 Dec 7;36(46):3258–64.

If anticoagulation is recommended, offer a direct oral anticoagulant (DOAC) (rivaroxaban, apixaban, dabigatran, edoxaban) first line. If contra-indicated, not tolerated, or unsuitable, offer warfarin.

If anticoagulation is not appropriate, left atrial appendage occlusion can be considered.

Patients who are taking long-term anticoagulation should be monitored and supported to improve any other risk factors for bleeding including uncontrolled hypertension, labile international normalized ratio (INR), interacting medications, excessive alcohol intake, and reversible causes of anaemia.

If the patient is at risk of falling or elderly, these reasons alone are not a justification for withholding anticoagulation.

Special considerations

Ablation

Ablation is considered when medical treatment has failed, is not appropriate, or concomitant heart failure is present. This can take the form of atrioventricular node ablation, left atrial catheter or surgical ablation.

Long-term anticoagulation should be considered if there is a risk of recurrence (see 'Long-term anticoagulation').

Postoperative atrial fibrillation

Rhythm control is preferred over rate control following cardiothoracic surgery.

Further reading

1. Kirchhof P, Benussi S, Kotecha D, et al. (2016). ESC Guidelines for the management of atrial fibrillation developed in collaboration with EACTS. *Eur Heart J*. 37:2893–962.
2. Scottish Intercollegiate Guidelines Network (2014). Prevention of stroke in patients with atrial fibrillation. Available at: https://www.sign.ac.uk/assets/af_publication.pdf
3. Royal College of Emergency Medicine Learning (2019). Atrial fibrillation. Available at: https://www.rcemlearning.co.uk/reference/atrial-fibrillation/

Chapter 5

Chronic heart failure

Guideline:
NICE NG106 (Chronic heart failure in adults: diagnosis and management): https://www.nice.org.uk/guidance/ng106

OUP disclaimer: Oxford University Press makes no representation, express or implied, that the drug dosages are correct and that the recommendations are an exclusive or mandatory course of care. All health professionals reading this text have a responsibility to evaluate its appropriateness and take the individual needs of the patient into account.

Local trust guidelines: please refer to your local guidelines as necessary.

Overview

The population of patients who suffer from chronic heart failure (CHF) is increasing. CHF may be divided into left- and right-sided failure. Left-sided failure often develops due to coronary heart disease and, as it worsens, can lead to right-sided failure. CHF may also be divided into heart failure with reduced ejection fraction (HFrEF) (ejection fraction <40%) and heart failure with preserved ejection fraction (HFpEF) (ejection fraction ≥40%).

Diagnosis

History

Symptoms include dyspnoea, orthopnoea, paroxysmal nocturnal dyspnoea, ankle swelling, and reduced exercise tolerance. Less commonly, patients may report nocturnal cough, wheezing, and weight gain.

The New York Heart Association (NYHA) classification divides CHF into four classes based on symptoms and functional limitation (Table 5.1).

Table 5.1 The NYHA functional classification system

Class	Description
I	No limitation
II	Slight limitation
III	Marked limitation
IV	Symptoms present at rest

Source: Dolgin M, New York Heart Association NYH, Fox AC, Gorlin R, Levin RI, New York Heart Association. Criteria Committee. Nomenclature and criteria for diagnosis of diseases of the heart and great vessels. 9th ed. Boston, MA: Lippincott Williams and Wilkins; March 1, 1994.

Examination

- **General signs:** cachexia, tachypnoea
- **Neck signs:** elevated JVP, hepatojugular reflux
- **Cardiac signs:** laterally displaced apex beat, S3, S4, gallop rhythm, pansystolic murmur
- **Respiratory signs:** bilateral coarse crepitations, pleural effusion (dull percussion, reduced air entry)
- **Abdominal signs:** hepatomegaly, ascites
- **Peripheral signs:** peripheral oedema (ankle, sacral).

Investigations

Bedside

Electrocardiography (ECG)

It is unusual to have CHF with a normal ECG. Pathological changes may include:

- Pathological Q waves (previous infarction)
- LBBB
- AF
- Non-specific ST/T wave changes.

Consider for evaluation of risk factors

- **Urinalysis:** may show glycosuria (diabetes) or proteinuria (renal disease)
- **Peak flow:** COPD.

Bloods

- FBC
- U&E (in anticipation of diuretic therapy)
- LFT (may be abnormal in right-sided heart failure or may indicate excessive alcohol intake which can lead to CHF)
- TFT (thyrotoxicosis and hypothyroidism are risk factors for CHF)
- HbA1c (diabetes is a risk factor for CHF)
- NT-proBNP or BNP (Box 5.1).

Box 5.1 NT-proBNP and BNP

The heart produces the hormones NT-proBNP and BNP when the ventricles are stretched. The serum levels of NT-proBNP and BNP have a high negative predictive value and are prognostic. They are used to stratify the urgency of investigations:

- **NT-proBNP <400ng/L (or BNP <100pg/mL):** CHF unlikely
- **NT-proBNP 400–2000ng/L (or BNP 100–400pg/mL):** TTE, specialist review within 6 weeks
- **NT-proBNP >2000ng/L (or BNP <400pg/mL):** TTE, specialist review within 2 weeks.

Note that levels may be lower in some people with obesity or African/African-Caribbean heritage or who are taking drugs such as ACE inhibitors. They may be higher in patients aged >70 years, or those with conditions such as COPD, renal disease, or diabetes.

Imaging

TTE should be performed in patients with raised NT-proBNP or an abnormal ECG to assess:

- Valvular function
- Systolic and diastolic ventricular function
- Intracardiac shunts (atrial or ventricular septal defects, or patent foramen ovale)
- Pulmonary artery systolic pressure (suggestive of right-sided heart failure if raised)
- Wall motion abnormalities (evidence of a previous cardiac event).

Cardiac MRI, transoesophageal echocardiography, or radionuclide angiography can be considered if TTE images are poor.

Chest X-ray is recommended to exclude other causes of dyspnoea. There may be evidence of cardiomegaly and other signs which are typically seen in acute heart failure (see Chapter 2).

Management

Lifestyle and simple interventions

Encourage patients to:

- Limit salt intake to <6 g/day (approximately 1.5 teaspoons). Salt substitutes are not advisable as they contain high levels of potassium
- Stop smoking
- Avoid excessive alcohol consumption
- Participate in an exercise-training programme (cardiac rehabilitation) if they have stable CHF (NYHA class II–III).

Psychological interventions

Depression is common in CHF and cognitive behaviour therapy (CBT) can be considered.

Pharmacological management

The pharmacological therapies in Fig. 5.1 have been shown to improve mortality in HFrEF (ejection fraction <40%).

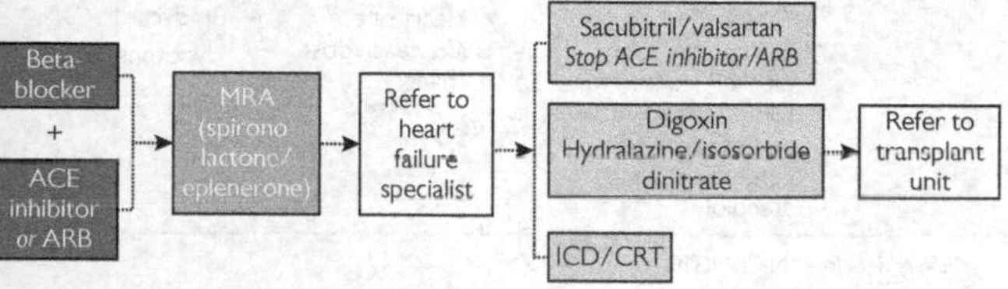

Fig. 5.1 Pharmacological treatment flowchart for heart failure with reduced ejection fraction. ACE, angiotensin-converting enzyme; ARB, angiotensin II receptor blocker; CRT, cardiac resynchronization therapy; ICD, implantable cardioverter defibrillator; MRA, mineralocorticoid receptor antagonist.

Prognostic therapy

First line therapy

All patients should be started on (Table 5.2):

1. ACE inhibitor, or an ARB if intolerant
2. Beta-blocker.

Second-line therapy

- Mineralocorticoid receptor antagonists are offered as an additional therapy if symptoms persist, e.g. spironolactone 25mg OD
- Contraindications include significant hyperkalaemia and renal dysfunction (stage 3 chronic kidney disease (CKD) or worse)
- Monitor U&E and blood pressure before starting and after every dose change. Monitor monthly for 3 months, and then twice a year.

Specialist medication

- Hydralazine or isosorbide dinitrate
- Sacubitril with valsartan
- Ivabradine
- Digoxin.

Table 5.2 First-line treatment for heart failure with reduced ejection fraction

Drug	How to use	Monitoring	Important side effects
ACE inhibitor	• Start with a low dose, e.g. ramipril 2.5mg OD • Increase dose every 2 weeks until maximum tolerated dose or maximum dose reached	• U&E 1–2 weeks after initiation and each titration • Blood pressure before and after each dose change • Review monthly for 3 months, then twice a year	• Angioedema • Cough • Electrolyte imbalance • Kidney injury • Hypotension
ARB	• Start with a low dose, e.g. losartan 12.5mg OD • Increase dose every 2 weeks until maximum tolerated dose or maximum dose reached		• Electrolyte imbalance • Kidney injury • Hypotension
Beta-blockers	• Start with a low dose, e.g. bisoprolol 2.5mg OD • Switch to a beta-blocker licensed for CHF if already on another type for comorbidity, e.g. atenolol	• As for ACE inhibitor/ARB • Heart rate after each dose change	• Worsening symptoms • Bradycardia • Hypotension

Source: data from NICE NG106.

Symptomatic therapy

Diuretics (usually loop, occasionally thiazides) are used to manage fluid overload or congestion, e.g. furosemide 40mg OD initially in patients with either HFrEF or HFpEF.

Surgical management

Cardiac resynchronization therapy (CRT) and implantable cardioverter defibrillator (ICD)

CRT and ICD therapy are indicated for patients who have HFrEF, with left ventricular ejection fraction ≤35%.

CRT encompasses CRT-D (with defibrillator) and CRT-P (pacing only). The choice between ICD, CRT-D, and CRT-P depends on the presence of LBBB, QRS duration, and NYHA class.

Valve replacement

Some patients may benefit from a transcatheter mitral valve repair[1] if:

- They have symptomatic heart failure despite maximal medical therapy **AND**

1 Stone GW, Lindenfeld JL, Abraham WT, et al. Transcatheter mitral valve repair in patients with heart failure. *N Engl J Med.* 2018; 379:2307–18.

- Moderate–severe or severe secondary MR (e.g. secondary to a myocardial infarction).

Cardiac transplantation

Patients with drug-refractory severe CHF and refractory cardiogenic shock should be referred to specialist CHF centres to be assessed for their suitability for transplantation.

Monitoring and follow-up

A minimum of 6-monthly clinical reviews should be offered.

Patients should be educated to monitor their weight at home, and to report any clinical deterioration (>1.5–2kg weight gain in 2 days) to expedite an early assessment.

Special considerations

Chronic kidney disease

Concomitant renal disease is common in CHF. This group of patients are at a higher risk of hyperkalaemia with ACE inhibitor, ARB, diuretic, and mineralocorticoid receptor antagonist use. Consider lower and/or slower titration of doses if eGFR is <45mL/min/1.73m^2, and liaise with the renal team if eGFR is <30mL/min/1.73m^2.

Heart failure with preserved ejection fraction

Empagliflozin has been demonstrated to reduce the risk of hospitalization and cardiovascular death due to HFpEF[2].

Further reading

1. Scottish Intercollegiate Guidelines Network (SIGN) (2016). *Management of Chronic Heart Failure*. Edinburgh: SIGN; 2016. Available at: https://www.sign.ac.uk/assets/sign147.pdf

2 Anker SD, Butler J, Filippatos G, et al. Empagliflozin in heart failure with a preserved ejection failure. *N Engl J Med*. 2021; 385:1451–61.

Chapter 6

Hypertension

Guideline:
NICE NG136 (Hypertension in adults: diagnosis and management): https://www.nice.org.uk/guidance/ng136

OUP disclaimer: Oxford University Press makes no representation, express or implied, that the drug dosages are correct and that the recommendations are an exclusive or mandatory course of care. All health professionals reading this text have a responsibility to evaluate its appropriateness and take the individual needs of the patient into account.

Local trust guidelines: please refer to your local guidelines as necessary.

Overview

Hypertension is known as the 'silent killer'. This is because it is most commonly asymptomatic but chronically, and occasionally acutely, it can lead to end-organ damage which is life-limiting. In the majority of cases, hypertension is primary (essential hypertension), but some cases may be due to a secondary cause (Table 6.1).

Table 6.1 Secondary causes of hypertension

Renovascular	Bilateral renal disease, e.g. glomerulonephritis, interstitial nephritis, diabetic nephropathy
	Renal artery stenosis
	Coarctation of the aorta
Endocrine	Thyrotoxicosis
	Conn's syndrome
	Phaeochromocytoma
	Acromegaly
	Cushing's syndrome
Drug induced	Ciclosporin, cocaine, contraceptives
Other	Obstructive sleep apnoea

Diagnosis

History

Patients with accelerated (malignant) hypertension (Box 6.1) may report headache or may have signs or symptoms of secondary causes of hypertension.

Examination

Feel the pulse prior to measuring blood pressure. Automated blood pressure machines should be avoided in patients with an irregular pulse.

If the blood pressure is raised in one arm and hypertension is suspected, measure the blood pressure in the other arm as well. If there is a difference in readings >15mmHg, repeat the measurements. If the difference of >15mmHg persists, use the arm with the higher reading in future to assess the blood pressure (Fig. 6.1). Consider pathological causes for blood pressure discrepancy >15mmHg between the arms, e.g. peripheral arterial disease, aortic dissection or aneurysm, Takayasu's arteritis, subclavian steal syndrome, and thoracic inlet syndrome.

If the blood pressure is >140/90mmHg on the first reading, repeat the measurement. If the second measurement is significantly different, perform a third measurement and use the lower blood pressure of the last two readings (Fig. 6.1).

Investigations

Diagnosis

See Table 6.2 and Box 6.1.

Ambulatory blood pressure monitoring (ABPM)

Two measurements should be taken per hour during waking hours, generating at least 14 measurements to diagnose hypertension.

Home blood pressure monitoring (HBPM)

This is an alternative for those unable to tolerate ABPM. Two measurements are taken twice daily for 4–7 days. Hypertension can be confirmed by averaging all the measurements (exclude measurements on day 1).

If stage 3 hypertension is accompanied by retinal haemorrhage or papilloedema, this is accelerated (malignant) hypertension and is a medical emergency (see Box 6.1).

Assessing cardiovascular risk

- Serum HbA1c, total cholesterol, and high-density lipoprotein cholesterol should be measured.

Assessing target organ damage

See Table 6.3.

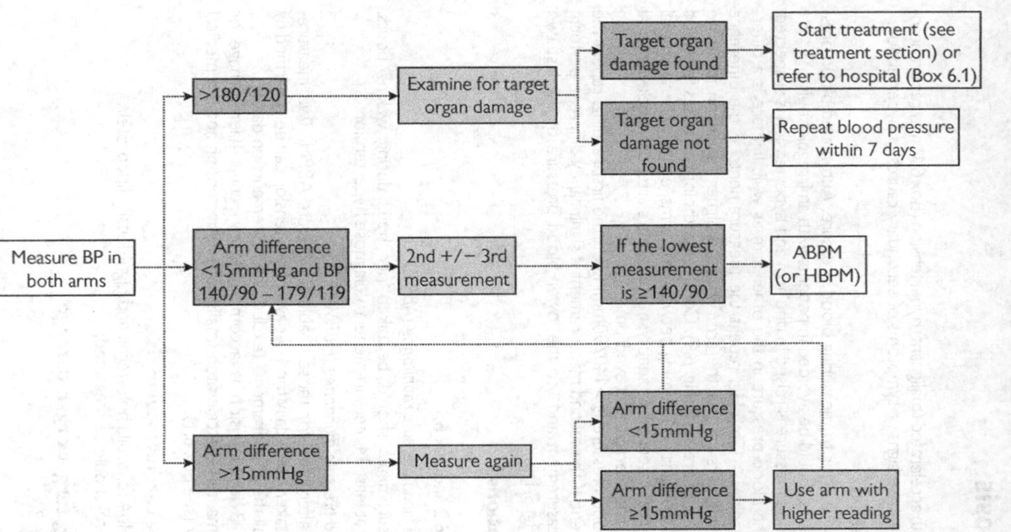

Fig. 6.1 Diagnosing hypertension. ABPM, ambulatory blood pressure monitoring; HBPM, home blood pressure monitoring.

Table 6.2 Definitions of hypertension (both required for diagnosis)

Stage	Clinic reading	ABPM or HPBM
1	≥140/90mmHg	≥135/85mmHg
2	≥160/100mmHg	≥150/95mmHg
3 (severe)	≥180mmHg systolic, or ≥120mmHg diastolic	N/A

Source: data from NICE NG136.

Box 6.1 Who to refer to hospital urgently (same day)

- Blood pressure >180/120mmHg and:
  - Signs of retinal haemorrhage or papilloedema (accelerated/ malignant hypertension) **OR**
  - New-onset confusion **OR**
  - Chest pain **OR**
  - Signs of heart failure **OR**
  - Acute kidney injury (AKI)
- Phaeochromocytoma is suspected (classic triad of symptoms is headache, palpitations, and sweating although the absence of these symptoms does not exclude it).

Source: data from NICE NG136.

Table 6.3 Investigating for target organ damage

Target organ	Investigation	Changes which may be seen due to hypertension
Eyes	Fundoscopy	Changes of hypertensive retinopathy, e.g. arteriovenous nipping, haemorrhage, cotton wool spots, papilloedema
Heart	12-lead ECG	Left ventricular hypertrophy
Kidneys	Urine analysis	Raised albumin:creatinine ratio (ACR), proteinuria Haematuria
	Bloods	Raised creatinine, reduced estimated glomerular filtration rate (eGFR)

Source: data from NICE NG136.

Chronic management

Patient education

Unwanted side effects of antihypertensive treatment are common. Information on the importance of good blood pressure control should be provided to patients to encourage compliance.

Lifestyle and simple interventions

Many simple lifestyle interventions, such as having a healthy balanced diet, can help to reduce blood pressure. Advice should include:

- Adequate exercise (minimum of 30 minutes of moderate intensity exercise, 5 days a week)[1]
- Avoiding excessive salt in the diet
- Avoiding excessive caffeine consumption
- Alcohol intake should be within recommended limits
- Smoking cessation is helpful in reducing overall cardiovascular risk.

Pharmacological management

Stage 1 or 2 hypertension may be diagnosed following a raised clinic blood pressure reading **AND** a raised ABPM or HBPM reading.

Treat if:

- Age <80 years, stage 1 hypertension, with:
  - Target organ damage (Table 6.2)
  - Established cardiovascular disease
  - Renal disease
  - Diabetes
  - ≥10% 10-year cardiovascular risk
- Stage 2 or 3 hypertension
- Target organ damage is found on examination (commence treatment prior to ABPM/HBPM result).

Consider drug treatment in stage 1 hypertension if:

- Age >80 years and blood pressure is >150/90mmHg
- Age <60 years and 10-year cardiovascular risk is estimated to be <10%

Choice of pharmacological therapy is summarized in Fig. 6.2.

Specialist referral

Evaluation of secondary hypertension by a specialist should be considered in patients <40 years with hypertension.

Complications

Hypertension is a common and major risk factor for cardiovascular diseases, CKD, and premature death.

Monitoring and follow-up

Target clinic blood pressure measurements are age dependent and as follows:

- Age <80 years: <140/90mmHg
- Age ≥80 years: <150/90mmHg.

1 NICE Clinical Knowledge Summaries. Obesity. Scenario: management. 2017. Available at: https://cks.nice.org.uk/obesity#!scenario

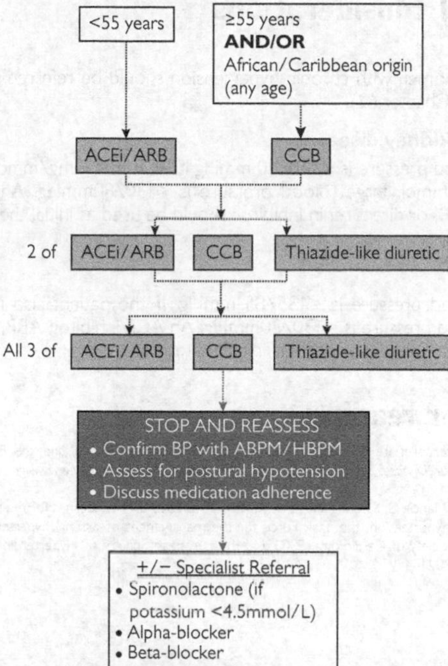

Fig. 6.2 Pharmacological treatment of hypertension. ACEi, angiotensin-converting enzyme inhibitor; ARB, angiotensin receptor blocker; BP, blood pressure; CCB, calcium channel blocker.

ABPM or HBPM can be considered if patient has significant 'white coat' hypertension, with the following targets:

- Age <80 years: <135/85mmHg
- Age ≥80 years: <145/85mmHg.

Review of blood pressure control and other cardiovascular risk factors should take place at least annually.

If an ACE inhibitor or an ARB are used concurrently with multiple diuretics, close monitoring (initially at 1 month) of electrolytes and renal function is required.

Special considerations

Pregnancy

Pregnant women with chronic hypertension should be referred to a specialist (see Chapter 62).

Chronic kidney disease

Target blood pressure is <140/90 mmHg if ACR is <70mg/mmol. If ACR is >70mg/mmol, target blood pressure is <130/80mmHg. An ACE inhibitor, ARB, or direct renin inhibitor should be used as initial therapy (see Chapter 47).

Diabetes

Target blood pressure is <135/85 mmHg. If the patient also has CKD, target blood pressure is <130/80mmHg. An ACE inhibitor, ARB, or direct renin inhibitor should be used as initial therapy.

Further reading

1. Scottish Intercollegiate Guidelines Network (2017). *Risk Estimation and the Prevention of Cardiovascular Disease*. Edinburgh: SIGN; 2017. Available at: https://www.sign.ac.uk/assets/sign149.pdf
2. Williams L, Mancia G, Spiering W, et al. (2018). 2018 ESC/ESH Guidelines for the management of arterial hypertension: the Task Force for the management of arterial hypertension of the European Society of Cardiology (ESC) and the European Society of Hypertension (ESH). *Eur Heart J*. 39:3021–4.

Chapter 7

Pericardial diseases

Guideline:
ESC (2015 ESC Guidelines for the diagnosis and management of pericardial diseases): https://academic.oup.com/eurheartj/article/36/42/2921/2293375

OUP disclaimer: Oxford University Press makes no representation, express or implied, that the drug dosages are correct and that the recommendations are an exclusive or mandatory course of care. All health professionals reading this text have a responsibility to evaluate its appropriateness and take the individual needs of the patient into account.

Local trust guidelines: please refer to your local guidelines as necessary.

Overview

Pericarditis, pericardial effusions, cardiac tamponade, and constrictive pericarditis are all forms of pericardial disease. The causes of pericardial disease include infection, myocardial infarction, uraemia, autoimmune disease, sarcoidosis, malignancy, and radiotherapy. Tuberculosis (TB) is a common cause in endemic countries.

Diagnosis

History/diagnostic criteria

Acute pericarditis

An inflamed pericardium usually causes pericarditic (pleuritic) chest pain, which is improved by sitting up and leaning forward. There may be symptoms suggesting the underlying aetiology, e.g. fever, weight loss, or cough. Viruses are a common cause of pericarditis. See Box 7.1 for diagnostic criteria.

Box 7.1 Diagnostic criteria for pericarditis (≥2 out of 4 criteria required)

- Pericarditic chest pain
- Pericardial rub
- ECG changes: new widespread ST elevation or PR depression
- Pericardial effusion (new or worsening).

Source: data from 2015 ESC Guidelines for the diagnosis and management of pericardial diseases.

Pericardial effusion and cardiac tamponade

Normally, pericardial fluid lubricates the pericardial layers. However, pathological accumulation of pericardial fluid can compress the heart causing dyspnoea, orthopnoea, and chest pain.

Cardiac tamponade is a medical emergency where rapid pericardial accumulation of fluid, pus, blood, or gas (e.g. from inflammation, trauma, rupture of the heart, or aortic dissection) compresses the heart to the point of cardiogenic shock and haemodynamic instability.

Constrictive pericarditis

A tight and fibrosed pericardium can constrict the heart, causing symptoms of right heart failure (e.g. peripheral oedema, breathlessness, and abdominal swelling) despite preserved right and left ventricular function. This can occur following any pericardial disease. The risk is low (<1%) following viral or idiopathic pericarditis and high (20–30%) following bacterial pericarditis.

Examination

Use an ABCDE approach to examine the patient and assess for haemodynamic instability. Table 7.1 describes signs associated with different pericardial diseases.

Look out for signs suggesting the underlying aetiology, e.g. crackles on auscultation of the chest, lymphadenopathy, or vasculitic rashes.

Investigations

Order investigations to confirm diagnosis of pericardial disease (Table 7.2) and assess for haemodynamic compromise. Look for aetiology of pericardial disease in all patients with ⚑ (Box 7.2).

Consider viral swabs, sputum cultures, blood cultures, autoimmune screen, or tumour markers based on history and examination findings.

Table 7.1 Cardiovascular signs associated with each pericardial disease

Pericarditis	Pericardial rub
Cardiac tamponade (or large pericardial effusion)	↑ heart rate ↓ blood pressure Pulsus paradoxus Raised JVP Muffled heart sounds
Constrictive pericarditis	Kussmaul sign (paradoxical rise in JVP in inspiration) Pericardial knock (high-pitched early diastolic added sound) Signs of right heart failure: • Peripheral oedema • Ascites • Hepatomegaly

Table 7.2 Investigations for the diagnosis of pericardial diseases

Category	Specific investigations	Indication
Bedside	ECG	Assess for: • New widespread ST elevation or PR depression (pericarditis) • Low QRS voltage with electrical alternans (pericardial effusion)
Bloods	White cell count, erythrocyte sedimentation rate (ESR), C-reactive protein (CRP)	To monitor disease activity and efficacy of therapy
	Creatine kinase/ troponin	Raised in myo(peri)carditis
	U&E, LFT, TFT	To assess baseline function and potential cause of pericarditis
Imaging	Chest X-ray	Enlarged cardiac silhouette with pericardial effusions >300mL May reveal cause of pericardial disease (e.g. TB, malignancy)
	TTE	Identify and assess pericardial effusions To assess left/right ventricular function
Other	CT scan	May show pericardial thickening/ calcification in constrictive pericarditis May reveal cause of pericardial disease (e.g. TB, malignancy)
	Cardiac MRI	To confirm myocarditis May show pericardial thickening/ calcification in constrictive pericarditis
	Coronary angiography	To exclude ACS if diagnosis unclear

Source: data from 2015 ESC Guidelines for the diagnosis and management of pericardial diseases.

Box 7.2 Red flags

- Fever >38°C
- Subacute onset of symptoms (often seen with malignant pericardial effusions)
- Large pericardial effusion or cardiac tamponade
- Lack of response after >1 week of medical therapy
- Myocardial involvement (elevated troponin, ventricular impairment)
- Immunosuppression
- Trauma
- Oral anticoagulant therapy.

Source: data from 2015 ESC Guidelines for the diagnosis and management of pericardial diseases.

Management

Acute management

Treat underlying cause of pericardial disease, e.g. give antibiotics in suspected bacterial infections.

Call for help?

If there is haemodynamic instability, contact a senior and request urgent cardiology input.

Unstable patients with cardiac tamponade need:

- Urgent pericardiocentesis (guided by echocardiography):
  - Aspirated fluid can be sent for cytology, culture, and biochemistry
- Urgent surgical drainage may be required if there is bleeding into the pericardium, e.g. following trauma or aortic dissection, or if percutaneous drainage is difficult or impossible.

Treatment after stabilization

Pericarditis

- Aspirin 750mg–1g TDS for 1–2 weeks, then decrease by 250–500mg every 1–2 weeks

  OR

  Non-steroidal anti-inflammatory drugs (NSAIDs), e.g. ibuprofen 600mg TDS for 1–2 weeks then decrease by 200–400 micrograms every 1–2 weeks
- Add in colchicine 500 micrograms OD (if weight <70kg) or BD (if weight >70kg) to improve response to medical management and prevent recurrence
- If no improvement is seen with these therapies or if they are contraindicated, low-dose prednisolone may be used (0.2–0.5mg/kg/day)
- Restrict physical activity until symptoms and investigations normalize.

Specialist treatment

Specialist opinion should be sought in pericardial disease that does not resolve or has sinister aetiology:

- In recurrent or chronic pericarditis consider:
  - IV immunoglobulin, anakinra, or azathioprine
  - Pericardiectomy
- In pericardial effusion consider:
  - Pericardiocentesis for persistent, large, or symptomatic effusions
  - Pericardiectomy (or pericardial window) for reaccumulating/loculated effusions or if biopsy is required
  - Surgical drainage in suspected bacterial and neoplastic pericarditis
- In constrictive pericarditis consider:
  - A trial of anti-inflammatories and conservative management for 2–3 months initially
  - Pericardiectomy in patients with chronic constrictive pericarditis (and NYHA class III or IV) but note it is associated with significant operative morbidity and mortality.

Special considerations

Pregnancy

- NSAIDs (>20 weeks' gestation) can constrict the ductus arteriosus and cause fetal renal impairment
- Colchicine is contraindicated.

Renal impairment

NSAIDs can exacerbate renal impairment.

Further reading

1. Ramrakha P, Hill J (eds) (2012). Pericardial diseases. In: *Oxford Handbook of Cardiology*, 2nd ed (pp. 327–56). Oxford: Oxford University Press. Available at: https://doi.org/10.1093/med/9780199643219.003.0009

Chapter 8

Stable angina

Guidelines:
NICE CG95 (Recent-onset chest pain of suspected cardiac origin: assessment and diagnosis): https://www.nice.org.uk/guidance/cg95

NICE CG126 (Stable angina: management): https://www.nice.org.uk/guidance/cg126

OUP disclaimer: Oxford University Press makes no representation, express or implied, that the drug dosages are correct and that the recommendations are an exclusive or mandatory course of care. All health professionals reading this text have a responsibility to evaluate its appropriateness and take the individual needs of the patient into account.

Local trust guidelines: please refer to your local guidelines as necessary.

Overview

Stable angina is intermittent, stable chest pain caused by flow-limiting disease in the epicardial coronary arteries, known as coronary artery disease (CAD). Unstable angina falls under the umbrella term ACS and is covered in Chapter 1.

Diagnosis

Diagnostic criteria

Stable angina may be diagnosed when there is anginal pain (see 'History'), **AND**

- There is significant CAD on CT coronary angiography or invasive coronary angiogram (see 'Other') **OR**
- There is reversible myocardial ischaemia during non-invasive functional imaging (see 'Other').

History

Cardiovascular risk factors are discussed in Box 8.1.

Anginal pain:

- Central, tightening pain in the chest, neck, shoulders, jaw, or arms
- Inducible by exertion
- Resolves with rest or GTN within about 5 minutes.

If the patient reports all three of the anginal pain characteristics, they have 'typical' angina. If they have two of the characteristics, they have 'atypical' angina, and if one or no characteristics, they have 'non-anginal pain'.

Unlikely angina:

- Continuous or prolonged pain **and/or**
- Pain unrelated to activity **and/or**
- Pleuritic pain **and/or**
- Pain associated with symptoms such as dizziness, palpitations, tingling, or difficulty swallowing.

Differentials:

- **Must exclude ACS!** (see Chapter 1)
- Hypertrophic cardiomyopathy
- Microvascular angina
- Gastro-oesophageal reflux (see Chapter 30).

Box 8.1 Cardiovascular risk factors

- Age (>45 years in men, >55 years in women)
- Smoking history
- Past medical history of diabetes, hypertension, dyslipidaemia, or previous CAD, e.g. myocardial infarction
- Family history of cardiovascular disease.

Examination

Check for:

- Indicators of elevated cardiovascular risk, e.g. obesity, diabetes or lipid deposits secondary to hypercholesterolaemia,
- Signs of other cardiac disease which might be causing anginal symptoms, e.g. ejection systolic murmur in aortic stenosis, left ventricular hypertrophy in hypertrophic cardiomyopathy, radial–femoral delay of aortic coarctation
- Signs of non-cardiac disease which might be causing acute chest pain, e.g. crackles in pneumonia, costochondral tenderness in costochondritis.

Investigations

Bedside

- Pulse oximetry, pulse, and blood pressure
- 12-lead ECG (check for pathological Q waves, LBBB, ST-segment and T wave flattening or inversion which would suggest underlying cardiovascular disease and check the underlying rhythm).

Bloods

- FBC:
  - Anaemia can exacerbate angina
  - A raised white cell count may indicate an infection and alternative cause of the chest pain
- U&E, LFT:
  - Baseline measurement before initiating therapy
- Glucose, HbA1c, and lipids:
  - To assess cardiac risk factors, e.g. diabetes mellitus and hypercholesterolaemia
- Troponin:
  - To exclude MI
- CRP:
  - Indicates infection or inflammation.

Imaging

- Chest X-ray to exclude other causes of chest pain.

Other

CT coronary angiography

- Patients should have a CT coronary angiogram if:
  - They have not been previously diagnosed with CAD and have a history consistent with 'typical' or 'atypical' angina **OR**
  - They have 'non-anginal pain' but their ECG has Q waves or ST–T changes
- Significant CAD found during CT coronary angiography is ≥70% diameter stenosis of at least one major epicardial artery segment or ≥50% diameter stenosis in the left main coronary artery.

Non-invasive functional imaging

Examples of non-invasive functional imaging include:

- Exercise testing
- Myocardial perfusion scintigraphy (MPS) with single-photon emission computed tomography (SPECT)
- Stress echocardiography (with exercise or dobutamine)
- Adenosine stress magnetic resonance perfusion.

These may be performed if:

- A patient has known CAD and it is unclear whether their symptoms are due to their existing diagnosis
- CT coronary angiography was not diagnostic.

Invasive coronary angiography

Performed to determine coronary anatomy:

- If functional imaging is indicative of ischaemia
- If functional imaging is not diagnostic
- If coronary intervention is being considered based on CT or functional imaging findings.

Management

Patient education

Explain:

- The long-term course and management of stable angina
- Factors that can induce angina, e.g. exertional activity, emotional stress, exposure to cold, eating a heavy meal
- The need to obtain medical help if symptoms start to occur more frequently or more severely than previously.

Lifestyle and simple interventions

- Advise on exercise, smoking cessation, diet, and weight control.

Pharmacological management

Antianginal drug treatment

Symptomatic relief

- GTN spray (Box 8.2).

Box 8.2 Glyceryl trinitrate

- Patients should know to use GTN prior to exertional activity
- They may experience flushing, headaches, or light-headedness due to the vasodilating properties and should sit down if they become light-headed
- If GTN is used because of an acute pain episode, patients should wait for 5 minutes before repeating the dose if the pain is still present. If the second dose does not cause the pain to resolve within 5 minutes, they should call an ambulance.

First-line preventative therapy

- Beta-blocker, e.g. bisoprolol 2.5mg OD, or a calcium channel blocker, e.g. amlodipine 5mg OD
- If ineffective, a combination of the two options may be tried.

Second-line/additional medical therapy

- Any of the following:
  - Isosorbide mononitrate, 20mg BD or TDS initially, then titrate dose upwards as required
  - Ivabradine 2.5–5mg BD initially (use 2.5mg if age >75 years)
  - Nicorandil 5–10mg BD initially
  - Ranolazine 375mg BD initially.

Prevention of cardiovascular disease

- Aspirin 75mg
- Statin therapy, e.g. atorvastatin 20mg OD
- Antihypertensive (see Chapter 6) and diabetic therapy if needed.

Surgical/interventional management

If medical therapy fails to control the symptoms, consider coronary artery bypass graft (CABG) or percutaneous coronary intervention (PCI). See Table 8.1 for a comparison of the interventions.

Table 8.1 Coronary artery bypass graft versus percutaneous coronary intervention

CABG	PCI
Potential survival advantage of CABG over PCI for people with multivessel disease and who: • Have diabetes **OR** • Are aged >65 years **OR** • Have anatomically complex three-vessel disease ± involvement of the left main stem	Avoids risks of open-heart surgery and general anaesthetic: • May be better tolerated by elderly and those with ↑ comorbidities

Source: data from NICE CG126.

Psychosocial considerations

- Impact on patient's quality of life: how does angina limit their daily living, work, and exercise?

Complications

- ACS: consider if sudden worsening in the frequency or severity of symptoms (see Chapter 1).

Further reading

1. Firth J, Conlon C, Cox T (eds) (2020). Management of stable angina. In: *Oxford Textbook of Medicine*, 6th ed (Chapter 16.13.3). Oxford: Oxford University Press. Available at: https://doi.org/10.1093/med/9780198746690.003.0366
2. Ramrakha P, Hill J (eds) (2012). Coronary artery disease. In: *Oxford Handbook of Cardiology*, 2nd ed (pp. 211–308). Oxford: Oxford University Press. Available at: https://doi.org/10.1093/med/9780199643219.003.0005

Chapter 9

Transient loss of consciousness

Guideline:
NICE CG109 (Transient loss of consciousness ('blackouts') in over 16s): https://www.nice.org.uk/guidance/cg109/

OUP disclaimer: Oxford University Press makes no representation, express or implied, that the drug dosages are correct and that the recommendations are an exclusive or mandatory course of care. All health professionals reading this text have a responsibility to evaluate its appropriateness and take the individual needs of the patient into account.

Local trust guidelines: please refer to your local guidelines as necessary.

Overview

Transient loss of consciousness (TLoC) is a common presentation and causes range from vasovagal syncope to more serious etiologies such as cardiac arrhythmias and epilepsy. A good history is essential in diagnosing the underlying pathophysiology.

Diagnosis

Differential diagnosis

- Neurocardiogenic:
  - Vasovagal (simple faint)
  - Situational syncope
- Orthostatic hypotension:
  - Antihypertensives or other medications which may cause hypotension
  - Hypovolaemia (e.g. dehydration, gastrointestinal (GI) bleed)
- Autonomic dysfunction/failure (e.g. autonomic neuropathy, Parkinson's disease)
- Cardiovascular:
  - Arrhythmia
  - Structural heart disease (e.g. AS, hypertrophic obstructive cardiomyopathy)
- Carotid sinus syncope
- Epileptic seizure
- Non-epileptic attack disorder (also known as psychogenic seizures or pseudosyncope)
- Unexplained syncope.

Remember, the syncopal episode may be multifactorial.

History

It is important to get a detailed history from the patient and any witnesses. Table 9.1 lists details that may be elicited in the history to help distinguish between different causes of TLoC. Box 9.1 describes the criteria for diagnosing uncomplicated vasovagal syncope.

Check:

- How the patient appeared and what they were doing before the TLoC
- How they appeared during TLoC and afterwards
- How long before the patient regained consciousness
- Did they sustain any injuries?
- Did they recall the events before and after the TLoC?
- Any previous episodes of TLoC?
- Past medical history (including if the patient has a pacemaker) and family history of cardiac disease, inherited cardiac conditions, or sudden death
- Medication history including any recent dosage changes.

Make a note of any medications which could cause hypotension. Common examples include diuretics, e.g. bendroflumethiazide, furosemide, and bumetanide and alpha-blockers, e.g. tamsulosin and doxazosin.

Examination

- Bedside observations including heart rate and lying and standing blood pressure
- General examination for injuries from fall, evidence of tongue biting, bladder or bowel incontinence
- Cardiac examination (evidence of arrhythmias or structural heart disease, e.g. AS)

Table 9.1 How to differentiate types of TLoC from the history

Type of TLoC	Salient details in the history

Vasovagal (simple faint)	• 3 Ps:
	  • Posture—prolonged standing
	  • Provoking factors—such as pain or a medical procedure
	  • Prodromal symptoms—e.g. feeling hot
	• Brief seizure-like activity can often occur
	• Immediate recovery of consciousness without confusion

Situational syncope	• Syncope occurs following straining during urination or after coughing or swallowing
Orthostatic hypotension	• Light-headedness/TLoC usually occurs when patient stands up from sitting • It is confirmed by a fall in blood pressure on standing of >20mmHg systolic and/or >10mmHg diastolic • Consider contributing drugs and if they can be stopped
Epileptic seizure (see Chapter 50)	• Pre-TLoC: prodromal déjà vu or jamais vu • During TLoC: tongue biting (biting the side of the tongue is particularly suggestive), head turned to one side, absence of pallor, abnormal posturing, limb shaking • Post TLoC: confusion, focal weakness (Todd's paresis), amnesia for events before and after TLoC
Non-epileptic attack disorder	• Repeated events without a consistent pattern • Multiple unexplained physical symptoms • Events are unusually prolonged • Can be difficult to differentiate from epileptic seizures, requiring specialist assessment
Carotid sinus syncope	• Triggered by head turning, tight-fitting collars, shaving (actions causing pressure on the carotid sinus)
Structural heart disease, e.g. hypertrophic cardiomyopathy, AS	• Exercise-induced syncope
Arrhythmic syncope	• Sudden onset, little warning • May present with facial injuries as no warning prior to TLoC • May be preceded by palpitations • Rapid recovery

Source: data from NICE CG109.

- Neurological examination (check for focal deficit which might be postictal if temporary or suggest chronic neurological pathology if permanent)
- Consider rectal examination if suspicion of upper GI bleed.

Call for help?

If the patient has not made a full recovery of consciousness, contact a senior clinician.

Box 9.1 Diagnosing uncomplicated vasovagal syncope

This can be done if:

- There is nothing in the history or examination to indicate an alternative cause
- TLoC occurred after standing or was provoked, e.g. by pain or a medical procedure and was preceded by prodromal symptoms.

In this situation, a patient should be advised to see their general practitioner (GP) for an ECG if one has not already been performed.

Note that syncope soon after **stopping** exercise is more likely to be due to a vasovagal syncope but syncope **during** exercise is more likely to have a cardiovascular cause.

Source: data from NICE CG109.

Investigations

Bedside tests

- ECG:
  - Conduction abnormality (e.g. right bundle branch block (RBBB)/ LBBB or heart block)
  - Long QT (QTc >450ms) or short QT (QTc <350ms) interval
  - ST segment or T wave abnormalities
  - Arrhythmia, e.g. bradycardia, Brugada syndrome, Wolff–Parkinson–White syndrome.

Bloods

- FBC (anaemia)
- U&E (AKI/dehydration/GI bleed)
- Glucose (hypoglycaemia)
- Venous blood gas (lactate often raised following seizures)
- Group and save if bleed is suspected.

Imaging

- Plain film X-rays to assess for any suspected fractures sustained in fall
- CT scan if head injury identified (see Chapter 120), or stroke suspected (see Chapter 56).

Other

- Echocardiogram if structural heart disease is suspected.

Acute management

Patient education

- Patients must not exercise until investigated/assessed unless diagnosed with a simple faint
- Offer safety advice for people who have had TLoC, advise them on what to do if they have another event (i.e. when to seek medical advice again) and strategies for avoiding their triggers
- Patients must not drive until assessed:
  - Following cardiology/neurology specialist assessment, patients must report the TLoC event to the Driver and Vehicle Licensing Agency (DVLA) (see Chapter 115)
- Some cardiac and neurological diseases limit people from certain occupations, e.g. professional athletes with cardiac syncope must be advised to stop exercising, heavy goods vehicle drivers can have their driving licences revoked by the DVLA.

Pharmacological management

- Consider stopping antihypertensives and prescribing IV fluids
- Treat any concurrent pathology (e.g. sepsis, GI bleed, aortic dissection).

Specialist referral

Cardiology

Investigations may be carried out as per Table 9.2.

Use the following criteria to consider whether the patient requires an urgent referral or not.

Urgent referral

- Pathological ECG findings
- Past history of heart failure or suggestive findings on examination
- Exertional TLoC
- Family history of sudden cardiac death in people aged <40 years and/or an inherited cardiac condition
- New or unexplained breathlessness
- A heart murmur.

Routine referral

- All patients with TLoC unless:
  - Already referred urgently to cardiology
  - Diagnosed with vasovagal (simple faint), situational syncope, or orthostatic hypotension
  - History is consistent with epilepsy.

Neurology

- Refer for neurology review if suspecting stroke, epileptic seizures, psychogenic non-epileptic seizures, or psychogenic pseudosyncope.

Some trusts have specialist syncope clinics—see local guidelines for further advice on referrals.

Table 9.2 Additional cardiovascular investigations in the assessment of TLoC

Type of investigation	Indications
Cardiac arrhythmia investigations	Ambulatory ECG (Holter monitoring): • If TLoC several times a week • If evidence of conduction abnormality on 12-lead ECG External event recorder (with facility for patient to indicate when a symptomatic event has occurred): • If TLoC once every 1–2 weeks Implantable event recorder: • If TLoC infrequent, i.e. less than once every 2 weeks
Exercise testing	Refer for exercise testing urgently (within 7 days) if TLoC occurred during exercise (unless contraindicated e.g. suspected AS or hypertrophic cardiomyopathy)
Tilt test	Perform if suspected vasovagal syncope but multiple episodes affect quality of life (check if syncope is accompanied by asystole)
Carotid sinus massage	Test in a safe room with ECG recording and resuscitation equipment: • Offer if suspecting carotid sinus syncope or unexplained syncope >60 years • Diagnose carotid sinus syncope if it reproduces syncope due to marked bradycardia/asystole/ hypotension

Source: data from NICE CG109.

Further reading

1. Katritsis D, Gersh B, Camm A (2016). Syncope. In: *Clinical Cardiology: Current Practice Guidelines* (pp. 743–57). Oxford: Oxford University Press. Available at: https://doi.org/10.1093/med/9780199685288.003.1517_update_004

Part 2

Care of the elderly

Chapter 10

Delirium

Guideline:
NICE CG103 (Delirium: prevention, diagnosis and management): https://www.nice.org.uk/guidance/cg103

OUP disclaimer: Oxford University Press makes no representation, express or implied, that the drug dosages are correct and that the recommendations are an exclusive or mandatory course of care. All health professionals reading this text have a responsibility to evaluate its appropriateness and take the individual needs of the patient into account.

Local trust guidelines: please refer to your local guidelines as necessary.

Overview

Delirium is a common neuropsychiatric syndrome that results in a sudden change in a person's mental state. Patients with delirium have longer hospital stays, increased mortality, and increased risk of requiring institutional placement. There is also a higher risk of hospital-acquired complications, such as pressure sores and falls. Delirium consists of three clinical subtypes:

- Hyperactive delirium (25%)—patients who have heightened arousal, restlessness, agitation, or aggression
- Hypoactive delirium (65%)—patients who become more sleepy, quieter, or withdrawn
- Mixed delirium (10%)—characterized by patients who move between the other two subtypes.

Clinical features of delirium

- May be reported by the patient, carer, or a relative
- Decline in cognitive function—worsened concentration, slow responses, disorganized thinking, confusion
- Altered perception—visual or auditory hallucinations
- Decline in physical function—reduced mobility, restlessness, agitation, changes in appetite
- Changes in social behaviour—lack of cooperation with reasonable requests, withdrawal, changes in mood or attitude
- Altered sleep–wake cycle.

Diagnosis

Risk factors

- Age ≥65 years
- Cognitive impairment and/or dementia
- Current hip fracture
- Severe illness.

History

- A collateral history is mandatory
- Ask about cognitive and functional baseline
- Ask about clinical features of delirium (listed earlier in topic)
- Ask about any possible precipitants such as falls, infection, urinary retention, constipation, dehydration, and pain
- Include drug history and alcohol history.

Examination

- Check consciousness level (Glasgow Coma Scale (GCS) or 'Alert, Voice, Pain, Unresponsive' (AVPU) scores)
- Screen for cognitive dysfunction using a tool such as the Abbreviated Mental Test Score (AMTS)[1]
- Assess for any sources of infection
- Perform rectal examination to assess for constipation and examine for urinary retention, e.g. palpable bladder, suprapubic tenderness
- Neurological examination.

Investigations

To rule out precipitating factors and differential diagnoses:

- Bedside: oxygen saturations, blood pressure, temperature, urinalysis, ECG
- Bloods: FBC, CRP, U&E, LFT, calcium, TFT, haematinics, glucose, blood cultures
- Imaging: chest X-ray. Consider a CT head to rule out differential diagnoses such as stroke, subdural haemorrhage, or a space-occupying lesion.

Clinical assessment

If indicators of delirium are identified, carry out a clinical assessment based on the Confusion Assessment Method (CAM)[2] where the following three points are needed to fulfil a diagnosis of delirium:

1. Acute onset and fluctuating course
2. Inattention and easily distractible
3. Disordered thinking or altered level of consciousness.

Diagnostic and Statistical Manual of Mental Disorders[3], fifth edition (DSM-5) criteria can also be used in the diagnosis of delirium.

1 Hodkinson HM Evaluation of a mental test score for assessment of mental impairment in the elderly. *Age and Ageing* 1972;1(4):233-8. PMID 4669880. http://ageing.oxfordjournals.org/cgi/reprint/1/4/233.

2 Inouye SK, van Dyck CH, Alessi CA, Balkin S, Siegal AP, Horwitz RI. Clarifying confusion: the confusion assessment method. A new method for detection of delirium. *Ann Intern Med.* 1990 Dec 15;113(12):941-8. doi:10.7326/0003-4819-113-12-941. PMID: 2240918.

3 American Psychiatric Association. *Diagnostic and statistical manual of mental disorders* (5th ed.). 2013 https://doi.org/10.1176/appi.books.9780890425596

Management

Observe patients daily for changes or fluctuations in their usual behaviour and be aware that distress is as common in patients with hypoactive delirium as those with hyperactive delirium.

Manage the underlying cause or combination of causes of their delirium (Table 10.1).

If the delirium does not resolve, re-evaluate for underlying causes, but also consider assessing for possible dementia.

Table 10.1 Management of underlying causes of delirium

Precipitating factors	Management
Environmental factors	• Avoid moving people between wards or rooms unless absolutely necessary • Provide appropriate lighting, a visible clock, and a calendar • Reorientate them, explaining where they are, why they are in hospital, and what your role is • Facilitate regular visits from family and friends • Encourage activities which are cognitively stimulating • Do not prevent sleep at night; reduce loud noises, bright lights, and medication rounds if possible
Fluid and electrolyte abnormalities	• Encourage oral intake • Keep a food and fluid chart • Perform a Malnutrition Universal Screening Tool (MUST)[4] score to assess nutritional status and involve dietetics if appropriate • Ensure dentures fit correctly • Consider electrolyte replacement or IV fluids if poor oral intake
Infection	• Assess daily for clinical signs of infection • Consider the use of bloods to monitor markers of inflammation • Avoid unnecessary urinary catheterization
Drugs	• Review and rationalize all medications
Urinary and faecal retention	• Catheterize if urinary retention >500mL • Consider laxatives if constipated • Keep a stool chart and fluid input/output chart
Pain	• Analgesia • Assess for non-verbal signs of pain if patients have difficulty communicating, e.g. Abbey pain score
Sensory impairment	• Remove ear wax, ensure hearing aids are working and fitted correctly • Ensure spectacles are within reach of the patient
Hypoxia	• Treat underlying cause of hypoxia and provide oxygen therapy if target saturations are not being met
Postoperative	• Encourage early supervised mobilization with appropriate mobility aids

4 https://www.bapen.org.uk/screening-and-must/must-calculator

Management of aggression and agitation in delirium

- First, identify and treat the underlying cause if possible
- Use verbal and non-verbal techniques to de-escalate the situation. Only consider medications if there is no effect with behavioural approaches
- If the patient is considered to be a risk to themselves or others, consider giving short-term antipsychotics (e.g. haloperidol orally (PO)/ intramuscularly (IM) 0.5–1mg hourly, maximum 3mg in 24 hours). Call for senior help if higher doses are required
- Avoid using antipsychotic drugs for people with:
    - Parkinson's disease
    - Lewy body dementia
    - Elongated QTc >470ms
    - Alcohol withdrawal

Instead consider giving a benzodiazepine (e.g. lorazepam 0.5–1mg PO/IM 1–2 hourly maximum 4mg daily)

- Always start with the smallest dose and titrate upwards until the desired sedation is achieved
- Check the ECG for a prolonged QTc interval before and after starting haloperidol
- Monitor sedated patients with regular observations, with particular attention being paid to respiratory rate and oxygen saturations.

Further reading

1. MacLullich AMJ, Marcantonio ER, Meagher DJ (2017). Delirium. In: Michel JP, Lynn Beattie B, Martin FC, et al. (eds) *Oxford Textbook of Geriatric Medicine*, 3rd ed. (pp. 363–72). Oxford: Oxford University Press. Available at: https://doi.org/10.1093/med/9780198701590.003.0049
2. Guys and St Thomas NHS Trust. Clinical Guidelines: The Prevention, Recognition and Management of Delirium in Adult In-Patients. Available at: https://www.guysandstthomas.nhs.uk/resources/our-services/acute-medicine-gi-surgery/elderly-care/delirium-adult-inpatients.pdf

Chapter 11

Dementia

Guideline:
NICE NG97 (Dementia: assessment, management and support for people living with dementia and their carers): https://www.nice.org.uk/guidance/ng97

OUP disclaimer: Oxford University Press makes no representation, express or implied, that the drug dosages are correct and that the recommendations are an exclusive or mandatory course of care. All health professionals reading this text have a responsibility to evaluate its appropriateness and take the individual needs of the patient into account.

Local trust guidelines: please refer to your local guidelines as necessary.

Overview

Dementia affects approximately 850,000 people in the UK, with one in six people over the age of 80 years having dementia. Dementia encompasses a wide range of progressive neurological disorders where there is a decline in cognitive function which impairs the memory, ability to reason, and ability to communicate. It can also cause personality changes. All the symptoms may impair activities of daily living.

Dementia subtypes

Alzheimer's disease (60% of cases)

- Excess deposition of beta-amyloid plaques causing progressive neuronal damage and loss of acetylcholine neurotransmitters
- Frontal and temporal lobes of the brain are particularly affected
- Early impairment of episodic memory (short-term memory loss, repeated questioning, difficulty learning new information).

Vascular

- Caused by cerebrovascular disease, with or without a clinical history of stroke
- Patients with cardiovascular risk factors are particularly at risk
- May have a stepwise progression in the severity of symptoms (may have focal neurological signs like hemiparesis or visual field defects).

Mixed

- A mixed picture of both Alzheimer's disease and vascular dementia—autopsy studies have revealed this to be more common than vascular aetiology alone.

Lewy body

- Deposits of alpha-synuclein protein (Lewy bodies) within neurons
- Repeated falls, visual hallucinations, and fluctuating cognition may occur
- Parkinsonian motor features and autonomic dysfunction (postural hypotension, difficulty swallowing, and incontinence/constipation).

Frontotemporal

- Significant frontotemporal brain atrophy on imaging
- Personality change and behavioural disturbance (apathy/social/sexual disinhibition) or aphasia
- Hyperorality and dietary changes, particularly with a preference for sweet foods, is common
- Other cognitive functions may be preserved—patients typically score well on neuropsychological tests early in the course of the disease.

Creutzfeldt–Jakob disease (CJD)

Consider if rapidly progressive dementia. Typical symptoms involve intellect and memory changes, speech, balance and personality changes, and abnormal jerking movements.

Diagnosis

History

- Elicit cognitive, behavioural, and psychological symptoms
- It is important to note the timeline of events and the impact of symptoms on daily life
- Collateral history is crucial.

Examination

- Look for signs of Parkinsonism suggestive of Lewy body dementia or focal neurological deficits suggestive of vascular dementia
- Cognitive testing (e.g. Montreal Cognitive Assessment or Addenbrooke's Cognitive Examination).

Investigations

Aim to rule out reversible causes of cognitive impairment.

Bedside

- Urine culture (infection).

Bloods

- FBC, U&E, LFT, calcium, magnesium, glucose, TFT (hypothyroidism), vitamin B_{12}, folate, HbA1c. Consider HIV and syphilis screening if high clinical suspicion.

Imaging

- Brain imaging with CT/MRI (structural abnormalities).

Other

- If reversible causes and drug causes of cognitive impairment have been excluded, refer the patient to a dementia diagnostic service for a formal diagnosis
- If the diagnosis remains unclear, specialist memory clinics may perform fluorodeoxyglucose positron emission tomography (FDG-PET), perfusion SPECT, or a lumbar puncture
- For hospitalized patients, a CAM can be used to help identify delirium (see Chapter 10).

Management

The management of dementia requires a multidisciplinary team, which may include old age psychiatrists, geriatricians, GPs, physiotherapists, occupational therapists, social services, specialist nurses, and community support groups.

Education

- Discuss with the patient and family members or carers about the diagnosis and progressive nature of the disease
- Discuss the effect the diagnosis may have on their occupation (if appropriate) and lifestyle, e.g. importance of notifying the DVLA (see Chapter 115) of a new diagnosis of dementia
- Discuss the possibility of participating in research studies.

Disease progression

Unfortunately, there are no disease-modifying drugs for dementia. However, acetylcholinesterase inhibitors and *N*-methyl-D-aspartic acid (NMDA) receptor agonists can be used for symptomatic treatment of cognitive and global functioning:

- Acetylcholinesterase inhibitors:
  - Donepezil, rivastigmine, and galantamine can be used as monotherapies for mild to moderate Alzheimer's or Lewy body dementia.
  - Common side effects of acetylcholinesterase inhibitors include diarrhoea and vomiting, and cramps. Hallucinations, peptic ulcer disease, and bradyarrhythmias can also occur
- NMDA receptor agonist:
  - Memantine is recommended for patients with moderate Alzheimer's disease who are intolerant to acetylcholinesterase inhibitors, or in established Alzheimer's disease
  - Common side effects of antiglutamatergic treatment include dizziness, hallucinations, and confusion
- Stop any medications with ↑ anticholinergic burden as this can worsen cognitive impairment
- Dosette boxes can help aid medication compliance.

Agitation and psychosis

- Address any underlying cause for their distress (e.g. pain, infection)
- Utilize non-pharmacological therapies
- Consider antipsychotics (lorazepam/haloperidol) if the patient is at risk of harming themselves or others, or if the agitation or psychosis is causing them distress. Avoid longer term use due to the risk of cerebrovascular side effects
- Antipsychotics may worsen motor symptoms in Lewy body dementia or Parkinson's disease dementia. This should be discussed with the patient and family and if commenced should be monitored closely.

Depression and anxiety

- Consider cognitive behavioural therapy
- Consider antidepressants in moderate to severe depression (see Chapter 38) and anxiety (see Chapter 40).

Sleep problems

- Consider a personalized multicomponent sleep management approach including sleep hygiene education, exposure to daylight, exercise, and personalized activities
- Do not routinely offer melatonin or other sedatives.

Pain

- If the patient is unable to reliably report pain, use an objective tool to monitor for pain, e.g. Abbey pain scale.

Advanced care planning

Offer opportunities for patients together with their family to discuss future plans including:

- Lasting power of attorney for health and welfare
- Advance statement about their wishes and preferences regarding any future ceilings of care
- Advanced decisions to refuse treatment and cardiopulmonary resuscitation status (see Chapter 114)
- Preferred place of care and death
- Consider palliative care input and prescribing anticipatory medications.

Further reading

1. Alzheimer's Society website. Available at: https://www.alzheimers.org.uk

Chapter 12

Falls

Guideline:
NICE CG161 (Falls in older people: assessing risk and prevention): https://www.nice.org.uk/guidance/cg161

OUP disclaimer: Oxford University Press makes no representation, express or implied, that the drug dosages are correct and that the recommendations are an exclusive or mandatory course of care. All health professionals reading this text have a responsibility to evaluate its appropriateness and take the individual needs of the patient into account.

Local trust guidelines: please refer to your local guidelines as necessary.

Overview

Falls and fall-associated injuries are common in older people (age >65 years). Falls may be a presenting symptom of acute illness, especially if they are of recent onset, or they can be a manifestation of underlying chronic disease. This chapter is also applicable to patients aged 50–64 years who have an underlying condition which puts them at a high risk of falls.

Diagnosis

Differential diagnosis

The differential diagnosis for the cause of a fall is wide and older people often have more than one underlying diagnosis (Table 12.1).

History

A general outline of an acute fall history should include:

- *Circumstances of the fall:*
  - Where, when, who was there, what was the patient doing at the time of the fall?
- *Before the fall:*
  - Any prodromal symptoms, e.g. light-headedness, palpitations, chest pain, nausea?
- *During the fall:*
  - Did anyone witness the fall? If there was a witness, take a collateral history
  - Was there any loss of consciousness (does the patient recall the fall itself, or just waking up after)?
  - Any signs of seizure activity (e.g. limb jerking/tongue biting or incontinence)?
  - Did the patient's appearance change (pale/flushed/blue)?
  - Was there any head injury?
  - Did they fall on an outstretched hand or backwards?
- *After the fall:*
  - Was there clear recollection of the fall or were they confused?
  - How soon were they able to resume normal activities?
  - Was there any speech difficulty or limb weakness?
- *Severity:* were there any injuries?
- *Chronicity:* how many times have they fallen in the last 6 months? Explore each episode and identify if there is a pattern
- Coexisting medical conditions and medications the patient is taking
- Alcohol consumption.

Examination

Examine using an ABCDE approach (Table 12.2). See ⚑ in Box 12.1.

Investigations

Not all of the investigations listed will be appropriate for all circumstances (e.g. some may only be relevant in acute falls or where a specific precipitant cause is suspected, or a specific injury is suspected secondary to the fall), so clinical judgement should be applied when deciding how to investigate.

Bedside

- Cognitive screening (4 'A's Test (4AT)/AMTS)
- Lying and standing blood pressure
- Blood glucose
- Urinalysis
- ECG.

Table 12.1 Differential diagnosis in a patient presenting with falls

	History of	Differential diagnosis
Medications	Recent change in medication or polypharmacy	Polypharmacy Psychotropic medications, e.g. benzodiazepines, antidepressants, antipsychotics Medications that cause orthostatic hypotension, e.g. alpha-blockers, ACE inhibitors, amitriptyline Medications that cause peripheral neuropathy, e.g. chemotherapy agents Medications that cause hypoglycaemia, e.g. insulin, sulphonylureas
Musculoskeletal	Joint buckling or instability	Arthritis or previous joint injury
	Lack of regular or adequate exercise	Deconditioning due to immobility
Neurology	Focal neurological symptoms	Stroke or TIA (see Chapter 56)
	Behavioural disturbances, cognitive or mood impairment	Dementia (see Chapter 11) Delirium (see Chapter 10) Depression (see Chapter 38)
	Witnessed history suggestive of seizure, prolonged postictal state	Seizure disorder (see Chapter 50)
	Head trauma or previous traumatic brain injury	Subdural haematoma
Gait disorders	Shuffling gait	Parkinson's disease (see Chapter 55)
	Abnormal gait—broad based, short stepping	Normal pressure hydrocephalus Cerebellar lesion
	High-stepping gait	Foot drop
	Positive Romberg's test	Peripheral neuropathy

Cardiovascular	TLoC without any warning symptoms	Tachy- or bradyarrhythmias Valvular heart disease
	(Pre-) Syncope precipitated by turning the head or wearing tight collars	Carotid sinus hypersensitivity
	(Pre-) Syncope precipitated by standing up or a brisk change in position	Orthostatic hypotension
Genitourinary	Urinary urgency or dysuria	Incontinence Urinary tract infection
Endocrine	History of diabetes	Hypoglycaemia (see Chapter 21)
	Chronic steroid use with sudden cessation of therapy	Adrenal insufficiency
Ear, nose, and throat (ENT)	Dizziness, vertigo, or imbalance	Benign paroxysmal positional vertigo (BPPV) Vestibular dysfunction
Environmental	A collateral history about the home environment is vital	Poor lighting, loose rugs, clutter, stairs, walking aids, unsuitable footwear
Other factors	Visual impairment Alcohol consumption Psychological factors, e.g. the fear of falling itself	

Table 12.2 ABCDE approach to an acute falls review

	Findings
B	Poor airway expansion and oxygen saturation due to rib fractures or signs of pneumonia
C	Tachy- or bradyarrhythmias, orthostatic hypotension, murmurs to suggest valvular heart disease
D	Assess level of alertness, hypo/hyperthermia, hypoglycaemia
E	*Chest:* rib tenderness/bruising suggestive of fractures
	Abdomen: abdominal tenderness/urinary retention to suggest urinary/intra-abdominal infection
	Musculoskeletal: look for signs of injury and assess for any evidence of fractures which includes C-spine tenderness, limb deformity, bruising
	Neurological: abnormalities in cranial nerves, e.g. visual impairment, upper or lower limb weakness, or sensory impairment (stroke/TIA); glove-and-stocking sensory impairment and Romberg's sign positive (peripheral neuropathy); ataxia (cerebellar pathology)
	ENT: Dix–Hallpike manoeuvre if symptoms suggestive of BPPV
	General: look for evidence of long lie such as pressure sores and hypothermia
	Gait, balance, and mobility: assess gait. Timed Up and Go test, Timed 180° Turn Test

Box 12.1 Red flags

The following require urgent assessment and consideration of further imaging:

- Acute change in level of consciousness, focal neurology, or head injury with concurrent anticoagulant or antiplatelet therapy use (perform CT head; see Chapter 121)
- Limb pain or inability to weight bear or anatomical abnormality that suggests a fracture (request X-rays and seek advice from orthopaedic team)

Bloods

- FBC (anaemia, infection)
- U&E (dehydration)
- Creatine kinase (rhabdomyolysis in long lie)
- LFT (chronic alcohol use)
- Bone profile including vitamin D (calcium abnormalities, electrolyte disturbance)
- CRP (infection)
- Vitamin B_{12}, TFT (peripheral neuropathy).

Imaging

- Chest X-ray (rib fractures, signs of pneumonia, haemothorax)
- CT head (acute or subacute intracranial bleed or infarct) and C-spine
- Echocardiogram (valvular heart disease)

Other

- 72-hour cardiac tape (arrhythmia)
- Carotid sinus massage
- Tests of autonomic function, e.g. tilt table testing to assess adrenergic response
- Electroencephalogram (EEG) if seizure disorder is suspected
- Dual-energy X-ray absorptiometry (DXA) for assessment of osteoporosis risk (see Chapter 24).

Acute management

Treat any underlying medical illness leading to the fall or occurring concurrently, i.e. infections, dehydration, electrolyte abnormalities, abnormal blood glucose levels, pressure-related injuries, and hypothermia.

Some trusts may have a post-falls protocol, which may include a post-falls assessment tool and guidelines on management after a fall, i.e. if CT head is indicated after head injury, duration of GCS monitoring, and referral to specialist falls services.

Chronic management

Patient education

Discuss individual risk factors for falling and provide information about measures to prevent further falls in the context of a falls prevention programme, and how to get help when they have fallen, e.g. pendant alarms. Educate family members and carers.

Lifestyle and simple interventions

- Strength and balance training
- Home hazard and safety assessment and intervention, e.g. microenvironments, crash mat alarms
- Vision and hearing assessments.

Psychological interventions

- Screen for mood disorders using the Hospital Anxiety and Depression scale and treat appropriately.

Pharmacological management

- Review medications that might have contributed towards the fall and discontinue if possible
- Commence bone protection if osteoporosis is diagnosed.

Psychosocial considerations

- Loss of mobility leading to social isolation, depression, increased dependence, and disability.

Specialist referral

Cardiac pacing should be considered in cardioinhibitory carotid sinus hypersensitivity.

Offer referral to a specialist falls service in older people for a multifactorial falls risk assessment. This will assess factors including:

- Polypharmacy
- Cognitive impairment
- Continence issues
- Previous falls
- Inappropriate footwear
- Comorbidities including syncope syndrome or concurrent medications which might affect balance
- Postural instability or mobility/balance issues
- Visual impairment.

Further reading

1. Wilcock G, Rockwood K (2011). Medicine in old age. In: Warrell DA, Cox TM, Firth JD (eds) *Oxford Textbook of Medicine*, 5th ed (Chapter 29.1). Oxford UK: Oxford University Press. Available at: https://doi.org/10.1093/med/9780199204854.003.2901_update_001

Chapter 13

Hip fractures

Guideline:
NICE CG124 (Hip fracture: management): https://www.nice.org.uk/guidance/cg124/

OUP disclaimer: Oxford University Press makes no representation, express or implied, that the drug dosages are correct and that the recommendations are an exclusive or mandatory course of care. All health professionals reading this text have a responsibility to evaluate its appropriateness and take the individual needs of the patient into account.

Local trust guidelines: please refer to your local guidelines as necessary.

Overview

Hip fractures commonly occur in the elderly population. The aetiology is often multifactorial, with contributing factors including osteoporosis and frailty. Mortality following hip fracture is up to 30% in the year following the fracture and up to 50% do not return to their baseline level of functioning.

Diagnosis

History

- History of fall in the elderly/severe trauma (road traffic accident, high-impact fall) in the young
- May be atraumatic in pathological fractures (secondary to primary bone tumour or metastatic deposits)
- Acute pain in the hip and/or groin area and may have referred pain to the knee
- Associated inability to weight bear on affected side.

Examination

- On inspection, affected leg is shortened, abducted, and externally rotated
- Tenderness on palpation of the greater trochanter and by rotation of the hip joint
- Assess neurovascular status of the affected limb
- Perform an ABCDE examination to identify any causes leading to the fall and other injuries or fractures
- Screen for cognitive impairment/acute confusion on admission and regularly reassess the patient for delirium (see Chapter 10) with AMTS and CAM or equivalent.

Investigations

Bedside

- Urinalysis and Bence Jones protein (if pathological fracture is suspected)
- ECG to investigate the cause of the fall (see Chapter 12).

Bloods

- FBC, U&E, coagulation profile, group and save, vitamin D, TFT, calcium
- Prostate-specific antigen (PSA) (in men) and serum electrophoresis if a pathological fracture is suspected
- Creatine kinase if history of long lie.

Imaging

- Anteroposterior (AP) pelvis (Fig. 13.1 and Table 13.1) and lateral hip radiographs
- Obtain full-length femoral views if pathological fracture is suspected
- Chest X-ray to investigate the cause of the fall
- If a hip fracture is suspected clinically despite negative hip radiographs of an adequate standard, offer further imaging, e.g. MRI, or CT if MRI is not available within 24 hours or is contraindicated.

Table 13.1 Classification of neck of femur fractures

Classification	Description		
Intracapsular	Garden I	Non-displaced	Impacted incomplete fracture
	Garden II		Non-displaced complete fracture
	Garden III	Displaced	Partially displaced complete fracture
	Garden IV		Fully displaced complete fracture
Extracapsular	Inter-trochanteric fracture		Fracture between the two trochanters
	Sub-trochanteric fracture		Fracture <5cm distal to the lesser trochanter

Source: data from The Journal of Bone and Joint Surgery. Vol. 43-B, No. 4, Low-angle fixation in fractures of the femoral neck, R. S. Garden, 1 Nov 1961.

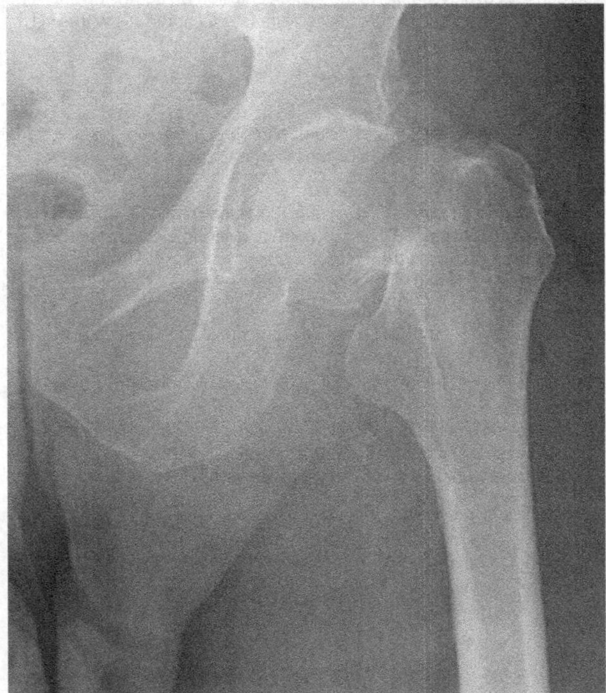

Fig. 13.1 A neck of femur fracture seen on an AP X-ray of the left hip.
Courtesy of The Norfolk and Norwich University Hospitals (NNUH) Radiology Dept.

Management

Multidisciplinary management

Offer patients a formal hip fracture programme which includes:

- Orthogeriatric assessment and continued multidisciplinary review
- Early optimization for surgery
- Early identification of individual goals for rehabilitation
- Involvement of related services including mental health, falls prevention, bone health, primary care, and social services.

Acute management

- Initial management should consist of an ABCDE approach to stabilize the patient
- Assess and treat pain immediately on presentation, 30 minutes after analgesia is administered and hourly thereafter until the patient is settled on the ward
- Prescribe according to the World Health Organization (WHO) analgesia ladder, starting with regular paracetamol, unless contraindicated. Opioids may also be required. NSAIDs are not recommended
- Consider a femoral nerve block if paracetamol and opioids do not provide sufficient analgesia
- Analgesia should be sufficient to allow small movements for imaging, nursing care, and rehabilitation
- Optimize comorbidities early to prevent delays to surgery such as anaemia, reversing anticoagulation, dehydration, electrolyte disturbance, glycaemic control, decompensated heart failure, cardiac arrhythmia or ischaemia, chest infection, or exacerbation of chronic chest conditions.

Surgical management

- Definitive management is surgical (Table 13.2). This should be done on the day of, or the day after, admission
- If the patient has a particularly complex or terminal illness, surgery should still be considered as a palliative measure to minimize pain. The multidisciplinary team (MDT) should consider the patient's priorities for rehabilitation and their wishes for end-of-life care.

Treatment after stabilization

- Mobilization should be attempted on day 1 postoperatively and daily thereafter with regular physiotherapy review
- Thromboprophylaxis
- Ongoing MDT approach with orthogeriatric involvement
- Review bone protection including calcium and vitamin D supplements, bisphosphonates, and consideration for DXA scanning
- If fracture was due to a fall, measure postural blood pressure postoperatively and review medications for iatrogenic causes (see Chapter 12)
- Consider continued rehabilitation in the community as part of early supported discharge or in a community hospital or residential care unit.

Table 13.2 Examples of surgical management of neck of femur fractures

Fracture type	Undisplaced intracapsular fractures (Garden I and II)	Displaced intracapsular fractures (Garden III and IV)	Extracapsular
Surgical option	Internal fixation with **dynamic hip screw** or **cannulated hip screws**	**Total hip replacement** is preferred in patients who were active, mobilizing independently, are not cognitively impaired, and are medically fit for anaesthesia and the procedure **Hemiarthroplasty** is often recommended in the elderly who do not meet the above-listed criteria	Trochanteric fractures above and including the lesser trochanter: extramedullary implants such as a **dynamic hip screw** Subtrochanteric fracture: **intramedullary nail** is usually preferred

Source: data from NICE CG124.

Special considerations

Complications of hip surgery include infection, bleeding, risk of thrombo-embolic events, avascular necrosis of femoral head and leg-length discrepancy. Long-term complications include joint dislocation, aseptic loosening, and periprosthetic fracture.

Further reading

1. Baldwin A (ed) (2020). Proximal femoral fractures. In: *Oxford Handbook of Clinical Specialties*, 11th ed. Oxford: Oxford University Press. Available at: https://doi.org/10.1093/med/9780198827191.003.0008
2. Baldwin A (ed) (2020). Hip fractures in the elderly. In: *Oxford Handbook of Clinical Specialties*, 11th ed. Oxford: Oxford University Press. Available at: https://doi.org/10.1093/med/9780198827191.003.0008

Part 3

Endocrinology

Chapter 14

Adrenal insufficiency

Guideline:
Society for Endocrinology Endocrine Emergency Guidance (Emergency management of acute adrenal insufficiency (adrenal crisis) in adult patients): https://ec.bioscientifica.com/view/journals/ec/5/5/G1.xml

OUP disclaimer: Oxford University Press makes no representation, express or implied, that the drug dosages are correct and that the recommendations are an exclusive or mandatory course of care. All health professionals reading this text have a responsibility to evaluate its appropriateness and take the individual needs of the patient into account.

Local trust guidelines: please refer to your local guidelines as necessary.

Overview

Chronic adrenal insufficiency may be primary (the adrenal gland is unable to produce cortisol) or secondary (the pituitary gland does not stimulate the adrenal gland to produce cortisol). The most common cause is iatrogenic secondary (sometimes called tertiary) adrenal insufficiency. See Box 14.1 for a list of causes.

Acute adrenal insufficiency may be the consequence of a missed diagnosis of chronic insufficiency. Alternatively, it may be due to abruptly stopping long-term steroid medication, or it may result from an ↑ body requirement for cortisol without adequate adjustment of medications, e.g. in acute illness or perioperatively.

Box 14.1 Causes of adrenal insufficiency

Primary

- Autoimmune (Addison's disease)
- Congenital adrenal hyperplasia
- Adrenal malignancy
- Deposits within the adrenal gland, e.g. sarcoidosis, amyloidosis, haemochromatosis
- Infection, e.g. TB
- Bleeding within the adrenal glands, e.g. following meningococcal septicaemia
- Surgical removal of the adrenal glands.

Secondary

- Hypopituitarism, e.g. tumour compressing the pituitary gland, infection, hypophysitis (particularly associated with checkpoint inhibitor treatment of malignancy, or postpartum), trauma, apoplexy
- Iatrogenic—following discontinuation of long-term steroid treatment where the dose of steroid is equivalent to >5mg prednisolone/day for >4 weeks.

Diagnosis

History

Chronic symptoms

The symptoms of adrenal insufficiency may develop slowly and are non-specific. Typical symptoms include:

- Fatigue
- Weight loss
- Dizziness and postural collapse (more commonly in primary insufficiency because of mineralocorticoid deficiency, which is not seen in secondary insufficiency)
- Abdominal pain
- Nausea and vomiting
- Fever
- Confusion
- Back and leg cramps
- Tanned appearance and/or pigmentation of scars, buccal mucosa, and skin creases (if primary adrenal failure).

If a patient has abdominal pain or is vomiting and the cause is not clear, consider adrenal insufficiency.

Ask whether the patient has any autoimmune conditions, e.g. vitiligo, T1DM (see Chapter 21), or any family history of these conditions. Ask about headaches and visual symptoms which might indicate a space-occupying lesion resulting in secondary insufficiency. In addition, it is also important to take a thorough drug history and ask specifically about steroid use, including IV, oral, topical, and inhaled formulations.

Acute symptoms

In an acute adrenal crisis, in addition to the symptoms previously listed, patients tend to be weak and clinically shocked, with an impaired mental state ranging from mild confusion to comatose.

If the patient is acutely unwell and adrenal insufficiency is suspected, proceed directly to management and *do not* wait for the results of investigations to confirm the diagnosis.

Examination

Fig. 14.1 shows the examination findings seen in chronic adrenal insufficiency. Fig. 14.2 shows the additional findings which may be seen in an acute adrenal crisis.

> Look in the palmar creases, at the nipples, at old scars, and in the mucous membranes for hyperpigmentation.

Investigations

Bedside

- Heart rate and ECG
- Lying and standing blood pressure.

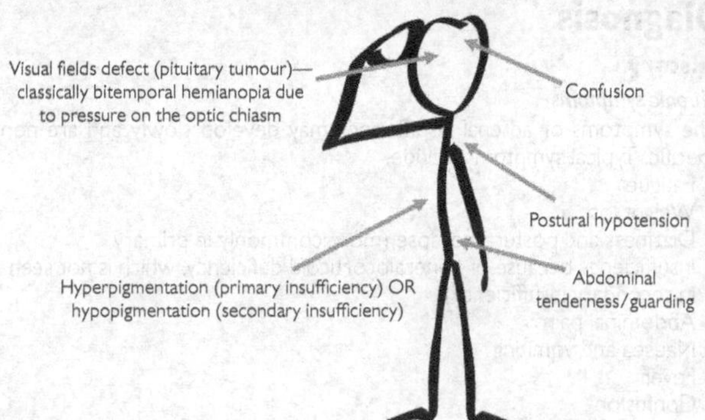

Fig. 14.1 Examination findings in chronic adrenal insufficiency.

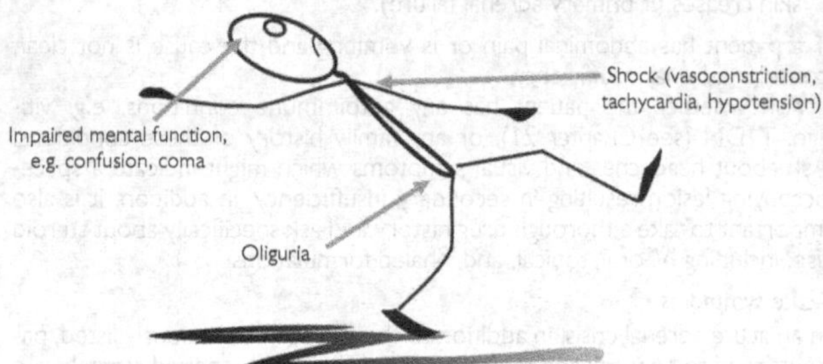

Fig. 14.2 Additional examination findings in an acute adrenal crisis.

Bloods

- FBC (normochromic anaemia and sometimes lymphocytosis and/or eosinophilia)
- U&E (kidney injury and hyponatraemia in primary and secondary insufficiency and hyperkalaemia in primary insufficiency)
- Calcium (low)
- Glucose (low)
- ESR (high)
- Cortisol (low) and adrenocorticotropic hormone (ACTH) levels (high in primary disease, low in secondary)—ideally at 9am. See Box 14.2.
- TFT (thyroid-stimulating hormone (TSH) may be high—seek specialist advice, or low). See Box 14.3.

Box 14.2 Adrenocorticotropic hormone testing

The ACTH samples should be taken at the same time as the serum cortisol, and should be taken directly to the laboratory. It is worthwhile calling the laboratory first to ask if they have any special containers, e.g. containing ice, in which to transport the ACTH sample.

Box 14.3 Thyroid function tests

Never treat thyroid abnormalities prior to correction of adrenal insufficiency as this may precipitate a crisis.

Other

- Short Synacthen test—if haemodynamically stable. See Box 14.4
- Serum aldosterone (low) and plasma renin (high) (if primary adrenal failure; this can be useful with the ACTH test to differentiate the underlying cause).

Box 14.4 Short Synacthen test

Useful if a 9am cortisol level is within the normal range but not >400nmol/L (excludes the diagnosis).

- Note history of asthma/allergic disorder and ensure resuscitation facilities are available for possible anaphylaxis
- Measure basal cortisol **FIRST** (this may be combined with testing ACTH if not already tested and if the test is performed at 9am)
- Administer 250 micrograms Synacthen™ IM
- Repeat serum cortisol measurements 30 minutes after the Synacthen injection
- Failure of the cortisol measurement to adequately rise (cut-offs depend on local laboratory but usually an incremental rise of 200nmol/L or 30 minute value >430nmol/L) suggests adrenal insufficiency. If cortisol is low, a raised ACTH measurement indicates primary insufficiency and a low ACTH measurement indicates secondary insufficiency.

Management

Acute management

DO NOT delay treatment while waiting for investigations.

Steroid

- Hydrocortisone 100mg IV/IM **immediately**:
  - After the stat dose give hydrocortisone 200mg as a continuous infusion every 24 hours **OR**
  - Hydrocortisone 50mg IV/IM four times daily (QDS).

Fluids

- 1L 0.9% sodium chloride rapidly over 1 hour unless contraindicated (caution if renal/cardiac impairment or elderly), and then continue fluids to treat dehydration.

Treatment after stabilization

Refer to the endocrinology team for advice about switching the patient to oral hydrocortisone, usually after 72 hours, commencing fludrocortisone (50–300 micrograms OD, required in primary insufficiency only) and identifying the cause of the adrenal insufficiency.

Arrange regular follow-up in the endocrine clinic.

Education

Prior to discharge:

- **Discuss** the need for lifelong steroid therapy and the risk of an acute crisis if the therapy is suddenly stopped or reduced
- **Signpost** to support organizations, e.g. Addison's self-help group (ADSHG; https://www.addisonsdisease.org.uk/)
- **Explain** the sick day rules (Box 14.5) and explain that failure to follow them may lead to an acute crisis
- **Explain** the need for ↑ hydrocortisone as perioperative treatment
- **Ensure** the patient has an adequate supply of oral hydrocortisone so that they will be able to double their dose if needed, and provide the patient with 100mg hydrocortisone IM for use in emergencies. Ensure they know how and when to administer the IM dose (Box 14.5)

Provide the patient with a steroid emergency card (see 'Further reading') which should be presented to any healthcare professional that the patient comes into contact with, and discuss the importance of medical alert devices (e.g. bracelets).

Box 14.5 Sick day rules

1. **Double** the dose of hydrocortisone if the patient is ill with a fever **OR** needs to take antibiotics
2. If oral hydrocortisone cannot be swallowed or metabolized, e.g. **vomiting (more than one episode) or diarrhoea**, the patient will need to have a dose of 100mg **IM hydrocortisone**, even if they have already had their regular oral dose, and they should seek medical help.

Source: data from Arlt W, et al. (September 2016) Society for Endocrinology Endocrine Emergency Guidance: Emergency management of acute adrenal insufficiency (adrenal crisis) in adult patients. Endocrine Connections 5(5): G1–G3.

Special considerations

Specialist advice should be sought in pregnancy. In general, the hydrocortisone dose will need to be ↑ in the third trimester and for delivery.

Further reading

1. Turner HE, Eastell R, Grossman A (eds) (2018). Adrenal gland. In: *Oxford Desk Reference: Endocrinology* (pp. 134–203). Oxford: Oxford University Press. Available at: https://doi.org/10.1093/med/9780199672837.003.0006
2. Society for Endocrinology (2020). New NHS Steroid Emergency Card. Available at: https://www.endocrinology.org/endocrinologist/137-autumn-20/society-news/new-nhs-steroid-emergency-card-available-to-order/

Chapter 15

Diabetic ketoacidosis

Guideline:
Joint British Diabetes Societies Inpatient Care Group (The management of diabetic ketoacidosis in adults): http://www.diabetologists-abcd.org.uk/JBDS/JBDS_IP_DKA_Adults_Revised.pdf

OUP disclaimer: Oxford University Press makes no representation, express or implied, that the drug dosages are correct and that the recommendations are an exclusive or mandatory course of care. All health professionals reading this text have a responsibility to evaluate its appropriateness and take the individual needs of the patient into account.

Local trust guidelines: please refer to your local guidelines as necessary.

Overview

Diabetic ketoacidosis (DKA) occurs most frequently, but not exclusively, in patients with type 1 diabetes mellitus (T1DM). It is a medical emergency which typically resolves within 24–48 hours if recognized and treated appropriately. The management of DKA in children is covered in Chapter 75.

Diagnosis

History

DKA may be the presenting finding of T1DM. Alternatively, it may develop due to an insulin deficiency (e.g. insufficient dosing of insulin), or due to an increased demand for insulin (e.g. infection, surgery, medications, pregnancy, or an inflammatory state).

Typically, patients can present with any of the following symptoms:

- Drowsiness/confusion
- Vomiting
- Abdominal pain
- Polyuria
- Polydipsia
- Lethargy
- Anorexia.

Diagnostic criteria

Diagnostic criteria for DKA are summarized in Fig. 15.1. Alternative presentations are discussed in Box 15.1.

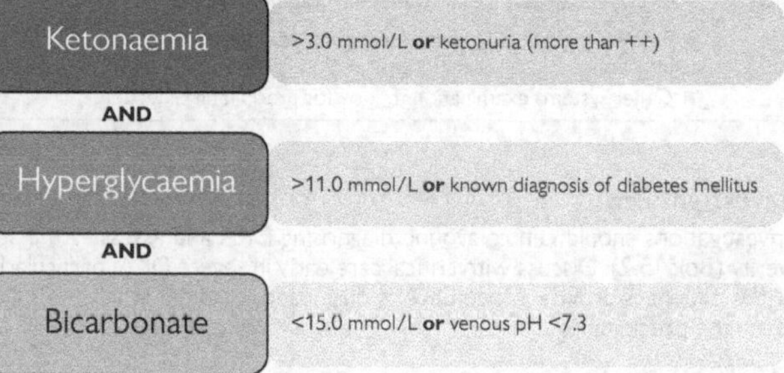

Ketonaemia
>3.0 mmol/L **or** ketonuria (more than ++)
AND
Hyperglycaemia
>11.0 mmol/L **or** known diagnosis of diabetes mellitus
AND
Bicarbonate
<15.0 mmol/L **or** venous pH <7.3

Fig. 15.1 Diagnostic criteria for diabetic ketoacidosis.

Box 15.1 Alternative presentations of DKA

Consider DKA in all unwell patients with an elevated glucose level, even in the absence of symptoms.

DKA should also be considered in unwell patients with type 2 diabetes mellitus (T2DM) who are taking SGLT2 inhibitors, e.g. dapagliflozin, empagliflozin, canagliflozin. These drugs can cause DKA with a **normal** glucose level (euglycaemic DKA).

Hyperglycaemic hyperosmolar state (HHS; see Chapter 18) is typically associated with dehydration and hyperglycaemia, **without** significant ketosis or acidaemia; however, it may also occur in combination with DKA.

Examination

The main examination finding is dehydration due to the combination of vomiting, and osmotic diuresis. Signs of DKA precipitants (e.g. infection) may also be found (Table 15.1).

Table 15.1 Possible examination findings in DKA

A	• May be compromised if ↓ GCS score
B	• Tachypnoea (attempted respiratory compensation for metabolic acidosis), progressing to Kussmaul's respiration (rapid and deep) • Oxygen saturation (may be ↓ if there is a chest infection) • Signs of chest infection, e.g. inspiratory crackles, wheeze
C	• Hypotension • Tachycardia • Prolonged capillary refill time • Reduced or absent jugular venous pulse • Reduced skin turgor and dry mucous membranes • Reduced urine output
D	• GCS/AVPU score (↓ in severe dehydration or sepsis)
E	• Fever (contributes towards causing dehydration and indicates infection) • Other systems examination to look for precipitating infection

Investigations

Investigations should centre around diagnosing DKA and assessing the severity (Box 15.2). Discuss with critical care early in severe DKA, particularly if the patient is drowsy. Once DKA is diagnosed, consider what may have been the precipitating cause.

Bedside

- Point-of-care capillary blood glucose (CBG)
- Point-of-care blood ketones
- ECG and continuous cardiac monitoring
- Urine:
  - Urinalysis, and send for microscopy, culture, and sensitivity (MC&S) if a urinary tract infection is suspected
  - Beta-human chorionic gonadotropin (βHCG) test for pregnancy
- Weight.

Bloods

- FBC
- U&E
- LFT
- Venous blood glucose
- Blood cultures
- Venous blood gas (VBG); alternatively arterial blood gas (ABG; if oxygen saturation is low and a chest infection is suspected).

Imaging

- Chest X-ray (if a chest infection is suspected).

Box 15.2 Severe DKA criteria

- Blood ketones >6mmol/L
- Bicarbonate <5mmol/L
- Blood pH <7.0
- Anion gap >16:
  - Equation = $(Na^+ + K^+) - (Cl^- + HCO_3^-)$
- Potassium <3.5mmol/L on admission
- GCS score <12/abnormal AVPU score
- Oxygen saturation <92% on air (if >94% is normal for the patient)
- Systolic blood pressure <90mmHg
- Pulse <60bpm or >100bpm.

Source: data from The Management of Diabetic Ketoacidosis in Adults. September 2013 – JBDS 02.

Management

Acute management

Patients with severe DKA (Box 15.2) should be reviewed by a senior clinician and may require higher dependency care.

> If the patient is drowsy, consider inserting a nasogastric tube to reduce the risk of aspiration.

IV fluids

Commence 0.9% saline **prior** to commencing a fixed rate insulin infusion (FRII).

> It is ideal to have at least one large-bore cannula in a large vein.

Hypotension (systolic blood pressure <90mmHg)

- Give 500mL 0.9% saline over 10–15 minutes
- Repeat if still hypotensive and then request urgent senior review.

Normotensive (systolic blood pressure ≥90mmHg)

Fluid should be administered aggressively unless the patient has risk factors (Box 15.3), in which case a more cautious approach may be needed (which may require higher dependency care):

- 1L 0.9% saline over 1 hour **AND THEN**
- 1L 0.9% saline with potassium chloride over 2 hours **AND THEN**
- 1L 0.9% saline with potassium chloride over 2 hours **AND THEN**
- 1L 0.9% saline with potassium chloride over 4 hours **AND THEN**
- 1L 0.9% saline with potassium chloride over 4 hours **AND THEN**
- 1L 0.9% saline with potassium chloride over 6 hours **AND THEN** continue monitoring as outlined under 'Potassium'.

Box 15.3 Risk factors where slower fluid may be required

- Age 18–25 years (careful fluid replacement to avoid cerebral oedema)
- Very elderly (to avoid fluid overload)
- Pregnant
- Cardiac or renal failure
- Another significant comorbidity.

Source: data from The Management of Diabetic Ketoacidosis in Adults. September 2013 – JBDS 02.

Potassium

Insulin treatment causes movement of potassium ions into cells which causes hypokalaemia. Potassium should therefore be checked prior to commencing each infusion of IV fluid. The result is then used to determine how much potassium chloride (KCl) should be added to the subsequent infusion.

- Potassium level >5.5mmol/L: no KCl in next infusion
- Potassium level 3.5–5mmol/L: 40mmol/L KCl
- Potassium level <3.5mmol/L: 40mmol/L KCl and request senior review.

Fixed rate insulin infusion

- Prescribe an insulin infusion of 50 units of short-acting insulin, e.g. Actrapid®, mixed with 50mL 0.9% saline
- The infusion rate should start at 0.1 units/kg/hour and should commence after the first bag of IV fluids has begun
- Continue any long-acting insulin that the patient is usually prescribed.

> IV fluids and insulin may be given through the same cannula, but **only** if it is a large-bore cannula **and** it is attached to a split connector with one-way valves.

Monitoring

General

- Regular routine observations and monitoring of GCS score
- Continuous cardiac monitoring if the patient has severe DKA (Box 4.2).

Bloods

- Check ABG and ketone levels hourly:
    - Aim for blood ketones to fall by at least 0.5mmol/L/hour (if ketone monitoring is unavailable, aim for bicarbonate level to rise by 3.0mmol/L/hour or blood glucose levels to fall by 3.0mmol/L/hour). If this is not achieved, call for senior help and consider increasing the FRII by 1mmol/hour.

> If the CBG machine is unable to calculate a precise measurement (because glucose is >27mmol/L), then use the glucose value from a serum sample processed in the laboratory or blood gas machine.
>
> If the glucose level is <14mmol/L, add a 10% glucose infusion at a rate of 125ml/hour. **Continue** the saline infusion and FRII; however, consider reducing the rate of the FRII to 0.05 units/kg/hour to reduce the risk of hypokalaemia and hypoglycaemia.

- VBG after 1 hour, after 2 hours, and then 2-hourly (record pH, potassium, and bicarbonate levels) during the first 6 hours, and then again at 12 hours.

Examination

- Reassess fluid status after 12 hours of IV fluids, or sooner if any clinical concern. Aim for a urine output of at least 0.5mL/kg/hour.

> If the patient is incontinent or anuric, consider catheterization to ensure accurate fluid balance assessment.

Treatment after stabilization

Ensure patients receive prophylactic LMWH (see Chapter 99) unless contraindicated.

Resolution

DKA has resolved when:

1. Blood ketones are <0.6mmol/L **AND**
2. Venous pH is >7.3 **OR** bicarbonate is >18mmol/L.
   - If the patient is not eating or drinking, continue IV fluids and switch to a variable rate insulin infusion (VRII)
   - If they are eating and drinking regular meals, restart the patient's insulin regimen (or start a new regimen under the guidance of an inpatient diabetes team if newly diagnosed). Give short-acting insulin just before a meal, and stop the FRII 1 hour after the meal.

All patients with DKA should be reviewed by the local diabetes team within 24 hours of admission. Consideration should be given to changing insulin dosages following resolution of DKA. All patients should be discharged with a care plan which should be copied to the GP. This should include specific advice about how to manage diabetes during illness, follow-up arrangements, and contact details for the diabetes team to help avoid further admissions.

Special considerations

Complications

Potassium imbalances

Hypokalaemia and hyperkalaemia are potential causes of mortality in patients with DKA.

Hypoglycaemia

There is a small risk of hypoglycaemia (<4mmol/L) during the treatment of DKA. This can be associated with cardiac arrhythmias, brain injury, and death.

Cerebral oedema

This is a rare complication in children and young adults and is associated with rapid administration of large volumes of IV fluids.

Pulmonary oedema

This may occur in patients at risk of fluid overload and reflects the need for caution with fluid replacement.

Further reading

1. Wass J, Owen K (eds) (2014). Diabetic hyperglycaemic emergencies. In: *Oxford Handbook of Endocrinology and Diabetes*, 3rd ed (pp. 683–4). Oxford: Oxford University Press. Available at: https://doi.org/10.1093/med/9780199644438.003.0013

Chapter 16

Hypercalcaemia

Guideline:
Society for Endocrinology Endocrine Emergency Guidance (Emergency management of acute hypercalcaemia in adult patients): https://ec.bioscientifica.com/view/journals/ec/5/5/G9.xml

OUP disclaimer: Oxford University Press makes no representation, express or implied, that the drug dosages are correct and that the recommendations are an exclusive or mandatory course of care. All health professionals reading this text have a responsibility to evaluate its appropriateness and take the individual needs of the patient into account.

Local trust guidelines: please refer to your local guidelines as necessary.

Overview

Hypercalcaemia is defined as a serum concentration of calcium >2.60mmol/L. Approximately 50% of extracellular calcium is bound to albumin, therefore total serum calcium levels require correcting for serum albumin concentration.

Calcium homeostasis is regulated through intestinal absorption, bone resorption, and renal tubular reabsorption. These are primarily controlled by parathyroid hormone (PTH) and vitamin D. Hypercalcaemia results from an abnormality of one or more of these processes.

Hypercalcaemia can be classified according to severity (Table 16.1).

Causes of hypercalcaemia are listed in Table 16.2.

Table 16.1 Severity of hypercalcaemia

Severity	Adjusted serum calcium (mmol/L)
Mild	2.6–3.0
Moderate	3.0–3.5
Severe	>3.5

Table 16.2 Causes of hypercalcaemia

Primary hyperparathyroidism[a]	• Adenoma (80–85%) • Hyperplasia • Carcinoma—rare • Multiple endocrine neoplasia
Malignancy[a]	• PTH-related peptide secreted by solid tumours (80%) • Osteoclast activating factors • Metastatic bone destruction
Granulomatous disorders	• Sarcoidosis • Granulomatosis with polyangiitis • TB • Histoplasmosis
Drugs	• Thiazide diuretics • Lithium • Vitamin A toxicity • Vitamin D toxicity • Theophylline toxicity
High bone turnover	• Paget's disease with immobilization • Thyrotoxicosis • Immobilization
Renal failure associated	• Tertiary hyperparathyroidism • Aluminium toxicity • Rhabdomyolysis (biphasic with initial hypocalcaemia and then hypercalcaemia can develop)

Table 16.2 *Continued*

Familial	• Familial hypocalciuric hypercalcaemia
Miscellaneous	• Adrenal insufficiency • Milk-alkali syndrome • Phaeochromocytoma

[a] Most common causes of hypercalcaemia, accounting for 90% of cases.

Diagnosis

History

Obtain a thorough history, including family history and signs of underlying malignancy. Patients with acute hypercalcaemia may present with the following:

- Polyuria and polydipsia
- Mood disturbances: depression, memory loss, confusion, coma
- Abdominal pain due to nephrolithiasis, nephrocalcinosis or constipation
- Muscle weakness and bone pain
- Proximal myopathy
- Nausea
- Symptoms due to arrhythmias, e.g. palpitations.

> A way to remember the typical symptoms of hypercalcaemia is 'painful bones, renal stones, abdominal groans, and psychic moans'.

Patients may have symptoms from the underlying cause of their hypercalcaemia, e.g. night sweats, weight loss, or anorexia secondary to an underlying malignancy.

They may also have symptoms from conditions that may develop *as a result* of hypercalcaemia (Box 16.1).

Box 16.1 Conditions that may develop as a result of hypercalcaemia

- Pancreatitis
- Peptic ulceration
- Cardiomyopathy
- Kidney disease.

Examination

Use the ABCDE approach to examine patients (Table 16.3).

Investigations

Bedside

- ECG: shortened QT interval, prolonged PR interval, and arrhythmias.

Bloods

- Calcium (Box 16.2), phosphate, PTH, vitamin D, U&E, and LFT (including albumin).

Imaging

- Chest X-ray may reveal underlying malignancy or granulomatous disease
- If evidence of primary hyperparathyroidism is present, further neck imaging (such as ultrasound or sestamibi scanning) is indicated.

Table 16.3 Findings suggestive of acute hypercalcaemia in an ABCDE examination

C	• Hypertension • Dehydration
D	• Confusion • Hyporeflexia • Hypotonia • Paresis • Coma
E	• Itching • Conjunctivitis • Renal angle tenderness (stones) • Corneal calcification • Fragility/pathological fractures

Box 16.2 Interpretation of bloods

- Avoid prolonged tourniquet application and repeat serum calcium to confirm diagnosis
- High calcium and high PTH = primary or tertiary hyperparathyroidism
- High calcium and low PTH = malignancy or other less common causes.

Management

Severe, symptomatic hypercalcaemia is life-threatening. The initial acute management of hypercalcaemia focuses on rehydration and stopping any causative medication. Diagnosis of the underlying disease is essential in order to reverse the mechanism of the impaired calcium balance.

Acute management

Vigorous rehydration

Since most patients with hypercalcaemia are dehydrated, 4–6L of 0.9% saline should be infused in 24 hours if there are no contraindications, e.g. congestive cardiac failure. Volume expansion with saline enhances urinary calcium excretion because calcium is coupled to sodium in the kidneys. After 24 hours of fluid resuscitation, recheck serum calcium level before considering administering bisphosphonates.

> Monitor fluid balance in the elderly and patients with renal impairment and considering giving furosemide if appropriate for overload only.

Intravenous bisphosphonates

These agents inhibit osteoclast activity; however, they may take 72 hours to reach full therapeutic effect. Commence once volume replete if calcium is still elevated and monitor serum calcium response. Occasionally a second dose is needed. Rarely, hypocalcaemia may develop if the patient is vitamin D deficient.

- Zoledronic acid 4mg over 15 minutes **OR**
- Pamidronate 30–90mg at 20mg/hour **OR**
- Ibandronic acid 2–4mg.

Second-line treatments

Glucocorticoids

Inhibit 1,25OHD production and are useful in hypercalcaemia caused by vitamin D intoxication, granulomatous disorders, and lymphoma. Prednisolone given at a dose of 40mg daily is usually effective within 72 hours.

Denosumab

Under strict specialist supervision.

Calcitonin

Works predominantly by inhibiting osteoclast bone resorption, while it also enhances calcium and phosphate urinary excretion.

Renal dialysis

May be indicated in severe renal failure and is a very effective method of treating hypercalcaemia should the above-mentioned measures not be successful.

Parathyroidectomy

Occasionally considered in the acute presentation of primary hyperparathyroidism, if resistant to pharmacological measures.

Further reading

1. NICE Clinical Knowledge Summaries (2019). Hypercalcaemia. Available at: https://cks.nice.org.uk/topics/hypercalcaemia/
2. Levi R, Silver J (2011). Hypercalcaemia. In: Wass JAH, Stewart PM, Amiel SA, Davies MJ (eds) *Oxford Textbook of Endocrinology and Diabetes*, 2nd ed (pp. 642–52). Oxford: Oxford University Press. Available at: https://doi.org/10.1093/med/9780199235292.003.0411

Chapter 17

Hyperglycaemia

Guidelines:
Joint British Diabetes Societies for Inpatient Care (Management of hyperglycaemia and steroid (glucocorticoid) therapy, 2021): https://abcd.care/sites/abcd.care/files/site_uploads/JBDS_08_Steroids_DM_Guideline_FINAL_28052021.pdf

Joint British Diabetes Societies for Inpatient Care (The use of variable rate intravenous insulin infusion (VRIII) in medical inpatients, 2014): https://abcd.care/sites/abcd.care/files/resources/JBDS_IP_VRIII.pdf

OUP disclaimer: Oxford University Press makes no representation, express or implied, that the drug dosages are correct and that the recommendations are an exclusive or mandatory course of care. All health professionals reading this text have a responsibility to evaluate its appropriateness and take the individual needs of the patient into account.

Local trust guidelines: please refer to your local guidelines as necessary.

Overview

Hyperglycaemia is defined as either fasting serum glucose >7mmol/L, or random glucose >11.1mmol/L. It is a common occurrence in diabetic and non-diabetic patients (stress hyperglycaemia), and is associated with prolonged hospital stays, worse outcomes, and increased mortality. In diabetic patients, hyperglycaemia can develop into the life-threatening emergencies of DKA (see Chapter 15) and HHS (see Chapter 18).

Diagnosis

CBG measurement is part of routine nursing care. History and examination are important in identifying the cause and context of the hyperglycaemia, and establishing how unwell the patient is.

History

Take a focused history to identify presenting features of hyperglycaemia including:

- Polyuria
- Thirst
- Urinary frequency
- Urinary urgency
- Vomiting
- Weight loss.

Ask about infective symptoms that may have caused hyperglycaemia, e.g. respiratory and urinary symptoms. Establish whether the patient is known to be diabetic and ask about alcohol intake and medication (including compliance with antiglycaemic drugs, recent medication changes, and steroid use). Ask about family history of diabetes (including age of onset), and in females ask about hyperglycaemia during previous pregnancies.

> The most common causes of hyperglycaemia are acute illness, non-compliance with diabetic medication, and alcohol.

Examination

Begin your examination with a general inspection. Signs such as vomiting, abdominal tenderness, and reduced consciousness should alert you to a possible diagnosis of DKA or HHS.

Perform a full physical examination looking for signs of infection. This should include listening to the chest, examining the abdomen, and assessing the skin for signs of cellulitis and ulcers.

Assess volume status; typically, hyperglycaemia will lead to dehydration and may present with clinical signs such as:

- Tachycardia
- Hypotension or postural hypotension
- Dry mucous membranes
- Raised capillary refill time >2 seconds
- Reduced skin turgor.

> Sweet 'pear-drop' breath suggests underlying ketosis and should heighten your suspicion of DKA.

Investigations

Bedside

- CBG
- Serum ketones should be measured in people with T1DM with persistent hyperglycaemia (>2 readings above 12mmol/L, at least 1 hour apart), or in **any** patient if unwell. Interpret as per Table 17.1

- Send urine for culture if urinary tract infection is suspected
- Sputum sample if the patient is producing purulent sputum
- Skin swabs if indicated.

Be aware that patients with T2DM taking SGLT inhibitors (e.g. dapagliflozin, empagliflozin, and canagliflozin) can present with euglycaemic DKA. In this situation, the CBG may be normal but the patient may have ketoacidosis. It is important to check blood ketone levels in these patients.

Table 17.1 Interpretation of serum ketones

Serum ketones (mmol/L)	Action to be taken
<0.6	Normal
0.6–1.4	Check in 2 hours
1.5–2.9	Check in 1 hour, consider DKA
>3	Perform VBG to check pH, consider treating as DKA

Note: urinary ketones are also used, a reading of >2+ should prompt the measurement of serum ketones and VBG.

Bloods

- FBC
- CRP
- U&E
- LFT
- Serum glucose
- HbA1c
- VBG
- Blood cultures if the patient is pyrexial.

Imaging

- Chest X-ray if chest infection is suspected.

Management

A single reading of elevated blood glucose in an otherwise well person may not require intervention. If an obvious cause of hyperglycaemia is identified (e.g. infection), this should be treated. If a patient is unwell, consider the need for a VRII (sometimes referred to as a 'sliding scale') and IV fluids.

Acute management

Persistent hyperglycaemia

If DKA (see Chapter 15) or HHS (see Chapter 18) are detected, these should be treated as per their guidelines.

The management of steroid-induced hyperglycaemia is covered later in this chapter.

A VRII is indicated in an unwell patient with a CBG >10mmol/L, without DKA or HHS, if they are not eating or drinking.

If a VRII is not indicated, and the patient is being treated with glucose-lowering medications, e.g. gliclazide, these should be optimized. If the patient is being treated with insulin, consider a 'correction' dose of short-acting insulin (2–4 units) if required or increase the insulin regimen.

Be careful to avoid overnight hypoglycaemia due to overtreatment of high blood glucose before bedtime.

Setting up VRIIs

This is an infusion of fast-acting or short-acting insulin (e.g. Actrapid®). The starting rate depends on the most recent CBG. Initially patients should be started on the standard-rate regimen (Table 17.2). If CBGs remain high despite the VRII (i.e. in insulin-resistant patients), the rates may be changed to an increased rate regimen. If the patient becomes hypoglycaemic or is known to be very insulin sensitive, it may be appropriate to use a reduced-rate regimen.

Table 17.2 Starting (standard) rate of VRII

Capillary blood sugar (mmol/L)	Starting rate (mL/hour)
<4	0
4.1–8.0	1
8.1–12.0	2
12.1–16.0	4
16.0–20.0	5
20.1–24.0	6
>24.0	8

Adapted under a Creative Commons Licence (CC BY-NC 4.0) from The use of variable rate intravenous insulin infusion (VRIII) in medical inpatients. October 2014. Joint British Diabetes Societies, Inpatient Care Group (JBDS 09).

Regular long-acting subcutaneous insulin should **always** be continued alongside a VRII.

Fluid resuscitation

If receiving a VRII, patients will require IV fluids as per local guidelines. Elderly patients at risk of fluid overload should receive 25–30mL/kg in 24 hours (usually approximately 2L). Patients who are dehydrated, e.g. vomiting, will require additional IV fluid to replace losses.

If a patient is at risk of fluid overload, e.g. heart failure, consider using smaller volumes of 10% glucose rather than greater volumes of a lower percentage glucose.

Insulin drives potassium (K^+) into cells, therefore consider concurrent potassium chloride (KCL) replacement depending on K^+ level:

- K^+ >5.5: no replacement required
- K^+ 3.5–5.5: supplement with 0.15% KCL (20mmol)
- K^+ <3.5: supplement with 0.3% KCL (40mmol).

If using 0.9% sodium chloride (NaCl) for IV fluid, when glucose levels are <14mmol/L, consider switching from NaCl to 5% dextrose to avoid hypoglycaemia.

Remember: while on a VRII it is important to regularly measure pH, glucose, K^+, and ketones to monitor clinical improvement.

Treatment after stabilization

Discontinuing VRIIs

When a patient is eating and drinking with stable blood sugar levels, consider stopping the VRII. Ensure they have eaten a meal at least 30 minutes before restarting oral hyperglycaemic medication. Measure CBG 1 hour after stopping the VRII, and four times over the next 24 hours to ensure that there is no rebound hyperglycaemia.

Consider a referral to the diabetes team of anyone who has required IV insulin treatment.

Special considerations

Steroid-induced hyperglycaemia

Steroids cause hyperglycaemia and glucose levels should be expected to rise 4–8 hours after an oral steroid dose, or sooner following a parenteral dose.

Often, but not always, glucose levels improve as the steroid dose is reduced or stopped; therefore, any treatment that has been initiated will need to be titrated down again.

If a patient has steroid-induced hyperglycaemia, they should be tested for diabetes (see Chapter 26) at least 6 weeks after their steroid course has completed.

Glucose monitoring frequency for patients on steroid therapy

- **Patients without a diabetes diagnosis:** OD. If >12mmol/L, escalate testing frequency to QDS
- **Patients with a diabetes diagnosis:** QDS testing.

Treating steroid-induced hyperglycaemia

If CBG is >12 mmol/L more than twice in 24 hours, commence treatment.

Insulin treatment may be more appropriate than oral treatment if hyperglycaemia persists throughout the day.

If the patient is acutely unwell, they should be started on a VRII pending specialist diabetes team review.

Options for treatment

Non-diabetic

- Sulfonylurea, e.g. gliclazide, starting dose 40mg OD
- 10 units of basal insulin to be given in the morning, e.g. Humulin® I, Insuman® Basal
- A multiple daily injection regimen may be required for steroid treatments involving multiple daily dosages.

T1DM

- Increase insulin dosages by 2 units every 24–48 hours and seek specialist diabetes team review.

T2DM not receiving insulin therapy

- Commence gliclazide 40mg OD or escalate current dose by 40mg if the patient is already taking it (maximum dose 240mg in the morning, maximum daily dose 320mg)
- Metformin, escalate dose to a maximum of 1g BD.

T2DM already on insulin therapy

- If taking basal insulin in the evening, consider switching the dose to morning.

Patients with diabetes who are undergoing surgery

This guidance is covered in Chapters 92 and 93.

Further reading

1. Raine T, Collins G, Hall C, et al. (2018). Hyperglycaemia. In: *Oxford Handbook for the Foundation Programme*, 5th ed (p. 330). Oxford: Oxford University Press.

Chapter 18

Hyperglycaemic hyperosmolar syndrome

Guideline:
Joint British Diabetes Societies Inpatient Care Group (The management of the hyperosmolar hyperglycaemic state (HHS) in adults with diabetes): https://abcd.care/sites/abcd.care/files/site_uploads/JBDS_Guidelines_Current/JBDS_06_The_Management_of_Hyperosmolar_Hyperglycaemic_State_HHS_%20in_Adults_FINAL_0.pdf

OUP disclaimer: Oxford University Press makes no representation, express or implied, that the drug dosages are correct and that the recommendations are an exclusive or mandatory course of care. All health professionals reading this text have a responsibility to evaluate its appropriateness and take the individual needs of the patient into account.

Local trust guidelines: please refer to your local guidelines as necessary.

Overview

Hyperglycaemic hyperosmolar state (HHS) is a medical emergency with a mortality of 10–20%.[1] It typically affects older patients, sometimes as a first presentation of T2DM and it develops over days, as compared with DKA (see Chapter 14) which develops over hours. HHS is characterized by severe dehydration along with hyperglycaemia which results in a hyperosmolar state. Treatment involves rehydration and restoration of electrolyte disturbances in a cautious manner that avoids rapid and dangerous cellular fluid shifts.

1 Pasquel FJ, Umpierrez GE. Hyperosmolar hyperglycemic state: a historic review of the clinical presentation, diagnosis, and treatment. *Diabetes Care*. 2014; 37:3124–31.

Diagnosis

History/diagnostic criteria

Diagnosis should be considered when the following features are present:

- Severe dehydration—indicated by hypovolaemia and hypernatraemia
- Marked hyperglycaemia (≥30mmol/L) **without** significant hyperketonaemia (<3mmol/L) or acidosis (pH >7.3, bicarbonate >15 mmol/L)
- Osmolality ≥320mOsm/kg.

Patients can present with a mixture of HHS and DKA. Consider in the presence of significant hyperketonaemia.

Examination

Systematically examine the patient using an ABCDE approach (Table 18.1). Hyperglycaemia results in an osmotic diuresis which causes dehydration.

Table 18.1 HHS examination findings

A	• Check for evidence of airway compromise due to reduced conscious level
B	• Hypoxia
C	• Tachycardia • Hypotension • JVP not visible • Cool peripheries • Prolonged capillary refill time
D	• ↓ GCS score is common when osmolality >330mOsm/kg • Limb weakness may be a sign of raised urea
E	• Sunken eyes and longitudinal furrows on the tongue suggest dehydration • Examine feet for ulceration

Call for help early in HHS patients

The patient usually has some impairment of conscious level due to significant metabolic derangement and they may be more dehydrated than they appear—water moves from cells into the extracellular space, temporarily preserving intravascular volume.

Investigations

Use biochemical parameters in conjunction with clinical findings. Look for precipitating factors, e.g. infection or a vascular event.

Bedside

- Point-of-care capillary glucose and ketones
- Urinalysis and MC&S
- ECG—cardiac events can be a precipitant or complication of HHS.

Bloods

- FBC
- U&E:
  - To calculate osmolality (Box 18.1)
  - If patients have acute or chronic kidney injury, this may be contributing to their acidosis and will need strict fluid balance management
- CRP
- VBG (including HCO_3^-/lactate)
- Serum glucose and ketones
- HbA1c
- Blood cultures.

Box 18.1 Osmolality calculation

$$2Na^+ + \text{glucose} + \text{urea}$$

Imaging

- Chest X-ray.

Escalation

Consider escalation to higher dependency care if any of the following are present:

- Serum pH <7.1 (DKA may coexist)
- Potassium derangement on admission
- GCS score <12
- Oxygen saturation <92% on air
- Signs of shock: systolic blood pressure <90mmHg, heart rate >100bpm or <60bpm, or hypothermia
- Signs of severe dehydration: osmolality >350mOsm/kg, sodium >160mmol/L, or creatinine >200µmol/L
- Macrovascular event, e.g. myocardial infarction or other serious comorbidity.

Management

Acute management

Correct biochemical abnormalities **slowly** to prevent vascular complications and avoid pathology caused by rapid cellular fluid shifts (e.g. sudden drop in blood pressure, cerebral oedema, central pontine myelinolysis).

After initial assessment, use the treatment algorithm (Fig. 18.1) to:

- Normalize osmolality (Box 18.1)
- Replace fluid/electrolyte losses (Box 18.2 and Table 18.2)
- Reduce glucose (aim to reduce to 10–15mmol/L).

Box 18.2 Expect an initial rise in sodium

- Serum osmolality reduces when blood glucose is lowered. Water shifts into the intracellular space, and serum sodium concentration rises
- A fall in glucose of 5.5mmol/L will cause a 2.4mmol/L rise in sodium. A rise greater than this indicates inadequate fluid resuscitation
- Rising sodium is only a concern if osmolality is not falling concurrently.

Source: The management of the hyperosmolar hyperglycaemic state (HHS) in adults. February 2022. Joint British Diabetes Societies, Inpatient Care Group (JBDS 06).

Table 18.2 Potassium replacement—aim to maintain within normal range

Potassium level in first 24 hours (mmol/L)	Potassium replacement in infusion solution
>5.5	Nil
3.5–5.5	40mmol/L
<3.5	Senior review—additional potassium required

Treatment after stabilization

- Check serum osmolality 2-hourly for the first 6 hours, and then 4-hourly (if improving) for the next 12 hours. After the first 24 hours, bloods can be checked daily if improving
- Blood glucose level should be checked hourly for the first 24 hours. Target: 10–15mmol/L in the first 24 hours
- Discontinue IV insulin when the patient is eating and drinking
- Continue to assess fluid balance—aim for 3–6L positive by 12 hours but check for signs of fluid overload or cerebral oedema
- Daily foot checks due to high risk of pressure ulceration. Consider using heel protectors
- It may take up to 72 hours for electrolytes and osmolality to return to within normal range
- Continue anticoagulation while patient is recovering
- Refer to specialist team.

Further reading

1. 'Hyperglycaemic Emergencies'—online lecture material by Dr S Nag for the Royal College of Physicians. Available at: https://www.rcplondon.ac.uk/file/6424/download?token=D9VhtcgX

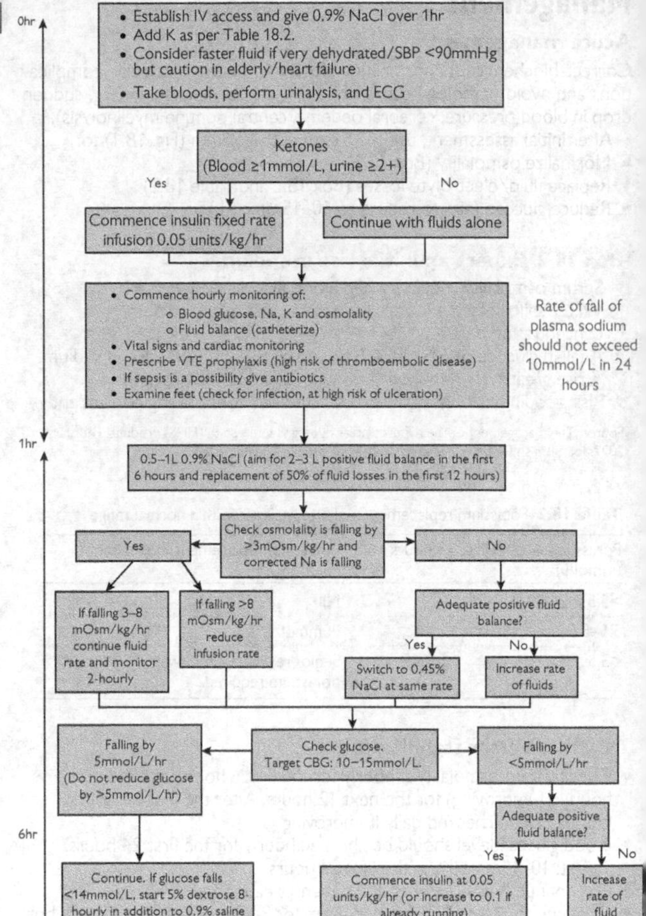

Fig. 18.1 Example treatment algorithm.
VTE, venous thromboembolism.

Chapter 19

Hyperthyroidism

Guideline:
NICE NG145 (Thyroid disease: assessment and management): https://www.nice.org.uk/guidance/ng145

OUP disclaimer: Oxford University Press makes no representation, express or implied, that the drug dosages are correct and that the recommendations are an exclusive or mandatory course of care. All health professionals reading this text have a responsibility to evaluate its appropriateness and take the individual needs of the patient into account.

Local trust guidelines: please refer to your local guidelines as necessary.

Overview

Hyperthyroidism is a common condition which affects approximately 2% of women and 0.2% of men in the UK and occurs due to an overproduction of thyroid hormones. Initially, symptoms may develop insidiously which can make diagnosis challenging. Untreated, symptoms become more severe and can become disabling and even life-threatening. In the long-term, untreated hyperthyroidism leads to increased cardiovascular morbidity and mortality and patients are at an increased risk of developing osteoporosis. It is therefore vital to recognise symptoms early in order to make a timely diagnosis and initiate management.

Diagnosis

Causes

Hyperthyroidism may be caused by:

- Graves' disease (75%)
- Toxic nodular hyperthyroidism—toxic adenoma and toxic multinodular goitre (15%)
- Thyroiditis (10%); silent, postpartum, subacute (viral)
- Drug induced (amiodarone, checkpoint inhibitors, interferon)
- Pituitary adenoma
- Other rare causes.

> It is essential to establish the cause so that appropriate management can be commenced.

History

Cardiovascular

- Palpitations
- ↑ perspiration
- Light-headedness.

Gastrointestinal

- ↑ appetite
- Diarrhoea
- Weight loss.

Neurological

- Difficulty sleeping
- Tremor
- Anxiety
- Irritability
- Hyperactivity
- Fatigue
- Heat intolerance.

Other

- Oligomenorrhea
- Thyroid eye disease (TED) in Graves' disease (Box 19.1)—red, gritty, bulging eyes, light sensitivity, double vision, loss of vision (⚑)—seek urgent expert advice
- Thyroiditis—fever, thyroid pain, malaise, recent viral illness, postpartum.

Box 19.1 Thyroid eye disease

TED is an autoimmune condition, most commonly associated with Graves' disease, which can lead to blindness. It can develop before or after thyroid symptoms develop and smoking increases the risk.

Examination

Red flags for possible thyroid malignancy are listed in Box 19.2.

Cardiovascular
- Warm, sweaty to touch
- Irregular pulse
- Tachycardia.

Thyroid
- Goitre—diffuse or nodular
- Tenderness (suggests thyroiditis)
- Thyroid bruit.

Neurological
- Tremor
- Proximal myopathy
- Hyperreflexia.

Other
- TED—exophthalmos, diplopia, lid lag
- Pretibial myxoedema
- Thyroid acropachy
- Thyrotoxic periodic paralysis.

Box 19.2 Red flags for thyroid malignancy
- Rapid nodular growth
- Shortness of breath
- Hoarse voice
- Swallowing difficulties.

Source: data from NICE NG145.

Investigations

The main aim of the investigations is to determine the aetiology as this determines the long-term management. It is important to differentiate between thyroiditis (usually transient and self-limiting) and other causes of hyperthyroidism that require definitive treatment. Interpretation of investigation findings are listed in Table 19.1.

Bedside
- ECG—AF or sinus tachycardia.

Bloods
- TSH (suppressed in primary and elevated in secondary hyperthyroidism)
- Free thyroxine (FT4)/triiodothyronine (FT3)
- FBC/U&E/LFT/CRP—to exclude other causes
- TSH-receptor antibodies (Graves' disease)
- ESR—raised in thyroiditis.

If a patient is acutely unwell with a non-thyroidal illness, do not routinely use TFT as the results may be unreliable.

Imaging

- Radioisotope scanning
- Ultrasound if palpable thyroid nodule.

Table 19.1 Investigation findings in different causes of hyperthyroidism

Investigation	Graves' disease	Toxic nodular hyperthyroidism	Thyroiditis
Bloods	TSH undetectable FT4 and FT3 raised Only FT3 raised in T3 toxicosis	TSH undetectable FT4 and FT3 raised Only FT3 raised in T3 toxicosis	TSH undetectable FT4 and FT3 raised Raised ESR/CRP
Antibodies	TSH-receptor antibodies raised TPO antibodies may be raised		TPO antibodies may be raised
Radioisotope scan	Diffuse uptake	Focal pattern of uptake	Minimal uptake

TPO, thyroid peroxidase.

Management

Refer all patients to an endocrinologist for further assessment.

Patient education

Discuss the function of the thyroid gland and the risks of over- and undertreatment. Explain the importance of treatment compliance even when asymptomatic to avoid long-term complications. Explain the need for routine monitoring. Risks of various management options are discussed in Table 19.2.

Lifestyle and simple interventions

- Smoking cessation (particularly if TED)
- Selenium supplements (particularly if TED).

Pharmacological management

- Thionamide:
  - Carbimazole is first line (propylthiouracil if pregnant)
    - Monotherapy (titrated dose of carbimazole) **OR**
    - 'Block and replace' (higher dose of carbimazole, add levothyroxine when needed)
- Radioiodine
- Beta-blockers for adrenergic symptoms.

Surgical management

- Thyroidectomy/hemithyroidectomy.

Graves' disease

- Radioiodine is usually recommended as first line but thionamides can be offered as first line in mild, uncomplicated disease or if radioiodine is unsuitable
- Thionamides may be given as a 12–18-month course

Table 19.2 Risks of hyperthyroidism management options

	Radioiodine	Surgery	Antithyroid drugs

Risks	• Long-term hypothyroidism likely
	• Short-term radiation protection required
	• Avoidance of pregnancy/fathering a child in near future
	• New or worsening thyroid eye disease particularly if untreated hypothyroidism
		• Invasive and requires general anaesthetic
		• Long-term hypothyroidism
		• Scarring
		• Swallowing and breathing difficulties
		• Voice change
		• Hypoparathyroidism
			• Long-term cure rate 50% Graves' disease (but lower for nodule/multinodular goitre)
			• Carbimazole:
			  • Agranulocytosis
			  • Pancreatitis
			  • Birth defects if taken in pregnancy
			• Propylthiouracil:
			  • Agranulocytosis
			  • Liver failure
			  • Need for regular bloods and follow-up appointments

Source: data from NICE NG145.

- If there are concerns about compression or malignancy, surgery should be offered first line (once euthyroidism is achieved with thionamide treatment).

Toxic nodular hyperthyroidism

- Radioiodine is first line unless unsuitable
- Surgical or long-term antithyroid medications are second line
- For cases of a single nodule, radioiodine or hemithyroidectomy are first-line options.

Thyroiditis

- Supportive management, e.g. simple analgesia.

Monitoring and follow-up

Thionamide therapy

- Check FBC and LFT before starting—only recheck if unwell
- Warn patient regarding risks and give written advice (1. agranulocytosis, 2. pancreatitis, 3. teratogenic)
- Stop therapy immediately if the patient develops agranulocytosis (⚑)
- Check TSH/FT4 every 6 weeks until TSH is within the reference range, titrating as appropriate to the lowest dose required to maintain TSH in reference range, then check TSH every 3 months until the therapy is stopped (12–18 months depending on regimen)
- After stopping therapy—measure TSH within 8 weeks of stopping, 3 monthly for a year, then annually thereafter or sooner if symptoms of recurrent hyperthyroidism.

> If receiving thionamides, a rise in TSH or fall in FT4 should lead to a reduction or withdrawal in thionamide dose.

Radioiodine therapy

- Check TSH/FT4/FT3 every 6 weeks for the first 6 months until TSH is within the reference range
- Warn and monitor for evidence of TED
- Measure TSH at 9 and 12 months and then every 6 months thereafter
- Offer levothyroxine to those who develop hypothyroidism
- If hyperthyroidism persists, offer antithyroid drugs and further radioiodine 6 months post treatment.

Surgical therapy

- Offer levothyroxine to all patients:
  - <65 years and no history of cardiovascular disease: starting dose 1.6 micrograms/kg/day, rounded to the nearest 25 micrograms
  - ≥65 years or history of cardiovascular disease: starting dose 25–50 micrograms/day
- Measure TSH postoperatively and then annually thereafter
- Measure calcium postoperatively and replace as required (may be short-term).

Special considerations

Subclinical hyperthyroidism

- Occurs when TSH is suppressed but T3/T4 levels are within the normal range (Box 19.3).

Box 19.3 Interpretation of TSH levels in subclinical hyperthyroidism

- A TSH level >0.1mIU/L is more likely to be related to non-thyroidal illness than hyperthyroidism
- A TSH level <0.1mIU/L is more likely to be due to mild hyperthyroidism.

Management

- Seek specialist advice if patient has two low TSH readings at least 3 months apart and evidence of thyroid disease
- If untreated and TSH persistently outside the reference range, consider testing TSH/FT4/FT3 every 6 months.

Amiodarone

- Amiodarone therapy may cause hyperthyroidism (amiodarone-induced thyrotoxicosis (AIT)) or hypothyroidism due to its high iodine content
- In patients with underlying hyperthyroidism (including latent Graves' disease), they may develop type 1 AIT after starting amiodarone. This requires thionamide therapy
- In previously euthyroid individuals who take amiodarone (often for several months/years), they may develop type 2 AIT caused by thyroiditis. Often patients recover after several months and may subsequently experience hypothyroidism before their thyroid hormone levels normalize. This type sometimes responds to steroid therapy.

Thyroid storm

- Thyroid storm manifests with signs of severe hyperthyroidism resulting in multisystem decompensation. This represents a life-threatening emergency and may be triggered in patients with hyperthyroidism (may be previously undiagnosed). Triggers include infection or surgery.

Secondary hyperthyroidism

- Secondary hyperthyroidism causes a normal or raised TSH level. This may be due to a pituitary tumour that produces TSH or resistance to pituitary hormones
- If secondary hyperthyroidism is suspected, it is important to check visual fields and request an MRI brain.

Elderly

- Often present with weight loss, depression, and cardiovascular features, such as AF and deterioration of pre-existing cardiac disease.

Pregnancy

- All pregnant patients with hyperthyroidism should see a specialist as they may need antithyroid drug dose reduction
- Patients on a 'block and replace' regimen should be switched to a maintenance regimen and patients on carbimazole should be switched to propylthiouracil
- During pregnancy, target FT4 levels should be at upper end of the reference range due to the risk hypothyroidism poses to the fetus and ↑ rates of miscarriage and premature delivery
- Hyperemesis gravidarum may be associated with thyrotoxic biochemistry but this resolves without treatment when hyperemesis settles.

Further reading

1. Boelaert K (2018). Thyroid hormone metabolism. In: Turner HE, Eastell R, Grossman A (eds) *Oxford Desk Reference: Endocrinology* (pp. 41–47). Oxford: Oxford University Press. Available at: https://doi.org/10.1093/med/9780199672837.003.0002
2. Newson L (2020). Hyperthyroidism. Patient. Available at: https://patient.info/doctor/hyperthyroidism
3. Wass JAH, Owen K (eds) (2014). Thyroid. In: *Oxford Handbook of Endocrinology and Diabetes*, 3rd ed (pp. 1–105). Oxford: Oxford University Press. Available at: https://doi.org/10.1093/med/9780199644438.003.0001

Chapter 20

Hypocalcaemia

Guideline:
Society for Endocrinology Endocrine Emergency Guidance (Emergency management of acute hypocalcaemia in adult patients): https://ec.bioscientifica.com/view/journals/ec/5/5/G7.xml

OUP disclaimer: Oxford University Press makes no representation, express or implied, that the drug dosages are correct and that the recommendations are an exclusive or mandatory course of care. All health professionals reading this text have a responsibility to evaluate its appropriateness and take the individual needs of the patient into account.

Local trust guidelines: please refer to your local guidelines as necessary.

Overview

Hypocalcaemia is defined as an adjusted calcium level <2.1mmol/L (ionized <0.9mmol/L). Hypocalcaemia raises the resting membrane potential of neurons, bringing them closer to the threshold potential for depolarization which may lead to spasm, tetany, or seizures and can be life-threatening. The commonest cause of hypocalcaemia is a total thyroidectomy which includes removal of the parathyroid glands.

- **Mild hypocalcaemia:** asymptomatic **AND** adjusted calcium 1.9–2.1mmol/L
- **Severe hypocalcaemia:** symptomatic **OR** adjusted calcium <1.9mmol/L.

'Adjusted' or 'corrected' calcium has been modified to take into account albumin levels (albumin is one of the primary calcium binding proteins). Only unbound ionized calcium is physiologically active and therefore it is important to use the adjusted figure. Exact reference ranges vary between laboratories, check locally.

Diagnosis

History

Establish any past medical history which might indicate an underlying cause of hypocalcaemia.

Causes

Usually due to the failure of PTH secretion (inappropriately low PTH) or an inability to release calcium from bone (elevated PTH).

- Hypoparathyroidism:
  - Surgical:
    - Post thyroidectomy (may be temporary/permanent)
    - Post selective parathyroidectomy (usually transient and mild)
  - Autoimmune
  - Radiation
  - Failure of development of the parathyroid glands
  - Magnesium deficiency
- Failure of calcium release from bone:
  - Severe vitamin D deficiency (dietary, malabsorption, low ultraviolet light exposure, chronic renal failure)
  - Cytotoxic medications (e.g. foscarnet, gadolinium)
  - Renal failure
  - Resistance to PTH (magnesium deficiency, pseudohypoparathyroidism)
- Complexing of calcium from circulation:
  - Pancreatitis
  - Large transfusions (transfused citrate 'chelates' calcium)
  - Rhabdomyolysis
- Multifactorial:
  - Sepsis
  - Burns.

Symptoms

Symptoms are more severe if there has been an acute drop in the adjusted calcium level.

- Perioral and/or digital paraesthesia
- Laryngospasm (temporarily difficult to speak or breathe due to spasm of vocal cords)
- Generalized weakness.

Examination

Central nervous system

- Trousseau's and Chvostek's signs (Box 20.1)
- Tetany, cramps, carpopedal spasm
- Focal or generalized seizures
- Altered mental state.

Cardiovascular system

- Arrhythmias (i.e. ventricular tachycardia)
- Reduced cardiac output leading to hypotension or heart failure
- Bradycardia.

Box 20.1 Eponymous clinical signs in hypocalcaemia

Trousseau's sign (more sensitive)

Inflate the blood pressure cuff to a level 10–20mmHg greater than the systolic blood pressure for 3 minutes. In hypocalcaemia this unmasks latent neuromuscular hyperexcitability, leading to carpal spasm.

Chvostek's sign

Twitching of facial muscles in response to tapping of the facial nerve (i.e. anterior to the tragus).

Investigations

Bedside

- ECG—prolonged PR and QT intervals, arrhythmias (i.e. ventricular tachycardia).

Bloods

- Adjusted calcium
- Phosphate and magnesium
- PTH
- U&E
- Vitamin D.

Other

- Amylase (if suspicion of pancreatitis)
- Creatine kinase (if suspicion of rhabdomyolysis).

Management

Acute management

Mild hypocalcaemia

- Oral supplements (e.g. Calvive® 1000, two tablets BD)
- Patient may be discharged when calcium level >2.1mmol/L
- If the calcium level remains 1.9–2.1mmol/L, increase the dose (e.g. Calvive® 1000, three tablets BD).

Severe hypocalcaemia

This is a **medical emergency**—get senior clinician help immediately. This patient may require critical care admission for cardiac monitoring ± inotropic support.

- Examine with an ABCDE approach
- Give 100% oxygen if significantly reduced GCS score or patient is seizing
- Start ECG monitoring
- **IV calcium gluconate bolus (Box 20.2):**
  - 10–20mL 10% calcium gluconate in 50–100mL 5% dextrose
  - Give over 10 minutes *with cardiac monitoring*
  - Repeat until asymptomatic
- **Followed by IV calcium gluconate infusion:**
  - 100mL 10% calcium gluconate in 1L 0.9% NaCl/5% dextrose
  - Infuse at 50–100mL/hour
  - Titrate until calcium levels have normalized.

Box 20.2 Use of calcium gluconate

- Calcium gluconate can cause transient but dramatic hypotension and arrhythmias
- It can also cause local vasoconstriction or ischaemia—ideally administer via a central line, otherwise into a large vein with fast running IV fluids
- Calcium infusions should be avoided in severe CKD (stage 3-5)—seek advice from nephrology.

Treatment after stabilization

Treat the cause

- Vitamin D deficiency:
  - 300,000 units of cholecalciferol **OR** 300,000 units of ergocalciferol split over 6–10 weeks
- Hypomagnesaemia:
  - Review medications that might cause hypomagnesaemia, e.g. omeprazole
  - Replace IV, e.g. 24mmol over 24 hours (as 6g $MgSO_4$ in 500mL 0.9% NaCl/5% dextrose)
  - Monitor serum magnesium
- Post thyroidectomy:
  - Recheck calcium levels after 24 hours
  - If severe hypocalcaemia or continues to have mild hypocalcaemia after 72 hours—get specialist advice: will require treatment with alfacalcidol or calcitriol.

Follow-up

- If the patient is started on alfacalcidol or calcitriol, recheck serum calcium at 1 week. If stable, recheck at 1, 3 and 6 months.
- These patients will likely need ongoing oral calcium supplementation and should have specialist follow-up.

Further reading

1. British Association of Endocrine and Thyroid Surgeons. Post thyroidectomy/parathyroidectomy guideline. Available at: https://www.baets.org.uk/wp-content/uploads/BAETS-Post-op-Hypocalcaemia-Guidance.pdf

Chapter 21

Hypoglycaemia

Guideline:
Joint British Diabetes Societies for Inpatient Care (The hospital management of hypoglycaemia in adults with diabetes mellitus, 5th edition): https://abcd.care/sites/abcd.care/files/site_uploads/JBDS_Guidelines_Current/JBDS_01_HypoGuideline%20_March_2022.pdf

OUP disclaimer: Oxford University Press makes no representation, express or implied, that the drug dosages are correct and that the recommendations are an exclusive or mandatory course of care. All health professionals reading this text have a responsibility to evaluate its appropriateness and take the individual needs of the patient into account.

Local trust guidelines: please refer to your local guidelines as necessary.

Overview

Hypoglycaemia refers to a CBG level <4.0mmol/L. Prolonged severe hypoglycaemia can lead to permanent neurological deficit and death. Patients who have had diabetes for a long time, particularly those with tight glycaemic control, are more likely to have poor hypoglycaemic awareness, increasing their risk of recurrent hypoglycaemia and a severe hypoglycaemic episode.

Diagnosis

History

Box 21.1 lists patients at higher risk of hypoglycaemia.

Box 21.1 Which patient groups are at risk of hypoglycaemia?

- Type 1 diabetics
- Type 2 diabetics on insulin treatment
- Long-term diabetics
- Those with poor glycaemic awareness
- Elderly people
- Those with renal impairment (due to reduced clearance of insulin)
- Those with hepatic impairment (due to reduced glycogen stores).

Source: data from The Hospital Management of Hypoglycaemia in Adults with Diabetes Mellitus. March 2022. JBDS-IP 04.

Causes

- Incorrect type/time/dose of insulin or oral hypoglycaemic agent e.g. gliclazide
- Missed/delayed meals, vomiting or prolonged starvation ('nil by mouth')
- Sepsis
- Alcohol excess
- Liver failure
- Cortisol insufficiency or abrupt cessation of long-term steroid therapy.

Symptoms

- Autonomic (sweating, shaking, palpitations and hunger)
- Neuroglycopenic (confusion, drowsiness, behavioural disturbance, speech difficulties, incoordination, seizures, and coma).

Examination

Table 21.1 lists possible ABCDE examination findings in hypoglycaemic patients.

Table 21.1 Potential examination findings in a patient with hypoglycaemia

C	• Tachycardia
D	• ↓ GCS score
E	• Confusion • Aggressive or altered behaviour • Speech difficulty • Incoordination • Sweating • Shaking • Seizure

Source: data from The Hospital Management of Hypoglycaemia in Adults with Diabetes Mellitus. March 2022. JBDS-IP 04.

It is vital to consider hypoglycaemia in any patient who presents with ↓ level of consciousness, with altered behaviour or who appears intoxicated.

Investigations

- CBG
- Consider the likely cause and investigate appropriately depending on the differential diagnosis, e.g. insulin and C-peptide levels (paired with glucose), urinary sulphonylurea levels, septic screen, 9am cortisol level
- Consider a CT head in those who have prolonged ↓ GCS score to exclude alternative pathology.

Acute management

- Initiate treatment without delay and escalate to a senior clinician if treatment fails in order to consider escalation to intensive care
- In all cases, stop any causal factor, e.g. IV insulin infusion or SC insulin pump

Mild hypoglycaemia (episode that can be self-treated)

1. Give quick acting carbohydrate (15–20g), e.g. 4–5 Glucotabs®/ 150–200mL fruit juice. Repeat CBG after 10–15 minutes to ensure improvement/resolution
2. Give additional short-acting carbohydrates if CBG remains <4.0mmol/L
3. If CBG remains <4.0mmol/L after three treatment cycles, escalate management to step 3 on severe hypoglycaemia protocol.

> For those with severe renal impairment, fruit juices should be avoided due to their potassium concentration

Severe hypoglycaemia (episode that requires third-party assistance to treat)

1. If confused but conscious and able to swallow, 2 tubes of glucose gel can be squeezed between teeth and gums
2. Repeat CBG in 10–15 minutes to ensure improvement/resolution and repeat step 1 up to two times if CBG <4.0mmol/L
3. If CBG still <4.0mmol/L or the patient's swallow is unsafe, (e.g. seizing or unconscious) give IV glucose over 15 minutes (200mL of 10% or 100mL of 20%) through a large-bore cannula
4. Repeat CBG in 10 minutes. Repeat IV glucose infusion if <4.0mmol/L.

> Where IV access is not available, 1mg IM glucagon can be administered **once only**. IM glucagon may be less effective in those with low glycogen stores (hepatic impairment/chronic malnourishment) and slower to work than IV glucose.
>
> IV glucose is recommended to be prescribed 'as required' (PRN) for all diabetic inpatients for use in case of emergency.

Treatment after stabilization

- When the CBG is ≥4.0mmol/L, give a long-acting carbohydrate, e.g. one slice of toast or two biscuits
- Do not omit regular long-acting insulin, but the dose may need adjustment
- Monitor CBG regularly for 24–48 hours to establish a trend and consider regimen alteration
- If nil by mouth, start a 10% glucose infusion, at a rate of 100mL/hour until eating normally again
- Consider diabetic specialist review
- Ask about frequency, severity, and awareness of hypoglycaemia.

Concurrent use of the following medications with antidiabetic agents can precipitate hypoglycaemic episodes: warfarin, quinine, salicylates, monoamine oxidase inhibitors, sulphonamides including co-trimoxazole, and NSAIDS.

If the hypoglycaemic episode was due to long-acting insulin or sulphonylurea therapy, hypoglycaemia may recur during the following 24–36 hours.

Further reading

1. Wilkinson IB, Raine T, Wiles K, et al. (2017). Hypoglycaemia. In: *Oxford Handbook of Clinical Medicine*, 10th ed (p. 214). Oxford: Oxford University Press. Available at: https://doi.org/10.1093/med/9780199689903.003.0005
2. Diabetes UK. Insulin wall chart. Available at: https://www.diabetes.org.uk/resources-s3/2017-11/wallchartinsulins.pdf

Chapter 22

Hyponatraemia

Guideline:
Society for Endocrinology (Emergency management of severe hyponatraemia in adult patients): https://ec.bioscientifica.com/view/journals/ec/5/5/G4.xml

OUP disclaimer: Oxford University Press makes no representation, express or implied, that the drug dosages are correct and that the recommendations are an exclusive or mandatory course of care. All health professionals reading this text have a responsibility to evaluate its appropriateness and take the individual needs of the patient into account.

Local trust guidelines: please refer to your local guidelines as necessary.

Overview

Hyponatraemia is diagnosed when serum sodium is <135mmol/L. It may be acute or chronic and has a variety of possible causes (Box 22.1).

Severe hyponatraemia is predominantly a clinical diagnosis, made on the basis of signs and symptoms and supported by the biochemical sodium measurement (<130mmol/L). If diagnosed, severe hyponatraemia is a medical emergency and should be treated promptly, regardless of the cause. This approach differs to the management of non-severe hyponatraemia which is detailed at the end of the chapter.

Box 22.1 Common causes of hyponatraemia

- Excessive bodily water, e.g. excessive oral intake, liver cirrhosis, heart failure, nephrotic syndrome, syndrome of inappropriate secretion of antidiuretic hormone (SIADH), or glucocorticoid insufficiency
- Sodium loss, e.g. renal disease, skin or GI losses
- Pseudohyponatraemia, e.g. lipaemia or proteinaemia
- Excess of solute, e.g. glucose, mannitol, or ethanol.

Diagnosis

History

- Onset of symptoms
- Recent diagnoses or other symptoms, e.g. GI infections, pancreatitis, malignancy
- Recent diet and fluid intake
- Past medical history, e.g. cardiac failure, liver failure, nephrotic syndrome, hypothyroidism, hypoadrenalism
- Drug history specifically asking about diuretics (particularly thiazides)
- Recreational drug use, e.g. ecstasy.

The symptoms that distinguish severe hyponatraemia from non-severe hyponatraemia include:

- Vomiting
- ↓ consciousness (GCS score ≤8)
- Seizures
- Cardiorespiratory arrest.

Other symptoms that commonly develop in both severe and non-severe hyponatraemia include nausea, confusion, and headache.

Examination

The clinical signs depend on the cause of the hyponatraemia and the speed with which it developed. Different causes may result in signs of hypervolaemia (e.g. raised JVP, oedema), hypovolaemia (e.g. dry mucous membranes, postural hypotension), or euvolemia.

The following observations should be measured:

- Temperature, respiratory rate, oxygen saturation, and heart rate
- Lying and standing blood pressure
- GCS score.

Hyponatraemia can develop secondary to other conditions (see Fig. 22.2 later in the chapter). Signs of these underlying conditions may be evident on examination.

Investigations

Bedside

- ECG.

Bloods

- FBC
- U&E
- LFT
- Bone profile
- Serum glucose
- TFT
- Serum osmolality (Fig. 22.1)
- 9am cortisol
- Amylase (if pancreatitis is suspected).

Other

- Urine osmolality (Fig. 22.1)
- Urine sodium (Fig. 22.1).

A serum sodium should be collected at the same time as the urine osmolality and sodium so that the measurements are 'paired' (Fig. 22.1).

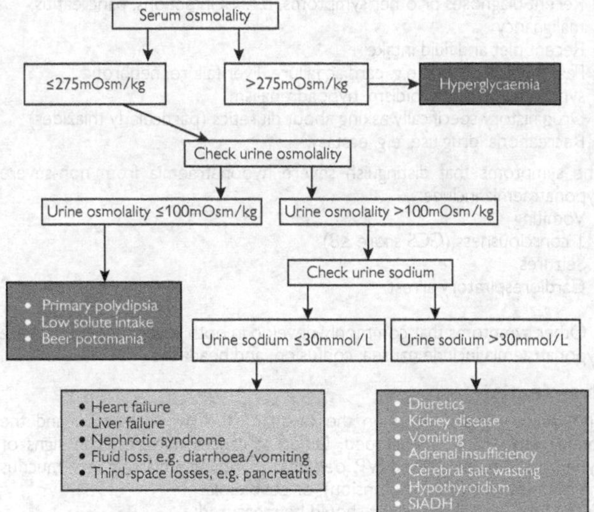

Fig. 22.1 Interpretation of paired osmolality testing and differential diagnosis.

If the patient has kidney disease or has been taking diuretics, all possible causes of hyponatraemia should be considered as a possible underlying diagnosis, regardless of the urine osmolality and urine sodium results.

Management of severe hyponatraemia

Acute management

Management steps are detailed in Fig. 22.2 and should be provided with senior supervision and with the patient connected to cardiac telemetry.

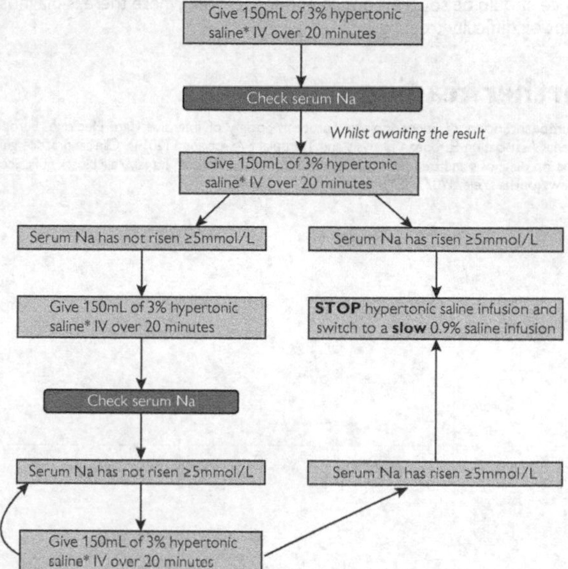

Fig. 22.2 Acute management of severe hyponatraemia. * Or equivalent concentration.

Treatment after stabilization

Target sodium level

The serum sodium level should not rise more than **10mmol/L** in the first 24 hours. From then onwards, the daily increase should not exceed **8mmol/L** until the level is 130mmol/L.

Request help from an endocrinologist, particularly if the daily threshold is exceeded.

A daily rise in sodium level beyond these thresholds risks the development of central pontine myelinolysis, which can cause neurological damage which may be permanent.

Monitoring frequency

- Serum sodium should be measured 6 hours after treatment has been given and then again at 12 hours. After this, serum sodium should be checked daily until stable.

Management of non-severe hyponatraemia

The management of non-severe hyponatraemia depends on treating the underlying cause, rather than actively attempting to correct the sodium. Advice should be sought from an endocrinologist where there is diagnostic doubt or difficulty treating.

Further reading

1. European Society of Endocrinology, European Society of Intensive Care Medicine, European Renal Association-European Dialysis and Transplant Association (2014). Clinical practice guideline on diagnosis and treatment of hyponatraemia. Available at: https://eje.bioscientifica.com/view/journals/eje/170/3/G1.xml

Chapter 23

Hypothyroidism

Guideline:
NICE NG145 (Thyroid disease: assessment and management): https://www.nice.org.uk/guidance/ng145

British Thyroid Association (UK guidelines for the use of thyroid function tests): https://www.british-thyroid-association.org/sandbox/bta2016/uk_guidelines_for_the_use_of_thyroid_function_tests.pdf

OUP disclaimer: Oxford University Press makes no representation, express or implied, that the drug dosages are correct and that the recommendations are an exclusive or mandatory course of care. All health professionals reading this text have a responsibility to evaluate its appropriateness and take the individual needs of the patient into account.

Local trust guidelines: please refer to your local guidelines as necessary.

Overview

Hypothyroidism is the clinical state that occurs as a result of impaired production of thyroid hormones: T4 and T3.

Hypothyroidism is common, affecting 1–2% of the population. Incidence increases with increasing age. It disproportionally affects females with a ratio of 10:1.

- Primary hypothyroidism (95%):
  - Atrophic autoimmune thyroiditis or goitrous autoimmune thyroiditis (Hashimoto's disease)—most common
  - Following destructive treatment to the thyroid or nearby tissue, e.g. radioiodine therapy, thyroidectomy, external beam radiotherapy
  - Drugs including amiodarone, interferon, and lithium
  - Congenital hypothyroidism (rare)
- Secondary hypothyroidism (5%):
  - The result of pituitary disease or damage causing reduced TSH production
- Subclinical hypothyroidism—a state where TSH is elevated, but T4 is normal. Symptoms may or may not be present.

Diagnosis

History

Symptoms can be vague and their onset insidious. Have a low threshold for checking TFT in patients presenting with non-specific symptoms.

Symptoms

- Low mood or cognitive impairment
- Hoarse voice
- Thinning hair
- Fatigue/lethargy
- Cold intolerance
- Dry or thinning skin
- Constipation
- Weight gain
- Irregular menstruation.

Examination

For clinical signs remember '**BRADYCARDIC**':

- **B**radycardia
- **R**eflexes relax slowly
- **A**taxia
- **D**ry, thin hair and skin
- **Y**awning/drowsy/coma
- **C**old hands
- **A**scites ± non-pitting oedema
- **R**ound, puffy face
- **D**efeated demeanour
- **I**mmobile ± ileus
- **C**ongestive cardiac failure.

Neuropathy, myopathy, and goitre may also be present.

Investigations

Bloods

- TFT:
  - When TSH is ≥10mU/L and T4 is below the reference range, this is overt hypothyroidism and should be treated
  - See Table 23.1 for interpretation
- FBC
- Cholesterol/lipid profile
- HbA1c/fasting blood glucose
- Vitamin D
- Calcium.

Antithyroid peroxidase antibodies may be tested to investigate for autoimmune causes of primary hypothyroidism. Although the results might not change the treatment, there is evidence to suggest that when patients understand the cause of their condition, this leads to increased treatment compliance.

Table 23.1 Interpretation of thyroid function tests in hypothyroidism

TFT results	Interpretation
TSH ↑ (≥10mU/L) T4 ↓	Primary hypothyroidism
TSH ↑ T4 ↔	Subclinical hypothyroidism
TSH ↓ T4 ↓	Secondary (central) hypothyroidism—rare

Source: data from UK Guidelines for the Use of Thyroid Function Tests. July 2006. British Thyroid Association.

Management

Management of overt and subclinical hypothyroidism is covered in Fig. 23.1.

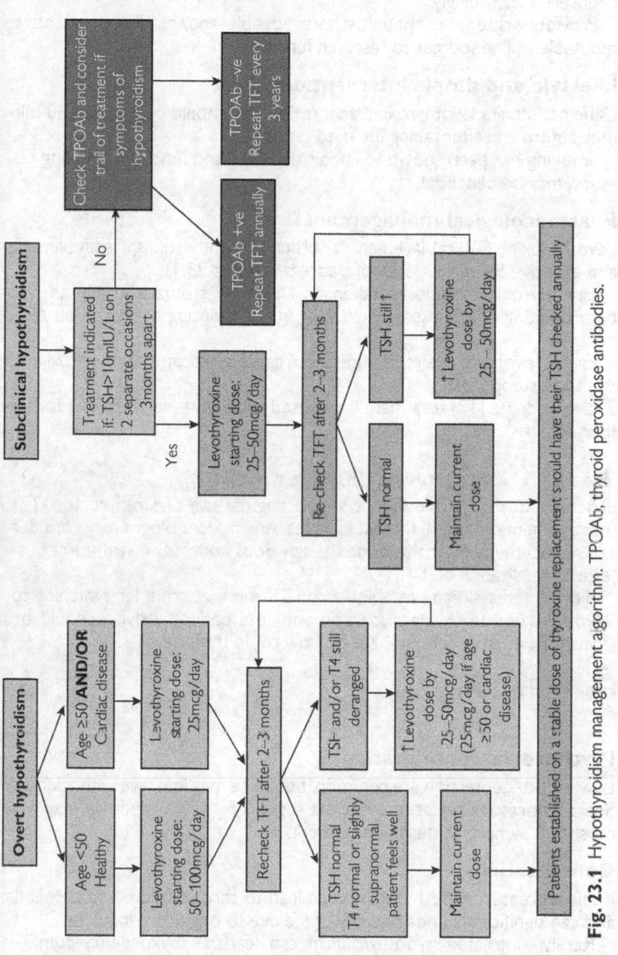

Fig. 23.1 Hypothyroidism management agorithm. TPOAb, thyroid peroxidase antibodies.

Patient education

Lifelong levothyroxine replacement is usually needed—patients should be counselled accordingly.

Provide written information where possible and/or direct patients to reputable online sources to research further.

Lifestyle and simple interventions

Caffeine impairs levothyroxine absorption and should be avoided 60 minutes before and after taking the medication.

Smoking has been shown to impair thyroid gland function; smoking cessation may be beneficial.

Pharmacological management

Levothyroxine (T4) replacement for primary hypothyroidism is simple, safe, and effective for the majority of patients (see Fig. 23.1).

Levothyroxine should be taken on an empty stomach ideally an hour before eating; this is usually first thing in the morning but it can be taken at night.

Excess levothyroxine replacement can cause symptoms of thyrotoxicosis, AF, and osteoporosis.

Liothyronine (T3) treatment is not used routinely—see Box 23.1 for further details.

Box 23.1 Liothyronine (T3) treatment

There is currently no evidence supporting the use of Liothyronine (T3) replacement or natural thyroid extracts. An endocrinologist *may* consider T3 replacement if levothyroxine therapy does not resolve symptoms despite normalization of TFT.

For patients already established on T3 therapy, consider switching to levothyroxine following discussion with the patient. Advice should be sought from an endocrinologist on how to do this safely.

Source: data from NICE NG145 and UK Guidelines for the Use of Thyroid Function Tests, July 2006, British Thyroid Association.

Psychosocial considerations

Low mood/depression are common, but these may improve with adequate thyroid hormone replacement. Data suggest 5–10% of patients may have persistent symptoms despite treatment.

Complications

If left untreated, hypothyroidism can lead to cardiac failure and dementia, and can significantly impair quality of life due to ongoing symptoms.

Rarely, untreated hypothyroidism can lead to myxoedema coma—a medical emergency characterized by hypothermia, hypoglycaemia, bradycardia, cardiac failure, cyanosis, seizures, and impaired consciousness.

After commencing levothyroxine or changing the dose, repeat testing should not occur for a minimum of 2 months as stable thyroid hormone levels will not have been achieved before this.

Monitoring and follow-up

TFT should be checked annually once the patient is established on a stable dose of levothyroxine—TSH monitoring in isolation is usually sufficient.

Patients who continue to experience symptoms despite adequate levothyroxine replacement should be investigated for alternative causes.

Where the diagnosis of hypothyroidism is in doubt, levothyroxine can be stopped and TFT rechecked 6 weeks later.

Where alternative causes cannot be identified and symptoms persist, endocrinology referral may be warranted in order to review ongoing management.

Special considerations

Pregnancy

Pregnancy increases thyroid hormone requirements; dose increases of 25–50% are usually needed from the first trimester.

Women with known hypothyroidism who are planning pregnancy should be referred to a specialist and have TFT checked prior to conception. They should be advised to delay conception if not euthyroid.

If already pregnant, TFT should be checked immediately and a specialist's advice sought regarding levothyroxine dose adjustment.

TFT should be checked every 6 weeks during pregnancy to ensure the patient remains euthyroid, minimizing the risk of obstetric and neonatal complications.

Further reading

1. BMJ Best Practice (2021). Primary hypothyroidism. Available at: www.bestpractice.bmj.com/topics/en-gb/535
2. Wass J, Owen K (eds) (2014). Thyroid. In: *Oxford Handbook of Endocrinology and Diabetes*, 3rd ed (pp. 1–105). Oxford: Oxford University Press. Available at: https://doi.org/10.1093/med/9780199644438.003.0001
3. Wilkinson IB, Raine T, Wiles K, et al. (2017). Endocrinology. In: *Oxford Handbook of Clinical Medicine*, 10th ed (pp. 202–41). Oxford: Oxford University Press. Available at: https://doi.org/10.1093/med/9780199689903.003.0005
4. Allahabadia A, Razvi S, Abraham P, et al. (2009). Diagnosis and treatment of primary hypothyroidism. *BMJ*. 338:b725.

Chapter 24

Osteoporosis

Guidelines:
NICE CG146 (Osteoporosis: assessing the risk of fragility fracture): https://www.nice.org.uk/guidance/cg146

National Osteoporosis Guideline Group (NOGG 2021: clinical guideline for the prevention and treatment of osteoporosis): https://www.nogg.org.uk/full-guideline

Endocrine Society (Pharmacological management of osteoporosis in postmenopausal women): https://www.endocrine.org/clinical-practice-guidelines/osteoporosis-in-postmenopausal-women

OUP disclaimer: Oxford University Press makes no representation, express or implied, that the drug dosages are correct and that the recommendations are an exclusive or mandatory course of care. All health professionals reading this text have a responsibility to evaluate its appropriateness and take the individual needs of the patient into account.

Local trust guidelines: please refer to your local guidelines as necessary.

Overview

Osteoporosis is a systemic skeletal disease, characterized by low bone mass and microarchitectural deterioration of bone tissue, leading to ↑ bone fragility and ↑ fracture risk[1]. Osteoporosis leads to >300,000 fragility fractures in the UK each year. These fractures occur from low-impact trauma, such as a fall from standing height. The prevalence of osteoporosis is 2% at age 50, and 25% at age 80 in women. There is a significant associated cost, mostly related to hip fracture care.

1 Consensus development conference: diagnosis, prophylaxis and treatment of osteoporosis. *Am J Med.* 1993; 94:646–50.

Diagnosis

History/diagnostic criteria

Fragility fractures result from a mechanical force that would not ordinarily result in fracture. They are associated with low bone mineral density (BMD) and occur most commonly in the vertebrae, proximal femur, and distal radius (also consider in the humerus, pelvis, and ribs). Hip and vertebral fractures are associated with reduced life expectancy.

Assessment criteria and risk factors for osteoporosis are summarized in Table 24.1.

Table 24.1 Assessment criteria and risk factors for osteoporosis

Age category	Assess if
Women ≥65 years Men ≥75 years	All should be assessed
Women 50–64 years Men 50–74 years	• History of fragility fracture • History of falls • Family history of hip fracture • Current or recent frequent use of steroids (≥7.5mg prednisolone/day for ≥3 months or equivalent) • BMI <18.5kg/m^2 • Smoker • Alcohol intake >14 units/week • Secondary causes of osteoporosis, e.g. hypogonadism, untreated premature menopause, hyperthyroidism, hyperparathyroidism, diabetes, inflammatory bowel disease (IBD), rheumatoid arthritis, COPD, chronic liver failure, CKD

Source: data from NICE CG146.

The patient groups listed in Table 24.1 should be assessed initially using a risk assessment tool (see 'Methods of risk assessment').

However, the following two groups should be referred for a DXA scan directly, without using a risk assessment tool:

- Patients aged >50 years **AND** a previous fragility fracture
- Patients aged <40 years **AND** current/recent high-dose steroid use for ≥3 months (equivalent to ≥7.5 mg prednisolone OD) **OR** previous fragility fracture.

Methods of risk assessment

Two risk assessment tools, FRAX® and QFracture®, are available for use in the UK to estimate the 10-year probability (as a percentage) of a major osteoporotic or hip fracture.

Both tools are designed to be used before DXA scanning and help to decide if a DXA scan is necessary (aside from the exceptions previously mentioned). Once a patient has had a DXA scan, the FRAX® score should be recalculated incorporating the DXA result.

FRAX®

FRAX[2] can be used for people aged 40–90 years, either with or without BMD values. It takes into account previous and family history of fractures, smoking, alcohol and steroid use, and risk factors for secondary osteoporosis. The result is plotted onto a graph (Fig. 24.1) provided by the National Osteoporosis Guideline Group (NOGG) which plots age against risk, and indicates whether the patient would benefit from treatment or not.

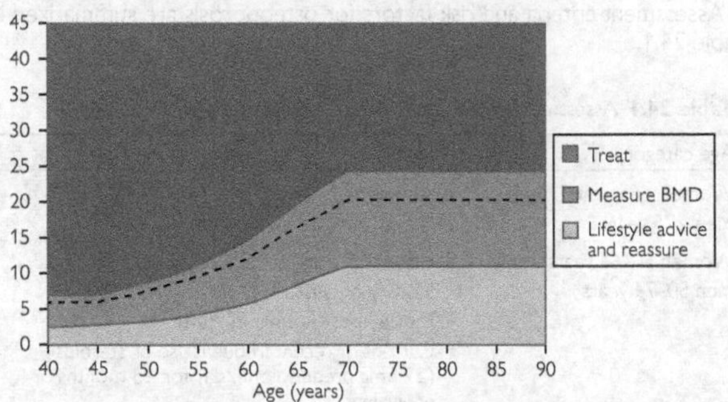

Fig. 24.1 Graph showing the 10-year probability (%) of a patient having a major (spine, hip, forearm, or humerus) osteoporotic fracture. The dotted line represents the intervention threshold based on the 10-year probability of a hip fracture. Patients in the lightest blue zone can be reassured. Patients in the darkest blue zone should be treated. Patients in the mid blue zone may be referred for BMD measurements in order to reassess their fracture probability, or may be directed to treatment if above the dotted line, depending on clinical judgement.

QFracture®

QFracture[3] can be used for people aged 30–99 years. BMD values cannot be incorporated into the algorithm. QFracture® considers more specific comorbidities such as chronic liver disease and dementia compared to FRAX®.

If treatment is advised after using the risk assessment tools, the patient should have a DXA scan prior to commencing treatment.

> Patients above the upper age limits defined by the tools are automatically considered to be at high risk. Remember that in patients >80 years, results should be interpreted cautiously as a 10-year score may underestimate their short-term risk.

2 FRAX® Fracture Risk Assessment Tool. Available at: http://www.sheffield.ac.uk/FRAX

3 QFracture®-2016 risk calculator. Available at: http://qfracture.org

Investigations

Bloods

- FBC
- U&E (CKD)
- CRP/ESR (chronic inflammatory disease)
- Calcium (hyper)
- LFT (chronic liver disease)
- TFT (hyperthyroidism).

Consider testing if clinical suspicion:

- Serum 25-hydroxyvitamin D (vitamin D deficiency)
- Myeloma screen
- PTH (hyperparathyroidism)
- Pituitary hormones (androgen deficiency in males, premature menopause in females, prolactinoma in both sexes)
- Tests for Cushing's syndrome
- Endomysial/tissue transglutaminase antibody (coeliac disease).

Imaging

DXA scan

DXA uses X-rays to non-invasively assess bone density at the hip and lumbar spine. The scan facilitates calculation of a T-score (comparison with the bone density of a 30-year-old, see Box 24.1) and a Z-score (age matched).

Box 24.1 T-scores

- Score ≥–1.0 = normal bone density
- Score –1.1 to –2.4 = osteopenia
- Score ≤–2.5 = osteoporosis

Source: data from Assessment of Fracture Risk and its Application to Screening for Postmenopausal Osteoporosis. Geneva 1994. WHO Technical Report Series 843.

Management

Lifestyle and simple interventions

Encourage patients to:

- Perform regular weight-bearing exercises
- Stop smoking
- Reduce alcohol consumption
- Eat foods with calcium regularly.

Pharmacological management

Calcium and vitamin D supplementation

If daily intake of calcium (700–1200 mg/day) or exposure to sunlight is inadequate, prescribe calcium and/or vitamin D supplementation, e.g. Adcal D3®, one tablet BD.

Bisphosphonates (first line)

For example, oral alendronate 10mg OD or 70mg once weekly, oral risedronate 5mg OD or 35mg once weekly.

Bisphosphonates block the action of inorganic pyrophosphate and this prevents bone resorption. Side effects include dyspepsia and bowel disturbance (Box 24.2). Osteonecrosis of the jaw and atypical femoral fractures are rare but important adverse effects to warn patients about.

Contraindications: hypocalcaemia (check prior to commencing treatment), severe renal impairment (GFR ≤35mL/min).

If oral treatment is not tolerated, patients may be referred to a specialist for consideration of an IV bisphosphonate infusion, e.g. zoledronic acid, or other specialist options (see 'Specialist treatments (non-bisphosphonate)').

Box 24.2 Patient instructions when taking bisphosphonates

Side effects such as dyspepsia and oesophagitis are common with bisphosphonates, but the risk is reduced when patients are taught the correct way to take the tablets.

1. Take on an empty stomach and at least 30 minutes before eating or drinking (except for water)
2. Swallow the tablet with a full glass of water (at least 200mL) while sitting or standing
3. Patients must not lie down for 30 minutes after they have the tablet.

Source: data from NOGG 2017: Clinical guideline for the prevention and treatment of osteoporosis.

Specialist treatments (non-bisphosphonate)

- Denosumab (monoclonal antibody against RANKL on osteoclasts, inhibiting activity):
  - 6-monthly SC injection
  - BMD falls with interruption of therapy
- Raloxifene (selective oestrogen receptor modulator):
  - May be considered in postmenopausal women if low risk of deep vein thrombosis (DVT) and/or high risk of breast cancer (reduces breast cancer risk)

- Hormone replacement therapy (HRT):
  - May be considered in women if aged <60 years, or <10 years after menopause if low risk of DVT and breast cancer
- Teriparatide (recombinant human PTH):
  - May be considered if very high risk of fractures. Can be prescribed for up to 2 years
- Romosozumab (sclerostin antagonist):
  - May be considered if very high risk of fractures. Can be prescribed for up to 1 year
  - Contraindicated if ischaemic heart disease/cerebrovascular disease.

Monitoring and follow-up

Patients who do not have osteoporosis on initial assessment should be re-assessed after 2 years, or sooner if their risk factors change.

Patients on bisphosphonates should be reviewed after 5 years (3 years if on zoledronic acid). They should have a reassessment of their fracture risk.

If they continue to be osteoporotic, or still fall within the treat section of the NOGG fracture probability table, consider whether to continue treatment for a maximum of another 5 years.

If they are no longer osteoporotic and fall below the NOGG intervention threshold, consider stopping the bisphosphonate for a 'drug holiday' and reassess after 1.5–3 years.

Special considerations

Pregnancy

Bisphosphonates are contraindicated in pregnancy and while breastfeeding.

Further reading

1. Tabernacle B, Honey M, Jinks A (eds) (2009). Osteoporosis. In: *Oxford Handbook of Nursing Older People*. Oxford: Oxford University Press. Available at: https://doi.org/10.1093/med/9780199213283.003.0017

Chapter 25

Type 1 diabetes mellitus

Guideline:
This chapter was based on: NICE NG17 (Type 1 diabetes in adults: diagnosis and management, updated December 2020): https://www.nice.org.uk/guidance/ng17. Since the chapter was written, the guideline has been updated to: NICE NG17 (Type 1 diabetes in adults: diagnosis and management, updated August 2022). Please see the approach to management and target blood pressure measurements in NG17, updated August 2022.

OUP disclaimer: Oxford University Press makes no representation, express or implied, that the drug dosages are correct and that the recommendations are an exclusive or mandatory course of care. All health professionals reading this text have a responsibility to evaluate its appropriateness and take the individual needs of the patient into account.

Local trust guidelines: please refer to your local guidelines as necessary.

Overview

T1DM is a condition caused by autoimmune destruction of the cells that synthesize insulin. Over time, high blood sugar levels due to a lack of insulin lead to tissue damage. If untreated or poorly treated, this can cause microvascular and macrovascular complications including retinopathy, nephropathy, neuropathy, cardiovascular, peripheral vascular, and cerebrovascular disease.

Diagnosis

Diagnostic criteria

- HbA1c ≥48mmol/mol (6.5%) **OR**
- Fasting glucose ≥7mmol/L **OR**
- Random glucose ≥11.1mmol/L.

In the absence of symptoms of hyperglycaemia, a second test should be performed on another day to confirm the diagnosis.

History

- Symptoms—polydipsia, polyuria, unexplained weight loss, lethargy (4 'T's—thirst, toilet, tiredness, thinner)
- Personal ± family history of T1DM or other autoimmune disease.

Examination

- Typical age <50 years and BMI <25kg/m² (but not always!)
- Signs of weight loss or dehydration
- Unwell if presenting with DKA.

Investigations

- Blood glucose—capillary and venous
- Blood ketones
- Antibodies—send to confirm diagnosis, particularly when there may be diagnostic doubt.

> Do not send C-peptide, unless there is diagnostic doubt.

Management

At diagnosis, a patient should undergo a thorough medical, environmental, emotional, cultural, and educational assessment in order to create an individualized holistic management plan. If the patient presents with DKA, refer to Chapter 15 for more information.

Patient education

Within 6–12 months of diagnosis, all adults with T1DM **must** be offered a structured education programme of proven benefit.

Lifestyle and simple interventions

Dietary

Must refer for dietician review. Key points to discuss include:

- Carbohydrate counting
- Weight control
- Effect of alcohol on glycaemic control
- Avoidance of hypoglycaemia.

Physical activity

Encourage physical activity, but ensure patients are aware of its effect on blood glucose levels and understand how to adjust nutritional intake and insulin doses appropriately.

Psychological interventions

Many people with T1DM will require additional psychological support. Diabetes can directly affect mental health, e.g. causing anxiety or depression. Mental health can also directly affect the ability of the person to manage their diabetes. Psychological support should be offered to all patients with T1DM.

Pharmacological management

Insulin

Multiple daily injection basal-bolus insulin regimens combining long-acting (basal) and rapid-acting (bolus) insulins are the first-line regimen for all adults with T1DM. Sample regimens are suggested in Table 25.1. If this type of regimen is not available or does not achieve good glycaemic control, other regimens (e.g. mixed insulins) should be considered.

See Box 25.1 for advice on insulin dose calculations.

Continuous subcutaneous insulin infusion (pump therapy)

- Consider[1] if:
  1. Escalating insulin doses to bring down HbA1c results in severe hypoglycaemia or
  2. HbA1c remains ≥69mmol/mol despite escalation of insulin doses.

Plasma glucose testing

- Encourage patients to test blood glucose at least four times a day. More often may be required—see Box 25.2. Some patients may be eligible for continuous glucose monitoring devices.

1 NICE. Continuous subcutaneous insulin infusion for the treatment of diabetes mellitus (TA151) 2008. Available at: https://www.nice.org.uk/guidance/ta151

Box 25.1 Insulin dose calculations

The insulin dose may be calculated from the total insulin required during the last 6 hours on a VRII. The total insulin should be divided by 6 to give the hourly insulin requirement and then multiplied by 20 to give the total daily insulin requirement. Alternatively, the dose may be estimated from the patient's weight (0.3 units/kg for newly diagnosed diabetes). Ask for specialist advice before commencing insulin.

For a basal-bolus regimen, 50% of the insulin is given as basal and the remainder divided into bolus doses. For a mixed regimen, 60% of the insulin is given at breakfast and 40% given in the evening.

Table 25.1 Sample basal-bolus insulin regimens

Long-acting		Rapid-acting (TDS with meals)
Detemir BD OD alternatives such as glargine or degludec may be preferable for patients who need help from carers to administer injections or with concerns about nocturnal hypoglycaemia	PLUS	Humalog® **OR** NovoRapid® **OR** Apidra®

- Targets:
  - **5–7mmol/L** fasting level on waking
  - **4–7mmol/L** before meals at other times of day
  - **5–9 mmol/L** before bedtime and at least 90 minutes after eating (if the patient chooses to monitor post-prandial levels).

Box 25.2 Patients who should test blood glucose up to ten times a day

- Target HbA1c not achieved
- Legal requirement, e.g. DVLA
- Before, during, and after sport
- Impaired awareness of hypoglycaemia
- Increasing frequency of hypoglycaemic episodes
- During illness
- Planning pregnancy, pregnancy, and breastfeeding
- High-risk activities.

Islet cell replacement

Islet cell or pancreas transplantation may be an option for those with recurrent severe hypoglycaemia or suboptimal control.

Complications

Hypoglycaemia

See Chapter 21 for more information.

- Adverse effect of insulin therapy
- Emergency treatment is with fast-acting glucose for those able to swallow and IM glucagon or IV dextrose in those with a ↓ GCS score
- Hypoglycaemia awareness is a key part of any diabetes education programme and this should be assessed at each annual review.

Labile glycaemic measurements

If levels are erratic, assess sites of insulin injection and technique. Reassess patient's understanding of insulin therapy and possible lifestyle causes or complications, e.g. gastroparesis.

Diabetic ketoacidosis

See Chapter 15.

Monitoring and follow-up

Key care processes

There are nine key care processes that patients with T1DM should receive at least yearly:

- Cholesterol test
- Creatinine test
- Smoking status discussion
- Body mass index (BMI) measurement
- Foot examination
- Blood pressure check
- HbA1c test
- Urine albumin test (ACR)
- Retinal screening.

HbA1c

- Check every **3–6 months**
- HbA1c targets are discussed in Box 25.3.

Box 25.3 HbA1c targets

HbA1c targets should be set individually based on lifestyle, occupation, risk of complications, comorbidities, and history of hypoglycaemia. An HbA1c level ≤48mmol/mol minimizes the risk of long-term vascular complications.

TSH

- Measure TSH levels annually.

Microvascular complications

- Nephropathy: perform ACR 5 years after diagnosis and then annually, along with serum creatinine. The first voided urine sample of the day should be tested:
  - Start a renin–angiotensin system (RAS) blocking drug if microalbuminuria or albuminuria is found, e.g. ramipril 2.5mg OD. If not tolerated, switch to an angiotensin-2 blocker, e.g. losartan 25mg OD

  - Refer to a nephrologist if glomerular filtration rate (GFR) <30mL/min/1.73m^2
- Neuropathy: examine feet at every diabetic review and ask about symptoms of gastroparesis and autonomic neuropathy, e.g. nocturnal diarrhoea, orthostatic hypotension, and erectile dysfunction
- Retinopathy: ensure patients have annual retinal screening. The first screening should be as soon as possible following diagnosis. Classification ranges from background retinopathy (least severe), to pre-proliferative retinopathy, proliferative retinopathy, and maculopathy (most severe).

Macrovascular complications

- Ischaemic heart disease and cerebrovascular disease may occur as a consequence of diabetes
- Vascular risk factors, including cholesterol levels and smoking status, should be assessed at clinical review and smoking cessation encouraged if appropriate
- Blood pressure target: <135/85mmHg or <130/80mmHg if albuminuria on ACR testing or two or more features of metabolic syndrome:
  - A RAS blocking drug is first line for treating hypertension, e.g. ramipril 2.5mg OD.

Special considerations

Hospital admission

- Allow patients with T1DM to self-administer SC insulin if willing and able and safe
- Aim for a plasma glucose level of 5–8mmol/L during surgery or acute illness
- Use an VRII ('sliding scale') if a patient is 'nil by mouth', unable to eat, or their illness is expected to lead to unpredictable blood glucose levels and insulin absorption
- Do not stop a patient's basal insulin, even when on a VRII.

Surgery

- See Chapters 92 and 93 for the management of diabetes in patients undergoing surgery.

Eating disorders

- Be alert to the possibility of bulimia, anorexia, and insulin dose manipulation in those who show excessive concern regarding their body shape and weight. Other risk factors include very low BMI, recurrent hypoglycaemia, and poor glucose control
- See also Chapter 39.

Pregnancy

See Box 25.2. Ensure the patient is booked into a high-risk multidisciplinary diabetes–obstetrics clinic.

For further details about diabetes in pregnancy, see Chapter 59.

Age >60 years

If age >60 years and presenting with new-onset diabetes and weight loss, consider the possibility of pancreatic cancer. See Chapter 110.

Further reading

1. NICE (2008). Continuous subcutaneous insulin infusion for the treatment of diabetes mellitus (TA151). Available at: https://www.nice.org.uk/guidance/ta151
2. NICE (2008). Allogeneic pancreatic islet cell transplantation for type 1 diabetes mellitus (IPG257). Available at: https://www.nice.org.uk/guidance/ipg257

Chapter 26

Type 2 diabetes mellitus and diabetic foot problems

Guidelines:
NICE NG28 (Type 2 diabetes in adults: management): https://www.nice.org.uk/guidance/ng28

NICE NG19 (Diabetic foot problems: prevention and management): https://www.nice.org.uk/guidance/ng19

OUP disclaimer: Oxford University Press makes no representation, express or implied, that the drug dosages are correct and that the recommendations are an exclusive or mandatory course of care. All health professionals reading this text have a responsibility to evaluate its appropriateness and take the individual needs of the patient into account.

Local trust guidelines: please refer to your local guidelines as necessary.

Overview

T2DM is a chronic metabolic condition affecting >285 million people worldwide. It is characterized by insulin resistance and a progressive lack of insulin production. T2DM is associated with obesity, hypertension, multimorbidity, sedentary lifestyles, and poor dietary habits, therefore its management requires multidisciplinary input. This chapter refers to T2DM in non-pregnant adults. T1DM in adults is covered in Chapter 25, diabetes in pregnancy is covered in Chapter 59, and diabetes in children is covered in Chapter 77.

Diagnosis

History

Identify patients with risk factors such as obesity, family history (heritability of T2DM is approximately 25%) or African, Afro-Caribbean, or South Asian ethnicity. Patients are often diagnosed through screening programmes or through coincidental investigations for tiredness or other illnesses.

Characteristic diabetes symptoms of polyuria, polydipsia, blurred vision, lethargy, and weight loss are not usually present in T2DM and would point to a diagnosis of T1DM.

Examination

Very few findings may be seen on diagnosis:

- Hypertension
- High BMI with concentration around the abdomen (central obesity)
- Signs of insulin resistance, e.g. acanthosis nigricans, *Candida* infections.

Later signs may include:

- Foot signs: dry feet, foot ulcers
- Peripheral neuropathy
- Peripheral vascular disease
- Diabetic retinopathy: haemorrhages, exudates, and neovascularization.

Investigations

Bedside

- Capillary blood glucose
- Urinalysis to assess for glucose, proteins, and ketones.

Bloods

- Diagnostic blood tests are discussed in Box 26.1.

Box 26.1 Diagnostic blood tests

- Fasting glucose ≥7mmol/L **OR**
- Random glucose ≥11.1mmol/L **OR**
- HbA1c ≥48mmol/mol **OR**
- 2 hour oral glucose tolerance test ≥11.1mmol/L
- In the absence of symptoms of hyperglycaemia, a second test should be performed on another occasion to confirm the diagnosis.

Management

The general approach to management of patients with T2DM is summarized in Fig. 26.1. HbA1c targets are listed in Table 26.1.

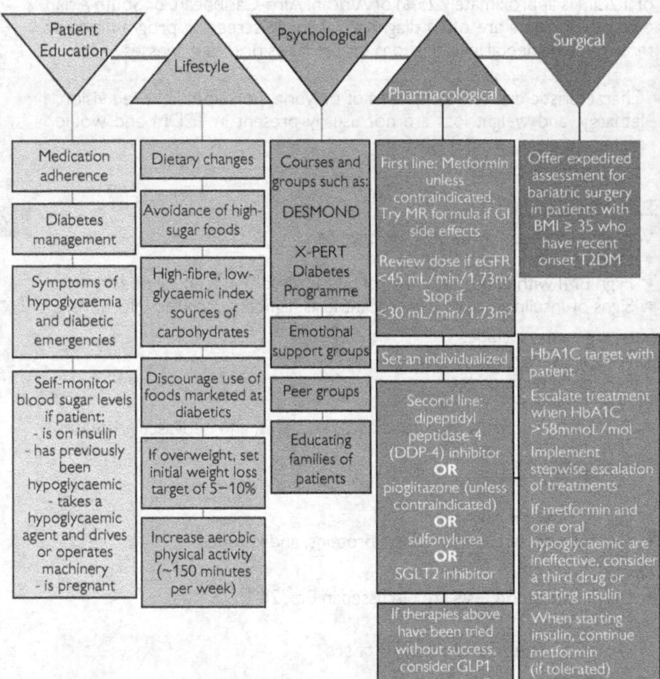

Fig. 26.1 Multifaceted management approach for patients with T2DM. MR, modified release.

Table 26.1 HbA1c targets

Management	Target HbA1c
Lifestyle and dietary **OR** single medication not associated with hypoglycaemia	48mmol/mol
Medication associated with hypoglycaemia	53mmol/mol

Source: data from NICE NG28.

Complications

- Macrovascular complications
- Autonomic and sensory neuropathy (Box 26.2) (see Chapter 25)
- Diabetic nephropathy
- Diabetic retinopathy (Box 26.2).

Box 26.2 Peripheral neuropathy

- Starts in the toes and soles of the feet and spreads up the shins symmetrically
- Results in ↓ vibration perception, fine touch, pin-prick, and temperature sensation
- ↓ vibration sensation and absent ankle reflexes are often first to appear
- More severe cases occur in the fingers and hands
- Painful neuropathy may occur with sharp, burning, stabbing pains.

Box 26.3 Diabetic retinopathy

- Upon T2DM diagnosis, patients should be referred for routine retinopathy screening
- In the event of sudden visual loss or acute visual symptoms, patients should have an emergency ophthalmology review.

Diabetic foot problems

The combination of neuropathy and peripheral vascular disease in T2DM leads to diabetic foot problems which are the leading cause of morbidity.

- Approximately 6000 people with diabetes undergo lower limb amputation annually, with diabetic foot ulceration preceding 80% of amputations
- Patients should be examined at diagnosis and at least annually thereafter, including on each new hospital admission
- Skin care and nail care should be discussed during clinical reviews to reduce the risk of foot problems developing
- The highest risk patients may need weekly foot checks.

Assessing risk of diabetic foot lesions

Examine feet for:

- Neuropathy (use 10g monofilament)
- Limb ischaemia (use ankle–brachial pressure index (ABPI))
- Ulceration
- Callus
- Inflammation or infected areas
- Deformity
- Gangrene
- Charcot arthropathy:
  - If a patient with T2DM fractures their foot or ankle, this may develop into Charcot's arthropathy
  - Suspect Charcot arthropathy if there is redness, warmth, or swelling, especially in the presence of renal failure and peripheral neuropathy.

Use Table 26.2 to assess the risk of developing a diabetic foot problem based on examination findings.

Table 26.2 Risk of developing a diabetic foot problem

Low risk	Moderate risk	High risk
No risk factors aside from callus	Foot deformity **OR**	Previous ulcer or amputation **OR**
	Neuropathy **OR**	On renal replacement therapy **OR**
	Non-critical limb ischaemia	Two of: neuropathy, callus/deformity, and non-critical limb ischaemia

Source: data from NICE NG19.

- If moderate or high risk of developing a diabetic foot problem, refer to a specialist team
- Diagnose an active diabetic foot problem if there is:
    - Ulceration **OR**
    - Spreading inflammation **OR**
    - Critical limb ischaemia **OR**
    - Gangrene **OR**
    - Suspicion of Charcot arthropathy
- The SINBAD scoring system (Fig. 26.2) may be used to classify the severity of a diabetic foot ulcer. Be alert to ⚑ of life- or limb-threatening problems in Box 26.4.

Management of diabetic foot ulcers

- Offload with non-removable casting for neuropathic, non-infected ulcers

SITE	Forefoot	0
	Mid/Hindfoot	1
ISCHAEMIA	Pedal blood flow intact, at least 1 pulse palpable	0
	Clinical evidence of reduced pedal blood flow	1
NEUROPATHY	Protective sensation intact	0
	Protective sensation lost	1
BACTERIAL INFECTION	None	0
	Present	1
AREA	Ulcer <1cm^2	0
	Ulcer ≥1cm^2	1
DEPTH	Ulcer confined to skin and subcutaneous tissue	0
	Ulcer reaching muscle, tendon or bone	1
		Total
	<3 = less severe ulcer, ≥3 = more severe ulcer	**/6**

Fig. 26.2 SINBAD scoring system to identify severity of diabetic foot ulcer.
Source: data from Ince P, et al (May 2008) Use of the SINBAD Classification System and Score in comparing outcome of foot ulcer management on three continents. Diabetes Care. 31(5): 964–967.

Box 26.4 Life- or limb-threatening diabetic foot problems

Look out for life- or limb-threatening diabetic foot problems which require immediate referral to acute services:

⚑ Ulceration with fever, signs of sepsis or limb ischaemia
⚑ Clinical concern of deep-seated soft tissue infection or osteomyelitis
⚑ Gangrene (with or without ulceration).

Source: data from NICE NG19.

- Treat infection or ischaemia
- Use pressure redistributing devices, e.g. inflatable foot protectors
- Wound debridement followed by negative pressure wound therapy
- Refer to MDT foot care service (this may include a podiatrist, nurse, orthotist, microbiologist, diabetologist, interventional radiologist, and vascular, orthopaedic, and plastic surgeons[1]).

Management of diabetic foot infection

- Suspect osteomyelitis even in the presence of normal inflammatory markers and X-ray
- Take cultures ideally from the base of a debrided wound
- Consider MRI to confirm osteomyelitis
- Follow local antibiotic guidelines—for mild infections, initially use oral antibiotics with Gram-positive cover. For moderate to severe infections, use antibiotics with Gram-positive, -negative, and anaerobic cover
- If osteomyelitis is present, the antibiotic course should be prolonged (6 weeks minimum).

Management of Charcot's arthropathy

- Refer to MDT foot care service within 1 working day of suspected diagnosis
- Offer non-weight-bearing device until diagnosis is confirmed
- Take weight-bearing X-ray of the foot and ankle
- Offer non-removable (if suitable) offloading device for treatment
- Continuous monitoring of treatment efficacy with temperature checks and serial X-rays.

Monitoring and follow-up

- A full diabetes review should take place at least annually including a foot examination

> If there is a sudden decrease in HbA1c to less than the target level, consider possible causes including improved diabetic control, deteriorating renal function, or sudden weight loss.

- If at moderate or high risk of a diabetic foot problem, reassess more frequently
- For patients on insulin therapy, review injection technique and confirm understanding of hypoglycaemia and hyperglycaemia and self-management of these conditions. Ensure the patient is aware of DVLA guidance (see Chapter 115)
- Measure HbA1c every 3–6 months until the HbA1c and doses of antidiabetic medication are stable. Measure HbA1c every 6 months thereafter.

Emergency referral

- Arrange emergency review by an ophthalmologist if there is sudden loss of vision, rubeosis iridis, preretinal or vitreous haemorrhage, or retinal detachment.

1 Huang DY, Wilkins CJ, Evan DR, et al. The diabetic foot: the importance of coordinated care. *Semin Intervent Radiol*. 2014; 31:307–12.

Special considerations

Pregnancy

For details about diabetes in pregnancy, see Chapter 59.

Surgery

See Chapters 92 and 93 for the management of diabetes in patients undergoing surgery.

Further reading

1. Wass J, Owen K (eds) (2014). Diabetes. In: *Oxford Handbook of Endocrinology and Diabetes*, 3rd ed (pp. 683–822). Oxford: Oxford University Press. Available at: https://doi.org/10.1093/med/9780199644438.003.0013
2. Diabetes UK (2019). Diabetes and emotional health. A practical guide for healthcare professionals supporting adults with type 1 and type 2 diabetes, 2nd ed. Available at: https://www.diabetes.org.uk/resources-s3/2019-03/0506%20Diabetes%20UK%20Australian%20Handbook_P4_FINAL_1.pdf

Part 4

Gastrointestinal

Chapter 27

Acute upper gastrointestinal bleeding and variceal bleeding

Guidelines:
NICE CG141 (Acute upper gastrointestinal bleeding in over 16s: management): https://www.nice.org.uk/guidance/cg141

Baveno VI Faculty (Expanding consensus in portal hypertension): https://www.journal-of-hepatology.eu/article/S0168-8278%2815%2900349-9/fulltext

British Society of Gastroenterology (UK guidelines on the management of variceal haemorrhage in cirrhotic patients): https://gut.bmj.com/content/64/11/1680.long

OUP disclaimer: Oxford University Press makes no representation, express or implied, that the drug dosages are correct and that the recommendations are an exclusive or mandatory course of care. All health professionals reading this text have a responsibility to evaluate its appropriateness and take the individual needs of the patient into account.

Local trust guidelines: please refer to your local guidelines as necessary.

Overview

An upper gastrointestinal bleed (UGIB) refers to bleeding from the oesophagus, stomach, or duodenum, and can range from minor to life-threatening in severity. A variceal bleed must always be considered in bleeding patients with chronic liver disease, as they require specific management and have a mortality rate of 10%. Causes of UGIB are listed in Box 27.1.

Box 27.1 Causes of UGIB

- Duodenal ulcer (prevalence 40%)
- Erosive gastritis/duodenitis (20%)
- Oesophageal varices (15–20%)
- Gastric ulcers (10–20%)
- Mallory–Weiss tear (5–10%).

Diagnosis

History

Presenting complaint

- Haematemesis
- 'Coffee-ground vomit': due to iron in haemoglobin being oxidized by gastric acid. Not all brown vomits are a GI bleed!
- Melaena: offensive, black, tarry stool
- Abdominal pain
- Symptoms of blood loss: syncope, fatigue, shortness of breath, chest pain.

Past medical history

- Gastric or duodenal ulcers, or previous bleed
- Liver disease.

Drug history

- NSAIDs
- Anticoagulants (warfarin, DOACs)
- Antiplatelets (aspirin, clopidogrel)
- Alcohol excess or IVDU

Examination

Initial examination should focus on vital signs, looking for signs of haemorrhagic shock (syncope, hypotension, pallor, tachycardia, tachypnoea, altered GCS score).

- **Blood pressure and heart rate:** in young patients, tachycardia (heart rate >100bpm) may be the only sign of blood loss
- **Temperature:** infection should always be suspected in a UGIB, particularly in patients with chronic liver disease
- **Digital rectal examination (DRE):** look for melaena and/or fresh blood
- **Signs of chronic liver disease:** e.g. finger clubbing, spider naevi, gynaecomastia, jaundice, and palmar erythema. These are suggestive of a variceal bleed being the underlying cause,

Investigations

- FBC: ↓ haemoglobin/↓ platelets (seen in alcohol excess, cirrhosis)
- U&E: ↑ urea:creatinine ratio (suggest bleeding into the upper GI tract as urea is produced from digested blood)
- LFT: chronic liver disease
- Coagulation profile: impairment implies possible liver disease, however needs to be interpreted with caution; INR is not a reliable indicator of coagulation profile status in cirrhosis.

Management

Fig. 27.1 is a flowchart providing an overview of management.

Calculate a Glasgow-Blatchford score for all patients on admission (see 'Further reading')[1]—patients with a score of 0 may be considered safe for discharge without further investigations. Careful safety netting is required.

Resuscitation

Table 27.1 describes the ABCDE approach to the resuscitation of a patient with UGIB or variceal bleeding.

Table 27.1 Resuscitation in acute upper gastrointestinal or variceal bleeding

A	Patients at risk of aspiration should be considered for early intubation for airway protection
C	Insert at least two large cannulae (consider a central line if difficult access) IV fluid resuscitation, aiming to maintain systolic blood pressure ≥100mmHg **Blood products (see Chapter 94):** • Patients with significant ongoing haemorrhage should be transfused in line with local protocols. Consider activating a major haemorrhage pathway • Give packed red blood cells as required, aiming for a haemoglobin of 70–80g/L. Over-transfusion of stable patients (i.e. >80g/L) has been shown to be harmful. Consider patient's age, cardiovascular disease, and whether bleeding is ongoing • Consider platelets if actively bleeding and platelet count <50 × 10^9/L • Consider fresh frozen plasma (FFP) if actively bleeding and prothrombin time (PT)/INR/activated partial thromboplastin time (APTT) >1.5× normal. If fibrinogen remains <1.5g/L despite FFP, give cryoprecipitate. Caution is advised with the use of FFP in variceal haemorrhage as excessive volume expansion can precipitate further bleeding • If taking warfarin, reversal is mandatory if actively bleeding. Follow local protocols which usually includes prothrombin complex concentrate and 10mg IV vitamin K • If taking DOACs, e.g. apixaban, rivaroxaban, dabigatran, and there is significant bleeding, use Beriplex® and specific reversal agents (e.g. idarucizumab) • For appropriate use of platelets, FFP, prothrombin concentrate, and other specific reversal agents, seek advice from a haematologist Balloon tamponade (Sengstaken–Blakemore tube) may occasionally be used in significant bleeds to temporarily stop bleeding and allow the patient to be stabilized

Source: data from NICE CG141.

Oesophagogastroduodenoscopy (OGD)

- Should occur immediately after resuscitation in unstable patients and within 24 hours for all UGIB
- Calculate a post-endoscopy Rockall score (calculates mortality risk following upper GI bleeding).[1] Variables include age, presence of shock, comorbidities, diagnosis on OGD, and whether there was evidence of bleeding in the stomach
- Do not give acid suppression drugs prior to endoscopy in non-variceal bleeds.

Pharmacological management

Non-variceal bleed

Give a proton pump inhibitor (PPI) to patients with non-variceal bleed **after** endoscopy, if evidence of recent haemorrhage is seen.

Variceal bleed

Terlipressin (2mg QDS IV)

- Terlipressin is a synthetic analogue of vasopressin which reduces portal blood flow and hence variceal pressure
- It should be started as soon as possible and continued for up to 5 days
- Terlipressin should be used with caution in patients with cardiovascular disease
- Treatment is often stopped after haemostasis, but this decision should be made by a gastroenterologist. Other vasoactive drugs which are sometimes used by specialists include somatostatin and octreotide.

Antibiotics (e.g. ceftriaxone 1g OD IV)

- Antibiotics in accordance with local protocols should be given on admission to all chronic liver disease patients with a suspected UGIB (whether variceal or due to another cause).

Prevention of hepatic encephalopathy

- Lactulose and enemas may be used acutely, and rifaximin long-term, for the prevention of hepatic encephalopathy. The dose of lactulose should be titrated to achieve two or three soft bowel movements per day.

Rebleeding after endoscopic treatment (requires senior review)

If a patient bleeds following maximal endoscopic therapy, other options may be required.

For uncontrolled non-variceal haemorrhage

CT angiogram plus vessel embolization

- If active bleeding seen on CT and available locally.

Surgery

- If embolization not possible.

1 Rockall TA, Logan RF, Devlin HB, et al. Risk assessment after acute upper gastrointestinal haemorrhage. *Gut*. 1996; 38:316–21.

For uncontrolled variceal haemorrhage

Balloon tamponade (Sengstaken–Blakemore tube)

- Temporarily stops bleeding in 90% of patients
- Only used for short-term control prior to definitive treatment. Balloon must be deflated within 24 hours due to risk of oesophageal ulceration and rupture
- Consider intubation and ventilation prior to insertion of a Sengstaken–Blakemore tube.

Transjugular intrahepatic portosystemic shunt (TIPSS)

- Consider for variceal bleeds that rebleed despite endoscopic therapy
- Aims to relieve portal hypertension by using a stent to shunt blood from the portal circulation to the hepatic vein, bypassing the cirrhotic liver
- Contraindications include heart failure, severe pulmonary hypertension, sepsis, and hepatic encephalopathy.

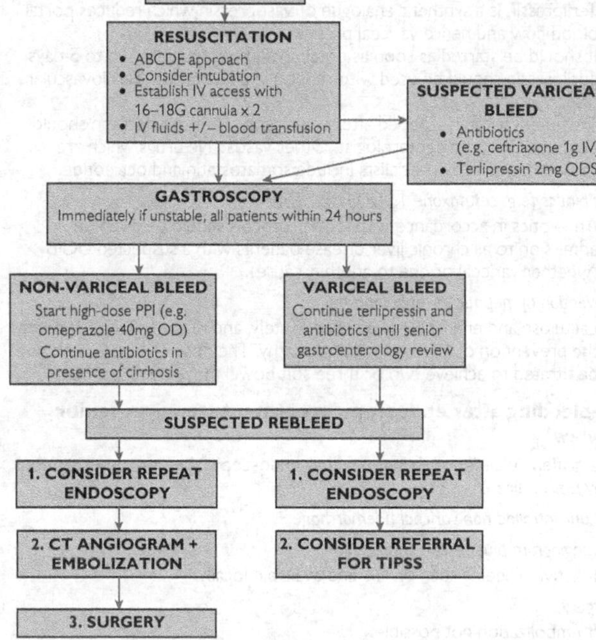

Fig. 27.1 Flowchart for management of an acute UGIB.

Considerations following haemostasis

Medication review

- Stop NSAIDs
- **Continue low-dose aspirin for secondary prevention of vascular events if haemostasis has been achieved**. Failure to restart aspirin leads to higher cardiovascular events and mortality
- Restarting other antiplatelet/anticoagulant medication should be discussed between the patient, endoscopist, and other relevant specialities. *Do not stop these medications long-term just because of a GI bleed!*

Prophylaxis for oesophageal varices

- Primary prophylaxis (varices which have **NOT** bled): non-cardioselective beta-blockers have been shown to reduce bleeding and mortality, e.g. carvedilol 6.25mg OD
- Secondary prophylaxis (postvariceal bleed): regular endoscopic band ligation plus non-cardioselective beta-blocker.

Further reading

1. Blatchford O, Murray WR, Blatchford M (2000). A risk score to predict need for treatment for upper gastrointestinal haemorrhage. *Lancet*. 356:1318–21. (Calculate score at: https://www.mdcalc.com/glasgow-blatchford-bleeding-score-gbs#evidence)
2. Chavez-Tapia NC, Barrientos-Gutierrez T, Tellez-Avila F, et al. (2011). Meta-analysis: antibiotic prophylaxis for cirrhotic patients with upper gastrointestinal bleeding – an updated Cochrane review. *Aliment Pharmacol Ther*. 34:509–18.
3. Marks D, Harbord M (2013). Acute upper gastrointestinal bleeding. In: *Emergencies in Gastroenterology and Hepatology* (pp. 1–20). Oxford: Oxford University Press. Available at: https://doi.org/10.1093/med/9780199231362.003.0001

Chapter 28

Coeliac disease

Guideline:
British Society of Gastroenterology (BSG guidelines on the diagnosis and management of adult coeliac disease): https://www.bsg.org.uk/clinical-resource/bsg-guidelines-on-the-diagnosis-and-management-of-adult-coeliac-disease/

OUP disclaimer: Oxford University Press makes no representation, express or implied, that the drug dosages are correct and that the recommendations are an exclusive or mandatory course of care. All health professionals reading this text have a responsibility to evaluate its appropriateness and take the individual needs of the patient into account.

Local trust guidelines: please refer to your local guidelines as necessary.

Overview

Coeliac disease is an autoimmune disorder where an inappropriate, T-cell-mediated immune response against gluten leads to malabsorption and an inflammatory response.

Diagnosis

History

The presentation of coeliac disease in part depends on the age of the patient. Children are more likely to present with GI symptoms and/or failure to thrive. A common presentation in adults is asymptomatic iron deficiency anaemia.

- Classical symptoms and signs of malabsorption:
  - Diarrhoea
  - Steatorrhoea
  - Weight loss or failure to thrive
  - Fatigue
  - Symptoms of specific nutrient deficiencies, e.g. fatigue due to iron deficiency anaemia
- Abdominal symptoms, e.g. nausea, vomiting, bloating, excessive flatus, pain, and cramping
- Asymptomatic and diagnosed through screening, or after a diagnosis of osteoporosis (see Chapter 24)
- Dermatological symptoms, e.g. dermatitis herpetiformis
- Hyposplenism leading to reduced immune function
- Neurological symptoms, e.g. peripheral neuropathy and paraesthesiae, ataxia, and balance difficulties.

Examination

There are few specific examination signs, so a high index of suspicion is needed. Common features include:

- Aphthous ulcers
- Signs of anaemia, e.g. conjunctival pallor, angular stomatitis, koilonychia
- Signs of vitamin B_{12} deficiency, e.g. ataxia, extensor plantars, absent knee/ankle reflexes
- Poorly fitting clothes due to weight loss
- Abdominal tenderness and distension
- Failure to thrive on height/weight charts
- Dermatitis herpetiformis (Fig. 28.1):
  - Cutaneous manifestation of coeliac disease
  - Extremely itchy bullous rash
  - Typically on buttocks, scalp, and extensor aspects of elbows and knees.

Investigations

See Fig. 28.2 for an algorithm for the diagnosis of coeliac disease.

Bedside

- Height and weight measurements.

Bloods

See Table 28.1 for a summary.

Other

- OGD with duodenal biopsy:
  - Must be done while the patient is on a gluten-containing diet for a definitive diagnosis
  - A positive biopsy will show signs of coeliac histology (Box 28.1)

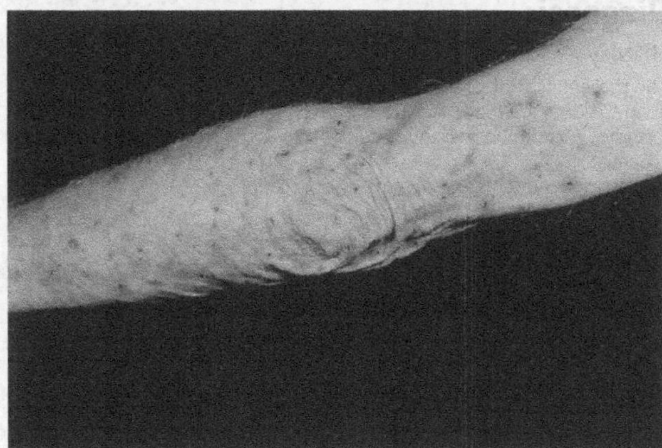

Fig. 28.1 Dermatitis herpetiformis.

Reproduced from Bloom S et al (2011) 'Oxford Handbook of Gastroenterology and Hepatology 2e' Oxford University Press: Oxford, with permission from Oxford University Press. See colour plate 1.

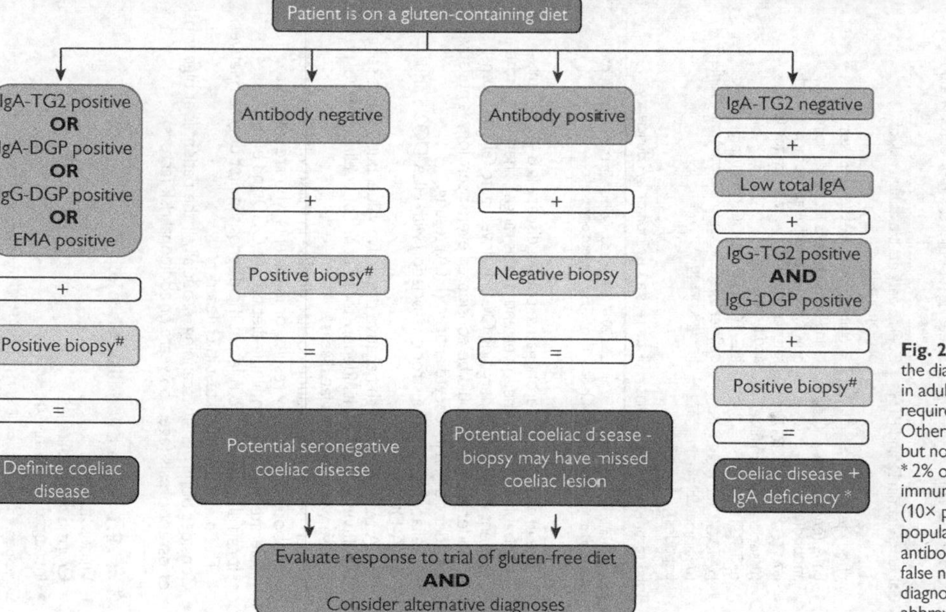

Fig. 28.2 Algorithm for the diagnosis of coeliac disease in adults. # Villous atrophy is required for a positive biopsy. Other features are supportive but not diagnostic.
* 2% of coeliac patients are immunoglobulin (Ig)-A deficient (10× prevalence general population), therefore IgA antibody testing may lead to false negatives and not be diagnostic. (See Table 28.1 for abbreviations.)

Table 28.1 Blood tests for the diagnosis of coeliac disease

Test	Rationale
FBC	Anaemia is common in coeliac disease
Iron studies and haematinics	Deficiencies in iron, vitamin B_{12} and folate are common, resulting in anaemias
LFT	Transaminases may be raised
Glucose and TFT	Screening for other common autoimmune diseases
Calcium, vitamin D, and PTH	Coeliac patients are at high risk of osteoporosis
Antibody testing: • EMA (endomysial antibodies) • IgA-TG2 and IgG-TG2 (tissue transglutaminase or TTG) • IgA-DGP and IgG-DGP (deamidated gliadin peptides)	Required for diagnostic purposes Using multiple tests increases sensitivity, however any positive antibody is enough for the patient to be referred for OGD and biopsy IgG-TG2 and IgG-DGP are useful in IgA-deficient patients as all the other antibodies are IgA based
Total serum immunoglobulins	If there is a suspicion of IgA deficiency

Source: data from Ludvigsson JF, et al (June 2014) Diagnosis and management of adult coeliac disease: guidelines from the British Society of Gastroenterology.

  - The prevalence of seronegative coeliac disease is 6–22% (but probably closer to the lower end of this range), therefore if the patient is already undergoing OGD to investigate GI symptoms, duodenal biopsy should be considered even if serology is negative
- Consider human leucocyte antigen (HLA) testing:
  - Coeliac disease has a strong association with HLA-DQ2.5 and HLA-DQ8
  - HLA testing has a high negative predictive value, but it is not specific. Positive genetic results identify those *at risk* of coeliac disease, not those who have coeliac disease
  - It can be used to exclude coeliac disease in those with equivocal antibody or histology results, or in patients who are unable to tolerate a gluten-containing diet before OGD and biopsy
  - It can also be used to rule out the diagnosis in first-degree relatives. This may be a useful test in children
- Consider bone density scanning, especially if the patient is at higher risk of osteoporosis (age >55 years or additional risk factors).

Box 28.1 Signs of coeliac histology
- Villous atrophy
- Crypt hyperplasia
- Intraepithelial lymphocytosis.

Source: data from Ludvigsson JF, et al (June 2014) Diagnosis and management of adult coeliac disease: guidelines from the British Society of Gastroenterology.

Management

Patient education

- Screening:
  - Strong genetic component: 10% prevalence in first-degree relatives, so consider offering screening
  - There is insufficient evidence for population screening
- Direct patients to support groups.

Lifestyle and simple interventions

- Must start a gluten-free diet with appropriate dietetic support.

Pharmacological management

- Must give calcium supplementation and bone protection if appropriate
- Pneumococcus vaccination must be given
- Consider haemophilus, meningococcus, and influenza vaccinations
- Dapsone is first line for dermatitis herpetiformis
- Immunosuppressive agents such as steroid, budesonide, azathioprine, and ciclosporin may be required in refractory disease.

Psychosocial considerations

- Living with a gluten-free diet:
  - Difficulty in obtaining, increased expense of, and increased time required to prepare gluten-free food
  - Impact on social life such as difficulty obtaining gluten-free food in restaurants
  - Impact on travel such as difficulty obtaining or explaining requirement for gluten-free food abroad
- Depression and fatigue are common.

Complications

- Flares:
  - If a patient has an unexpected flare, a dietary review must be carried out to check for accidental gluten exposure
  - Consider testing for associated conditions, e.g. lactose intolerance, pancreatic exocrine insufficiency
- Consequences of nutrient deficiencies
- Increased risk of osteoporosis and bone fracture
- Hyposplenism and reduced immunity
- Enteropathy-associated T-cell lymphoma (EATL)
- Infertility and poor fetal outcome.

Monitoring and follow-up

- Patients must be followed up annually
- All of the following must be done:
  - Check height and weight
  - Discuss symptom control
  - Review adherence to gluten-free diet, preferably with dietician input
  - Bloods monitoring: FBC, ferritin, folate, vitamin B_{12}, LFT, glucose, TFT, calcium, and coeliac autoantibodies
- Consider DXA scanning and starting bone protection

- Duodenal biopsy does not need to be regularly repeated, but one repeat duodenal biopsy >6 months after starting gluten-free diet is often recommended in adults to confirm resolution of epithelial damage.

Further reading

1. Wilkinson IB, Raine T, Wiles K, et al. (2017). Coeliac disease. In: *Oxford Handbook of Clinical Medicine*, 10th ed (p. 266). Available at: https://doi.org/10.1093/med/9780199689903.003.0006
2. Simon C, Everitt H, van Dorp S, et al. (2020). Coeliac disease. In: *Oxford Handbook of General Practice*, 5th ed (pp. 382–3). Available at: https://doi.org/10.1093/med/9780198808183.003.0012
3. Bloom S, Webster G, Marks D (2011). Coeliac disease. In: *Oxford Handbook of Gastroenterology*, 2nd ed (p. 259). Available at: https://doi.org/10.1093/med/9780199584079.003.0169
4. American College of Gastroenterology (2013). ACG clinical guidelines: diagnosis and management of celiac disease. Available at: https://gi.org/guideline/diagnosis-and-management-of-celiac-disease/
5. NICE (2015). Coeliac disease: recognition, assessment and management (NG20). Available at: https://www.nice.org.uk/guidance/ng20

Chapter 29

Crohn's disease

Guidelines:

European Crohn's and Colitis Organisation (3rd European evidence-based consensus on the diagnosis and management of Crohn's Disease 2016: part 1: diagnosis and medical management): https://academic.oup.com/ecco-jcc/article/11/1/3/2456546

European Crohn's and Colitis Organisation (3rd European evidence-based consensus on the diagnosis and management of Crohn's disease 2016: part 2: surgical management and special situations): https://academic.oup.com/ecco-jcc/article/11/2/135/2456548

OUP disclaimer: Oxford University Press makes no representation, express or implied, that the drug dosages are correct and that the recommendations are an exclusive or mandatory course of care. All health professionals reading this text have a responsibility to evaluate its appropriateness and take the individual needs of the patient into account.

Local trust guidelines: please refer to your local guidelines as necessary.

Overview

Crohn's disease (CD) is a lifelong, idiopathic, autoimmune disorder that can cause inflammation of any part of the GI tract, although it most frequently affects the terminal ileum, colon, and perianal areas. It is estimated to affect at least 115,000 people in the UK and typically follows a relapsing–remitting pattern of disease.

Diagnosis

Diagnosis is made through clinical history and examination, combined with evidence from biochemical, endoscopic, histological, and radiological investigations. CD may be classified as mild, moderate, or severe (Box 29.1)

Box 29.1 Severity of Crohn's disease

Classified into mild, moderate, or severe disease although these categories are not precisely defined.

The Crohn's Disease Activity Index (CDAI)[1] classifies active disease as a score >150, with severe disease >300.

NICE[2] defines severe active CD as very poor general health with one or more of weight loss, fever, severe abdominal pain, and frequent (3–4/day) diarrhoeal stools present.

History

- GI symptoms:
  - Chronic diarrhoea (present in >80% patients)
  - Abdominal pain (80%)
  - Blood/mucus in stool (40–50%)
  - Perianal fistula (4–10%)
- Systemic symptoms: weight loss (60%), fever
- Extraintestinal manifestations: joints, skin, and eyes (see following section)
- Recent travel history focusing on GI infections
- Country of origin (focusing on TB endemic regions) and family history of TB (intestinal TB can mimic CD leading to diagnostic confusion and some CD treatments, e.g. anti-TNF, increase the risk of developing active TB)
- Risk factors for CD: current smoker, family history of inflammatory bowel disease (IBD)
- Medication history, especially NSAIDs (Box 29.2).

Box 29.2 NSAIDs

Excessive use may cause NSAID enteropathy or colopathy which can mimic CD, or exacerbate existing CD. Frequent use is also a minor risk factor for CD.

Extraintestinal manifestations of Crohn's disease

Up to 35% of patients have extraintestinal manifestations of CD (Table 29.1), which can precede GI symptoms.

1 https://www.mdcalc.com/crohns-disease-activity-index-cdai

2 https://www.nice.org.uk/guidance/ng129/chapter/Recommendations

Table 29.1 Extraintestinal manifestations of Crohn's disease

Related to disease activity	Not related to disease activity
Peripheral large joint arthritis	Pyoderma gangrenosum
Erythema nodosum	Uveitis
Oral aphthous ulcers	Axial arthropathy (sacroiliitis or spondylitis)
Episcleritis	Small joint peripheral arthritis
	Primary sclerosing cholangitis (uncommon in CD)

Source: data from European Crohn's and Colitis Organisation Part 2.

Examination

- General health and appearance
- BMI
- Blood pressure, heart rate, and temperature
- Abdominal tenderness or distension
- Palpable abdominal masses
- Inspection of the perianal area (fistulas) and oral cavity (ulcers)
- DRE.

Investigations

Bedside

- Faecal calprotectin:
  - Not diagnostic
  - Typically used in primary care for its good negative predictive value
- Stool tests to exclude infectious diarrhoea (*Clostridium difficile*, MC&S based on travel history).

Bloods

- FBC (↑ platelets, ↓ haemoglobin)
- CRP/ESR (↑)
- Low albumin is a sign of severe inflammation, sepsis, or NSAID use
- Iron studies (including transferrin saturation), vitamin B_{12}, and folate.

Imaging

Allows staging of disease and may detect possible complications (fistula, obstruction, abscess). Consider patient age and likely location of disease when requesting.

- MRI small bowel: more sensitive than CT at diagnosing inflammation
- CT abdomen/pelvis: usually readily available, first line for suspected abscess or obstruction, but consider radiation exposure
- Abdominal ultrasound scan (USS): reasonable sensitivity in detecting bowel inflammation, but may give an incomplete picture of extent of disease. Needs an experienced operator and not available in every centre
- Small bowel capsule endoscopy (SBCE): generally reserved for high clinical suspicion of CD but MRI/CT/colonoscopy negative. High negative predictive value for excluding CD if normal.

Endoscopy and histology

- Ileo-colonoscopy with biopsies is typically the first-line diagnostic procedure
- Flexible sigmoidoscopy is preferable if severe active disease, as bowel preparation may not be tolerated and there is a higher risk of perforation with colonoscopy
- Endoscopic signs of CD: patchy inflammation; 'skip lesions' (inflammation between normal mucosa); longitudinal ulcers; cobblestone appearance of ileum/colon; fistulas and strictures
- Consider OGD in patients with symptoms such as vomiting and dyspepsia, to investigate the upper GI tract.

Management

Patient education

Information must be appropriate for the patient's age, literacy level, and cultural background and should cover prognosis, likely treatment side-effects, cancer risk, nutrition, and contact details for support groups.

Lifestyle and simple interventions

Smoking increases CD activity. All patients should be strongly encouraged to stop smoking, with active cessation programmes recommended.

Pharmacological management

- Treatment must be led by a gastroenterologist experienced in managing IBD. Basic principles are highlighted in Fig. 29.1
- Some CD patients will have a mild–moderate pattern of disease, with little or no requirement for steroids
- Reduction of steroid use is a key aim of good CD management.

Surgical management

Up to 75% of CD patients will require surgery. Indications for surgery include:

Obstructive symptoms

- Small bowel strictures: strictureplasty or bowel resection
- Colonic strictures: endoscopic dilatation (high risk for perforation particularly if active inflammation) or segmental/total colonic resection.

Abscess

- Urgent surgical or percutaneous drainage plus antibiotics.

Fistula

- Exclude presence of concurrent abscess with pelvic MRI
- Management using examination under anaesthetic (EUA), abscess drainage ± seton placement. Antibiotics may be needed as an adjunctive measure.

Isolated ileocaecal disease

- Laparoscopic ileocaecal resection should always be considered in patients with isolated terminal ileal disease. Current evidence suggests this compares favourably with medical therapy and therefore a careful discussion with the patient is important.

Psychosocial considerations

Offer multidisciplinary support to deal with psychological concerns about CD, including body image, living with a chronic illness, and effect on school/work.

Complications

- Colorectal cancer: the overall risk is low, but surveillance colonoscopy is required for patients who have been symptomatic for a decade and have colitis which affects more than one segment of colon.[3]

3 NICE CG118; https://www.nice.org.uk/guidance/cg118/

INDUCE REMISSION

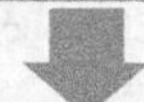

PO/IV corticosteroids

9mg budesonide OD, typically 8-week course[a]

OR

40mg prednisolone OD, reducing over 8 weeks[b]

OR

100mg hydrocortisone QDS (inpatient care only)[b]

Steroids should only be used in short courses, not for maintenance of remission

Consider Biologic if incomplete response to steroids and/or severe disease[c]

Infliximab

OR

Adalimumab

OR

Ustekinumab

Consider Surgery

Surgery is an option for induction therapy

For inflammatory disease, surgery is most commonly used if medical therapy fails to control disease

Surgery may be the primary treatment modality especially for bowel obstruction, fistula, and perforating disease.

MAINTAIN REMISSION

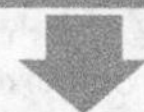

Immunomodulator

Azathioprine or mercaptopurine[d]

OR

Methotrexate

Immunomodulators are typically used as monotherapy for those with steroid-responsive disease, or as concommittant therapy with anti-TNF biologic

Continue or commence Biologic

Infliximab[e]

OR

Adalimumab[e]

OR

Ustekinumab

OR

Vedolizumab

Review at least annually

[a]Preferred for mild/moderate ileocaecal flare.

[b]Preferred for severe flares, small bowel or colonic disease.

[c]Severe disease features include: perianal disease, multifocal small bowel disease, upper GI disease, deep ulcers, profound weight loss.

[d]Check thiopurine methyltrasferase (TPMT) activity before starting. Do not give azathioprine or mercaptopurine if TPMT activity is very low/deficient.

[e]Anti-TNF therapy is typically used in conjunction with an immunomodulator to reduce the risk of anti-drug antibody formation.

Fig. 29.1 Basic management principles of CD.

- Metabolic bone disease: give calcium and vitamin D supplementation if using steroids for >6 weeks
- ↑ risk of venous thromboembolic events in active CD: in-hospital thromboprophylaxis essential
- Complications of therapy:
  - Azathioprine: lymphoma, non-melanoma skin cancers, immunosuppression
  - Anti-tumour necrosis factor (TNF): infusion reactions, reactivation of latent TB, infection, *possible* risk of lymphoproliferative disorders or malignancy
  - Anti- interleukin (IL)-12p40 (ustekinumab): injection site reactions, low risk of infection
  - Anti-α4β7 (vedolizumab): gut-specific agent with very low frequency of side effects
  - Steroids: Cushing's syndrome.

Monitoring and follow-up

CD patients must have regular follow-up, and assessment of disease activity. The mode of assessment will depend on the individual patient.

Special considerations

Pregnancy

- Fertility is typically unaffected by well-controlled CD
- Patients conceiving during inactive disease have a similar risk of relapse to non-pregnant patients
- For the majority of CD medications there is no evidence of harm during pregnancy and breastfeeding, although pregnancy must be avoided if the patient is taking methotrexate
- Investigation during pregnancy should always be considered carefully and discussed with the patient:
  - Colonoscopy is not performed during pregnancy
  - There is no evidence of harm with flexible sigmoidoscopy, although this should be avoided if possible.

Further reading

1. Crohn's Disease Activity Index (CDAI). Available at: https://www.mdcalc.com/crohns-disease-activity-index-cdai
2. Colombel J, Sandborn W, Reinisch W, et al. (2010). Infliximab, azathioprine or combination therapy for Crohn's disease. *N Engl J Med*. 362:1383–95.
3. NICE (2011). Colorectal cancer prevention: colonoscopic surveillance in adults with ulcerative colitis, Crohn's disease or adenomas (CG118). Available at: https://www.nice.org.uk/guidance/cg118/
4. NICE (2019). Crohn's disease management (NG129). Available at: https://www.nice.org.uk/guidance/ng129/
5. Feuerstein JD, Cheifetz AS (2017). Crohn disease: epidemiology, diagnosis and management. *Mayo Clin Proc*. 92:1088–103.

Chapter 30

Gastro-oesophageal reflux disease and dyspepsia

Guideline:
NICE CG184 (Gastro-oesophageal reflux disease and dyspepsia in adults: investigation and management): https://www.nice.org.uk/guidance/cg184

OUP disclaimer: Oxford University Press makes no representation, express or implied, that the drug dosages are correct and that the recommendations are an exclusive or mandatory course of care. All health professionals reading this text have a responsibility to evaluate its appropriateness and take the individual needs of the patient into account.

Local trust guidelines: please refer to your local guidelines as necessary.

Overview

Dyspepsia is an umbrella term for a cluster of non-specific symptoms (see 'History'). If present for at least 4 weeks, dyspepsia may signify underlying upper GI tract pathology, e.g. gastro-oesophageal reflux disease (GORD). Causes of dyspepsia are listed in Box 30.1.

Box 30.1 Causes of dyspepsia

- Functional (most common)
- GORD or gastritis
- *Helicobacter pylori* infection and peptic ulcer disease
- Symptom of cardiac or biliary disease
- Drugs, e.g. calcium channel blockers, nitrates, theophyllines, bisphosphonates, steroids, NSAIDs
- Cancer, e.g. oesophageal.

Source: data from NICE CG184.

Diagnosis

History

Dyspepsia symptoms:

- Recurrent epigastric pain/discomfort
- Acid reflux/heartburn
- The above-mentioned symptoms may be accompanied by nausea, vomiting, or bloating
- GORD may also present with a chronic cough, hoarseness, and 'water brash' where acid reflux mixes with excessively produced saliva in the throat
- Patients with a hiatus hernia are more likely to develop GORD.

Examination

Involves assessment of the underlying cause of dyspepsia:

- Cachexia
- Conjunctival pallor
- Epigastric/upper abdominal tenderness
- Melaena.

Investigations

Bloods

- FBC, U&E, LFT, and coagulation profile.

H. pylori testing

There are multiple tests available for *H. pylori*. Options are listed in Table 30.1.

Table 30.1 Options for *H. pylori* testing

	Demonstrates active infection	Unable to distinguish between active and past infection
Invasive tests	OGD with CLO (*Campylobacter*-like organism or rapid urease) test OGD with gastric biopsies (for histology)	
Non-invasive tests	Carbon-13 (C13) urea breath test Stool antigen test	H. *pylori* serology

Patients on PPIs should have a 2-week washout period prior to *H. pylori* testing with stool antigen, breath test, or CLO test to prevent false-negative results.

Upper gastrointestinal endoscopy

- Identifies presence of peptic ulcer disease, GORD, oesophagitis, and Barrett's oesophagus

- Perform within 2 weeks if:[1]
  - Dysphagia **OR**
  - Age ≥55 with weight loss **AND** upper abdominal pain **OR** reflux **OR** dyspepsia

> If dyspepsia is accompanied by significant upper GI tract bleeding, refer the same day for urgent endoscopy.

- Perform non-urgently if ≥55 years with:
  - Treatment resistant dyspepsia **OR**
  - Dyspepsia with raised platelet count **OR**
  - Dyspepsia with nausea/vomiting.

Oesophageal pH monitoring ± manometry

- Confirms diagnosis in patients with refractory symptoms despite treatment and patients without evidence of reflux on endoscopy despite classical symptoms of GORD

1 Suspected cancer: recognition and referral, NICE NG12; https://www.nice.org.uk/guidance/ng12

Management

Step-wise approach as laid out in the following sections. Patients with classical GORD symptoms without ⚑ symptoms/signs may only require lifestyle interventions and a short 4-week course of acid suppression therapy. If symptoms resolve following this, no further investigation is required.

Patient education

- Encourage the patient to identify triggers that provoke their symptoms.

Lifestyle and simple interventions

- Weight loss
- Reduction in alcohol consumption
- Smoking cessation
- Avoid specific food triggers, e.g. spicy food
- Avoid large meals for a few hours before going to bed
- Elevate head of bed.

Pharmacological management

Stop culprit medications (if possible)

- NSAIDs, steroids, and bisphosphonates increase risk of damaging upper GI tract mucosa
- Nitrates and calcium channel blockers and anticholinergics reduce lower oesophageal sphincter pressure.

Symptomatic relief

- Antacids/alginates can be used as short-term treatment for symptomatic relief.

Acid suppression therapy

Uninvestigated dyspepsia or GORD

- Offer full-dose PPI for 4 weeks if dyspepsia is not investigated or 4–8 weeks if GORD is diagnosed, e.g. omeprazole 20mg OD or lansoprazole 30mg OD
- Offer lowest tolerated dose of PPI for symptom recurrence following initial treatment
- If there is inadequate response to PPI, offer a histamine-2 receptor antagonist.

Peptic ulcer disease (without H. pylori infection)

- Offer full-dose PPI for 4–8 weeks, e.g. omeprazole 20mg OD or lansoprazole 30mg OD, or a histamine-2 receptor antagonist, e.g. ranitidine 150mg BD.

Functional dyspepsia

- Use low-dose PPI, e.g. omeprazole 10mg OD or lansoprazole 15mg OD.

Severe oesophagitis

- Provide full-dose PPI for 8 weeks and consider long-term maintenance therapy
- If treatment failure, consider switching PPI or escalating to a high dose, e.g. omeprazole 40mg BD, lansoprazole 30mg BD.

H. pylori eradication therapy

Consult with local antibiotic protocols if these are available. If unavailable, recommended regimens are as follows:

- First line:
  - 7 days of PPI, e.g. omeprazole 20–40mg BD
  - **PLUS** amoxicillin 1g BD
  - **AND EITHER** clarithromycin 500mg BD **OR** metronidazole 400mg BD
- Second line:
  - Repeat first-line course but switch clarithromycin or metronidazole to the alternative, whichever was not used first line
  - If previously exposed to both clarithromycin and metronidazole, switch to a quinolone, e.g. levofloxacin 250mg BD **OR** tetracycline 500mg QDS
- Penicillin allergy:
  - First line:
    - 7 days of PPI, e.g. omeprazole 20–40mg BD
    - **PLUS** clarithromycin 500mg BD
    - **AND** metronidazole 400mg BD
  - Second line:
    - Switch clarithromycin to levofloxacin 250mg BD
    - **OR** if previously exposed to a quinolone, switch clarithromycin to tetracycline 500mg QDS **AND** bismuth 240mg BD
  - If penicillin allergy and previous clarithromycin exposure:
    - 7 days of PPI, e.g. omeprazole 20–40mg BD
    - **PLUS** metronidazole 400mg BD
    - **AND** tetracycline 500mg QDS
    - **AND** bismuth 240mg BD.

Surgical management

Fundoplication may be considered in patients with severe symptoms or ongoing oesophageal insult (oesophagitis, stricture, or Barrett's metaplasia) despite maximal medical therapy. This procedure involves 'tightening' the lower oesophageal sphincter leading to ↑ lower oesophageal sphincter pressure which reduces acid reflux.

Complications

- Barrett's oesophagus
- Severe erosive oesophagitis
- Oesophageal stricture.

Monitoring and follow-up

- None if symptoms respond to lifestyle interventions or pharmacological management. Consider repeat testing for *H. pylori* if ongoing symptoms despite eradication therapy using C13 urea breath test
- Repeat endoscopy in 6–8 weeks to ensure healing if severe oesophagitis or gastric ulcer
- Regular follow-up endoscopy may be required if Barrett's oesophagus has been diagnosed (to monitor for malignant changes).

Special considerations

Referral to specialist services should be considered in:

- Refractory symptoms of GORD unresponsive to maximal medical therapy or if the symptoms are unexplained
- Refractory *H. pylori* infection (resistant to second-line treatment)
- For surgical management of GORD.

Further reading

1. Wilkinson IB, Raine T, Wiles K et al. (2017). Dyspepsia and peptic ulcer disease. In: *Oxford Handbook of Clinical Medicine*, 10th ed (pp. 252–3). Oxford: Oxford University Press. Available at: https://doi.org/10.1093/med/9780199689903.003.0006
2. Wilkinson IB, Raine T, Wiles K et al. (2017). Gastro-oesophageal reflux disease (GORD). In: *Oxford Handbook of Clinical Medicine*, 10th ed. (p. 254–5). Oxford: Oxford University Press. Available at: https://doi.org/10.1093/med/9780199689903.003.0006
3. Bloom S, Webster G, Marks D (2011). Dyspepsia and gastro-oesophageal reflux. In: *Oxford Handbook of Gastroenterology and Hepatology*, 2nd ed (pp. 52–8). Oxford: Oxford University Press. Available at: https://doi.org/10.1093/med/9780199584079.003.0012

Chapter 31

Irritable bowel syndrome

Guideline:
NICE CG61 (Irritable bowel syndrome in adults: diagnosis and management): https://www.nice.org.uk/guidance/cg61

OUP disclaimer: Oxford University Press makes no representation, express or implied, that the drug dosages are correct and that the recommendations are an exclusive or mandatory course of care. All health professionals reading this text have a responsibility to evaluate its appropriateness and take the individual needs of the patient into account.

Local trust guidelines: please refer to your local guidelines as necessary.

Overview

Irritable bowel syndrome (IBS) is a condition of unclear aetiology which presents with a combination of abdominal symptoms. It has a female predominance and usually occurs in a relapsing–remitting pattern.

Diagnosis

The key to approaching and diagnosing IBS is a clear history and the absence of positive examination findings and investigations. Based on the patient's symptoms, IBS can be divided into categories of diarrhoea predominant, constipation predominant, or mixed IBS symptoms.

History/diagnostic criteria

A minimum of 6 months' history of **A**bdominal pain, **B**loating, or **C**hanging bowel habit (diarrhoea, constipation, or alternating between both) should prompt a consideration of IBS. The abdominal pain does not usually have a fixed site.

Diagnosing IBS requires the presence of abdominal pain/discomfort which improves with defecation or occurs alongside a change in bowel frequency or stool consistency. These symptoms should **coexist** with two or more of the following symptoms:

- Symptoms worse with eating
- Bloating or distension of the abdomen
- Passing mucus per rectum
- Change in stool passage (feeling of incomplete evacuation, urgency or straining).

Other common symptoms include:

- Lethargy
- Nausea
- Back pain
- Symptoms related to the bladder (urinary urgency, nocturia)
- Faecal incontinence (ask specifically, as patients may not disclose this voluntarily).

Examination

- In most cases, there is no abnormality
- General tenderness may be elicited on palpation of the abdomen
- If required, based on symptoms, carry out a rectal examination to rule out other pathology
- Features of weight loss, aphthous ulcers, abdominal mass, rectal bleeding, or pallor if elicited should prompt consideration of other diagnoses.

Investigations

The aim of investigations is to exclude other disorders.

Bloods

- FBC
- ESR
- CRP
- Tissue transglutaminase (to exclude coeliac disease, especially in patients with mixed symptoms or predominance of diarrhoea).

Other

Abdominal ultrasound, endoscopy, barium enema, TFT, hydrogen breath test, faecal ova/parasite testing, and faecal occult blood are **NOT** recommended to diagnose IBS.

Management

Patient education

- Empower patients with IBS to manage their condition by providing information leaflets which illustrate the significance of self-help
- Increase amount of physical activity and relaxation
- Support groups:
  - The IBS Network—national charity with website providing information for self-help and networking with local support groups.

Lifestyle and simple interventions

- Eat regularly (avoid skipping meals) and without rushing
- Reduce intake of fibre (especially insoluble fibre such as bran) and resistant starches, e.g. pulses, reheated potato
- Increase fluid intake (aim for 8 cups a day at least) but reduce consumption of caffeine, alcohol, and fizzy drinks
- Maximum three portions of fresh fruit per day
- For symptoms of bloating, oats and linseeds may help
- If patients would like to try probiotics, a minimum trial period of 4 weeks is recommended whilst monitoring symptoms
- If the above-listed dietary interventions have not helped symptoms, patients should receive dietetic advice, including advice on exclusion diets such as a low-'FODMAP' diet (Box 31.1).

Box 31.1 Low-FODMAP diets

- FODMAP stands for fermentable oligosaccharides, disaccharides, monosaccharides, and polyols
- Foods with high FODMAPs are thought to increase symptoms of bloating and pain, secondary to poor absorption in the small intestine which leads to bacterial fermentation in the large intestine
- Some patients with IBS are very sensitive to FODMAPs but others are not, so eliminating FODMAPs will not always work
- The usual approach is to eliminate high-FODMAP foods for 4–8 weeks before gradually reintroducing different foods to find which are the worst triggers.

Pharmacological management

- Main aim is targeted symptom relief, if dietary and lifestyle interventions are ineffective
- Abdominal pain:
  - Consider antispasmodic agents such as hyoscine butylbromide (10–20mg TDS–QDS) or mebeverine (200mg BD)
- Diarrhoea:
  - Antimotility agents for symptoms of diarrhoea (loperamide 2mg, maximum 16mg a day) is the first choice
- Constipation:
  - Consider laxatives for constipation (except lactulose which can worsen bloating)
  - Linaclotide (290 micrograms OD) can be considered for patients who experience at least 12 months of constipation despite trials of multiple laxatives. Review after 3 months to assess response.

Second-line agents

- Tricyclic antidepressants can be considered if the above medications fail to improve symptoms
- Commence at low dose (e.g. amitriptyline 5–10mg OD) with gradual titration and regular review
- Selective serotonin reuptake inhibitors (SSRIs) should be considered if TCAs do not provide adequate clinical response, are poorly tolerated, or are contraindicated
- Follow up patients who have been started on TCAs or SSRIs after 4 weeks and 6–12 months.

Psychological interventions

- In patients with refractory IBS (no improvement in symptoms after 12 months of pharmacological management) consider referral for psychological interventions
- These include cognitive behavioural therapy (CBT), hypnotherapy, or psychological therapy.

Monitoring and follow-up

- Further investigation is required if new ⚑ symptoms develop.

Further reading

1. Bloom S, Webster G, Marks D (2011). Irritable bowel syndrome. In: *Oxford Handbook of Gastroenterology and Hepatology*, 2nd ed (pp. 373–6). Oxford: Oxford University Press. Available at: https://doi.org/10.1093/med/9780199584079.003.0220
2. The IBS Network website. Available at: https://www.theibsnetwork.org/

Chapter 32

Ulcerative colitis

Guidelines:
European Crohn's and Colitis Organisation, European Society of Gastrointestinal and Abdominal Radiology (ECCO-ESGAR guideline for diagnostic assessment in IBD part 1: initial diagnosis, monitoring of known IBD, detection of complications): https://academic.oup.com/ecco-jcc/article/13/2/144/5078195

European Crohn's and Colitis Organisation, European Society of Gastrointestinal and Abdominal Radiology (ECCO-ESGAR guideline for diagnostic assessment in IBD part 2: IBD scores and general principles and technical aspects): https://academic.oup.com/ecco-jcc/article/13/3/273/5078200

European Crohn's and Colitis Organisation (Third European evidence-based consensus on diagnosis and management of ulcerative colitis. Part 2: current management): https://academic.oup.com/ecco-jcc/article/11/7/769/2962457

OUP disclaimer: Oxford University Press makes no representation, express or implied, that the drug dosages are correct and that the recommendations are an exclusive or mandatory course of care. All health professionals reading this text have a responsibility to evaluate its appropriateness and take the individual needs of the patient into account.

Local trust guidelines: please refer to your local guidelines as necessary.

Overview

Ulcerative colitis (UC) is a chronic inflammatory condition of unknown aetiology which is thought to occur secondary to environmental triggers in genetically susceptible individuals.

UC occurs in the rectum and colon, unlike CD (see Chapter 29) which can occur in any part of the GI tract. UC can be further categorized according to the distribution of colonic inflammation: proctitis (limited to rectum), left-sided (up to the splenic flexure), and extensive colitis (proximal to splenic flexure).

Diagnosis

History

Diagnosis is achieved through a combination of history alongside biochemical, endoscopic, stool, and histological findings. Common history findings include:

- Rectal bleeding
- Diarrhoea
- Increase in bowel frequency
- Urgency, tenesmus, and incontinence
- Abdominal pain (typically cramps related to the need to defecate)
- Constitutional symptoms, e.g. fatigue
- In severe disease, systemic symptoms may manifest, e.g. fever and anorexia. Weight loss is relatively uncommon and typically occurs in late presentations of extensive disease.

Also ask about:

- Recent travel history regarding GI infections
- Smoking history: typically ex- or never-smokers
- Family history of IBD.

Examination

- May have no specific signs in patients with mild to moderate disease
- Abdominal tenderness (especially during acute flare)
- Extraintestinal manifestations (Box 32.1)
- Signs of anaemia, e.g. conjunctival pallor, koilonychia
- Rectal examination is usually unnecessary since the patient will need endoscopic investigation
- **Acute severe flare of UC**: tachycardia (>90bpm) and/or pyrexia (>37.8°C).

Box 32.1 Extraintestinal manifestations of ulcerative colitis

- Erythema nodosum
- Pyoderma gangrenosum
- Uveitis
- Finger clubbing
- Arthropathy: large joint arthritis and sacroiliitis
- Primary sclerosing cholangitis (PSC).

Investigations

Bedside

- Pulse rate and temperature
- Stool chart—monitor bowel frequency, stool consistency, and presence of blood with stool.

Bloods

- FBC: low haemoglobin, raised leucocytes and platelets
- CRP or ESR (the latter is rarely performed)
- Electrolytes: for baseline level

- LFT: alanine aminotransferase (ALT) and alkaline phosphatase (ALP) may be ↑ if concomitant PSC. Albumin may be low in more severe disease
- Iron studies.

Imaging

- Abdominal X-ray—to check for toxic megacolon in acute severe flare of UC (internal colon diameter ≥5.5cm)
- CT if suspected perforation (more severe persistent abdominal pain, and/or sepsis).

Other

- Stool sample:
    - Faecal calprotectin (FC)—marker of colon inflammation (↑). Useful for monitoring of disease activity. Not useful as a diagnostic tool, but typically used in primary care for its good negative predictive value (i.e. to exclude inflammatory bowel disease)
    - Microbiology analysis to rule out infective causes of bloody diarrhoea, especially *Clostridium difficile*
    - Test for ova, cysts, and parasites depending on the patient's demographics and travel history
- Lower GI endoscopy—ileo-colonoscopy or flexible sigmoidoscopy:
    - Continuous inflammation visualized in the rectum and extending proximally (unlike CD which has 'skip' lesions)
    - Mucosa—loss of vascular pattern, bleeding and friability, erosions, and/or ulcers. Larger (>5mm) and/or deep ulcers are typically representative of more severe disease
    - Biopsy—colonic and rectal biopsies should be taken. Histological features of UC are listed in Box 32.2
    - Flexible sigmoidoscopy is preferred in severe active disease as bowel preparation may not be tolerated, and there is a higher risk of perforation with colonoscopy.

Box 32.2 Histological features of ulcerative colitis

- Basal plasmacytosis (earliest feature)
- Crypt distortion
- Crypt abscesses
- Mucosal atrophy
- Absence of granuloma (granulomas seen in CD)
- Continuous colonic involvement with clear demarcation of inflammation plus rectal involvement.

Source: data from Maaser C, et al (August 2018) ECCO-ESGAR Guideline for Diagnostic Assessment in IBD Part 1: Initial diagnosis, monitoring of known IBD, detection of complications. Journal of Crohn's and Colitis 13(2): 144–164K.

Management

Guided by disease severity and distribution of UC. Truelove and Witts' criteria are predominantly used to assess disease severity in acute flares (Table 32.1).

Table 32.1 Assessing severity in UC flares
(Truelove and Witts' criteria modified to include CRP)

Variable	Mild UC	Moderate UC	Severe UC
Motions/day	<4	4–6	>6
Rectal bleeding	Small	Moderate	Large
Temperature	Apyrexial	37.1–37.8°C	>37.8°C
Resting pulse (bpm)	<70	70–90	>90
Haemoglobin (g/L)	>110	105–110	<105
ESR/CRP	<30		>30

Source: data from Truelove SC, et al (October 1955) Cortisone in Ulcerative Colitis. British Medical Journal 2(4947): 1041–8.

Patient education

- Patient to monitor symptoms and contact IBD team/nurse if they develop persistent changes in symptoms.

Pharmacological management

Acute flare

- Mild–moderate UC:
  - For proctitis alone, topical 5-aminosalicyclic acid (5-ASA) is first line (can be combined with topical steroids or oral 5-ASA for greater effectiveness)
  - Oral 5-ASA in combination with topical 5-ASA for left-sided and extensive disease
  - Oral steroids such as budesonide MMX® (Cortiment®) or prednisolone should be considered in cases refractory to 5-ASA
- Severe UC: indication for admission to hospital in those patients fulfilling Truelove and Witts' criteria. This means >6 bloody stools/day plus **one or more** of the criteria (temperature >37.8°C, pulse rate>90bpm, haemoglobin <105 g/L, CRP >30mg/L):
  - Treat with IV steroids, thromboprophylaxis, and IV rehydration with electrolyte replacement (will typically require potassium >60mmol/day)
  - Maintain haemoglobin of >8g/dL with transfusion
  - Consider medical rescue therapy with infliximab or ciclosporin if no or incomplete response to steroid by day 3. **Day 3 criteria are** >8 stools/day, **or** 3–8 stools/day and CRP >45mg/L
  - If no response to rescue therapy after 4–7 days, colectomy is recommended.

Thromboprophylaxis

Inpatients with UC should be prescribed thromboprophylaxis given their ↑ risk of thromboembolism, despite bloody diarrhoea.

Chronic management

Patients should remain on long-term maintenance treatment with the aim of achieving steroid free remission.

- Steroid-sparing therapy:
  - Patients requiring steroids despite 5-ASA treatment, and with steroid-responsive disease, should be commenced on thiopurines in the first instance. Evidence suggests there is little role for methotrexate as monotherapy in UC, but it does still have use as a concomitant immunomodulator with anti-TNF therapy
  - For those with active disease despite 5-ASA and thiopurines, or those with steroid-refractory disease, there are now a number of medical options. These include anti-TNF agents (e.g. infliximab, adalimumab), anti-integrin therapy (vedolizumab), JAK inhibitors (tofacitinib), and anti-IL-12p40 (ustekinumab)
  - Special considerations for prescribing steroid-sparing treatments are listed in Table 32.2.

Table 32.2 Prescribing thiopurines, anti-TNF agents, vedolizumab, and tofacitinib

	Thiopurines	Anti-TNF	Vedolizumab	Tofacitinib
Before starting	Check thiopurine methyltransferase (TMPT) levels Check baseline FBC, U&E, LFT Check serology for: Hepatitis B/C, HIV. Vaccinate/ treat if appropriate	Check serology for: Hepatitis B/C, HIV, varicella-zoster virus (VZV) Also perform TB testing as per local guidelines. Vaccinate/ treat if appropriate	No specific checks	Check serology for: Hepatitis B/C, Epstein–Barr virus, HIV, VZV Vaccinate/treat if appropriate Check fasting lipids Shingles vaccine if possible Consider risk of DVT and pulmonary embolism (PE). Use alternative agent if possible if additional VTE risks

Table 32.2 *Continued*

	Thiopurines	Anti-TNF	Vedolizumab	Tofacitinib
Monitoring	FBC and LFT every other week for 1 month, then every 3 months	Check anti-TNF trough levels if incomplete or loss of response, and at least every 6–12 months in stable patients	No specific monitoring	Check fasting lipids at 8 weeks Check FBC and LFT at 4 and 8 weeks, and then every 3 months
Cautions	Patient should have a low threshold for seeking medical attention if they develop fever/infection	Patient should have a low threshold for seeking medical attention if they develop fever/infection	No specific cautions	Patient should have a low threshold for seeking medical attention if they develop fever, shingles, or symptoms of DVT/PE

Source: data from the BNF.

Surgical management

- Subtotal colectomy with ileostomy may be required after failure of medical treatment or due to complications (e.g. colonic perforation)
- Subsequent completion proctectomy and permanent ileostomy, or formation of ileo-anal pouch, is a decision to be taken after full recovery from subtotal colectomy.

Psychosocial considerations

- Living with symptoms of ↑ bowel frequency and urgency:
  - Feelings of social embarrassment
  - Adolescents at ↑ risk of social isolation and depression
- Psychological impact of stoma formation
- Direct patients to stoma specialist nurses and support groups to help with the above points.

Complications

- Strictures
- Fibrosis
- Toxic colonic dilatation
- Bowel perforation
- ↑ risk of colorectal cancer
- Thromboembolism.

Monitoring and follow-up

- Most patients will require long-term maintenance treatment, usually with 5-ASA/mesalazine
- Follow up with IBD team at intervals appropriate for disease activity. This will include a review of symptoms, serum inflammatory markers, ± faecal calprotectin ± endoscopic assessment
- Patients on thiopurines or anti-TNF agents should have their drug levels monitored.

Endoscopy

- If patients are asymptomatic at follow-up but have abnormal inflammatory markers and/or faecal calprotectin, consider endoscopy to assess for active disease
- Monitor mucosal healing with endoscopy or faecal calprotectin 3–6 months after commencing treatment in patients who improve clinically with pharmacological treatment
- If new symptoms, poor response to treatment, or severe relapse, repeat endoscopy
- Surveillance colonoscopy should be carried out (between 5-yearly and annually, depending on risk stratification) due to ↑ risk of colorectal cancer associated with UC. Surveillance should be more frequent in patients with concurrent PSC.

Special considerations

Pregnancy

- Fertility is unaffected by well-controlled UC
- Patients conceiving during inactive disease have similar risk of relapse to non-pregnant patients
- For the majority of UC medications there is no evidence of harm during pregnancy and breastfeeding, although pregnancy must be avoided if the patient is taking methotrexate or tofacitinib
- Investigation during pregnancy should always be considered carefully and discussed with the patient. There is no evidence of harm with flexible sigmoidoscopy, although this is avoided if possible, particularly in the first trimester given the natural frequency of miscarriage in this stage of pregnancy. MRI is typically only performed in the second and third trimesters.

Further reading

1. Wilkinson IB, Raine T, Wiles K, et al. (2017). Ulcerative colitis. In: *Oxford Handbook of Clinical Medicine*, 10th ed (pp. 262–3). Oxford: Oxford University Press. Available at: https://doi.org/10.1093/med/9780199689903.003.0006

Part 5

Hepatobiliary

Chapter 33

Acute liver failure

Guideline:
European Association for the Study of the Liver (EASL Clinical Practical Guidelines on the management of acute (fulminant) liver failure): https://www.journal-of-hepatology.eu/article/S0168-8278(16)30708-5/fulltext

OUP disclaimer: Oxford University Press makes no representation, express or implied, that the drug dosages are correct and that the recommendations are an exclusive or mandatory course of care. All health professionals reading this text have a responsibility to evaluate its appropriateness and take the individual needs of the patient into account.

Local trust guidelines: please refer to your local guidelines as necessary.

Overview

Acute liver failure (ALF) refers to an acute episode of liver dysfunction in a patient without previously diagnosed liver disease, resulting in coagulopathy and hepatic encephalopathy (HE). ALF typically begins with an acute liver injury, suggested by deranged liver function and coagulopathy.

Diagnosis

The diagnosis of ALF is dependent on:

- Acute liver injury—a 2–3× increase in transaminases (ALT and aspartate aminotransferase (AST))—**and** impaired liver function evidenced by jaundice and coagulopathy
- The presence of HE.

Coagulopathy is defined as INR >1.5 and/or prolonged PT. Depending on the time of onset of HE from the time jaundice was noted, ALF can be further divided into hyperacute (7 days), acute (8–28 days), and subacute (5–12 weeks). The timeframe can help to suggest the potential cause of ALF (Table 33.1).

HE is necessary for a diagnosis of ALF. Its absence in the presence of newly deranged liver function and coagulopathy suggests an acute liver injury, but **not** ALF.

History

A focused history will help make a prompt diagnosis of ALF and give clues to the aetiology, guiding management and allowing prognostication. Ask about onset of symptoms and signs suggestive of liver dysfunction such as:

- Jaundice
- Confusion
- Atraumatic/spontaneous bleeding
- General malaise
- Nausea or vomiting
- Abdominal swelling (ascites is more typical of chronic liver disease but can occur in Budd–Chiari syndrome)
- Right upper quadrant (RUQ) pain.

Take a thorough social history, including foreign travel, occupation, alcohol use, and drug use. Be sure to ask about regular and acute medications, including over-the-counter and herbal medications! HE can be subtle so it helps to have a collateral history. Consider the timeframe of symptoms as this may provide a clue to the diagnosis (Table 33.1).

The most common causes of ALF worldwide are hepatitis A, B, and E. In Europe, drug-induced ALF is the most common cause.

Examination

Begin with a general inspection, looking in particular for jaundice, ascites, and evidence of HE. Take note of clues that may point to specific causes of ALF, including evidence of self-harm (overdose), tattoos or injection sites (hepatitis B), Kayser–Fleischer rings (Wilson disease), combination of RUQ pain, hepatomegaly, and ascites (typical triad of Budd–Chiari syndrome).

Signs of liver failure include:

- Asterixis
- Jaundice (examine skin and sclera)
- Ascites
- Bruising or bleeding
- HE (Table 33.2).

Table 33.1 Timeframe of different ALF presentations

Aetiologies which may also present hyperacutely are *italicized*.

Category	Acute	Acute and subacute
Viral	*Hepatitis A and E* Hepatitis B CMV HSV VZV Dengue	
Drugs or toxins	*Ecstasy* Chemotherapy NSAIDs Antiepileptics, e.g. phenytoin, carbamazepine Statins Flucloxacillin Anti-TB treatments	*Paracetamol overdose*
Vascular	Hypoxic hepatitis	Budd–Chiari syndrome
Pregnancy	Pre-eclampsia HELLP Fatty liver of pregnancy	
Other		Wilson disease Autoimmune Malignancy, including lymphoma

CMV, cytomegalovirus; HELLP, haemolysis, elevated liver enzymes and low platelets (syndrome); HSV, herpes simplex virus.

Reproduced from Wendon J, Cordoba J, Dhawan A, Larsen FS, Manns M, Samuel D, Simpson KJ, Yaron I, Bernardi M. EASL Clinical Practical Guidelines on the management of acute (fulminant) liver failure. J Hepatol. 2017 May;66(5):1047–1081 with permission from Elsevier.

Table 33.2 Grades of hepatic encephalopathy

Grade	Presentation
Grade 1	Altered mood, reduced attention span, sleep disturbance
Grade 2	Increasing drowsiness, time disorientation, personality change, asterixis, inappropriate behaviour
Grade 3	Stupor, bizarre behaviour, significant confusion
Grade 4	Coma

Source: data from Hepatic Encephalopathy in Chronic Liver Disease: 2014 Practice Guideline by the European Association for the Study of the Liver and the American Association for the Study of Liver Diseases (September 2014) Clinical Practice Guidelines 61(3): 642–659.

Investigations

Use investigations to decide on appropriate treatment and whether referral to a specialist centre is required (Table 33.3).

Bedside

- Urinalysis
- ECG.

Bloods

- FBC, U&E, LFT, coagulation profile (INR and/or PT, fibrinogen), glucose
- ABG (monitor for acidosis and lactate level)
- Arterial ammonia (sample often requires delivery to laboratory on ice)
- Paracetamol level
- Viral screen (hepatitis B surface antigen (HBsAg), anti-hepatitis B core (HBc) IgM (consider hepatitis B virus DNA), anti-hepatitis A virus IgM, anti-hepatitis E virus IgM, anti-HSV IgM, anti-VZV IgM, CMV, HSV, EBV, parvovirus, and VZV polymerase chain reaction (PCR))
- Autoimmune screen (antinuclear antibody (ANA), anti-smooth muscle antibody (SMA), anti-soluble liver antigen (SLA), anti-liver kidney microsomal antibody (LKMA), immunoglobulin profile, antineutrophil cytoplasmic antibody (ANCA), HLA typing)
- Blood cultures.

Imaging

- Chest X-ray (baseline)
- Ultrasound liver with Doppler examination of hepatic vessels
- CT abdomen may be required for further liver characterization.

Other

- Ascitic tap if ascites present (>250 neutrophils/mm^3 suggests spontaneous bacterial peritonitis)
- Liver biopsy may be useful to exclude cirrhosis, malignancy, or alcohol-induced acute liver injury.

Table 33.3 Criteria for referral to a specialist centre

ALF secondary to paracetamol overdose, or hyperacute presentation	ALF secondary to any other cause
pH <7.3 or HCO_3 <18	
Hypoglycaemia	
INR >3 on day 2, or INR >4 after day 2	INR >1.8
Oliguria and/or raised creatinine	Oliguria, renal failure, or Na <130mmol/L
Change in level of consciousness	Encephalopathy
High lactate not responding to fluids	Metabolic acidosis
	Bilirubin >300µmol/L
	Decreasing liver size

Reproduced from Wendon J, Cordoba J, Dhawan A, Larsen FS, Manns M, Samuel D, Simpson KJ, Yaron I, Bernardi M. EASL Clinical Practical Guidelines on the management of acute (fulminant) liver failure. J Hepatol. 2017 May;66(5):1047–1081 with permission from Elsevier.

Management

Acute management

The acute management of liver failure requires a systemic approach, reflecting the broad presentation and multiorgan involvement (Table 33.4). Consider ICU referral early.

Table 33.4 Acute management of ALF

A	• Protect airway if necessary due to HE or reduced consciousness (HE grade 3 or above is typically an indication for intubation)
C	• Patients are usually volume depleted • Consider IV fluid resuscitation and urinary catheterization to accurately measure fluid input and output • If blood transfusion is required, aim for a target haemoglobin of 70g/L
D	• Monitor neurological status 2-hourly for signs of worsening HE. Development of HE grade 2 or more should lead to ICU transfer • Do not give sedative agents • Patients should have 2-hourly CBG monitoring • Consider IV dextrose to avoid hypoglycaemia (commonly associated with ALF, especially paracetamol overdose)
E	• **Antibiotics:** low threshold if haemodynamically unstable, or worsening HE which might have an infective cause • ***N*-acetylcysteine:** give even in non-paracetamol cases • **Nutrition:** involve dieticians early, ideally continue enteral feeding but may require parenteral supplementation. Replace depleted electrolytes • **Medication review:** avoid drugs that are hepatically metabolized • **Alcohol withdrawal:** if concerned about alcohol withdrawal, try to use alternatives to chlordiazepoxide, e.g. oxazepam or lorazepam • **Renal replacement therapy (RRT):** consider need for RRT if worsening AKI, hyperammonaemia, hyponatraemia, or persistent acidosis • **Coagulopathy:** LMWH may be continued but should be regularly reviewed along with bleeding risk. Hepatic coagulopathy is associated with ↑ thrombosis rather than bleeding risk, but consider need for vitamin K and platelets if actively bleeding

Discuss other management with a hepatology specialist including whether to start steroids in suspected autoimmune hepatitis. Pregnancy-related ALF may require prompt delivery of the baby by an obstetrician.

Special considerations

Liver transplant

Early assessment of the patient for liver transplant is important. The King's College criteria for transplant (Table 33.5) are widely accepted.

Table 33.5 King's College criteria for liver transplant

ALF secondary to paracetamol	ALF secondary to a cause other than paracetamol
Arterial pH <7.3 after resuscitation (>24 hours since ingestion) **OR** All 3 of: HE grade 3 or 4 **AND** Serum creatinine >300µmol/L **AND** INR >6.5	INR >6.5 **OR** Any 3 out of 5 variables: • Indeterminate aetiology or drug-induced hepatitis • Age <10 years or >40 years • Interval between jaundice and encephalopathy onset >7 days • Bilirubin >300µmol/L • INR >3.5

Source: data from O'Grady JG, Alexander GJ, Hayllar KM, Williams R. Early indicators of prognosis in fulminant hepatic failure. Gastroenterology. 1989 Aug;97(2):439–45. doi: 10.1016/0016-5085(89)90081-4. PMID: 2490426.

Further reading

1. European Association for the Study of the Liver and the American Association for the Study of Liver Diseases (2014). Hepatic encephalopathy in chronic liver disease: 2014 practice guideline by the European Association for the Study of the Liver and the American Association for the Study of Liver Diseases. Available at: https://www.journal-of-hepatology.eu/article/S0168-8278(14)00390-0/fulltext
2. Bloom S, Webster G, Marks D (2011). Acute liver failure (ALF). *Oxford Handbook of Gastroenterology and Hepatology*, 2nd ed (pp. 572–7). Oxford: Oxford University Press. Available at: https://doi.org/10.1093/med/9780199584079.003.0150

Chapter 34

Alcohol-related liver disease

Guideline:
European Association for the Study of the Liver (EASL clinical practice guidelines: management of alcohol-related liver disease): https://www.journal-of-hepatology.eu/article/S0168-8278(18)30214-9/fulltext

OUP disclaimer: Oxford University Press makes no representation, express or implied, that the drug dosages are correct and that the recommendations are an exclusive or mandatory course of care. All health professionals reading this text have a responsibility to evaluate its appropriateness and take the individual needs of the patient into account.

Local trust guideline: please refer to your local guidelines as necessary.

Overview

Alcohol misuse is a major cause of preventable liver disease worldwide. Alcohol-related liver disease (ArLD) represents a spectrum from simple steatosis to liver cirrhosis which can lead to liver failure and hepatocellular carcinoma (HCC). The course of ArLD can be affected by inherited and environmental causes. The coexistence of other factors can accelerate liver injury, such as metabolic syndrome, iron overload, and chronic hepatitis virus.

The successful management of ArLD is dependent on reducing alcohol consumption and the secondary prevention of alcohol-associated complications.

Liver terminology

- **Alcoholic hepatitis:** recent onset of jaundice with or without other signs of hepatic decompensation, due to prolonged, excessive consumption of alcohol
- **Alcohol-related liver disease (ArLD):** umbrella term to include all liver disease secondary to excess alcohol intake
- **Cirrhosis:** advanced fibrotic chronic liver disease characterized histologically by bands of bridging fibrosis and the presence of regenerative nodules of hepatocytes
- **Compensated chronic liver disease (CLD):** CLD (>6 months) with maintained liver function. The Child–Pugh score for patients with CLD is based on biochemical and clinical features and predicts prognosis
- **Decompensated CLD:** development of features of liver failure including jaundice, ascites and/or encephalopathy in a patient with CLD
- **Acute-on-chronic liver failure:** Acute worsening of liver function with decompensation and multiple organ failure in a patient with CLD.

Diagnosis

History

- Most are asymptomatic, therefore any high-risk patient should undergo screening
- ArLD is suggested by:
  - Hazardous or harmful alcohol consumption (see Chapter 35)
  - Presence of clinical and/or biological abnormalities suggestive of liver disease
  - Imaging findings
- Alcoholic hepatitis is suggested by:
  - Recent-onset progressive jaundice, with or without decompensation
  - May be associated with fever (even if there is no infection), malaise, and weight loss.

Examination

- May range from normal to signs suggestive of cirrhosis
- Most physical signs are not specific of the aetiology:
  - Jaundice
  - Right upper quadrant pain
  - Abdominal distension due to ascites
  - Palmar erythema
- Signs of alcohol withdrawal/delirium tremens
- Signs suggestive of harmful alcohol intake:
  - Bilateral parotid gland hypertrophy
  - Muscle wasting
  - Malnutrition
  - Dupuytren's contracture
  - Symmetrical peripheral neuropathy
  - Splenomegaly
  - Gynaecomastia
  - Extensive spider angiomas
  - Caput medusae.

Investigations

Bloods

There are a number of prognostication tools that can be used in ArLD based on biochemical and clinical parameters.

Alcoholic hepatitis

- Glasgow alcoholic hepatitis (GAH) score
- Maddrey's Discriminant Function (MDF).

These predict mortality and guide which patients may benefit from steroid therapy.

Chronic liver disease or suspected cirrhosis

- Child–Pugh score
- United Kingdom Model for End-Stage Liver Disease (UKELD) score.

Table 34.1 Bloods in ArLD

Test	Significance
FBC	• Macrocytic anaemia • Thrombocytopaenia • Lymphopenia • Needed for GAH score
U&E	• Sodium and renal function monitoring in ascites/hepatorenal syndrome • Urea in GI bleed • Needed for GAH score
LFT	• Raised GGT, AST, ALT • Hyperbilirubinaemia and hypoalbuminaemia in advanced ArLD • Inverted AST:ALT of approximately 2:1 in ArLD • Needed for GAH and MDF scores
Carbohydrate deficient transferrin (CDT)	• May be useful in patients where alcohol history is unclear • Positive when ethanol intake of 50–80g/day is sustained over 1–2 weeks, normalizes after 2–3 weeks of abstinence
Magnesium, calcium, phosphate, and glucose	• Refeeding bloods • Hypoglycaemia can be a complication of alcohol withdrawal
PT and INR	• Indicative of liver synthetic function—both may be prolonged, but does not imply increased bleeding risk • Needed for GAH and MDF scores

Before attributing liver disease to alcohol misuse alone, perform a non-invasive liver screen to exclude alternative causes/hepatic comorbidity. See Table 36.1 in Chapter 36.

Ascitic tap

- When ascites is present on admission, an ascitic tap should always be performed to confirm that it is related to portal hypertension and to exclude spontaneous bacterial peritonitis:
  - Neutrophil count and culture (in blood culture bottles) should be performed to exclude spontaneous bacterial peritonitis (SBP)
  - Neutrophil count >250 cells/mm^3 is diagnostic of SBP. See Chapter 36.
- Calculate serum-ascites albumin gradient (SAAG) when investigating the cause of ascites:
  - >11g/L is indicative of portal hypertension as a cause of ascites
- Cytology should be performed on presentation to differentiate between malignant and non-malignant ascites.

Imaging

- Contributes to assessment but cannot confirm alcohol as the underlying cause
- Liver disease may be suggested by USS, CT, or MRI
- Transient elastography ('Fibroscan®') uses liver stiffness measurement to assess for fibrosis although it is not technically possible in the context of ascites.

Liver biopsy

- Invasive procedure with potential for severe complications in approximately 1:300–1:500 (such as intra-abdominal bleeding, pneumothorax)
- Consider if doubt regarding underlying diagnosis or to determine the presence of cirrhosis
- Percutaneous approach is appropriate in most patients; a transjugular approach is safer if low platelets/prolonged PT, and allows the assessment of portal hypertension by measurement of the hepatic venous pressure gradient.

Upper gastrointestinal endoscopy

- If evidence of cirrhosis, consider screening for oesophageal varices.

Management

Lifestyle and simple interventions

- Abstinence:
  - The most important intervention in ArLD
  - Improves survival at all stages in the ArLD spectrum
- Nutrition:
  - Protein malnutrition is associated with increased risk of complications
  - Get early dietetic input. Consider enteral nutrition in severe alcoholic hepatitis: protein-caloric intake often difficult to achieve orally.

Psychological interventions

- Brief interventions:
  - Attempt to increase awareness of the problems, consequences, and risks of alcohol consumption
  - Five As model:
    - **A**sk about use
    - **A**dvice to quit or reduce
    - **A**ssess willingness
    - **A**ssist to quit or reduce
    - **A**rrange follow-up.

Pharmacological management

- Treatment of alcohol withdrawal with benzodiazepines should be guided by objective scoring (e.g. Clinical Institute Withdrawal Assessment for Alcohol (CIWA-Ar)) (see Chapter 35)
- All patients with ArLD should be given thiamine (see Chapter 35); in practice, parenteral high-dose thiamine is given initially in patients admitted with ArLD
- Suspected alcoholic hepatitis—discuss with hepatology for consideration of possible corticosteroid therapy.

Surgical management

- Liver transplantation:
  - Consider in patients with:
    - ArLD Child–Pugh C (poorest prognosis) **OR**
    - Model for End-Stage Liver Disease (MELD) ≥15 **OR**
    - UKELD score of ≥49
- Liaise with local hepatology team
- Sustained abstinence from alcohol is essential prior to consideration of transplantation
- Once on the transplant waiting list, assess regularly for ongoing abstinence with questionnaire and laboratory tests (measurement of ethyl glucuronide in urine or hair).

Psychosocial considerations

- ArLD should be considered a dual pathology—liver disease and a disease of addiction
- There is a high prevalence of comorbid psychiatric orders and developing other addictions.

Complications

- Alcohol withdrawal (see Chapter 35):
  - Occurs in alcohol-dependent patients who suddenly decrease or stop alcohol intake
  - Usually develops within 6–24 hours after last alcoholic drink
- Alcoholic hepatitis
- Decompensated liver cirrhosis:
  - Ascites
- Complications of ascites including spontaneous bacterial peritonitis:
  - GI bleeding
  - Bacterial infections
  - AKI
- Hyponatraemia
- Hepatorenal syndrome:
  - Acute-on-chronic liver failure
- Relative adrenal failure
- Cirrhotic cardiomyopathy
- Hepatopulmonary syndrome
- Portopulmonary hypertension:
  - Coagulopathy
  - HE

Monitoring and follow-up

- Clinical, biochemical, and ultrasound surveillance is indicated for all patients with cirrhosis:
  - HCC screening should be performed in liver cirrhosis using ultrasound every 6 months
  - Biomarkers (i.e. AFP) are not recommended for routine surveillance of HCC.

Special considerations

Most drugs commonly prescribed in ArLD, including benzodiazepines, will need dose adjustment in accordance with the severity of liver impairment (see Chapter 35).

Further reading

1. European Association for the Study of the Liver (2018). EASL Clinical Practice Guidelines for the management of patients with decompensated cirrhosis. Available at: https://www.journal-of-hepatology.eu/article/S0168-8278(18)31966-4/fulltext

Chapter 35

Alcohol use disorders

Guidelines:
NICE CG100 (Alcohol-use disorders: diagnosis and management of physical complications): https://www.nice.org.uk/guidance/cg100

NICE CG115 (Alcohol-use disorders: diagnosis, assessment and management of harmful drinking (high-risk drinking) and alcohol dependence): https://www.nice.org.uk/guidance/cg115

OUP disclaimer: Oxford University Press makes no representation, express or implied, that the drug dosages are correct and that the recommendations are an exclusive or mandatory course of care. All health professionals reading this text have a responsibility to evaluate its appropriateness and take the individual needs of the patient into account.

Local trust guidelines: please refer to your local guidelines as necessary.

Overview

Approximately 25% of adults drink a hazardous or harmful volume of alcohol. Many of these individuals are alcohol dependant and suffer from withdrawal symptoms if their level of intake falls. Stigma and discrimination are common, so the patient may try to downplay their level of dependence to avoid perceived judgement. Patients should therefore be reassured that the discussions are confidential.

Diagnosis

Always assess:

- How much alcohol the patient typically consumes (Box 35.1)
- Whether the patient is misusing alcohol (using a tool such as the Alcohol Use Disorders Identification Test (AUDIT))—see Fig. 35.1
- Whether alcohol intake is hazardous or harmful
- The severity of alcohol dependence
- Risk to self (including unplanned withdrawal, suicidality, and neglect) and risk to others (including violence)
- Extent of any associated mental or physical health and social problems:
    - Those with harmful alcohol intake should be risk stratified for the presence of liver cirrhosis (see Chapter 34).

> If there is uncertainty regarding weekly alcohol intake, consider a retrospective drinking diary and if possible, take a collateral history.

Hazardous alcohol intake

- Level of alcohol intake that puts the individual at risk of alcohol-related harm, typically 14–35 units/week for a woman and 21–50 units/week for a man.

Harmful alcohol intake

- Level of alcohol intake that causes harm to the individual, typically >35 units/week for a woman and >50 units/week for a man.

Alcohol dependence

- Characterized by craving and having a preoccupation with alcohol, and continuing to drink alcohol despite potentially causing harm
- Severity of dependence can be assessed using the Alcohol Dependence Questionnaire (SADQ) (Table 35.1).

Referral criteria for specialist assessment

- Those scoring >15 on the AUDIT.

Referral for hospital admission

- People in acute alcohol withdrawal or those assessed to be at high risk of developing seizures or delirium tremens must be offered admission to hospital
- Have a lower threshold for admitting vulnerable patients (e.g. frail, cognitively impaired, lack of social support, learning difficulties, and homeless)
- If admission is declined, or there is insufficient capacity, the patient must be advised not to suddenly reduce their alcohol intake and they should seek help from a local alcohol support service.

Investigations

Bedside

- Perform bedside cognitive testing to screen for possible alcohol-related cognitive impairment (see Chapter 10) including Wernicke's encephalopathy and Korsakoff's syndrome (Box 35.2)
- Use the revised Clinical Institute Withdrawal Assessment of Alcohol Scale (CIWA-Ar) (Fig. 35.2) to assess the severity of withdrawal.

The Alcohol Use Disorders Identification Test: Interview Version

Read questions as written. Record answers carefully. Begin the AUDIT by saying "Now I am going to ask you some questions about your use of alcoholic beverages during this past year." Explain what is meant by "alcoholic beverages" by using local examples of beer, wine, vodka, etc. Code answers in terms of "standard drinks". Place the correct answer number in the box at the right.

1. How often do you have a drink containing alcohol?
   (0) Never [Skip to Qs 9-10]
   (1) Monthly or less
   (2) 2 to 4 times a month
   (3) 2 to 3 times a week
   (4) 4 or more times a week

2. How many drinks containing alcohol do you have on a typical day when you are drinking?
   (0) 1 or 2
   (1) 3 or 4
   (2) 5 or 6
   (3) 7, 8, or 9
   (4) 10 or more

3. How often do you have six or more drinks on one occasion?
   (0) Never
   (1) Less than monthly
   (2) Monthly
   (3) Weekly
   (4) Daily or almost daily

   Skip to Questions 9 and 10 if Total Score for Questions 2 and 3 = 0

4. How often during the last year have you found that you were not able to stop drinking once you had started?
   (0) Never
   (1) Less than monthly
   (2) Monthly
   (3) Weekly
   (4) Daily or almost daily

5. How often during the last year have you failed to do what was normally expected from you because of drinking?
   (0) Never
   (1) Less than monthly
   (2) Monthly
   (3) Weekly
   (4) Daily or almost daily

6. How often during the last year have you needed a first drink in the morning to get yourself going after a heavy drinking session?
   (0) Never
   (1) Less than monthly
   (2) Monthly
   (3) Weekly
   (4) Daily or almost daily

7. How often during the last year have you had a feeling of guilt or remorse after drinking?
   (0) Never
   (1) Less than monthly
   (2) Monthly
   (3) Weekly
   (4) Daily or almost daily

8. How often during the last year have you been unable to remember what happened the night before because you had been drinking?
   (0) Never
   (1) Less than monthly
   (2) Monthly
   (3) Weekly
   (4) Daily or almost daily

9. Have you or someone else been injured as a result of your drinking?
   (0) No
   (2) Yes, but not in the last year
   (4) Yes, during the last year

10. Has a relative or friend or a doctor or another health worker been concerned about your drinking or suggested you cut down?
   (0) No
   (2) Yes, but not in the last year
   (4) Yes, during the last year

Record total of specific items here

If total is greater than recommended cut-off, consult User's Manual.

Fig. 35.1 Alcohol Use Disorders Identification Test (AUDIT).

Reprinted from Babor T et al (2001). 'AUDIT: the Alcohol Use Disorders Identification Test: guidelines for use in primary health care.' WHO: Geneva, with permission from the World Health Organization.

Box 35.1 Alcohol content of different drinks

- 1 unit of alcohol = 8g or 10mL of pure alcohol
- 1 unit = 0.5 pints (284mL) of lager/beer/cider (alcohol by volume (ABV) 3.6%)
- 1 unit = 1 small shot measure (25mL) of spirits (ABV 40%)
- 1.5 units = 1 small glass (125mL) of wine (ABV 12%).

Table 35.1 SADQ score

Section 1: think of a typical period of heavy drinking in the last 6 months. **Add the scores according to frequency of each of the items: almost never = 0, sometimes = 1, often = 2, nearly always = 3**	
Physical	• Wake up feeling sweaty • Wake up drenched in sweat • Wake up with hands shaking • Wake up with body shaking
Affective	• Dread waking in the morning • Dread meeting someone first thing in the morning • Waking up feeling despairing • Waking up feeling frightened
Craving	• Wanting to drink first thing in the morning • Drinking first alcoholic drink as quickly as possible • Strong craving for drink on waking
Daily alcohol intake	• Drinking >0.25 bottle of spirits **OR** 1 bottle of wine **OR** 7 beers in a day • Drinking >0.5 bottle of spirits **OR** 2 bottles of wine **OR** 15 beers in a day • Drinking >1 bottle of spirits **OR** 4 bottles of wine **OR** 30 beers in a day • Drinking >2 bottles of spirits **OR** 8 bottles of wine **OR** 60 beers in a day
Dependence	• Drinking more alcohol to avoid shakes
Section 2: imagine you have stopped drinking completely for a few weeks, and then you drink very heavily for 2 days. How would you feel the next morning? **Add the scores according to frequency of each of the items: not at all = 0, slightly = 1, moderately = 2, quite a lot = 3**	
	• I would be sweaty • My hands would shake • My body would shake • I would be craving a drink
Interpretation of SADQ score: 0–15 = mild dependence 16–30 = moderate dependence 31–60 = severe dependence.	

Patient:______________ **Date:** ______________ **Time:** ______________ (24 hour clock, midnight = 00:00)

Pulse or heart rate, taken for one minute:______________ **Blood pressure:**______

NAUSEA AND VOMITING -- Ask "Do you feel sick to your stomach? Have you vomited?" Observation.
0 no nausea and no vomiting
1 mild nausea with no vomiting
2
3
4 intermittent nausea with dry heaves
5
6
7 constant nausea, frequent dry heaves and vomiting

TACTILE DISTURBANCES -- Ask "Have you any itching, pins and needles sensations, any burning, any numbness, or do you feel bugs crawling on or under your skin?" Observation.
0 none
1 very mild itching, pins and needles, burning or numbness
2 mild itching, pins and needles, burning or numbness
3 moderate itching, pins and needles, burning or numbness
4 moderately severe hallucinations
5 severe hallucinations
6 extremely severe hallucinations
7 continuous hallucinations

TREMOR -- Arms extended and fingers spread apart. Observation.
0 no tremor
1 not visible, but can be felt fingertip to fingertip
2
3
4 moderate, with patient's arms extended
5
6
7 severe, even with arms not extended

AUDITORY DISTURBANCES -- Ask "Are you more aware of sounds around you? Are they harsh? Do they frighten you? Are you hearing anything that is disturbing to you? Are you hearing things you know are not there?" Observation.
0 not present
1 very mild harshness or ability to frighten
2 mild harshness or ability to frighten
3 moderate harshness or ability to frighten
4 moderately severe hallucinations
5 severe hallucinations
6 extremely severe hallucinations
7 continuous hallucinations

PAROXYSMAL SWEATS -- Observation.
0 no sweat visible
1 barely perceptible sweating, palms moist
2
3
4 beads of sweat obvious on forehead
5
6
7 drenching sweats

VISUAL DISTURBANCES -- Ask "Does the light appear to be too bright? Is its color different? Does it hurt your eyes? Are you seeing anything that is disturbing to you? Are you seeing things you know are not there?" Observation.
0 not present
1 very mild sensitivity
2 mild sensitivity
3 moderate sensitivity
4 moderately severe hallucinations
5 severe hallucinations
6 extremely severe hallucinations
7 continuous hallucinations

ANXIETY -- Ask "Do you feel nervous?" Observation.
0 no anxiety, at ease
1 mild anxious
2
3
4 moderately anxious, or guarded, so anxiety is inferred
5
6
7 equivalent to acute panic states as seen in severe delirium or acute schizophrenic reactions.

HEADACHE, FULLNESS IN HEAD -- Ask "Does your head feel different? Does it feel like there is a band around your head?" Do not rate for dizziness or lightheadedness. Otherwise, rate severity.
0 not present
1 very mild
2 mild
3 moderate
4 moderately severe
5 severe
6 very severe
7 extremely severe

AGITATION -- Observation.
0 normal activity
1 somewhat more than normal activity
2
3
4 moderately fidgety and restless
5
6
7 paces back and forth during most of the interview, or constantly thrashes about

ORIENTATION AND CLOUDING OF SENSORIUM -- Ask "What day is this? Where are you? Who am I?"
0 oriented and can do serial additions
1 cannot do serial additions or is uncertain about date
2 disoriented for date by no more than 2 calendar days
3 disoriented for date by more than 2 calendar days
4 disoriented for place/or person

Total **CIWA-Ar** Score ______
Rater's Initials ______
Maximum Possible Score 67

*The **CIWA-Ar** is not* copyrighted and may be reproduced freely. This assessment for monitoring withdrawal symptoms requires approximately 5 minutes to administer. The maximum score is 67 (see instrument). Patients scoring less than 10 do not usually need additional medication for withdrawal.

Fig. 35.2 Clinical Institute Withdrawal Assessment of Alcohol Scale, Revised (CIWA-Ar).

Reprinted from Sullivan JT et al (1989). Assessment of alcohol withdrawal: The revised Clinical Institute Withdrawal Assessment for Alcohol scale (CIWA-Ar), British Journal of Addiction 84:1353–1357.

Box 35.2 Wernicke's encephalopathy and Korsakoff's syndrome

- In harmful drinking, alcohol intake can occur at the expense of healthy nutrition. Malnourishment leads to deficiency of thiamine, which is essential for neuronal function
- Wernicke's encephalopathy is characterized by a triad of: (1) confusion, (2) ophthalmoplegia, and (3) ataxia. Urgent treatment with IV thiamine is required
- Korsakoff's syndrome occurs in around 80% of patients with WE[1] and is characterized by amnesia, confabulation, lack of insight, and apathy.

Bloods

- FBC (macrocytic anaemia)
- LFT and coagulation profile studies (ArLD)
- Ca, Mg, phosphate (nutritional deficiencies due to alcohol intake)
- Blood sugar level (hypoglycaemia).

If ArLD is suspected, see Chapter 34 to guide investigations.

1 Victor M, Adams RD, Collins GH. The Wernicke-Korsakoff syndrome: a clinical and pathological study of 245 patients, 82 with post-mortem examinations. *Contemp Neurol Ser*. 1971; 7:1–206.

Management

Drinking >15 units alcohol/day OR score >20 on AUDIT AND no patient safety concerns

- Consider community-based assisted withdrawal.

Drinking >30 units alcohol/day OR score >30 on SADQ OR significant physical or psychiatric comorbidities OR patient safety concerns (e.g. experience of withdrawal-related seizures or delirium tremens during previous assisted withdrawal programmes)

- Consider inpatient-based withdrawal.

Patient education

- Agree a target. Abstinence is usually most appropriate, but some patients may prefer to moderate their intake. Always consider outcomes of any previous treatment.

Lifestyle and simple interventions

- Provide information about self-help groups (e.g. Alcoholics Anonymous or SMART Recovery)
- Consider residential rehabilitation.

Psychological interventions

- Consider cognitive behavioural or social therapies.

Pharmacological management

Community

- Use a benzodiazepine such as chlordiazepoxide, or carbamazepine, using a fixed-dose weaning regimen
- Titrate initial dose to severity of dependence/consumption
- Monitor the patient every other day and prescribe no more than 2 days of medication at one time
- Gradually reduce benzodiazepine doses over 7–10 days
- A family member or carer should preferably oversee the administration of medication
- Adjust the dose if severe withdrawal symptoms or oversedation occurs.

Inpatient

- Use a benzodiazepine such as chlordiazepoxide using either fixed-dose or symptom-led regimens (based on CIWA-Ar score) and using local protocol
- Gradually reduce the dose over 5–10 days.

Alcohol withdrawal seizures

- Use a rapidly acting benzodiazepine, e.g. 4mg IV lorazepam
- Review the withdrawal regimen to reduce the chance of further seizures.

Delirium tremens (acute confusion with hallucinations, usually within 3 days of alcohol withdrawal)

- First-line management: lorazepam (parenteral if oral is declined), e.g. 1–4mg orally in divided doses (0.5–2mg in divided doses if elderly)

- Second-line management: parenteral haloperidol
- If delirium tremens develops during treatment for acute alcohol withdrawal, review the patient's withdrawal drug regimen.

Wernicke's encephalopathy

- Prescribe parenteral thiamine, e.g. Pabrinex®, 2–3 pairs of ampoules, TDS for 3–5 days and then 1 pair of ampoules OD for a further 3–5 days
- Oral thiamine treatment should follow parenteral therapy.

Both community and inpatients

Adjuncts to aid reduction in alcohol intake (if >15 on SADQ)

- After successful withdrawal, consider acamprosate or oral naltrexone alongside a psychological intervention
- Caution with naltrexone (opioid antagonist) if patient is taking opioid therapies
- Prescribe for up to 6 months and monitor monthly
- Disulfiram can be used as an alternative but is contraindicated in pregnancy or if the patient has a severe mental health or cardiovascular disorder
- Alcohol, including the amount included in some foods, interacts with disulfiram which may cause complications including arrhythmias
- Disulfiram may also rarely cause hepatotoxicity. Check LFT and U&E prior to prescribing.

Nutritional supplementation

Offer prophylactic oral thiamine to harmful or dependent drinkers when they:

- Are malnourished or at risk of malnourishment
- Have decompensated liver disease
- Are in acute alcohol withdrawal or about to start a withdrawal programme.

Psychosocial considerations

Consider referral to the psychiatry team for those patients with a significant comorbid mental health disorder and those assessed to be at high risk of suicide.

> If a patient is malnourished or has decompensated alcoholic liver disease and they are admitted to hospital with an acute illness, they should be given parenteral thiamine initially, followed by oral thiamine.

Complications of harmful alcohol intake

- Wernicke–Korsakoff syndrome (Box 35.2)
- Alcoholic cardiomyopathy
- Renal failure (IgA-induced nephropathy)
- Nervous system (central and peripheral neuropathy)
- Chronic pancreatitis
- ArLD (see Chapter 34).

Special considerations

Family

- Recognize the impact on family members; provide information on alcohol misuse and how to support their relative
- Consider the effect of a parent's drinking on any child who is in their care and discuss with social services if there are safeguarding concerns.

Pregnancy and breastfeeding

- Alcohol in pregnancy can affect fetal development and can also cross into breast milk.

Further reading

1. Sher KJ, Talley AE, Littlefield AK, et al. (2011). Alcohol use and alcohol use disorders. In: Friedman HS (ed) *The Oxford Handbook of Health Psychology* (pp. 686–737). Oxford: Oxford University Press. Available at:https://www.oxfordhandbooks.com/view/10.1093/oxfordhb/9780195342819.001.0001/oxfordhb-9780195342819-e-028
2. NICE. Alcohol use disorders overview. Available at: https://pathways.nice.org.uk/pathways/alcohol-use-disorders

Chapter 36

Liver cirrhosis

Guidelines:

European Association for the Study of the Liver (EASL Clinical Practice Guidelines for the management of patients with decompensated cirrhosis): https://www.journal-of-hepatology.eu/article/S0168 8278(18)31966-4/fulltext

NICE NG50 (Cirrhosis in over 16s: diagnosis and management): https://www.nice.org.uk/guidance/ng50

Baveno VI Faculty (Expanding consensus in portal hypertension): https://www.journal-of-hepatology.eu/article/S0168-8278%2815%2900349-9/fulltext

European Association for the Study of the Liver, American Association for the Study of Liver Diseases (Hepatic encephalopathy in chronic liver disease: 2014 Practice Guideline): https://www.journal-of-hepatology.eu/article/s0168-8278(14)00390-0/fulltext

OUP disclaimer: Oxford University Press makes no representation, express or implied, that the drug dosages are correct and that the recommendations are an exclusive or mandatory course of care. All health professionals reading this text have a responsibility to evaluate its appropriateness and take the individual needs of the patient into account.

Local trust guidelines: please refer to your local guidelines as necessary.

Overview

Liver cirrhosis is characterized by progression from a stable, asymptomatic state of 'compensated' disease, to a 'decompensated' phase marked by the clinical consequences of liver failure. This transition represents a sharp decline in prognosis, with a reduction in median survival from 12 to 2 years. Many patients attending hospital acutely with complications of liver disease have features of decompensation.

Diagnosis

Decompensated cirrhosis is usually clear from the patient's history, examination, and biochemistry. Imaging may help confirm the diagnosis.

Consider using an admission checklist such as the 'BSG-BASL Decompensated Cirrhosis Care Bundle—First 24 Hours' (see Further reading) to ensure timely and comprehensive management for any patient admitted as an emergency with decompensated cirrhosis.

History

Consider risk factors for cirrhosis, including:

- Alcohol excess
- Hepatitis B or C
- Obesity (non-alcoholic fatty liver disease (NAFLD))
- T2DM.

Rarer causes include haemochromatosis, Wilson's disease, PSC, primary biliary cirrhosis, and autoimmune hepatitis.

Consider symptoms that may reflect decompensation:

- Jaundice
- Abdominal swelling
- Altered mental state
- Overt GI bleeding.

If decompensation is evident, consider possible triggers:

- Infection
- GI bleed
- Recent alcohol excess
- Constipation or dehydration
- Drugs (diuretics, opiates).

Examination

- **Hands:** clubbing, palmar erythema, Dupuytren's contracture
- **Asterixis ('liver flap'):** look for 'flapping' of hands when wrists are hyperextended
- **Face:** xanthelasma, yellow sclera
- **Limbs and body:** sarcopenia (loss of muscle bulk)
- **Chest:** gynaecomastia, spider naevi
- **Abdomen:** ascites, hepatomegaly, splenomegaly
- **Legs:** peripheral oedema
- **DRE:** melaena.

Investigations

Bedside

- Diagnostic paracentesis ('ascitic tap')
  - If ascites is present, perform ASAP
  - Send for neutrophil count, culture, albumin, and total protein
  - Do not wait for bloods results (including the coagulation profile) before obtaining the diagnostic tap
- Weight/BMI.

Bloods

- FBC:
  - ↓ haemoglobin (GI bleed, anaemia)
  - ↓ platelets (hypersplenism from portal hypertension)
  - ↑ white cell count (infection)
- ↑ CRP (infection):
  - CRP response may be attenuated in patients with severe liver dysfunction
- Renal function:
  - AKI—see 'Hepatorenal syndrome'
  - ↑ urea:creatinine ratio (GI bleed)
- LFT:
  - ↑ bilirubin, ↑ ALP, ↓ albumin (impaired liver function)
  - ↔/↑ ALT/AST (indicate liver inflammation, can be normal in cirrhosis)
- Coagulation profile:
  - ↑ PT/INR (impaired liver function)
- Blood cultures
- Consider a non-invasive liver screen if first presentation of cirrhosis (Table 36.1).

Table 36.1 Components of a non-invasive liver screen

Test	Disease
HBsAg	Hepatitis B
Anti-hepatitis C antibodies	Hepatitis C
Ferritin (*check transferrin saturations if ferritin elevated*)	Haemochromatosis
Alpha-1 antitrypsin level	Alpha-1 antitrypsin deficiency
Fasting glucose/high-density lipoprotein/triglyceride	Metabolic syndrome/NAFLD
Liver autoantibody screen	Primary biliary cirrhosis (*anti-mitochondrial antibody*) Autoimmune hepatitis (*ANA*) *SMA (anti-SMA)* *LKMA (anti-LKMA)*
Immunoglobulins	Autoimmune liver disease
Caeruloplasmin ± serum copper (*usually only if age <40 years, results may be misleading in decompensated liver disease*)	Wilson's disease

Imaging

Transient elastography ('Fibroscan®')

- Uses ultrasound to measure liver stiffness
- <10kPa plus absence of clinical signs: excludes cirrhosis
- >15kPa: ↑ probability of cirrhosis
- Not technically feasible if patient has significant ascites.

Ultrasound

- Can demonstrate fatty liver/cirrhosis and liver lesions (including HCC)
- Detects portal or hepatic vein thrombosis.

CT liver with triple phase contrast or MRI liver

- Detailed delineation of vascular anatomy
- Characterization of liver lesions.

Other

- Liver biopsy:
  - Invasive procedure
  - Used to clarify diagnosis if aetiology or severity of disease is unclear.

Management

Patient education

- Educate patients on the cause, prognosis, and potential complications of cirrhosis, and lifestyle factors that may affect the disease (e.g. alcohol excess, IV drug use, obesity).

Lifestyle and simple interventions

- If possible, the aetiological factor(s) causing liver injury should be removed or treated:
  - Cessation of alcohol use and treatment of viral hepatitis is associated with improved survival and lower risk of decompensation
- Ensure good nutrition:
  - Malnutrition leads to poorer prognosis and higher risk of complications
  - Dietician assessment
  - Encourage frequent, small meals.

Psychological interventions

- Alcohol abstinence:
  - Refer to hospital alcohol care team if available or community alcohol services
  - Motivational interviewing to encourage patient's belief in their ability to change
  - Consider CBT or referral to community support groups (e.g. Alcoholics Anonymous).

Pharmacological management

- Avoid NSAIDs, sedatives, and opioid analgesia where possible
- Daily multivitamin tablet.

Interventional radiology

Transjugular intrahepatic portosystemic shunt (TIPSS)

- Radiologically placed stent inserted between portal and hepatic veins, creating a shunt that reduces portal hypertension
- Indications:
  - Refractory ascites
  - Uncontrolled or recurrent variceal bleeding
- Contraindications: right-sided heart failure, pulmonary hypertension, active sepsis, hepatic encephalopathy, extensive HCC.

Surgical management

Liver transplantation

- Definitive treatment of decompensated cirrhosis and selected cases of HCC where the length or quality of life with transplantation is expected to exceed that without; average 5-year survival following liver transplantation is in excess of 80%
- Indications for liver transplantation in cirrhosis are patients with complications of cirrhosis in the context of a qualifying UKELD score (prognostic score used in CLD to predict the need for transplant):
  - Refractory ascites

- Recurrent, overt hepatic encephalopathy
- Other complications of portal hypertension not responsive to other therapy
- Prioritized in UK based on clinical need, stratified by UKELD
- Contraindications include extrahepatic malignancy, severe cardiorespiratory disease, systemic sepsis, expected non-compliance with drug therapy, ongoing alcohol consumption.

Psychosocial considerations

- If required, attempts should be made to help patients find stable accommodation, attend appointments, and manage addictive behaviours.

Complications

Gastric or oesophageal varices

- Diagnosis:
  - Patients with cirrhosis should be risk stratified for the presence of clinically significant varices:
    - Baveno VI criteria include liver stiffness <20kPa and platelet count >150 × 10^9/L. Patients who satisfy these criteria have a very low risk of having clinically significant varices and therefore screening endoscopy is not required
- Management and prophylaxis:
  - For treatment and prophylaxis of acute variceal bleeds, see Chapter 27.

Ascites

See Table 36.2.

Spontaneous bacterial peritonitis

- Diagnosis:
  - Ascitic neutrophil count > 250/mm^3
  - Perform diagnostic tap ASAP for patients admitted with ascites; delay associated with 3× ↑ in mortality
  - Blood plus ascitic fluid cultures
- Management:
  - Early treatment with broad-spectrum antibiotics as per local guidelines
  - Give 1.5g/kg 20% human albumin solution (HAS) at diagnosis (day 1) and 1g/kg at day 3
- Repeat diagnostic paracentesis at 48 hours: look for ↓ in neutrophil count of >25% to indicate effective treatment
- Secondary prophylaxis (e.g. ciprofloxacin 500mg OD) following an episode of spontaneous bacterial peritonitis should be offered. Obtain local microbiology advice
- Primary prophylaxis of spontaneous bacterial peritonitis can be considered in specific circumstances.

Acute kidney injury including hepatorenal syndrome

- Diagnosis:
  - AKI with reference to baseline creatinine (often low in patients with cirrhosis and low muscle bulk)
  - Hepatorenal syndrome comprises a minority of cases of AKI in cirrhosis and may be diagnosed in the absence of another cause

Table 36.2 Ascites grading and management

Grade	Definition	Management
Grade 1	Only detectable by ultrasound	• No treatment
Grade 2	Moderate ascites on examination	• No added salt in diet • Start *spironolactone 100mg OD*; ↑ by 100mg every 72 hours to max. 400mg • If not responding, add *furosemide 40mg OD*; ↑ by 40mg to max 160mg • Aim for 0.5–1kg/day weight loss • Monitor electrolytes • Reduce diuretics when ascites resolved
Grade 3	Large ascites + marked abdominal distension	• Large volume paracentesis: if >5L drained/expected, give 100mL 20% human albumin solution (HAS) for every 2L drained to prevent post-paracentesis circulatory dysfunction • Continue maximum tolerated diuretics
Refractory ascites	Does not respond to maximum diuretics	• Median survival of 6 months • Stop diuretics unless urinary sodium >30mmol/day • Consider referral to a tertiary liver unit for TIPSS or liver transplantation

  - Exclude: hypovolaemia, infection, diuretics, nephrotoxic drugs, parenchymal renal diseases
- Management:
  - Fluid resuscitation to achieve euvolaemia (5% HAS or crystalloid)
  - Monitor blood pressure, urine output, and fluid balance
  - Hold diuretics and any potential nephrotoxic medications
  - Septic screen and treat any infection
  - Consider terlipressin if no response to previous measures:
    - Start at 1mg QDS and gradually ↑ if no improvement
    - Give with 100mL 20% HAS BD
  - Up to 50% of patients demonstrate a gradual improvement, over 1–2 weeks.

Hepatic encephalopathy

- Diagnosis:
  - Altered mental state in a patient with liver cirrhosis, with no clear alternative cause found (*diagnosis of exclusion*)
    - Exclude: hypo/hyperglycaemia, alcohol intoxication, drugs, neurological infection, electrolyte disorders, intracranial bleed/stroke/neoplasm, severe systemic medical stress, dementia, psychiatric disorders
    - Ammonia: high levels do not confirm diagnosis or add prognostic value, but if normal make HE unlikely

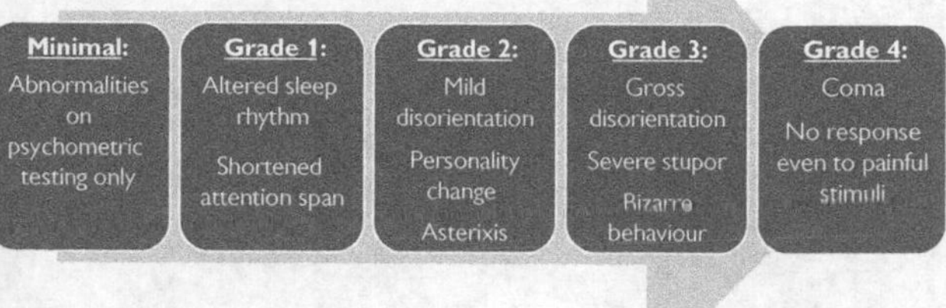

Fig. 36.1 Progression and classification of hepatic encephalopathy.

- Identify precipitants including infection; sedative medications; GI bleeding; dehydration/electrolyte disturbance; constipation; worsening underlying liver disease.
- Management:
  - Only overt HE requires treatment (grades 2–4, see Fig. 36.1)
  - Identify, exclude, and treat all other causes for brain dysfunction
  - Lactulose 25mL BD—aim for two or three soft bowel motions/day, continue after remission
  - Rifaximin 550mg BD—used for prevention of HE if further episode while on lactulose.

Monitoring and follow-up

Patients admitted with hepatic decompensation should be referred to a hepatology/gastroenterology service for specialist management and follow-up.

Patients with compensated cirrhosis should be reviewed clinically every 6 months, including:
- USS (screening for HCC)
- Calculation of risk stratification tool such as Child–Pugh score, MELD, or UKELD.

Further reading

1. British Society of Gastroenterology. BSG-BASL decompensated cirrhosis care bundle—first 24 hours. Available at: https://www.bsg.org.uk/clinical-resource/bsg-basl-decompensated-cirrhosis-care-bundle-first-24-hours/
2. Model for End-Stage Liver Disease (MELD) Score. Calculate score at: https://www.mdcalc.com/meld-score-model-end-stage-liver-disease-12-older
3. Wilkinson IB, Raine T, Wiles K, et al. (2017). Cirrhosis. In: *Oxford Handbook of Clinical Medicine*, 10th ed (pp. 276–7). Oxford: Oxford University Press. Available at: https://doi.org/10.1093/med/9780199689903.003.0006

Part 6

Mental health

Chapter 37

Bipolar disorder

Guideline:
NICE CG185 (Bipolar disorder: assessment and management):
https://www.nice.org.uk/guidance/cg185

OUP disclaimer: Oxford University Press makes no representation, express or implied, that the drug dosages are correct and that the recommendations are an exclusive or mandatory course of care. All health professionals reading this text have a responsibility to evaluate its appropriateness and take the individual needs of the patient into account.

Local trust guidelines: please refer to your local guidelines as necessary.

Overview

Bipolar disorder is characterized by episodes of mania/hypomania interspersed with episodes of depression:

- Mania: elevated mood/irritability with severe functional impairment for >7 days
- Hypomania: elevated mood/irritability with ↓/↑ function for >4 days, **BUT** not severe enough to cause a marked impairment in social or occupational functioning and **WITHOUT** psychosis.

Diagnosis

History

Include:

- Assessment of mood
- Detailed history of current manic/hypomanic/depressi ve episode:
  - For mania or hypomania, look for ≥3 of: heightened self-esteem or grandiosity, ↓ need for sleep, ↑ talkativeness, flight of ideas or racing thoughts, high distractibility, ↑ activity or agitation, ↑ high-risk behaviours
  - For depression, look for ≥5 of: depressed mood, lack of interest or pleasure, weight or appetite change, insomnia or hypersomnia, psychomotor agitation or retardation, fatigue, feelings of worthlessness or guilt, difficulty concentrating or making decisions, recurrent thoughts of death or dying
- History of any previous episodes including triggers, and treatments or interventions used
- Physical and mental health history
- Medication history (prescription and non-prescription)
- History of substance abuse, smoking, and alcohol consumption
- Family history
- Collateral history if possible
- Social history including psychosocial stressors, e.g. work, relationships
- History of self-neglect, self-harm, or suicidal thoughts.

Patients should always be asked about potential manic/hypomanic episodes when presenting with depression. If they describe overactivity or disinhibited behaviour lasting >4 days, consider referral to secondary care.

Refer urgently to secondary care if mania or severe depression is suspected, or if the patient is potentially a risk to themselves or to others.

> **DSM-5 criteria**[1]
> - Bipolar 1 = mania + depression
> - Bipolar 2 = hypomania + depression.

Examination

No specific examination is required. However, the examination components required before specific medications are started are discussed in Table 37.1.

Investigations

No specific investigations are required. However, the investigations which are required before specific medications are started are discussed in Table 37.1.

1 American Psychiatric Association. (2013). Diagnostic and statistical manual of mental disorders (5th ed.). https://doi.org/10.1176/appi.books.9780890425596

Management

Most patients are initially managed in secondary care but need ongoing monitoring in the community.

Lifestyle and simple interventions

- Develop a collaborative risk management plan, including:
  - Identifying triggers
  - Coping strategies and medication titration
  - Who to contact in a crisis
- Ensure patients with mania or hypomania can access a calming environment
- Offer a healthy eating and physical activity programme.

Psychological interventions

Depression

- CBT/interpersonal therapy/behavioural couples therapy **OR** specific evidence-based psychological therapy for bipolar disorder.

Pharmacological management

Acute management

Primary care

- Do not routinely start medications in primary care
- Some medications such as lithium can be restarted or commenced under a shared care plan.

Secondary care

Mania or hypomania

- If taking an antidepressant, consider stopping if it was recently started, the dose was recently adjusted, or there are probable issues of compliance
- Start an antipsychotic, e.g. haloperidol, olanzapine, quetiapine, or risperidone, if not already taking mood stabilizers/antipsychotics. If the first choice is not tolerated, trial a second choice
- Consider adding lithium if not responding to two different antipsychotics at the maximum tolerated dose
- If lithium is not suitable or unsuccessful, consider adding valproate instead (**NOT** suitable for women of childbearing age—see 'Prescribing and monitoring tips')
- If already taking lithium, check levels are within the therapeutic range. If levels are optimal, consider adding an antipsychotic
- If already taking valproate/mood stabilizer, consider increasing the dose and adding an antipsychotic
- Review treatment 4 weeks after symptoms have resolved to decide if long-term treatment is appropriate. Review again at 3–6 months if treatment is continued.

Prescribing and monitoring tips

- Lithium:
  - Fluid balance is important due to lithium's narrow therapeutic range—advise patient to be careful if usual habits change (e.g. going on holiday, exercising more) and to seek medical attention if they have diarrhoea or vomiting
  - Monitor for neurotoxicity at every appointment: ataxia, cognitive impairment, paraesthesia, tremor. These can occur at therapeutic levels
  - Many medications interact with lithium. In particular, patients should know to avoid NSAIDs which can increase serum lithium concentrations
- Valproate:
  - Ensure patients are aware of the signs/symptoms of blood and liver disorders which can develop with valproate use
  - Valproate must only be prescribed to women of childbearing age if other options are unsuitable **AND** they have a pregnancy prevention programme in place (see 'Further reading')
- Lamotrigine:
  - Patients taking lamotrigine should seek urgent medical help if they develop a rash or become pregnant.

Depression

- Medication options:
  - Fluoxetine plus olanzapine **OR**
  - Olanzapine alone **OR**
  - Lamotrigine alone **OR**
  - Quetiapine alone
- If already on lithium or valproate, check levels and increase if necessary
- If lithium/valproate is at maximum dose and cannot be increased, add a medication (above).

Chronic management

- Bipolar disorder is a chronic relapsing–remitting condition and it is important to follow up stable patients every 3–6 months
- Once stable, the need for continued psychological interventions should be discussed as well as whether medications should be reduced, stopped, or continued long-term
- Consider:
  - Which medications were successful in an acute setting
  - Medication side effects
  - Potential benefits of stopping medication, e.g. safe to conceive
  - Risk of relapse
- If stopping treatment, stop gradually (over at least 4 weeks) and monitor for relapse for 2 years.

Interactions

Be aware that many psychiatric medications interact with each other, e.g. valproate and lamotrigine—always check in the BNF before adding in a second medication.

Psychosocial considerations

- Family intervention should be considered if appropriate
- Support patients with education, employment, and financial issues
- Support carers and direct them to appropriate resources.

Monitoring and follow-up

Routine review

Monitor annually:

- Pulse
- Blood pressure
- Weight/BMI
- Diet and nutritional status
- Level of physical activity
- Bloods:
  - Glucose
  - HbA1c
  - Lipid profile
  - LFT
  - U&E
  - TFT
  - Calcium (if taking lithium).

Drug-specific monitoring

Drug specific monitoring should be performed as per Table 37.1.

Table 37.1 Parameters for initiating and monitoring psychiatric medications

Test	Antipsychotics	Lithium	Valproate	Lamotrigine
Pulse and blood pressure	At initiation and at every dose change		Every 6 months and then annually	At initiation
Weight/ BMI	At initiation, then weekly for 6 weeks, then at 12 weeks	At initiation, then every 6 months	At initiation, after 6 months, and then annually	
Blood glucose/ HbA1c/ lipids	At initiation, then 12 weeks after starting			

Table 37.1 *Continued*

Test	Antipsychotics	Lithium	Valproate	Lamotrigine
Drug levels		Initiation: • 1 week after starting • 1 week after every dose change • Weekly until levels are stable Monitoring: • Every 3 months for 1 year, then every 6 months • Alternatively, every 3 months if high risk of toxicity, e.g. elderly, taking interacting medications, impaired renal or thyroid function	Only if evidence of toxicity or ineffective-ness	Only if evidence of toxicity or ineffective-ness
FBC		At initiation	At initi-ation, after 6 months, and then annually	At initiation
LFT			At initi-ation, after 6 months, and then annually	At initiation
U&E/ eGFR		At initiation, then every 6 months		At initiation
TFT and calcium		At initiation, then every 6 months		
ECG	At initiation if cardiovas-cular risk, inpatient, or recom-mended by manufacturer	At initiation if cardiovascular risk		

Special considerations

Electroconvulsive treatment

- Should be considered for severe mania that has not responded to other treatments.

Young people under the age of 18

- Should be managed by a specialist CAMHS service.

Further reading

1. Medicines and Healthcare products Regulatory Agency (2018, updated 2021). Valproate use by women and girls. Available at: https://www.gov.uk/guidance/valproate-use-by-women-and-girls

Chapter 38

Depression

Guideline:
This chapter was based on: NICE CG90 (Depression in adults: recognition and management): https://www.nice.org.uk/guidance/cg90. Since the chapter was written, the guideline has been updated and replaced with on NICE NG222 (Depression in adults: treatment and management): https://www.nice.org.uk/guidance/ng222. Please see the approach to management in NG222.

OUP disclaimer: Oxford University Press makes no representation, express or implied, that the drug dosages are correct and that the recommendations are an exclusive or mandatory course of care. All health professionals reading this text have a responsibility to evaluate its appropriateness and take the individual needs of the patient into account.

Local trust guidelines: please refer to your local guidelines as necessary.

Overview

Depression is the most common psychiatric disorder. It is frequently managed by non-specialists, so a good understanding of symptoms and basic management is important for all medical professionals.

Diagnosis

History/diagnostic criteria

Use the following screening questions to start an assessment:

- Have you felt depressed, low in mood, or hopeless in the last month?
- Have you had little pleasure or interest in doing things in the past month?

If the answer to either question is yes, the patient should be assessed more fully.

Consider using a validated measure such as the PHQ-9 questionnaire (available at https://www.mdcalc.com/phq-9-patient-health-questionnaire-9).

History should consider symptoms, duration of symptoms, and the extent of functional impairment that the symptoms are causing.

Symptoms:

- Persistent low mood
- Loss of interest/pleasure
- Fatigue
- Worthlessness or excessive guilt
- Suicidal thoughts
- Poor concentration or indecision
- Psychomotor retardation or agitation
- Insomnia or hypersomnia
- Changes in appetite or weight
- Psychotic symptoms.

Consider whether the patient has any history of mood elevation, i.e. whether the depression may actually be part of bipolar disorder (see Chapter 37).

Severity of depression

- Subthreshold = fewer than five symptoms, no clear functional impairment
- Mild = approximately five symptoms, only mild functional impairment
- Moderate = symptoms and impairment between mild and severe
- Severe = most symptoms, marked functional impairment, with or without psychotic symptoms.

The history should also include:

- Previous history of depression and treatments trialled
- Psychiatric and medical history
- Interpersonal relationships
- Social circumstances
- Alcohol and drug abuse
- Risk of suicide and self-harm (see Chapter 44).

If the patient is at immediate risk of suicide or self-harm, refer urgently to specialist services.

Examination

- A mental state examination may reveal the symptoms listed previously.
- A general physical examination should also be performed to consider alternative explanations for depression, e.g. hypothyroidism (see Chapter 23), hypoadrenalism (see Chapter 14), hypercalcaemia (see Chapter 16).

Investigations

- No specific investigation is required, although some investigations may be useful to help eliminate differential diagnoses, e.g. TFT, calcium levels.

Management

Management stages

- **Stage 1:** any presentation of depression:
  - Identification, assessment, education, active monitoring
- **Stage 2:** persistent subthreshold or mild–moderate depression:
  - Low-intensity psychological interventions
- **Stage 3:** depression with poor response to stage 2 management **OR** moderate–severe depression:
  - High-intensity psychological interventions and/or pharmacological treatment
- **Stage 4:** severe depression **OR** high risk of self-harm or self-neglect **OR** complex comorbidities:
  - specialist treatment.

Patient education

- Give patients details of self-help and support groups
- Ensure patients and carers are both aware of how to access help when needed e.g. crisis teams
- St John's wort is not recommended due to a risk of serious interactions, and a lack of evidence regarding dosing.

Lifestyle and simple interventions

- Sleep hygiene, e.g. establishing regular sleep and wake times, avoiding alcohol before sleep.

Stage 1

- Active monitoring should be considered for patients who refuse intervention, or who may recover without intervention
- Provide information and review in 2 weeks
- Ensure contact is made if patient fails to attend follow-up.

Psychological interventions

Stage 2

If no improvement with stage 1, offer one or more of the following low-intensity psychological interventions:

- Self help
- Group or computerized CBT
- Structured group physical activity programme.

Stage 3

The following high-intensity psychological interventions should be used in conjunction with medication. They should also be used if stage 2 treatments were unsuccessful:

- CBT
- Interpersonal therapy
- Behavioural activation (a form of functional analytic psychotherapy)
- Behavioural couples therapy.

Pharmacological management

Pharmacological management is used for stage 3 patients, in conjunction with a high-intensity psychological intervention. It should also be considered for:

- Stage 2 patients with a history of moderate–severe depression
- Long-term (>2 years) subthreshold patients
- Stage 2 patients who have not responded to other interventions.

Antidepressant prescribing

SSRIs (e.g. fluoxetine, paroxetine, sertraline, citalopram) are first line. Considerations when picking and prescribing a medication include the following:

- Interactions—fluoxetine and paroxetine are more likely to cause interactions than other SSRIs
- Discontinuation symptoms—more likely with paroxetine
- Side effects:
  - Consider the likelihood of the patient stopping the drug due to side effects
  - Sometimes it may be helpful to co-prescribe a benzodiazepine for up to 2 weeks to help with the initial side effects of anxiety and agitation
  - SSRIs increase the risk of GI bleeding, so co-prescribing gastroprotection should be considered
- Monitoring requirements, e.g. monitoring for hypertension with venlafaxine and duloxetine
- Time to effect—the patient should be made aware that it takes time for the full effect to be achieved, usually at least 2 weeks
- Alternative options, e.g. tricyclic antidepressants (TCA). Combinations of medication may be considered on the advice of a consultant psychiatrist.

Consider toxicity in the event of overdose when prescribing, and whether the quantity of drug supplied at any given time should be limited in the interests of patient safety.

Switching antidepressants

If a switch is needed, it is preferable to switch to another SSRI. The second-line option is to switch to an antidepressant of a different class, e.g. serotonin and noradrenaline reuptake inhibitors (SNRIs), TCAs, or monoamine oxidase inhibitors (MAOIs).

The following medications require **particular caution** when switching between them:

- Fluoxetine to any other antidepressant—fluoxetine has a long half-life
- Fluoxetine/paroxetine to a TCA—both medications inhibit the metabolism of TCAs, so a lower starting dose should be used
- Switching to serotonergic antidepressants or MAOIs—risk of serotonin syndrome
- Switching from non-reversible MAOIs—long washout period. Other antidepressants should be avoided for 2 weeks.

Electroconvulsive therapy

Indications:

- Severe or life-threatening depression, where a rapid response is required, or other treatments have failed
- Moderate depression which has not responded to multiple drug treatments or psychological therapies
- Previous good response to electroconvulsive therapy or patient choice.

Important considerations:

- Comorbidities and anaesthetic risk
- Side effects: there is some evidence regarding cognitive impairment as an adverse effect, especially in the elderly. This should be reassessed regularly
- Consider whether the patient has capacity to give informed consent under the Mental Capacity Act and whether the Mental Health Act is relevant (see Chapter 112 for consent and capacity)
- If the patient responds well, an antidepressant (± a mood stabilizer such as lithium) should be started for relapse prevention.

Psychosocial considerations

- Support carers and encourage them to be alert to mood changes and suicidal ideation in the patient
- Befriending and rehabilitation programmes may be helpful for patients with long-standing moderate or severe depression.

Monitoring and follow-up

If not at high risk of suicide

- Follow up after 2 weeks
- If responding, follow up 2–4-weekly for the first 3 months
- After 3 months, increase intervals as appropriate.

If at high risk of suicide or age <30 years

- Follow up after 1 week, then as frequently as is appropriate.

Treatment monitoring

- If no improvement at 2–4 weeks, review medication compliance
- If minimal improvement at 3–4 weeks of using a therapeutic dose, consider increasing the dose or switching the medication, and providing additional psychological support
- If there is some improvement at 4 weeks, continue the treatment for a further 2–4 weeks. Consider switching if inadequate response or unable to tolerate side effects.

Stopping medication

- Medication should be used for at least 6 months post remission, or at least 2 years if high risk of relapse (usually at treatment dose)
- Inform patient about possible discontinuation symptoms, e.g. insomnia, sweating, restlessness
- Gradually stop the medication over at least 4 weeks (longer if the medication has a long half-life)
- If discontinuation symptoms are significant, it may be necessary to restart the medication and titrate it down even more gradually
- Aim for the patient to be stable on as little medication as possible (which may be none at all).

Chapter 39

Eating disorders

Guideline:
NICE NG69 (Eating disorders: recognition and treatment): https://www.nice.org.uk/guidance/ng69

OUP disclaimer: Oxford University Press makes no representation, express or implied, that the drug dosages are correct and that the recommendations are an exclusive or mandatory course of care. All health professionals reading this text have a responsibility to evaluate its appropriateness and take the individual needs of the patient into account.

Local trust guidelines: please refer to your local guidelines as necessary.

Overview

The topic of eating disorders includes anorexia, bulimia, and binge eating. Eating disorders involve the patient developing a set of negative beliefs around food, weight, and body shape, leading to inappropriate behaviours. These behaviours may have serious consequences, such as osteoporosis and growth stunting, so early recognition and treatment is important.

Diagnosis

History/diagnostic criteria

- Eating disorders can develop at any age, but the risk is highest between 13–17 years
- High-risk groups include fashion models, dancers, and professional sportspeople
- Symptoms may include:
  - Excessively fast weight loss
  - Restrictive eating patterns or altered eating behaviour, e.g. refusing to eat certain foods/food groups, binging
  - Food-related social withdrawal
  - Disproportionate concern about weight or shape
  - Problems managing a chronic illness where dietary alteration is part of the management, e.g. coeliac disease, T1DM
  - Menstrual disturbance
  - Dizziness, fainting, or palpitations
  - Compensatory behaviours, e.g. laxative abuse, forced vomiting
  - Unexplained abdominal pain
- A full psychiatric and medical history should be taken
- Discuss substance and alcohol abuse and the risk of self-harm.

Examination

Examination is intended to investigate the consequences and complications of malnutrition or the compensatory behaviours the patient is displaying. Findings may include:

- Anorexia:
  - Reduced muscle power
  - Poor peripheral circulation
  - Pallor
  - Peripheral oedema
  - Lanugo
  - Stunted growth or puberty
- Bulimia:
  - Unexplained dental erosion
  - Russell's sign (calluses on the knuckles due to recurrent damage from the teeth when trying to induce vomiting)
  - Swollen parotid glands.

Investigations

Bedside

- Basic observations may show:
  - Bradycardia
  - (Postural) Hypotension
  - Low temperature
- Weight:
  - Particularly high or low BMI for age
- ECG:
  - An ECG should be done if any of the following apply:
    - Very rapid weight loss
    - Excessive exercise

- Severe purging behaviour
- Current bradycardia or previous arrhythmias
- Hypotension
- High caffeine intake or use of other medications
- Muscular weakness
- Electrolyte imbalance

- Common abnormalities include bradycardia, ↑ QTc, and changes related to hypokalaemia (↑ amplitude and width of P waves, PR elongation, T wave flattening and inversion, ST depression, and U waves).

Bloods

- A full electrolyte panel including sodium, potassium, calcium, glucose, magnesium, and phosphate should be checked. Common abnormalities include:
  - Hyponatraemia
  - Hypokalaemia
  - Hypoglycaemia
- Impaired renal function and raised transaminases are also common.

Management

Consider whether the patient has capacity to make their own decisions (see Chapter 112). Use of the Mental Health Act may be required if the patient is refusing treatment and has significant impairment of decision-making abilities.

Consider whether the patient needs an urgent referral to specialist services, or if they require acute medical care due to electrolyte imbalances or dehydration.

Patient education

- Explain to the patient about the nature of the disorder, and the risks and benefits of treatments
- Patients should be advised that laxatives and diuretics will not aid weight loss.

Lifestyle and simple interventions

- If vomiting, advise:
  - Regular dental reviews
  - Avoid immediate teeth brushing after vomiting
  - Avoid acidic mouthwashes, foods, or drinks.

Psychological interventions

- Consider structured self-help, structured specialist therapy programmes, or CBT.

Pharmacological management

- Medication alone should not be used as a treatment for any eating disorder
- Medication should only be prescribed under specialist guidance
- Consider likely compliance and medication risks which may be exacerbated due to malnutrition
- Ensure ECG monitoring is carried out if a medication could affect cardiac function as patients are prone to arrhythmias secondary to malnutrition
- Oral supplementation is preferable for the treatment of electrolyte imbalance, unless there is very severe imbalance or the patient is unable to absorb enterally.

Psychosocial considerations

- Be aware of potential social and family issues such as bullying and abuse
- Patients and family may feel guilty and this needs to be addressed for treatment to be successful
- Eating disorders are often heavily stigmatized and this may cause patients to avoid accessing treatments
- Eating disorders often affect young people so psychological interventions need to be age appropriate.

Complications

- Request specialist paediatric/endocrine advice if physical growth and development has been affected
- Consider bone mineral density scanning after 1 year of being underweight if age <18 years, or after 2 years if age >18 years. Scan earlier if recurrent fractures or bone pain. Repeat annually if ongoing concerns. If abnormal, the patient may require hormonal or bisphosphonate treatment from a (paediatric) endocrinologist.

Monitoring and follow-up

- If the patient declines treatment and the issues are not complex or severe: consider discharging to primary care and re-referring as needed
- If the patient declines treatment and has issues which are complex or severe: continue to support with input from eating disorder services
- Monitor weight/BMI, blood pressure, bloods, and ECG at least annually. The assessment should include a risk assessment and a discussion of ongoing treatment options
- Monitor growth and development in children and young people.

Further reading

1. Royal College of Psychiatrists (2014). MARSIPAN: management of really sick patients with anorexia nervosa, 2nd ed (CR189). Available at: https://www.rcpsych.ac.uk/docs/default-source/improving-care/better-mh-policy/college-reports/college-report-cr189.pdf?sfvrsn=6c2e7ada_2

Chapter 40

Generalized anxiety disorder

Guideline:
NICE CG113 (Generalised anxiety disorder and panic disorder in adults: management): https://www.nice.org.uk/guidance/cg113

OUP disclaimer: Oxford University Press makes no representation, express or implied, that the drug dosages are correct and that the recommendations are an exclusive or mandatory course of care. All health professionals reading this text have a responsibility to evaluate its appropriateness and take the individual needs of the patient into account.

Local trust guidelines: please refer to your local guidelines as necessary.

Overview

The main feature of generalized anxiety disorder (GAD) is excessive worry regarding multiple things, associated with ↑ tension.

Diagnosis

History/diagnostic criteria

Consider GAD if recurrent primary care attendances, with significant worry or anxiety over a range of issues. It tends to present in those who have chronic physical health problems and/or regularly need reassurance on various symptoms.

Ask about:

- Current and past physical and psychiatric history
- Previous treatments trialled
- Comorbid substance abuse.

DSM-5 criteria[1]

- Extreme/disproportionate anxiety or worry, occurring on most days, regarding multiple events
- Occurs for >6 months
- Difficulty controlling worry
- Additional symptoms—three or more of:
    - Feeling restless or 'on edge'
    - Becoming fatigued easily
    - Difficulty in concentrating
    - Irritability
    - Muscular tension
    - Sleep disruption
- Clinically significant distress or functional impairment
- Symptoms cannot be attributed to another cause or disease.

Examination

- No specific examination required.

Investigations

- No specific investigation required.

1 American Psychiatric Association. (2013). Diagnostic and statistical manual of mental disorders (5th ed.). https://doi.org/10.1176/appi.books.9780890425596

Management

Management stages

- **Stage 1:** any presentation of GAD:
  - Identification, assessment, education, active monitoring
- **Stage 2:** GAD not improved with stage 1 management:
  - Low intensity psychological interventions
- **Stage 3:** GAD with poor response to stage 2 management **OR** GAD with marked functional impairment:
  - High-intensity psychological interventions **OR** pharmacological treatment
- **Stage 4:** treatment refractory GAD **OR** high risk of self-harm or self-neglect **OR** complex comorbidities:
  - Specialist treatment.

Patient education

- Inform the patient regarding the diagnosis and treatment options
- Patients should be made aware of the lack of evidence for over-the-counter medications, and also the risk of drug interactions when using them.

Lifestyle and simple interventions

- Avoid caffeine, excess alcohol, and illicit drugs.

Psychological interventions

If no improvement with stage 1, offer one or more of the following (stage 2 treatments):

- Individual non-facilitated self-help
- Individual guided self-help
- Psychoeducational groups.

If poor response to stage 2, or marked functional impairment (i.e. stage 3 disease), and the patient wishes to use a psychological intervention, offer either:

- CBT **OR**
- Applied relaxation.

If the patient does not respond to this or does not wish to use psychological interventions, progress to pharmacological management.

Pharmacological management

If a patient at stage 3 chooses pharmacological management:

- SSRIs are first line e.g. escitalopram 10mg OD. Note that they may take a week to reach full anxiolytic effect
- Second line: serotonin–noradrenaline reuptake inhibitor (SNRI), or alternative SSRI
- Avoid benzodiazepines, aside from in an acute crisis.

When prescribing, consider:

- Risk of withdrawal syndrome
- Side effect profile (Table 40.1)
- Potential drug interactions
- Risk of suicide and toxicity in overdose. Inform patients aged <30 years of the small risk of suicidal ideation/self-harm when using SSRIs/SNRIs.

Table 40.1 Side effects of medications used in GAD

Common side effect/risk	Example of causative medication
Risk of withdrawal syndrome	Paroxetine, venlafaxine
Risk of suicide and toxicity in overdose	All SSRIs and SNRIs, especially venlafaxine
↑ anxiety/agitation/insomnia	All SSRIs and SNRIs
↑ risk of bleeding	SSRIs
↑ risk of suicidal thinking and self-harm in those aged <30 years	All SSRIs and SNRIs

Psychosocial considerations

- Support carers where appropriate.

Monitoring and follow-up

- Review medications every 2–4 weeks for the first 3 months, and then 3-monthly
- If the medication is ineffective or not tolerated, consider an alternative drug and offer the patient a high-intensity psychological intervention. If the patient partially responds to medication, consider adding a high-intensity psychological treatment
- Medications should be taken for at least 1 year before attempting to wean, to reduce the risk of relapse.

Special considerations

Patients with stage 4 GAD (treatment refractory/high risk of self-harm or self-neglect/complex comorbidities) should be offered a specialist assessment.

Chapter 41

Panic disorder

Guideline:
NICE CG113 (Generalised anxiety disorder and panic disorder in adults: management): https://www.nice.org.uk/guidance/cg113

OUP disclaimer: Oxford University Press makes no representation, express or implied, that the drug dosages are correct and that the recommendations are an exclusive or mandatory course of care. All health professionals reading this text have a responsibility to evaluate its appropriateness and take the individual needs of the patient into account.

Local trust guidelines: please refer to your local guidelines as necessary.

Overview

The main feature of panic disorder is repeated, unpredictable episodes of panic, followed by persistent concern regarding future panic attacks and the consequences of this.

Diagnosis

History/diagnostic criteria

DSM-5 criteria[1]

Panic attack

A sudden surge of intense fear or discomfort which reaches a peak within a few minutes, including ≥4 of the following:

- Chest pain or discomfort
- Derealization or depersonalization
- Dizziness or faintness
- Fear of dying
- Fear of loss of control, or fear of going crazy
- Feeling hot or cold
- Nausea or abdominal distress
- Numbness or tingling
- Sensation of choking
- Sensation of shortness of breath or feeling smothered
- Shaking or trembling
- Sweatiness
- Tachycardia or palpitations.

Panic disorder

- Recurrent panic attacks
- ≥1 panic attack followed by ≥1 month of persistent concern about future attacks, or concern about the implications of attacks or a significant change in behaviour related to attacks.

> Remember panic attack ≠ panic disorder.

In the past medical history, ask about depression and substance abuse as these are common comorbidities.

Examination

A mental status examination may reveal the symptoms previously listed.

A general physical examination should also be performed to consider alternative explanations for the symptoms of panic disorder.

Investigations

No specific investigations are required, although they may be useful to eliminate other possible differential diagnoses, e.g. ECG, urine toxicology, cardiac enzymes, FBC, U&E, glucose, TFT, and D-dimer.

1 American Psychiatric Association. (2013). Diagnostic and statistical manual of mental disorders (5th ed.). https://doi.org/10.1176/appi.books.9780890425596

Management

At presentation:

- Check if the patient is already receiving treatment for panic disorder
- Only perform investigations which are required to exclude acute physical pathology
- Avoid admitting the patient if possible, as many patients are better managed in primary or community care.

Patient education

Inform (including written information) about panic disorder and treatment options, including support groups if available.

Lifestyle and simple interventions

Exercise as part of a healthy lifestyle.

Psychological interventions

- Individual non-facilitated or facilitated self-help (if mild to moderate)
- CBT (if moderate to severe).

Pharmacological management

For moderate to severe patients, if CBT is not suitable or desired:

- First line: any SSRI licensed for panic disorder, e.g. sertraline 25mg OD for 1 week, then ↑ to 50mg, then ↑ further if required to maximum 200mg/day
- Second line: tricyclic antidepressants, e.g. imipramine or clomipramine
- **Avoid** benzodiazepines, sedating antihistamines, and antipsychotics.

Prescribing tips

- Warn patients that their anxiety level may increase briefly when they start treatment
- Patients should also be aware of other side effects and withdrawal symptoms and should know not to stop medications suddenly
- Take into account the likelihood of accidental overdose or deliberate self-harm (overdose or otherwise) when prescribing (consider weekly dispensing); the risk is highest with tricyclic antidepressants
- If there is no improvement after 12 weeks, try an alternative medication or therapy
- If a treatment is effective, it can be used long-term.

Monitoring and follow-up

- For psychological interventions, progress should be reviewed at 4–8 week intervals
- For pharmacological interventions review within 2 weeks, then at 4, 6, and 12 weeks. If at 12 weeks it is decided to continue, review at 8–12 week intervals. Continue for at least 6 months after the optimum dose is reached if effective.

Special considerations

Refer to specialist services if significant symptoms remain after trialling two treatments.

Further reading

1. Baldwin A (ed) (2020). Psychiatry. In: *Oxford Handbook of Clinical Specialities*, 11th ed (pp. 682–773). Oxford: Oxford University Press. Available at: https://doi.org/10.1093/med/9780198827191.003.0012
2. Simon C, Everitt H, von Dorp F, et al. (2020). Oxford Handbook of General Practice, 5th ed (pp. 963–96). Oxford: Oxford University Press. Available at: https://doi.org/10.1093/med/9780198808183.003.0027

Chapter 42

Post-traumatic stress disorder

Guideline:
NICE NG116 (Post-traumatic stress disorder): https://www.nice.org.uk/guidance/ng116

OUP disclaimer: Oxford University Press makes no representation, express or implied, that the drug dosages are correct and that the recommendations are an exclusive or mandatory course of care. All health professionals reading this text have a responsibility to evaluate its appropriateness and take the individual needs of the patient into account.

Local trust guidelines: please refer to your local guidelines as necessary.

Overview

Post-traumatic stress disorder (PTSD) is an anxiety disorder which can develop after experiencing or witnessing a traumatic event. The condition is thought to result from inadequate memory processing and results in symptoms that can be disabling.

Diagnosis

History

Assess for possible triggers of PTSD, i.e. discuss whether the patient has ever experienced or witnessed any single, repeated, or multiple traumatic events, such as:

- Serious accidents
- Physical, sexual, or domestic assault or abuse
- War, conflict, or torture
- Serious physical health problems or traumatic childbirth experiences.

Ask about the following:

- Flashbacks—intrusive memories or mental imagery, recurrent nightmares
- Avoidance of triggers, i.e. any stimulus that provokes recollection of the trauma
- Hyperarousal, including hypervigilance, anger, and irritability
- Negative changes to mood and thinking
- Numbing of emotions
- Dissociation (feeling disconnected from yourself, your thoughts, feelings, or memories)
- Difficulty in regulating emotions
- Problems maintaining relationships
- Negative perception of oneself, including feeling worthless or defeated.

Ask about any associated functional impairment.

Conduct a risk assessment and consider suicide risk.

Management

Patient education

Provide patients and families/carers with verbal and written information regarding symptoms, treatment options, and support groups. Good sources of written information are http://www.mind.org.uk/information-support, http://www.nhs.uk/conditions or http://www.rcpsych.ac.uk/mental-health.

Reassure patients that PTSD is treatable.

> **Improving Access to Psychological Therapies (IAPT) programme**
>
> In England, IAPT services offer psychological therapies for depression and anxiety disorders, including trauma-focused therapies for PTSD. Patients can generally self-refer or be referred by a professional. IAPT services will be appropriate for most patients with PTSD, although referral to secondary care may be necessary for ↑ complexity, severity, or risk. More information on IAPT services can be found at: https://www.england.nhs.uk/mental-health/adults/iapt/

Psychological interventions

Options include:

- Trauma-focused CBT
- Trauma-focused computerized CBT
- Eye movement desensitization and reprocessing (EMDR)

In the case of persistent symptoms after trauma-focused therapy, consider CBT targeted at specific symptoms (e.g. sleep disturbance). This can also be considered for patients who are unable or unwilling to engage in trauma-focused therapy.

Pharmacological management

- Only offer drug treatment to patients with a diagnosis of PTSD (i.e. do not use for prevention)
- Only consider if the patient prefers drug treatment to psychological interventions
- Consider a SSRI, such as sertraline 25mg OD. Venlafaxine may also be considered as an alternative (off-label use)
- Consider antipsychotics such as risperidone, in addition to psychological therapies if:
  - The patient has disabling symptoms and behaviours, (e.g. psychotic symptoms) **AND**
  - Their symptoms have not responded to other drug or psychological treatments
- Antipsychotic treatment should only be initiated by a specialist.

Psychosocial considerations

Take these factors into account and help the patient to manage them (this may involve referring to other services/agencies for support).
Examples include:

- Safeguarding concerns
- Homelessness
- Social isolation
- Substance abuse
- Financial hardship
- Interpersonal difficulties.

Complications

- **Drug or alcohol misuse:** additional support may be required from specialist addiction services
- **Depression:** treating PTSD first will often lead to an improvement in depressive symptoms. However, if the depression is severe enough to make PTSD treatment problematic, or if there is a significant risk of harm, it is preferable to treat the depression first.

Monitoring and follow-up

- All drug treatments should be reviewed regularly by a specialist.

Further reading

1. Ehlers A (2012). Post-traumatic stress disorder. In: Geddes JR, Andreasen NC, Lopez-Ibor J, et al.(eds) *New Oxford Textbook of Psychiatry*, 2nd ed (chapter 93). Oxford: Oxford University Press. Available at https://academic.oup.com/book/24770/chapter/188331538

Chapter 43

Psychosis and schizophrenia

Guideline:
NICE CG178 (Psychosis and schizophrenia in adults: prevention and management): https://www.nice.org.uk/guidance/cg178

OUP disclaimer: Oxford University Press makes no representation, express or implied, that the drug dosages are correct and that the recommendations are an exclusive or mandatory course of care. All health professionals reading this text have a responsibility to evaluate its appropriateness and take the individual needs of the patient into account.

Local trust guidelines: please refer to your local guidelines as necessary.

Overview

This chapter covers the prevention and management of schizophrenia, schizoaffective disorder, schizophreniform disorder, and delusional disorder (this excludes psychosis secondary to bipolar affective disorder or depressive disorder). These disorders are characterized by psychotic symptoms.

Assessment

Psychotic symptoms

Psychosis may manifest subtly with a change in mood or with depressive symptoms. More overt psychotic symptoms can broadly be divided into hallucinations and delusions. Hallucinations are the experience of a sensory perception in the absence of an external stimulus. Delusions are false beliefs which the patient holds despite clear evidence to the contrary. Common symptoms include:

- Auditory hallucinations:
  - Hearing voices arguing or a running commentary on their actions
- Delusions:
  - Persecutory delusions, e.g. fear of being hurt or killed, fears of being stalked or conspired against
  - Delusions of grandeur, e.g. believing themselves to have a special talent or to be a millionaire
  - Delusional jealousy, e.g. belief that a partner is being unfaithful
  - Nihilistic delusions, e.g. believing that they do not exist or are dead, their loved ones are dead, the world no longer exists, or that their actions may destroy the world
- Disorders of thought:
  - Thought echo: patient hears their thoughts spoken aloud shortly after thinking them
  - Thought insertion: the patient believes that someone is putting thoughts into their brain
  - Thought withdrawal: the patient believes that someone is removing thoughts from their brain
  - Thought broadcasting: the patient believes that their thoughts are being broadcasted so others can hear them.

History

Cover the following:

- Psychiatric history and risk assessment
- Prescribed medication and recreational drug history
- Medical history and full physical examination (to identify physical illness, including organic brain disorders, and prescribed drug treatments that may result in psychosis)
- Lifestyle (including weight, smoking, alcohol, nutrition, physical activity, and sexual health)
- Psychosocial including social networks, relationships, and trauma (assess for PTSD; see Chapter 42)
- Developmental history
- Social history, including cultural issues, leisure activities, and caring responsibilities
- Occupational and educational history, and financial status.

Preventing psychosis

A first episode of psychosis is typically preceded by a prodromal period, lasting from a few days to 18 months. A person should be considered at risk of developing psychosis if they meet the criteria in Table 43.1.

Table 43.1 Prodromal criteria for patients at risk of developing psychosis

Distressed	+	Decline in social functioning	+	At least one of the following:
				• Transient or attenuated psychotic symptoms
				• Other experiences or behaviour suggestive of possible psychosis
				• A first-degree relative with psychosis or schizophrenia

If patients fit these criteria, they should be referred for urgent assessment by a consultant psychiatrist.

Patients with prodromal symptoms should be offered:

- CBT ± family intervention
- Treatment for any comorbid psychiatric disorder, including substance misuse.

They should not be given antipsychotic medication initially.

If the patient is not formally diagnosed with psychosis but symptoms persist, continue monitoring for signs of emerging psychosis for up to 3 years.

Management

Patient education

- Make patients and their carers aware of appropriate peer support and self-management programmes
- Ensure they have received appropriate instruction of what to do/who to call in a crisis.

Lifestyle and simple interventions

- Facilitate education/occupational activities
- Support patients to stop smoking. Use medications such as bupropion and varenicline cautiously as they may worsen psychiatric symptoms.

Psychological interventions

- Offer CBT and family therapy
- Consider offering art therapy (particularly for negative symptoms)
- If patients choose to try psychological intervention without medication, advise them that this is less effective than combined therapy
- Monitor regularly and review treatment within a month.

Pharmacological management

Offer antipsychotic medication (combined with psychological interventions—see 'Psychological interventions') to all patients with psychosis, guided by a consultant psychiatrist. Discuss the following with the patient and their carer:

- Response to previous antipsychotic medication
- Expected benefits
- Potential side effects (Table 43.2).

Table 43.2 Potential side effects of antipsychotics

Type of side effect	Example	Antipsychotics likely to cause these side effects
Metabolic	Weight gain, diabetes	Clozapine, olanzapine, quetiapine
Extrapyramidal	Akathisia, dyskinesia, dystonia	Typical antipsychotics (e.g. haloperidol)
Cardiovascular	Prolonged QT interval	Haloperidol, pimozide
Hormonal	Hyperprolactinaemia	Amisulpride, risperidone, paliperidone

Baseline tests

Baseline investigations before starting an antipsychotic:

- Weight
- Waist circumference
- Pulse and blood pressure
- Fasting blood glucose
- HbA1c
- Lipid profile

- Prolactin levels
- Assessment of any movement disorders
- Assessment of nutritional status, diet, and level of physical activity.

Perform a baseline ECG if:

- Using haloperidol, clozapine, or chlorpromazine (manufacturer requirement)
- A physical examination indicates cardiovascular risk (e.g. hypertension) or there is a history of cardiovascular disease.

Antipsychotic prescribing

- Start at the lower end of the therapeutic range and titrate upwards as needed
- Monitor for side effects and adverse effects
- If tolerated, trial the medication at the optimum dose for 4–6 weeks
- Do not combine antipsychotics (apart from short-term when switching)
- There is no specific order in which antipsychotics should be tried. It will depend on patient and doctor preference. All patients will respond to and tolerate medications differently, therefore there is no first-line medication which will be suitable for all patients. However, clozapine should not be used initially
- Examples of antipsychotics which could be tried initially include:
  - First-generation (typical) antipsychotics: chlorpromazine, flupentixol, haloperidol
  - Second-generation (atypical) antipsychotics: olanzapine, risperidone, quetiapine.

Treatment resistance

For patients who do not respond to treatment:

- Check adherence
- Check that the dose and duration were adequate
- Check that psychological therapies have been offered and engaged with
- Consider if there could be concurrent substance abuse, interacting medications, or physical illness
- Review the diagnosis.

Clozapine should be offered to people with schizophrenia who have failed to respond to separate trials (at adequate duration and dose) of at least two different antipsychotics, one of which must be a non-clozapine atypical antipsychotic.

If symptoms do not respond adequately to clozapine, check plasma clozapine levels.

If necessary, consider adding another antipsychotic.

Depot/long-acting injectable antipsychotic medication

Consider using depot medications if:

- This is the patient's preference
- There is a risk of non-adherence to medication.

Monitoring and stopping antipsychotics

- Inform patients that if they stop medication within 1–2 years their risk of relapse is high
- Review medication annually as a minimum

- Stop medication gradually and monitor closely for signs of relapse for at least 2 years.

Patients taking antipsychotic medication should continue to have their physical health monitored in secondary care (in accordance with Table 43.3) for at least 1 year, or until their condition has stabilized.

Table 43.3 Recommended physical health monitoring for patients using antipsychotic medications

Weight	Weekly for 6 weeks, at 12 weeks, at 1 year, and then annually
Waist circumference	Annually
Pulse, blood pressure, fasting glucose, HbA1c, lipid profile	At 12 weeks, at 1 year, and then annually

Violence, aggression, and self-harm

Patients with schizophrenia or psychosis may become violent or aggressive. For details on management of violence and aggression see Chapter 45. For concerns regarding self-harm, see Chapter 44.

Further reading

1. Barnes T (2011). Evidence-based guidelines for the pharmacological treatment of schizophrenia: recommendations from the British Association for Psychopharmacology. *J Psychopharmacol*. 25:567–620.
2. Joint Formulary Committee. Psychoses and related disorders. In: *British National Formulary*. Available at: https://bnf.nice.org.uk/treatment-summary/psychoses-and-related-disorders.html

Chapter 44

Self-harm

Guidelines:
This chapter was based on the following guidelines: NICE CG16 (Self-harm in over 8s: short-term management and prevention of recurrence): https://www.nice.org.uk/guidance/cg16

NICE CG133 (Self-harm in over 8s: long-term management): https://www.nice.org.uk/guidance/cg133. Since the chapter was written, the guidelines have been updated with minor changes and combined into: NICE NG225 (Self-harm: assessment, management and preventing recurrence): https://www.nice.org.uk/guidance/ng225

OUP disclaimer: Oxford University Press makes no representation, express or implied, that the drug dosages are correct and that the recommendations are an exclusive or mandatory course of care. All health professionals reading this text have a responsibility to evaluate its appropriateness and take the individual needs of the patient into account.

Local trust guidelines: please refer to your local guidelines as necessary.

Overview

Self-harm includes all self-poisoning or injury regardless of intention. Self-harm is common, with 25.7% of women and 9.7% of men aged 16–24 reporting that they have self-harmed previously.[1] Overall, the prevalence is estimated to be 0.5% across all age groups. The risk of suicide is 49× greater over a 12-month period if an individual has self-harmed, as compared with the rest of the population.[2] It is therefore essential to carefully and compassionately assess the complex issues that lie behind self-harm and to ensure that a plan is put in place to try and avoid morbidity and mortality.

1 McManus S, Bebbington P, Jenkins R, et al. Mental health and wellbeing in England: Adult Psychiatric Morbidity Survey 2014. Leeds. 2016. Available at: https://assets.publishing.service.gov.uk/government/uploads/system/uploads/attachment_data/file/556596/apms-2014-full-rpt.pdf

2 Hawton K, Bergen H, Cooper J, et al. Suicide following self-harm: findings from the Multicentre Study of Self-Harm in England, 2000–2012. *J Affect Disord.* 2015; 175:147–51.

Diagnosis

Triage in the emergency department:

- Assess risk to physical health
- Assess emotional and mental state
- Consider using the 'Australian Mental Health Triage Scale' (see 'Further reading')
- Conduct a preliminary psychosocial assessment, to include:
  - Mental capacity
  - Willingness to remain for further psychosocial assessment
  - Level of distress
  - Evidence of mental illness
- Ask the patient if they would prefer to be assessed by a male or female doctor, if it is possible to comply with their request
- If the patient needs to wait for treatment, provide a quiet space, with supervision to ensure safety.

History

The patient may be able to provide a history but if not, ask a collateral witness and/or paramedic.

In particular, ask about the following:

- Nature and timing of overdose or injuries
- Whether it was planned or spontaneous
- Substances/medications found at the scene
- Information about the home environment
- Social and family support network
- History leading to self-harm
- Initial emotional state and level of distress
- How the patient feels now
- Previous interactions with the mental health team
- The risk of further self-harm or suicide.

> LGBTQ+ people are at a higher risk of self-harm compared to the rest of the population.[3] Be aware of the need to use the person's preferred pronouns.

Examination

A full psychosocial assessment should be completed, usually by a specialist mental health liaison professional (Box 44.1). Ideally this should be held with the patient alone to facilitate confidentiality, and in case there are issues with carers that the patient wishes to discuss.

The psychosocial assessment should take place in parallel with medical treatment if needed (as long as the patient is in a fit condition to be interviewed).

Ensure that all of the assessment is fully documented and that a copy is sent to the patient's GP.

3 King M, Semlyen J, See Tai S. A systematic review of mental disorder, suicide, deliberate self-harm in lesbian, gay and bisexual people. *BMC Psychiatry*. 2008; 8:70.

Box 44.1 Mental health liaison teams

Most general hospitals have mental health liaison teams which are often staffed by experienced mental health nurses and social workers with some psychiatry input. They carry out psychosocial assessments for patients presenting with self-harm.

Gather information and perform a thorough triage before referring to the mental health liaison team.

Investigations

In the event of overdose, follow recommendations from TOXBASE and the National Poisons Information Service (NPIS) regarding what samples to collect (for link see 'Further reading').

Measure plasma paracetamol concentrations (Box 44.2) in all patients with confirmed or suspected paracetamol overdose or opioid poisoning, as well as in an unconscious, collapsed patient where drug overdose is possible.

Box 44.2 Paracetamol levels

Paracetamol levels taken 4–15 hours after ingestion can be used to assess risk and guide treatment, using a treatment graph which is available from TOXBASE or the BNF.

Management

Acute management

Assess the patient using an ABCDE approach.

For the treatment of poisoning, follow the guidance outlined in TOXBASE. General principles of the treatment of common poisons are outlined in Table 44.1.

Always consider the possibility of a mixed overdose.

Consider oral activated charcoal treatment for those who present within 2 hours of overdose, are conscious, have a protected airway, and are at risk of significant harm from poisoning (but check if already given by paramedics/pre-hospital).

See Table 44.1 and Box 44.3 regarding the use of flumazenil or naloxone.

The following should **not** be offered unless specifically recommended by TOXBASE or the NPIS:

- Multiple doses of activated charcoal
- Emetics
- Cathartics
- Gastric lavage
- Whole bowel irrigation.

Table 44.1 Basic management of specific poisons (for further details, please refer to TOXBASE)

Agent	Management and considerations
Paracetamol	IV acetylcysteine: • Can cause anaphylactoid reactions
Benzodiazepines	Flumazenil (Box 44.3): • Avoid if there is an ↑ risk of seizures, e.g. ingested proconvulsant such as tricyclic antidepressant or history of epilepsy or dependence on benzodiazepines • Give if the patient can protect their airway but there is respiratory depression which, if left untreated, will likely require invasive ventilation • May be given only by clinicians who have been trained in its use and if resuscitation equipment is available
Opioids	Naloxone (Box 44.3): • Use if impaired consciousness or respiratory depression, e.g. respiratory rate ≤8 • Use minimum effective dose to reverse respiratory depression • An IV infusion may be required

Box 44.3 Using flumazenil or naloxone

When using flumazenil or naloxone, be prepared to deal with prompt withdrawal including agitation, aggression, and violence. Patients will also require close monitoring for re-sedation as the effect of the antidotes wears off. In particular, monitor the respiratory rate and oxygen saturation.

Treatment after stabilization

Physical health

Ensure that the patient is stable from a physical health perspective. Admit for monitoring and consider the need for further treatment of the physical consequences of self-harm.

Mental Health Act

Assess if the patient continues to be a danger to themselves or others. If there are concerns, they should be assessed for sectioning under the Mental Health Act (see 'Further reading').

Coping strategies

Harm minimization strategies are not an option for people who repeatedly self-harm as there are no safe limits. If the patient is usually prescribed long-term medications, consider prescribing the least dangerous option and consider prescribing a reduced quantity of tablets, e.g. weekly or even daily dispensing. This strategy may also need to be extended to relatives who live in the same home and are prescribed long-term medications.

Consider discussing alternative coping strategies for people who repeatedly self-injure, e.g. methadone in heroin addiction, information about how to clean wounds. Consider providing information on dealing with scarring, if appropriate. The patient may require a short admission, particularly if a full assessment has not been possible due to patient distress or intoxication, or if the home environment is unsafe.

Referral for further assessment or treatment

It is essential to find out if the patient has a Responsible Clinician as often these patients' circumstances are complex. They can be challenging to manage due to the risk they pose to themselves but there may already be a care plan in place which will help guide decision-making. If in doubt, discuss with a senior member of staff.

The need for referral will be based on the psychosocial assessment, with the aim of addressing the underlying problems or mental disorder rather than just addressing the self-harming behaviour.

Longer-term care plans are made by adult mental health services, liaison psychiatry, CAMHS, or intellectual disability services. They aim to:

- Reduce self-harm
- Reduce risks arising from self-harm
- Reduce or stop other risk behaviours
- Improve social or occupational functioning
- Improve quality of life
- Treat the associated mental disorder.

Care plans should be multidisciplinary, collaborative, and reviewed at regular intervals. They should include a crisis plan so that the patient is able to obtain help in the event that other strategies have failed.

Consider offering 3–12 sessions of structured psychological therapy with the specific aim of reducing self-harm. This should be tailored to individual needs and could include CBT, psychodynamic, or problem-solving elements.

Do not offer drug treatment specifically to reduce self-harm. However, drug treatment may be appropriate to treat associated mental disorders. Consider the toxicity of prescribed drugs in overdose (e.g. SSRIs are less toxic than other antidepressants; see Chapter 38).

Special considerations

Children and young people (<16 years)

All under 16s should be assessed in the paediatric section of the emergency department. They should be admitted to a paediatric ward overnight and fully assessed the following day by the CAMHS team.

It is necessary to obtain consent from the parent or legally responsible adult before carrying out an assessment. An understanding is required of the issues relating to capacity and consent in this age group.

Learning disability

Consider any issues of capacity and consent and include a parent or legally responsible adult in the decision-making process. If admission is necessary, then liaise with and arrange a rapid review by the learning disability team.

Older people (>65 years)

There is a higher risk of self-harm and suicide in this age group, and all acts of self-harm should be regarded as evidence of suicidal intent until proven otherwise.

Further reading

1. Australian Government Department of Health. Mental health triage tool. Available at: https://www1.health.gov.au/internet/publications/publishing.nsf/Content/triageqrg~triageqrg-mh
2. National Poisons Information Service. TOXBASE. Available at: https://www.toxbase.org/
3. Joint Formulary Committee. Poisoning, emergency treatment. In: *British National Formulary*. Available at: http://www.medicinescomplete.com
4. NHS (2019). Mental Health Act. Available at: https://www.nhs.uk/using-the-nhs/nhs-services/mental-health-services/mental-health-act/

Chapter 45

Violence and aggression

Guideline:
NICE NG10 (Violence and aggression: short-term management in mental health, health and community settings): https://www.nice.org.uk/guidance/ng10

OUP disclaimer: Oxford University Press makes no representation, express or implied, that the drug dosages are correct and that the recommendations are an exclusive or mandatory course of care. All health professionals reading this text have a responsibility to evaluate its appropriateness and take the individual needs of the patient into account.

Local trust guidelines: please refer to your local guidelines as necessary.

Overview

Violence and aggression includes any action or behaviour which leads to injury or harm to another person.

Diagnosis

History

Taking a multidisciplinary approach, assess the risk of aggression and violence, considering the following factors:

- History of violence and aggression
- Psychiatric history
- Severity of illness and current symptoms
- Incidents between patients (e.g. teasing, bullying, unwanted physical or sexual contact, miscommunication)
- The impact of being subject to restriction (e.g. being detained, being denied leave)
- The impact of the physical environment (e.g. access to belongings and space)
- Personal factors (e.g. family disputes or financial difficulties)
- The approach of staff to the patient (should be positive and encouraging)
- Cultural factors
- Access to psychological therapies and activities.

Involve the patient and carer in the risk assessment wherever possible (try to obtain consent from the patient before involving the carer).

Examination

Conduct a mental state examination (Table 45.1). Focus on factors that may lead to violence and aggression.

Table 45.1 Mental state examination findings relevant to the risk of aggression and violence

Appearance and behaviour	High levels of arousal, agitation, violent or aggressive acts to other persons or environment, threatening or intimidating manner, evidence of drug or alcohol use
Speech	Aggressive or threatening tone or content, communication difficulties
Mood	Anxiety, disappointment, jealousy, frustration, anger
Thoughts	Persecutory thought content, passivity phenomena, violent ideation or intent
Perceptions	Command hallucinations
Cognition	Cognitive impairment, poor executive function
Insight	Lack of insight into mental disorder, risk of violence, and need for treatment

Investigations

Risk prediction instruments can be used to aid clinical judgement, e.g. Brøset Violence Checklist or Dynamic Appraisal of Situational Aggression—Inpatient Version.

Management

Acute management

Risk assessment

Involving the MDT, formulate a risk management plan based on your risk assessment. Take into account advanced directives and consider what measures and approaches have helped in the past.

De-escalation

Take the following approach with patients at risk of aggression or violence:

- Separate agitated patients from others where safe to do so. Use a designated quiet area of the ward for this if possible
- One staff member should take the primary role in communicating with the patient, but do not isolate a single staff member with the patient
- Seek clarification from the patient
- Negotiate to resolve the situation non-confrontationally
- Be mindful of your own non-verbal communication (avoid expressing anxiety or frustration—try to appear calm)
- Consider offering PRN medications (e.g. promethazine 25–50mg PO or lorazepam 1–2mg PO).

Restraint

Only use restrictive interventions (e.g. seclusion, restraint) if the above-listed measures fail and there is a risk of harm to the patient or others if this action is not taken. Ensure that restrictive interventions are:

1. Proportionate to the level of risk
2. The least restrictive option
3. Used for the shortest possible duration
4. Used in accordance with the patient's preferences if possible
5. Appropriate to the patient's developmental age, physical health, and frailty.

Mechanical restraint (e.g. handcuffs) should **only** be used in high-security settings, and only as an option of last resort.

Seclusion

Seclusion means confining a patient within a room for the protection of others. If necessary, it should take place within a designated room, and the patient should be under continuous observation. It should take place for the shortest duration possible and reviews should take place at least every 2 hours to consider whether the seclusion can be terminated.

Legal status

Use of restrictive interventions should prompt an urgent review of the patient's legal status. For informal patients (voluntary admission) who are secluded as an emergency, the need to use powers to detain under the Mental Health Act should be assessed urgently.

Rapid tranquillization

This is the use of parenteral (usually IM) medication for urgent sedation.

For adults use either **lorazepam 1–2mg IM** *or* **haloperidol 5mg IM + promethazine 25–50mg IM**.

When choosing, consider the patient's preferences, physical health problems, possible intoxication, previous response, possible interactions, and total daily dose (including regular medications). If there is insufficient information, use lorazepam.

Avoid haloperidol and promethazine if there is no ECG available (risk of dangerous QT prolongation) or if there is evidence of cardiovascular disease.

Review after the first dose. If there is a partial response, consider giving another dose. If there is no response, consider using another agent (e.g. if no response to lorazepam, then consider haloperidol/promethazine).

A daily medication review by a senior doctor is necessary if the patient is requiring rapid tranquillization. For patients who do not respond to rapid tranquillization, get urgent senior advice.

Following rapid tranquillization, ensure that the following are monitored at least every hour: pulse, blood pressure, temperature, hydration level, level of consciousness, and side effects, until there are no further concerns regarding the patient's physical health. These should be monitored every 15 minutes if any of the following apply:

- Doses of medication are given exceeding BNF limits
- The patient is asleep or sedated
- The patient has also been using drugs or alcohol
- The patient has a pre-existing physical health problem
- The patient has been harmed because of a restrictive intervention.

Treatment after stabilization

Pharmacological

There should be an agreed 'pharmacological strategy' for patients at risk of violence and aggression, including the use of regular and PRN medication. This should be formulated as soon as possible following admission.

Review this strategy at least once a week. If rapid tranquillization is being used, a senior doctor should review this at least once a day.

When reviewing medication, consider the following:

- What is the therapeutic aim?
- How long should the medication take to work?
- What is the total dose of medication prescribed and administered, including PRN?
- Have any doses been missed and why?
- Has there been a therapeutic response?
- Are there any side effects?

When prescribing PRN medication:

- Ensure that the MDT (particularly nursing staff) agree under which circumstances the medication should be administered
- Ensure that it is necessary (PRN medications should not be routinely prescribed, although they will be necessary for many patients who are at risk of aggression and violence)
- Check that the total dose of regular and PRN medication does not exceed BNF limits, especially if a regular daily dose is also being used (BNF maximum daily dose for haloperidol is 20mg/day)
- Consider stopping PRN medication that isn't being used. Review at least weekly.

> Doses above the BNF maximum should only be prescribed following discussion with a senior doctor. Clearly document the rationale for this decision in the patient's notes and be aware that these patients will require closer monitoring.

Psychosocial

Consider offering a psychological intervention to enable the patient to develop skills aimed at reducing the risk of future violence and aggression.

Observation

The observation level is the frequency with which staff will observe the patient to ensure their safety. Agree the level of observation for each patient with the MDT according to the risk assessment. The following observation levels are usually found on psychiatric inpatient wards:

- Low-level intermittent (30–60 minutes): for lower-risk patients
- High-level intermittent (15–30 minutes): for patients at ↑ but not immediate risk
- Continuous observation (i.e. 'one to one'): kept at eyesight or arm's length of a designated staff member—for patients who are at continuous risk
- Multiprofessional continuous observation (e.g. 'two to one'): these patients are at highest risk and require continuous observation from more than one member of staff.

Special considerations

Emergency departments

Violence or aggression as symptoms of a known or suspected mental health problem should be managed as a psychiatric emergency. Refer urgently to the mental health liaison team who should assess within 1 hour.

Further reading

1. Ogloff JR, Daffern M (2006). The dynamic appraisal of situational aggression: an instrument to assess risk for imminent aggression in psychiatric inpatients. *Behav Sci Law*. 24:799–813.
2. Woods P, Almvik R (2002). The Broset violence checklist (BVC). *Acta Psychiatr Scand*. 106:103–5.

Part 7

Nephrology

Chapter 46

Acute kidney injury

Guideline:
NICE NG148 (Acute kidney injury: prevention, detection and management): https://www.nice.org.uk/guidance/ng148

OUP disclaimer: Oxford University Press makes no representation, express or implied, that the drug dosages are correct and that the recommendations are an exclusive or mandatory course of care. All health professionals reading this text have a responsibility to evaluate its appropriateness and take the individual needs of the patient into account.

Local trust guidelines: please refer to your local guidelines as necessary.

Overview

Acute kidney injury (AKI) is defined as an abrupt (within 7 days) loss in kidney function, which may occur in the context of pre-existing kidney disease or completely normal renal function.

Diagnosis

History/diagnostic criteria

Factors known to precipitate AKI include acute illness, surgery, and receiving iodinated contrast. Particular care should be taken in patients with underlying risk factors for developing AKI, which include:

- CKD
- Heart failure
- Liver disease
- Age ≥65 years
- Diabetes
- History of AKI
- Hypovolaemia or sepsis
- Use of drugs that can cause or exacerbate kidney injury (including diuretics, ACE inhibitors, ARBs, NSAIDs, and aminoglycosides).

AKI can be detected and stratified according to severity using the criteria listed in Table 46.1.

Table 46.1 AKI severity classification criteria (from RIFLE, AKIN, and KDIGO systems)

AKI stage	Serum creatinine criteria	Urine output criteria
1	• Creatinine rise of ≥26µmol/L within 48 hours **OR** • Creatinine rise of 1.5–1.99× baseline within 7 days	• Urine output <0.5mL/kg/hour for >6 hours (in adults)
2	• Creatinine rise of 2–2.99× baseline within 7 days	• Urine output <0.5mL/kg/hour for >12 hours
3	• Creatinine rise of 3× or more from baseline within 7 days **OR** • Creatinine rise to ≥354µmol/L **OR** • New requirement for renal replacement therapy	• Urine output <0.3mL/kg/hour for >12 hours

AKIN, Acute Kidney Injury Network; KDIGO, Kidney Disease: Improving Global Outcomes; RIFLE, Risk, Injury, Failure, Loss of kidney function, and End-stage kidney disease.

AKI itself will not cause symptoms unless very severe. In this case, patients may present with nausea and vomiting, fatigue, shortness of breath (due to pulmonary oedema), peripheral oedema, and symptoms of uraemia (e.g. itch, chest pain due to pericarditis, or behavioural disturbances due to encephalopathy).

Examination

AKI examination findings are listed in Table 46.2.

Table 46.2 AKI examination findings

B	• Bibasal coarse crepitations
C	• Cool peripheries • Prolonged capillary refill time • ↑ JVP • Tachycardia
D	• Drowsiness
E	• Pitting oedema • Palpable distended bladder • Renal angle tenderness

Investigations

Investigations that should be carried out in AKI are listed in Table 46.3.

Table 46.3 Causes of AKI and appropriate investigations

Type	Causes	Investigations
Prerenal (reduction in blood supply to kidneys)	• Dehydration • Sepsis (see Chapter 122) • Shock	• ECG • Bloods including FBC, U&E, LFT, bone profile, CRP, blood cultures, VBG • Chest X- ray
Intrinsic (direct damage to kidneys)	• Acute glomerulonephritis • Drugs • Toxins including iodinated contrast • Reduced blood supply • Pyonephrosis (infected and obstructed kidney) • Myeloma • Rhabdomyolysis	• Urinalysis—check for (proteinuria and/or haematuria) • FBC • Serum electrophoresis, immunoglobulins, serum free light chains • Creatine kinase • Vasculitis screen if blood/ protein on urinalysis or otherwise unexplained AKI (ANCA, complement C3/ 4, ANA, anti-glomerular basement membrane antibodies, antistreptolysin O titres)
Postrenal (obstruction of urinary flow)	• Obstructing renal calculi • Bladder malignancy • Enlarged prostate • Retroperitoneal fibrosis • Pelvic malignancy • Urethral stricture	• Ultrasound of urinary tract

Start with simple investigations to identify a cause before considering performing a vasculitis screen or electrophoresis/immunoglobulins/serum free light chains, **unless** there are particular reasons to suspect specific conditions.
Ultrasound is **not** required if the cause has been identified and treated.
If the cause of AKI is not identified, consider a renal tract ultrasound.
If pyonephrosis is suspected, ultrasound should be performed within 6 hours.

Management

The management of AKI largely depends on the underlying cause. Call for help from a senior clinician if there are any clinical concerns or a high early warning system score. General principles include:

Acute management

- **IV fluids:** if the patient is hypovolaemic
- **Monitor:** U&E and urine output. Urinary catheterization may be required
- **Antibiotics:** if sepsis is suspected. Ensure choice of antimicrobial agent and dose are adjusted to renal function as per local guidelines/BNF/ Renal Drug Database.
- **Medications review:** stop nephrotoxics if indicated and antihypertensives if the patient is hypotensive. Note that some drugs that are metabolized by the kidney may require dosage alterations according to eGFR or creatinine clearance to avoid toxicity, e.g. digoxin
- **Renal replacement therapy:** should be considered immediately if any of the following are not responding to medical therapy:
  - Hyperkalaemia (see Chapter 48)
  - Metabolic acidosis
  - Symptomatic uraemia (e.g. tremor, cognitive impairment, coma, fits)
  - Fluid overload
  - Pericarditis
  - Pulmonary oedema
  - Anuria.

Treatment after stabilization

Referral to the urology team is indicated in cases of upper urinary tract obstruction.

Refer immediately if suspecting pyonephrosis, obstructed solitary kidney, bilateral upper urinary tract obstruction, or complications of AKI caused by urological obstruction. Nephrostomy or stenting should be undertaken as soon as possible, and within 12 hours of diagnosis.

Referral to the nephrology team is indicated if considering renal replacement therapy, in patients with a renal transplant, where the cause of AKI is uncertain or if specialist management of the cause is needed. If any of the following are present, discuss with a nephrologist as soon as possible, and within 24 hours:

- A diagnosis requiring specialist treatment (e.g. vasculitis, glomerulonephritis, myeloma)
- AKI with no clear cause
- Inadequate response to treatment
- Complications associated with AKI
- Stage 3 AKI
- Renal transplant
- Pre-existing CKD stage 4 or 5.

Once the AKI has resolved, consider a referral to nephrology if eGFR remains <30mL/min/1.73m^2.

Special considerations

Contrast-induced AKI

This is defined as AKI occurring within 48 hours of a patient receiving iodinated contrast. As such, the following may be considered when managing a patient at high risk of contrast-induced AKI:

- Discuss patients at high risk of contrast-induced AKI with a nephrologist to assess the benefits and risks of proposed imaging, but **do not** delay emergency imaging
- Unenhanced or alternative scanning techniques in patients with risk factors
- Consider withholding nephrotoxic medications pre and post scan
- Encourage oral hydration pre and post scan
- Volume expansion with IV normal saline or isotonic sodium bicarbonate at 1mL/kg/hour for 12 hours pre and post procedure if the patient is high risk, e.g. eGFR <30mL/min/1.73m^2, they have a renal transplant, a large volume of contrast is due to be used, or the contrast will be injected intra-arterially with first-pass renal exposure.

Further reading

1. Hertzberg D, Rydén L, Pickering JW, et al. (2017). Acute kidney injury—an overview of diagnostic methods and clinical management. *Clin Kidney J*. 10:323–31.
2. Steddon S, Ashman N, Chesser A, et al. (2014). Acute kidney injury (AKI). In: *Oxford Handbook of Nephrology and Hypertension*, 2nd ed (pp. 87–190). Oxford: Oxford University Press. Available at: https://doi.org/10.1093/med/9780199651610.003.0002

Chapter 47

Chronic kidney disease

Guidelines:
NICE NG203 (Chronic kidney disease: assessment and management): https://www.nice.org.uk/guidance/ng203

UK Kidney Association (Anaemia of chronic kidney disease): https://ukkidney.org/sites/renal.org/files/Updated-130220-Anaemia-of-Chronic-Kidney-Disease-1-1.pdf

UK Kidney Association (Sodium-glucose co-transporter-2 (SGLT-2) inhibition in adults with kidney disease): https://ukkidney.org/sites/renal.org/files/UKKA%20guideline_SGLT2i%20in%20adults%20with%20kidney%20disease%20v1%2018.10.21.pdf

OUP disclaimer: Oxford University Press makes no representation, express or implied, that the drug dosages are correct and that the recommendations are an exclusive or mandatory course of care. All health professionals reading this text have a responsibility to evaluate its appropriateness and take the individual needs of the patient into account.

Local trust guidelines: please refer to your local guidelines as necessary.

Overview

Chronic kidney disease (CKD) refers to an abnormality of renal function or structure, present for >3 months. The underlying cause of CKD should be established to ensure optimal management.

Terminology

- **eGFR:** this refers to estimated glomerular filtration rate, which is the standardized result calculated by laboratories when a serum creatinine level is requested
- **GFR category:** this refers to the internationally approved GFR categories of CKD which are explained in Fig. 47.1.

Diagnosis

History/diagnostic criteria

The causes of CKD are broad and the symptoms may be non-specific. Diagnoses that increase the risk of CKD include:

- Diabetes mellitus (DM)
- Hypertension
- Previous AKI in the last 3 years
- Cardiovascular disease
- Structural renal tract disease, recurrent renal calculi, or prostatic hypertrophy
- Multisystem disease with potential for renal involvement, e.g. systemic lupus erythematosus
- Gout
- Family history of end-stage kidney disease (GFR category G5) or hereditary kidney disease, e.g. polycystic kidney disease
- Incidental finding of haematuria or proteinuria.

All patients with these risk factors should be tested for CKD at presentation.

Patients on nephrotoxic drugs (e.g. ciclosporin, tacrolimus, lithium, NSAIDs) should have their eGFR monitored at least annually.

CKD is classified according to eGFR and ACR (Fig. 47.1):

- ↑ ACR and ↓ eGFR are independently associated with adverse outcomes
- Interpret the eGFR with caution at extremes of muscle mass (↓ muscle mass leads to overestimation of the eGFR and the converse is true of ↑ muscle mass)
- Patients with DM, CKD, or suspicion of CKD should be monitored for proteinuria
- Use urine ACR to detect proteinuria (>3mg/mmol):
  - If initial ACR is 3–70mg/mmol, confirm with an early morning sample
  - If initial ACR is >70mg/mmol, a repeat sample is not required

Examination

The patient may have examination findings related to the underlying cause, signs related to management, or stigmata of complications of CKD:

- Signs related to the underlying cause:
  - Polycystic kidney disease (MR, bilateral palpable flank masses with hepatomegaly if liver cysts)
  - Obstructive uropathy (palpable, distended bladder)
- Signs related to management:
  - Cushingoid from steroids
  - Peritoneal dialysis catheter
  - Fistula or vascular access route for haemodialysis
  - Parathyroidectomy scar; abdominal scar or palpable transplanted kidney from transplant
- Signs related to complications:
  - Anaemia: pallor, angular stomatitis, koilonychia
  - Fluid status: signs of peripheral or pulmonary oedema
  - Uraemia: excoriations, Lindsay's nails (proximal half of the nail appears white while the distal half appears reddish brown with a sharp demarcation between the halves)
  - Cachexia or malnutrition.

Prognosis of CKD by GFR and Albuminuria categories: KDIGO 2012			Persistent albuminuria categories Description and range		
			A1	A2	A3
			Normal to mildly increased	Moderately increased	Severely increased
			<30 mg/g <3 mg/mmol	30–300 mg/g 3–30 mg/mmol	>300 mg/g >30 mg/mmo
GFR categories (ml/min/1.73m^2) Description and range					
G1	Normal or high	≥90			
G2	Mildly decreased	60–89			
G3a	Mildly to moderately decreased	45–59			
G3b	Moderately to severely decreased	30–44			
G4	Severely decreased	15–29			
G5	kidney failure	<15			

Low risk (if no other markers of kidney disease, no CKD)
Moderately increased risk   High risk   Very high risk

Fig. 47.1 Classification of CKD and risk of adverse outcome.

Reprinted with permission from Kidney Disease: Improving Global Outcomes (KDIGO) CKD Work Group. KDIGO 2012 Clinical Practice Guideline for the Evaluation and Management of Chronic Kidney Disease. Kidney inter., Suppl. 2013; 3: 1–150.

Investigations

Bedside

- Blood pressure
- Urine (urinalysis, MC&S, ACR, Bence Jones protein).
- If proteinuria is found incidentally on urinalysis, calculate eGFR and check urine ACR:
  - Persistent microscopic haematuria (1+ or greater) should raise a suspicion of urinary tract malignancy and be followed up annually.

Bloods

See Table 47.1.

Imaging

Consider renal ultrasound if:

- Symptoms of obstructive uropathy
- Macroscopic, or persistent microscopic, haematuria
- Accelerated progression of CKD:
  - Decrease in eGFR of ≥25% and a change in GFR category within 12 months **OR**
  - Sustained decrease in eGFR of 15mL/min/1.73m^2 per year

- Family history of polycystic kidney disease and aged >20 years
- eGFR <30mL/min/1.73m²
- Renal biopsy is considered necessary:
  - Progressive disease, nephrotic syndrome, systemic disease, AKI not improving.

Table 47.1 Rationale for bloods for diagnosis and assessment of CKD

Test	Rationale
FBC	Anaemia is common in CKD. Screen 6–12-monthly
Iron studies and haematinics; tests for haemolysis; serum electrophoresis and free light chains	Important in the differentiation of the cause of anaemia Anaemia should be investigated if Hb <110g/L, or if the patient is symptomatic CKD should always be considered as a possible cause of anaemia when eGFR <60mL/min/1.73m²
Creatinine and urea	For diagnosis and monitoring
LFT	ALP may be ↑ in renal osteodystrophy
HbA1c	Diabetes is a risk factor for CKD
Calcium, phosphate, vitamin D, PTH, and calcidiol	Identifies mineral disturbances and vitamin D and PTH derangement
C-reactive protein	Assesses for inflammation
ANA, ANCA, anti-glomerular basement membrane, complement	Assesses for autoimmune causes of CKD

Management

Patient education

Patients should be prepared for the possibility of needing renal replacement therapy in progressive CKD.

Lifestyle and simple interventions

- Exercise
- Achieve a healthy weight
- Stop smoking
- All patients should receive dietary advice about potassium, phosphate, salt, and calorie intake. Patients with GFR category G4–5 should be seen by a specialist renal dietician to receive individualized information and support on dietary phosphate and protein management.

Pharmacological management

General

- Review potentially nephrotoxic medication and avoid NSAIDs
- Statin therapy, e.g. atorvastatin 20mg OD, and low-dose aspirin (75mg OD) in all patients with CKD
- Offer annual influenza and 23-valent polysaccharide pneumococcal vaccination with a booster every 5 years[1]
- Give a vitamin D supplement (cholecalciferol) if deficient.

Blood pressure control

- Use an ACE inhibitor, ARB, or direct renin inhibitor to control blood pressure in patients with any of the following:
  - CKD, hypertension, and ACR ≥30mg/mmol
  - CKD, diabetes, and ACR ≥3mg/mmol
  - CKD and ACR ≥70mg/mmol
- Blood pressure targets:
  - <140mmHg systolic, <90mmHg diastolic
  - If diabetic **OR** ACR ≥70mg/mmol, use target <130mmHg systolic, <80mmHg diastolic
- If patients do not fall into any of these categories, follow standard hypertension guidelines (see Chapter 6)
- Monitor eGFR and potassium before starting, 1–2 weeks after starting, and after each dose increase
- Do not use these medications if pre-treatment potassium >5mmol/L
- Stop medications if potassium >6mmol/L.

Electrolyte imbalances

- Hyperphosphataemia in patients with GFR category G4–5 should be managed with phosphate binders such as calcium acetate, 1 tablet with every meal
- Consider sodium bicarbonate if GFR category G4–5 and serum bicarbonate <20mmol/L.

SGLT2 inhibitors

- Start an SGLT2 inhibitor, e.g. dapagliflozin 10mg, if ACR ≥25

1 NICE Clinical Knowledge Summaries. Immunizations – pneumococcal: summary. 2016. Available at: https://cks.nice.org.uk/immunizations-pneumococcal#!topicSummary

- If commenced, patients should be monitored for hypovolemia and worsening of eGFR
- Advise that the medication should be held if the patient feels unwell, becomes dehydrated, or has reduced food intake. This is due to the risk of euglycaemic DKA.

Psychosocial considerations

- Anxiety, depression, and fatigue are common.

Complications

- Acute-on-chronic kidney disease
- Cardiovascular disease:
  - ↑ mortality associated with worsening renal function is largely secondary to cardiovascular disease
- Anaemia:
  - If eGFR is <60mL/min/1.73m^2, CKD may be the cause but other causes of anaemia should also be considered
  - Treat iron deficiency; oral iron supplements are usually sufficient if the patient is not on dialysis
  - Offer erythropoietin stimulating agents if the patient is likely to benefit in terms of quality of life and physical function
  - Avoid blood transfusion, particularly if transplantation is a treatment option, due to the risk of allosensitization
- Renal mineral and bone disorder:
  - Disturbance in vitamin D, calcium, PTH, and phosphate metabolism due to dysregulated homeostasis
- Peripheral neuropathy and myopathy (due to uraemia)
- Malignancy:
  - The exact cause is unknown, but end-stage kidney disease patients may have an ↑ risk of malignancy, particularly renal and thyroid
- Renal replacement therapy:
  - Dialysis or transplantation.

Monitoring and follow-up

- Monitor CKD with eGFR and ACR at least annually:
  - Monitor multiple times a year if high risk or very high risk (Fig. 47.1)
- Screen for anaemia at least annually in patients with GFR category G3 and at least biannually in patients with GFR category G4–5 not on dialysis
- Monitor serum potassium 2–4 times a year.[2] Also check before starting an ACE inhibitor, 1–2 weeks later and after every dose change
- Monitor calcium, phosphate, ALP, PTH, and 25-hydroxyvitamin D (calcidiol) levels if GFR G4–5.

2 UK Kidney Association. Clinical practice guidelines: treatment of acute hyperkalaemia in adults. 2020. Available at: https://ukkidney.org/sites/renal.org/files/RENAL%20ASSOCIATION%20HYPERKALAEMIA%20GUIDELINE%202020.pdf

Specialist renal referral

Refer if CKD with:

- eGFR reduction ≥25% causing a change in eGFR category in the last year
- eGFR falling ≥15mL/min/1.73m^2 per year
- ACR ≥70mg/mmol (unless secondary to diabetes)
- ACR ≥30mg/mmol with haematuria
- Resistant hypertension (poorly controlled on at least four antihypertensive medications)
- Rare or genetic cause
- Suspected renal artery stenosis.

Specialist urology referral

Refer if CKD with:

- Renal outflow obstruction

Special considerations

Pregnancy and breastfeeding

Many drugs may not be suitable for use in pregnancy and breastfeeding, while others require dose adjustment. See Table 47.2.

Table 47.2 Summary of safety of drugs used in CKD in pregnancy and breastfeeding

Drug	Safe in pregnancy?	Safe in breastfeeding?
Angiotensin-2 receptor antagonists and ACE inhibitors	Avoid in pregnancy unless essential	Information is limited; not recommended in breastfeeding
SGLT2 inhibitors	Avoid	Avoid
Statins	Avoid in pregnancy (discontinue 3 months prior to attempting to conceive)	Manufacturer advises to avoid; no information available
Antiplatelet medication (aspirin)	Use doses with caution during third trimester Avoid analgesic doses if possible in last few weeks	Avoid; possible risk of Reye's syndrome
Vitamin D supplement (cholecalciferol)	High doses teratogenic in animals but therapeutic doses unlikely to be harmful	Caution with high doses; may cause hypercalcaemia in infant—monitor serum calcium concentration
Vaccinations	Inactivated vaccines not known to be harmful	Inactivated vaccines not known to be harmful

Hepatic and renal impairment

Be aware that most drugs will need dose adjustment in accordance with the severity of impairment. The Renal Drug Handbook/Database is a key resource for safe prescribing in CKD; most hospitals will have this, usually via the pharmacy or the renal team.

Further reading

1. NICE Clinical Knowledge Summaries (2021). Chronic kidney disease: background. Available at: https://cks.nice.org.uk/chronic-kidney-disease#!background
2. The Renal Drug Database. Available at: https://renaldrugdatabase.com
3. KDIGO (2012). 2012 Clinical Practice Guideline for the evaluation and management of chronic kidney disease. Available at: https://kdigo.org/wp-content/uploads/2017/02/KDIGO_2012_CKD_GL.pdf

Chapter 48

Hyperkalaemia

Guideline:
UK Kidney Association (Treatment of acute hyperkalaemia in adults): https://ukkidney.org/sites/renal.org/files/RENAL%20ASSOCIATION%20HYPERKALAEMIA%20GUIDELINE%202020.pdf

OUP disclaimer: Oxford University Press makes no representation, express or implied, that the drug dosages are correct and that the recommendations are an exclusive or mandatory course of care. All health professionals reading this text have a responsibility to evaluate its appropriateness and take the individual needs of the patient into account.

Local trust guidelines: please refer to your local guidelines as necessary.

Overview

Hyperkalaemia is potentially a life-threatening emergency. Common underlying causes include acute or chronic renal impairment, inappropriate potassium supplementation, and drug side effects. In severe cases, urgent treatment is required to prevent arrhythmias.

Diagnosis

History/diagnostic criteria

The severity of hyperkalaemia can be categorized according to serum potassium levels and the presence of ECG changes (Table 48.1). In an emergency, a quick estimation of serum potassium can be achieved with blood gas testing, but a laboratory specimen should always be sent for confirmation.

Patients with hyperkalaemia may be asymptomatic, or the following symptoms and signs may be present:

- Arrhythmias
- Muscular weakness
- Paraesthesiae
- Chest pain
- Palpitations
- Syncope
- Breathlessness.

Table 48.1 Severity of hyperkalaemia according to serum potassium level

Mild	5.5–5.9mmol/L
Moderate	6.0–6.4mmol/L
Severe	≥6.5mmol/L

Predisposing factors

- CKD
- Dialysis patients; non-compliance, missed or inadequate dialysis sessions
- AKI
- Nephrotoxic medications (ACE inhibitor, e.g. ramipril; ARBs, e.g. losartan; NSAIDs, e.g. ibuprofen)
- Cardiac failure
- Diabetes mellitus (use of ACE inhibitors, diabetic ketoacidosis)
- Liver disease (use of aldosterone antagonists, hepatorenal failure)
- Adrenal insufficiency.

Examination

Systematically examine the patient using an ABCDE approach (Table 48.2).

Investigations

- **ECG:** all patients with moderate or severe hyperkalaemia should have a 12-lead ECG (Fig. 48.1).

The ECG may be normal, even in severe hyperkalaemia.

- **Bloods:**
  - Stratify severity by serum potassium concentration (see Table 48.1)
  - U&E, LFT, creatine kinase, bone profile, and magnesium; VBG for acid–base assessment.

Table 48.2 Hyperkalaemia examination findings

B	• Pulmonary oedema (secondary to renal disease) • Hyperventilation and Kussmaul's breathing (secondary to acidosis)
C	• Irregular pulse • Third heart sound • Raised JVP
E	• Pitting oedema • Arteriovenous fistula or other evidence of CKD, such as transplant scarring or ballotable kidneys • Stigmata of chronic liver disease

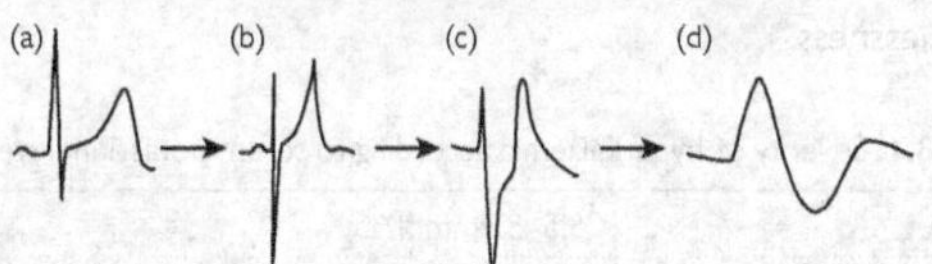

Fig. 48.1 Typical ECG changes in hyperkalaemia. (a) A normal complex. (b) Absence of P waves, tenting of T waves. (c) Broadening of the QRS complex. (d) Sine wave appearance. These changes typically follow a progressive pattern as the severity of hyperkalaemia increases.

Pseudohypokalaemia

- Sample haemolysis and long processing times can cause falsely high potassium results. To prevent this, take blood from large veins, avoid small needles and extended tourniquet time, and process the sample promptly
- A high platelet or cell count may also cause pseudohyperkalaemia. Repeat the bloods using a lithium-heparin tube (plasma sample) to check. A plasma value ≥0.4mmol/L lower than serum suggests the diagnosis.

Call for help?

Any clinical concerns should be escalated immediately to senior medical staff as patients may require referral to high dependency care.

Management

- **Mild hyperkalaemia without ECG changes:** step 5 only
- **In all other cases:** treat urgently starting from step 1.

Acute management

Step 1: protect the heart if there are ECG changes of hyperkalaemia

- 10mL 10% calcium chloride IV over 5–10 minutes **OR**
- 30mL 10% calcium gluconate IV over 5–10 minutes.

IV calcium salts antagonize cardiac membrane excitability and protect against arrhythmias. The dose can be repeated after 5–10 minutes if changes persist. The duration of action is 30–60 minutes.

> It is important that patients have ongoing cardiac monitoring during the calcium injection to monitor for arrhythmias.

Step 2: shift potassium into cells

- 10 units IV short-acting insulin (e.g. Actrapid®) in either:
  - 50mL 50% dextrose **OR**
  - 125mL 20% glucose
- Give over 15–30 minutes via a large vein
- Check CBG prior to the treatment. If <7mmol/L start an infusion of 10% dextrose at a rate of 50mL/hour for 5 hours. Monitor for hypoglycaemia by testing CBG at 0, 15, 30, 60, 120 minutes, and then monitor for up to 12 hours post infusion.
- In severe cases, a 10–20mg salbutamol nebulizer may be considered as an *additional* treatment. This therapy is effective within 30–60 minutes and lasts for 4–6 hours.

> Insulin-dextrose is maximally effective within 45–180 minutes. A repeat potassium level should therefore be checked between 60 and 180 minutes after the drugs are given. A reduction of approximately 1.0mmol/L is expected.

Step 3: remove potassium from the body

- Consider the need for a cation-exchange resin such as calcium resonium 15g orally or 30g rectally (do not use in severe cases due to slow onset of action)
- Refractory cases may require haemofiltration or dialysis, which may also be considered during a cardiac arrest suspected to be due to hyperkalaemia.

Treatment after stabilization

Step 4: monitor serum potassium levels

- After the effect of treatment has subsided, hyperkalaemia may recur. It is therefore advisable to monitor serum potassium levels regularly

- Patients with severe hyperkalaemia, or hyperkalaemia accompanied by ECG changes should have (at least) three-lead cardiac monitoring and consideration of transfer to a higher dependency unit.

Step 5: prevent recurrence

- Review potential causative agents and monitor renal function in patients being treated with drugs that can cause hyperkalaemia
- Request a dietician review.

Special considerations

Renal patients

If the patient is receiving regular dialysis, has advanced CKD, or severe AKI (especially if oligo-/anuric), urgently inform the local renal team (or intensive care, depending on local availability) in case emergency dialysis is required.

> If the patient is receiving sodium bicarbonate as part of their renal management, do not give sodium bicarbonate through the same IV line as calcium due to the risk of insoluble calcium salts forming in the bloodstream.

Further reading

1. UK Kidney Association (2020). Emergency management of hyperkalaemia in adults (algorithm, appendix 6). Available at: https://ukkidney.org/sites/renal.org/files/RENAL%20ASSOCIATION%20HYPERKALAEMIA%20GUIDELINE%202020.pdf

Part 8

Neurology

Chapter 49

Acute encephalitis

Guideline:
Association of British Neurologists, British Infection Association (Management of suspected viral encephalitis in adults): https://www.journalofinfection.com/article/S0163-4453(11) 00563-9/pdf

OUP disclaimer: Oxford University Press makes no representation, express or implied, that the drug dosages are correct and that the recommendations are an exclusive or mandatory course of care. All health professionals reading this text have a responsibility to evaluate its appropriateness and take the individual needs of the patient into account.

Local trust guidelines: please refer to your local guidelines as necessary.

Overview

Acute encephalitis refers to inflammation of the brain parenchyma. Causes include:

- Infectious: viral, bacterial, fungal, parasitic
- Post-infectious e.g. acute disseminated encephalomyelitis (ADEM)
- Antibody mediated e.g. by voltage-gated potassium channel (VGKC) antibodies.

HSV is the most commonly diagnosed cause of encephalitis and this presumed diagnosis should be treated in the immediate management of suspected infectious encephalitis. Untreated, HSV encephalitis mortality is >70%, but this reduces to 20–30% with IV aciclovir treatment.

Diagnosis

History

- Febrile or flu-like illness (often prodromal)
- Headache
- Altered/bizarre behaviour
- Change in cognition
- Change in personality
- ↓ GCS score
- Seizures
- Focal neurology.

Important points to elicit in history

- History of Immunocompromise/HIV status
- Travel and vaccination history
- Bites and animal contact
- Unwell contacts
- Collateral history if patient is cognitively impaired or has a ↓ GCS score.

Examination

Examine the patient using an ABCDE approach (Table 49.1). A mini mental state examination or other form of cognitive assessment is also important.

Table 49.1 Acute encephalitis examination findings

A/B/C	• Signs of septic shock, e.g. tachycardia, hypotension
D	• Meningism, e.g. neck stiffness, positive Kernig's sign, positive Brudzinski's sign (see Chapter 52) • Focal neurology (often upper motor neuron) • ↓ GCS score • Pyrexia
E	• Papilloedema • Bites • Rashes • Needle track marks

Investigations

Bedside

- Viral swabs:
  - Swab vesicles if rash present
  - Consider throat/rectal swab for enterovirus.

Bloods

- FBC, U&E, LFT, CRP, and coagulation profile
- Blood cultures
- Serum glucose and protein (paired with CSF)
- HIV testing in all patients.

Imaging

- CT head:
  - If ↑ intracranial pressure is suspected clinically, a CT head must be performed prior to lumbar puncture (LP).

Other

- LP:
  - Should be done as soon as possible but do not delay treatment if it cannot be done immediately
  - Ensure adequate reversal of anticoagulation prior to performing
  - Include viral PCR for HSV1, HSV2, VZV, and enterovirus:
    - These tests will identify 90% of cases of viral encephalitis
    - Cerebrospinal fluid (CSF) PCR for HSV has a sensitivity and specificity >95% if done between days 2 and 10 of the illness in immunocompetent adults
  - Consider further viral and antibody testing as per the advice of local microbiology/infectious disease/neurology teams
  - See Table 49.2.

Table 49.2 LP interpretation in viral encephalitis

Test	Result suggestive of viral encephalitis
CSF opening pressure	↔ or ↑
CSF colour	Clear
CSF protein	Mildly ↑
CSF/serum glucose ratio	↔
CSF white cell count	Moderately ↑
CSF lactate	<2mmol/L rules out a bacterial cause
Bacterial cultures	No growth

Normal CSF does **not** rule out HSV encephalitis—up to 10% of initial LPs are normal. If clinical suspicion is high, the LP should be repeated within 24–48 hours.

- MRI brain:
  - Within 24–48 hours if diagnosis is uncertain—more sensitive and specific than CT
  - Cingulate gyrus and medial temporal lobe oedema ± haemorrhage or restricted diffusion are suggestive of HSV encephalitis
  - If unable to tolerate MRI, perform a CT head with contrast
- EEG:
  - If considering a possible psychiatric diagnosis, encephalopathic changes on EEG may help to differentiate
  - Subclinical seizure activity will also show on EEG.

Management

Acute management

IV aciclovir

- Must give empirical treatment of IV aciclovir 10mg/kg TDS if:
  - Initial CSF or imaging results suggest viral encephalitis
  - Results will not be available within 6 hours
  - The patient is very unwell or deteriorating
- Continue IV aciclovir for 14–21 days, then repeat the LP to confirm CSF is negative for HSV PCR
- If HSV PCR is still positive, continue IV aciclovir and repeat LP weekly until negative.

Steroids

- Steroids should not be used routinely in HSV encephalitis
- However, there is an overlap between the presentations of encephalitis and meningitis, and many patients are given steroids (and antibiotics) as empirical treatment for meningitis (see Chapter 52).

Supportive management

- IV fluids and correction of electrolyte imbalances
- Seizure control (see Chapter 50).

Referrals

- Urgent intensive therapy unit (ITU) review if decreasing GCS score
- Neurology review within 24 hours
- Notify infectious disease team if an infectious cause is suspected.

Treatment after stabilization

- Must have outpatient neurology follow-up with ongoing rehabilitation and therapy input
- Make patient aware of support provided by voluntary sector organizations, e.g. Encephalitis Society

Special considerations

Returning traveller

- If returning from malaria endemic areas, do rapid malaria antigen testing and three thick and thin blood films
- Get advice from infectious disease team early as the patient may require additional investigations.

Immunocompromised

- Encephalitis should always be considered in immunocompromised patients with an altered mental state, even if the features seem atypical
- It may be appropriate to do a CT scan before the LP, as severely immunocompromised patients may have lesions on CT without focal neurology. An MRI should also be done urgently
- Consider that atypical pathogens may be responsible for encephalitis in an immunocompromised patient, e.g. *Cryptococcus neoformans* or *Toxoplasma gondii*; therefore, discuss with microbiology **prior** to sending CSF as additional tests may be needed.

Antibody mediated

No pathognomonic signs, however the following should raise suspicion and lead to a discussion with neurology:

- Subacute presentation (weeks–months)
- Orofacial dyskinesia (involuntary movements of the mouth or face)
- Choreoathetosis (rapid or slow involuntary movements)
- Faciobrachial dystonia (involuntary jerking of the arm and the same side of the face)
- Hyponatraemia
- Intractable seizures.

Further reading

1. BMJ Best Practice (2020). Encephalitis. Available at: https://bestpractice.bmj.com/topics/en-uk/436

Chapter 50

Epilepsy

Guideline:
NICE CG137 (Epilepsies: diagnosis and management): https://www.nice.org.uk/guidance/cg137

OUP disclaimer: Oxford University Press makes no representation, express or implied, that the drug dosages are correct and that the recommendations are an exclusive or mandatory course of care. All health professionals reading this text have a responsibility to evaluate its appropriateness and take the individual needs of the patient into account.

Local trust guidelines: please refer to your local guidelines as necessary.

Overview

Epilepsy is a neurological disorder characterized by recurrent unprovoked seizures. Although common, the diagnosis can be difficult to make, with up to 30% of patients incorrectly labelled with epilepsy. Epilepsy can cause status epilepticus which is a medical emergency. This is defined as a seizure lasting >5 minutes or when a patient has more than one seizure within 5 minutes, without regaining full or baseline consciousness.

Diagnosis

History

First seizure

Any patient who presents to the emergency department with a suspected seizure needs to be assessed to rule out other causes of TLoC (see Chapter 9), such as vasovagal or cardiac syncope, or non-epileptic attack disorder (also known as psychogenic seizures or pseudosyncope).

- Establish if loss of consciousness occurred and the duration
- Get a clear picture of the events before, during, and after the seizure, obtaining information from any eyewitnesses as necessary. For example, in tonic–clonic seizures:
  - Before: any warning signs, abnormal sensations, automatisms, or emotional change (aura if followed by a focal seizure)
  - During: ↑ tone and shaking of the upper and lower limbs, urinary incontinence (may also occur in non-epileptic events), and tongue biting
  - After: period of confusion or ↓ GCS score
- Check for precipitating factors such as alcohol or drug abuse, or infections.

Known epilepsy

- Usual seizure type and frequency, usual antiepileptic medications, and any recent changes
- Description of events pre, during, and post seizure. Was this a typical seizure for the patient?
- Establish any precipitating factors. In particular, check compliance with medication.

Examination

All patients presenting with a seizure should undergo a cardiovascular, neurological, and mental state examination.

Investigations

Investigations aim to rule out reversible causes of seizures (such as infection, hypoglycaemia, electrolyte disturbance or drug misuse) and reduce diagnostic uncertainty.

Bedside

- ECG to screen for common causes of cardiac syncope
- Urinary drug screens should be considered where appropriate.

Bloods

- FBC
- U&E
- Creatine kinase
- Bone profile
- Magnesium
- Glucose
- CRP
- Lactate (VBG)—raised lactate can be supportive in the diagnosis of seizures.

Imaging

- Consider chest X-ray to check for signs of aspiration
- Consider CT head, particularly if first seizure, to rule out acute intracranial pathology such as haemorrhage.

If the diagnosis is not clear from the history or eyewitness account, the following can be considered in specialist clinics as part of the patient's follow-up:

Other

EEG

- Should only be carried out to support a suspected diagnosis of epilepsy. It should not be used in isolation to confirm or refute the diagnosis, or if the history suggests the patient had a syncopal event, due to the likelihood of a false-positive result
- If a standard EEG has not been helpful in contributing to the diagnosis, a sleep-deprived EEG should be carried out in preference to repeat EEGs
- Longer-term ambulatory monitoring or video-telemetry can be considered if despite performing EEG the diagnosis remains uncertain.

MRI brain

Useful in identifying structural abnormalities.
It is particularly recommended in:

- New-onset seizures in an adult
- Patients aged <2 years
- Focal-onset seizures
- Continuation of seizures despite first-line investigations.

Classification

Seizures are typically classified in accordance with the area of onset, level of awareness (in focal seizures), and presence of motor symptoms. See Table 50.1.

Table 50.1 Seizure classification

Type of seizure		Symptoms
Focal (Awareness unimpaired)	Motor	*Automatisms:* lip smacking, chewing movements *Atonic:* sudden loss of tone in one part of the body *Clonic:* jerking movements of one part of the body *Myoclonic:* brief shock-like jerks of a muscle group *Tonic:* sudden increase in tone, stiffness of one part of the body
	Non- motor	Abnormal feelings or sensations such as an abdominal rising, déjà vu, sudden intense emotions, unusual tastes or smells, visual disturbances such as hallucinations or flashing lights or feelings of numbness or tingling
	Focal to bilateral	Previously termed secondary generalized seizures, typically present with an aura followed by a tonic–clonic seizure
Generalized (Awareness impaired)	Motor	*Tonic–clonic:* loss of consciousness with stiffness, generalized limb jerking, followed by a post ictal phase *Clonic/tonic/myoclonic/atonic:* as described above but affecting the entire body
	Non- motor	*Absence:* cease activity, appear blank as if they are daydreaming or staring, lasting a few seconds

Management

Acute epileptic seizure

Community

General management

- Do not restrain the patient
- Move anything which may be potentially dangerous, e.g. hot drinks, to prevent the patient from harming themselves as they fit
- Try to protect their head with a pillow or towel if possible, and loosen any clothing around their neck
- Once the seizure terminates, place the patient in the recovery position to await transfer to hospital. Record the length of the seizure.

If the patient is not known to have epilepsy

- Call an ambulance

Patient with epilepsy in status epilepticus

- If seizures are prolonged (continuing for >5 minutes) or repeated (≥3 seizures within 1 hour), give 10mg buccal midazolam or 10mg rectal diazepam. These doses may be repeated after 10 minutes if needed
- Call an ambulance if:
  - Seizure continues 5 minutes after medication has been given **OR**
  - The patient often has repeated seizures **OR**
  - The patient has previously had status epilepticus **OR**
  - This is the first time that antiseizure rescue medication has been given **OR**
  - There is any concern about the patient's clinical state.

Hospital

Patients in hospital with self-terminating seizures may not require any specific management. For the management of status epilepticus, see Table 50.2. **Contact an anaesthetist early for support**.

Table 50.2 ABCDE approach to the inpatient management of status epilepticus

A	Airway management with anaesthetic support
B	Measure respiratory rate and oxygen saturations Give 100% oxygen
C	Measure pulse and blood pressure Gain wide-bore IV access and send bloods for FBC, U&E, LFT, glucose, CRP, and VBG
D	Check CBG Measure temperature
E	Give IV lorazepam 4mg (dose can be repeated after 10–20min) IV diazepam can be used if lorazepam is unavailable, or buccal midazolam if IV access has not been possible If no improvement, commence a phenytoin infusion (20mg/kg, maximum 2g) at a rate of 50mg/min If ineffective, consider general anaesthesia If there is evidence of alcohol excess or malnutrition, prescribe 50mL 50% dextrose and/or IV thiamine (Pabrinex®)

Treatment after stabilization

- Perform investigations as described previously if not already completed
- All patients who have had a suspected first seizure should be seen urgently by a neurologist—usually as a referral to the 'first fit' clinic
- Information on minimizing the risk of future seizures and safety advice should be given prior to referral.

An eyewitness account is essential. If referring to a 'first fit' clinic, the patient should be advised that it is preferable for the eyewitness to accompany them.

Patient education

Safety advice

Should be discussed with all patients:

- Driving (see Chapter 115):
  - First seizure: do not drive for 6 months
  - Established epilepsy: should be seizure free for 1 year before driving may be considered
- Injury prevention: advice on water safety (patients should shower rather than take baths and should swim only if epilepsy is well controlled and a lifeguard is present), taking care with heights (e.g. using ladders), and not locking doors.

Other important information

Usually discussed in specialist clinics:

- Diagnosis, medication, and side effects, including the importance of family planning
- Trigger avoidance such as sleep deprivation, stress, alcohol, and drugs
- Sudden unexplained death in epilepsy, how to minimize the risk through optimum seizure control
- Voluntary organizations and further sources of support.

Psychological interventions

- CBT and relaxation therapies can be used as adjuncts to antiepileptic drug (AED) treatment.

Pharmacological interventions

- AED treatment should be initiated by specialists, and should be individualized according to seizure type, the patient, and their comorbidities. First-line treatment options are listed in Table 50.3
- AED therapy should be commenced only after the second seizure, unless:
  - EEG shows epileptic activity
  - The patient has a neurological deficit
  - The patient (or their carer) finds the risk of a second seizure unacceptable
  - Neuroimaging shows a structural abnormality
  - The first seizure was status epilepticus which required AED therapy to control
- AED monotherapy is ideal, following the guidance in Table 50.3. When switching AED, the second AED should be escalated to a tolerated adequate dose, before the first is withdrawn

- Withdrawal of AEDs should be undertaken only under the guidance of specialists, with patients fully informed of the risks and benefits, and only in those who have been unprovoked seizure free for >2 years.

Table 50.3 AED therapy of choice by seizure type

Seizure type	First-line treatment options	
Focal	Carbamazepine Lamotrigine	
Generalized tonic–clonic	Sodium valproate Lamotrigine	Carbamazepine Oxcarbazepine
Absence	Ethosuximide Sodium valproate	
Myoclonic	Sodium valproate Topiramate	Levetiracetam
Tonic/atonic	Sodium valproate	Lamotrigine

Monitoring and follow-up

All patients should be reviewed at least annually.

Special considerations

Contraception

- Female patients with epilepsy should be counselled on the possible interactions of their AED with contraception. Emphasis should also be placed on the importance of using barrier protection in addition to oral hormonal therapy.

Pregnancy

- High-dose folic acid (5mg OD) is recommended in all women planning a pregnancy when using AEDs
- Sodium valproate should be avoided in women of childbearing age, unless alternatives are not available, due to the high risk of teratogenicity
- Breastfeeding while taking AEDs is usually safe. The risk of each AED to the baby should be considered and a discussion should be held with the patient regarding the specific risks and benefits.
- Clinicians should not forget to give additional safety advice to parents with epilepsy regarding safety precautions when caring for their newborn.

Further reading

1. International League Against Epilepsy website. Available at: https://www.ilae.org/
2. Epilepsy Society website. Available at: http://www.epilepsysociety.org.uk
3. Epilepsy Action website. Available at: http://www.epilepsy.org.uk

Chapter 51

Headache

Guideline:
NICE CG150 (Headaches in over 12s: diagnosis and management): https://www.nice.org.uk/guidance/cg150

OUP disclaimer: Oxford University Press makes no representation, express or implied, that the drug dosages are correct and that the recommendations are an exclusive or mandatory course of care. All health professionals reading this text have a responsibility to evaluate its appropriateness and take the individual needs of the patient into account.

Local trust guidelines: please refer to your local guidelines as necessary.

Overview

Headache is the commonest neurological symptom which presents to both primary and secondary care. The causes can be classified into primary (underlying aetiology unknown) and secondary (when attributed to an underlying disease or disorder).

Diagnosis

Differential diagnosis

- Primary headache disorders
  - Migraine
  - Tension-type headache
  - Cluster headache and other trigeminal autonomic cephalalgias
- Secondary headache disorders
  - Iatrogenic
    - Medication overuse headache
  - Inflammatory conditions
    - Giant cell arteritis
  - Raised intracranial pressure
    - Tumour/metastatic disease
    - Abscess
    - Benign intracranial hypertension
  - Central nervous system infections
    - Meningitis
    - Encephalitis
  - Vascular disorders
    - Haemorrhage: extradural/subdural haematoma/subarachnoid haemorrhage
    - Thrombosis: cortical vein thrombosis, venous sinus thrombosis, stroke.

Table 51.1 Clinical features of key differential diagnoses for a headache

	Tension type	Migraine	Cluster	Medication overuse headache
Site	Bilateral	Unilateral or bilateral	Unilateral (around/above the eye)	Variable
Character	Mild–moderate band like pressure or tight sensation	Moderate to severe pulsating pain	Severe or very severe pain of a variable nature—may be burning, throbbing or sharp	Variable
Duration	30 minutes - continuous	4–72 hours	Up to 2 hours, but usually 30–90 minutes	Variable
Associated symptoms	Does not interfere with daily activities	Sensitivity to light/sound Nausea/vomiting Preceding aura (even without a headache)—lasting 5–60 minutes, with reversible symptoms such as: • Flashing lights, flickering spots/lines, or visual loss • Numbness or pins and needles • Speech disturbance	Autonomic symptoms on the same side as the headache such as nasal congestion or runny nose, red or watering eye, swollen eyelid, forehead sweating, miosis, and ptosis Patient is agitated and restless due to the pain	Headache developed/worsened after taking regular analgesics Triptans/ergots/opioids >10 days/month NSAIDs/paracetamol/aspirin >15 days/month
Subtypes	Chronic: 15 days per month for >3 months	Menstrual: migraines 2 days prior to, or within 3 days of starting menstruation for at least 2 out of 3 consecutive cycles Chronic: 15 days per month for >3 months		

History

Careful history taking is key to identifying the underlying cause

- Presenting complaint: headache features (Table 51.1)
- Past medical history
  - Previous headache disorders
  - Intracranial bleeds or thromboses
  - Procoagulant risk factors, e.g. cancer, factor V Leiden deficiency
  - Previous intracranial surgery
- Medications
  - Evidence of medication overuse. Ask particularly about:
    - Paracetamol, aspirin, and NSAIDs
    - Triptans
    - Opioids
    - Ergots, e.g. dihydroergotamine and ergotamine
    - Combination analgesics, e.g. co-codamol
  - Anticoagulants or antiplatelets increasing the risk of bleeding
  - Any regular medications the patient may use where headache is a side effect
- Family history
- Social history
  - Alcohol history (abuse can increase risk of traumatic haemorrhage)
  - Illicit drug use (could the headache be withdrawal related?)
  - Effect of headaches on activities of daily living
- Consider asking the patient to use a headache diary (minimum of 8 weeks) to look for patterns which may point towards a particular diagnosis. The diary should document frequency, duration, and severity of headache, associated symptoms, possible triggers, analgesia used, and any relationship of the headaches to the menstrual cycle.

Pain history

Don't forget the acronym 'SOCRATES':

- **S**ite: unilateral? Bilateral?
- **O**nset: sudden (thunderclap)? Gradual?
- **C**haracter: throbbing? Stabbing? Dull ache?
- **R**adiation: neck? Occiput? Eye?
- **A**ssociated symptoms: ⚑ symptoms? Nausea? Aura?
- **T**ime: duration? Episodic or continuous? Frequency? Relationship to menstrual cycle?
- **E**xacerbating and alleviating factors
- **S**everity: score out of 10.

Red flags

Beware of the following features in the history of a new-onset headache that can point towards a sinister underlying cause, for which you should consider urgent investigation or onward referral:

- ⚑ Fever, rash, or neck stiffness (suggestive of meningitis or infection; see Chapter 52)
- ⚑ Sudden-onset, reaching maximum intensity within 5 minutes (suggestive of subarachnoid haemorrhage)

- ⚑ New neurological or cognitive deficit, personality change, or ↓ level of consciousness (suggestive of intracranial haemorrhage, stroke, or space-occupying lesion; see Chapter 56)
- ⚑ Recent trauma (suggestive of traumatic haemorrhage, within the last 3 months)
- ⚑ Headache worsening with cough, sneeze, Valsalva, or posture (suggestive of ↑ intracranial pressure)
- ⚑ Severe eye pain or temporal artery tenderness (suggestive of other secondary headaches such as glaucoma or giant cell arteritis; see Chapter 84)
- ⚑ Vomiting
- ⚑ History of immunocompromise, previous or current malignancy (increases suspicion of intracranial infection or malignancy).

Examination

- A full neurological examination must be performed to elicit any focal deficits
- Assessment of cognitive function
- Ophthalmoscopy should assess for papilloedema
- If the history is suggestive, look for evidence of meningeal irritation (Kernig's or Brudzinski's signs; see Chapter 52) and a rash.

Investigations

Suspected primary headache disorders

Imaging

- Neuroimaging may be considered for a first bout of cluster headaches.

Suspected secondary headache disorders

Bedside

- Pyrexia, tachycardia, or hypotension may point towards meningitis.

Bloods

- FBC, CRP—elevated in infection
- ESR—elevated in temporal arteritis
- U&E and LFT function if prescribing antibiotics for suspected intracranial infection
- Coagulation profile—particularly if a patient is on anticoagulants and an intracranial haemorrhage is suspected.

Imaging

- CT head should be considered for anyone with ⚑ symptoms to assess for intracranial pathology.

Other

- LP as guided by specialists or senior clinicians:
  - Send for cell count, protein, glucose, Gram stain, and viral PCR in cases of suspected intracranial infection
  - Measure opening pressure
  - Xanthochromia if suspected subarachnoid haemorrhage.

Management

Primary headache disorders

Patient education

- In the management of all patients with headaches, ensure that the patient and their relatives are informed of the diagnosis, reassured that other pathology has been excluded, and given options for management
- Try to provide written information as well as details of support organizations
- Recommend to keep a headache diary.

Pharmacological management

See Table 51.2.

Table 51.2 Management of primary headache disorders

	Acute	Prophylactic
Tension	Aspirin/paracetamol/NSAIDs **Do not** offer opioids	Acupuncture (10 sessions over 5–8 weeks)
Migraine	Oral triptan, e.g. zolmitriptan 2.5mg + NSAID **OR** Oral triptan + paracetamol If the patient is able to tolerate only a single agent, consider triptan, high-dose aspirin (900mg), NSAID, or paracetamol If oral agents are not tolerated, consider IM metoclopramide or prochlorperazine +/- IM NSAID or nasal triptan Consider antiemetics in all patients	First line: topiramate (initial dose 25mg OD then titrated) or propranolol (80–240mg OD in divided doses) Second line: amitriptyline (initial dose 10–25mg OD then titrated) ± Riboflavin 400mg OD—can reduce migraine severity and frequency ± Acupuncture (10 sessions over 5–8 weeks) Review after 6 months of treatment
Menstrual-related migraine	Trial the above-listed migraine treatments	If acute treatments are ineffective, consider frovatriptan (2.5mg BD PO) or zolmitriptan (2.5mg BD–TDS PO) on the days of expected migraine If difficult to predict exact date of migraine onset, use for 2 days before menstruation is predicted to start, until 3 days after start of menstruation
Cluster	Oxygen (100% with a flow of at least 12L/min via a non-rebreathe mask, can be provided at home) SC (e.g. sumatriptan 6mg) or nasal (e.g. zolmitriptan 5mg) triptans	Verapamil—under the guidance of a specialist

Secondary headache disorders

Principles of management

- Stabilize the patient using an ABCDE approach, particularly if the GCS score is reduced, due to the risks of respiratory compromise. Involve higher level care if necessary
- Call for help: many secondary headaches are emergencies so ensure early escalation to a senior clinician and involve relevant specialities (e.g. neurosurgery, ophthalmology) as soon as possible
- Specific management will depend upon the identified underlying cause of the headache, and may include lifestyle advice, pharmacological interventions, or even surgery.

Medication overuse headache

- Advise the patient to stop taking the overused medication abruptly for at least 1 month
- Inform them that symptoms of headache may initially worsen before they improve
- Review after 4–8 weeks.

Special considerations

Specialist referral

- Migraine with any of the following atypical aura symptoms:
  - Motor weakness
  - Double vision
  - Unilateral visual symptoms
  - Poor balance
  - ↓ GCS score
  - Prolonged aura (>1 hour)
- For management of migraine prophylaxis in pregnancy
- For advice on cluster headache prophylaxis
- If patients have any ⚑ which might point towards a sinister underlying cause
- If medication overuse headache is due to opioid use
- Chronic migraine refractory to first-line treatments.

Pregnancy and women of childbearing age

Dosage adjustments may be necessary as per the BNF. Key points to remember include:

- Topiramate is teratogenic and may impair the effectiveness of some hormonal contraceptives. Women should receive careful counselling regarding appropriate contraception
- In the acute management of migraines, paracetamol is a safe treatment in pregnancy, but if this is ineffective, the risks of triptans and NSAIDs should be discussed and can be offered
- Seek specialist advice in pregnancy with the use of all prophylactic agents for the treatment of migraine
- Combined hormonal contraception is contraindicated for women who have migraine with aura.

Further reading

1. Manji H, Connolly S, Kitchen N, et al. (2014). Topics on headache. In: *Oxford Handbook of Neurology*, 2nd ed (Chapter 5). Oxford: Oxford University Press. Available at: https://doi.org/10.1093/med/9780199601172.003.0005_update_001

Chapter 52

Meningitis

Guideline:
British Infection Association (The UK joint specialist societies guideline on the diagnosis and management of acute meningitis or meningococcal sepsis in immunocompetent adults): https://www.journalofinfection.com/article/s0163-4453(16)00024-4/fulltext

OUP disclaimer: Oxford University Press makes no representation, express or implied, that the drug dosages are correct and that the recommendations are an exclusive or mandatory course of care. All health professionals reading this text have a responsibility to evaluate its appropriateness and take the individual needs of the patient into account.

Local trust guidelines: please refer to your local guidelines as necessary.

Overview

Meningitis is inflammation of the meninges which can be secondary to bacterial, viral, or fungal infection. Although rare, it is important to recognize and treat early, as patients can rapidly deteriorate. Meningococcal meningitis is one of the most severe forms, and is often associated with meningococcal septicaemia, characterized by a petechial rash and sepsis secondary to *Neisseria meningitides*. Other forms of meningitis are summarized in Table 52.1.

Table 52.1 Common causes of meningitis and populations most affected

Common causes of meningitis	Population most affected
HSV-1 and -2, enteroviruses, and VZV	Young adults
Neisseria meningitides	Young adults or immunocompromised
Streptococcus pneumoniae (pneumococcus)	Age >50 or immunocompromised
Listeria	Age >60 or immunocompromised (includes relative immunocompromise caused by alcohol dependence, diabetes mellitus, or malignancy)
Haemophilus influenzae	Immunocompromised
Cryptococcus	HIV-positive patients
TB	HIV-positive patients

Diagnosis

History

Patients with meningitis may present with an acute history of:

- Meningism characterized by a headache, neck stiffness, and photophobia
- Altered conscious level or focal neurology including seizures
- Fevers and rigors
- Non-blanching petechial rash (Fig. 52.1).

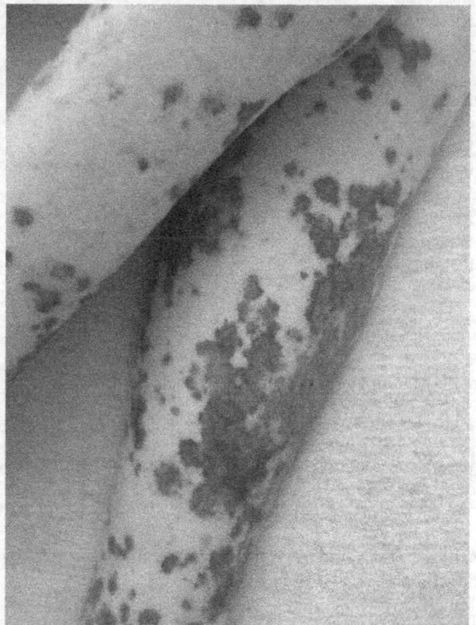

Fig. 52.1 Non-blanching petechial rash.

See colour plate 2.

Examination

All patients should be examined using the ABCDE approach. Findings are shown in Table 52.2.

Investigations

Investigations aim to diagnose infectious meningitis and to identify the organism responsible:

- **Nasopharyngeal swab** for meningococcal culture and enterovirus PCR
- **Bloods:** FBC, procalcitonin (if available—useful as it is specific for bacterial infections, if unavailable use CRP), LFT, U&E, coagulation profile, glucose, pneumococcal and meningococcal PCR, VBG with lactate and blood cultures

Table 52.2 Examination findings

A	Consider airway compromise if GCS score drops below 8		
C	Signs of septic shock (see Chapter 122): Hypotension Tachycardia Weak and thready pulse Prolonged capillary refill time Cool extremities		
D	↓ GCS score or coma		
	Motor M6 Obeys commands M5 Localizes to pain M4 Withdrawal from pain M3 Flexion to pain M2 Extension to pain M1 No motor response	*Verbal* V5 Orientated V4 Confused V3 Inappropriate words V2 Incomprehensible sounds V1 No verbal response	*Eyes* E4 Open spontaneously E3 Open to verbal command E2 Open to pain E1 No eye opening
E	Non-blanching petechial rash Fever Meningism (headache, neck stiffness, and photophobia) often with associated nausea and vomiting Kernig's sign (with the hip and knee flexed, extension at the knee causes pain and resistance) *and/or* Brudzinski's sign (when the neck is flexed the patients hips and knees flex due to neck stiffness)—both are highly specific signs but poorly sensitive		

- **CT head:** should be undertaken prior to LP if any of the following (indicating ↑ intracranial pressure) are present:
  - Focal neurology
  - Papilloedema
  - Seizures
  - GCS score <12
- **LP:** ideally within an hour of presentation **AND** prior to antibiotic administration **UNLESS**:
  - It is not possible to perform within an hour of admission **OR**
  - There is evidence of respiratory or cardiac compromise **OR**
  - Presence of severe sepsis or a rapidly evolving rash **OR**
  - There is infection at the site of LP **OR**
  - There is coagulopathy (see Box 52.1).

The following must be measured in the CSF:

- Opening pressure
- Glucose
- Protein
- Lactate (if antibiotics have not been given yet)

- MC&S
- PCR for pneumococci and meningococci
- PCR for enteroviruses, HSV-1 and -2, and VZV.

Table 52.3 shows LP findings in meningitis.

Table 52.3 Lumbar puncture findings in meningitis

	Normal	Bacterial	Viral	TB
Appearance	Clear	Turbid	Clear	Cloudy
Opening pressure (mmHg)	10–20	High	Normal/high	High
White blood cell count (cells/μL)	0–5	>100	10–1000	50–500
Cell type		Polymorphs	Lymphocytes	Lymphocytes
CSF protein	<45mg/dL	High	High	Very high
CSF glucose	>60% serum	Low	Normal	Low

Adapted from Table 19.4 from Wilkinson I et al (2018) Oxford Handbook of Clinical Medicine. Oxford: Oxford University Press, with permission from Oxford University Press.

Box 52.1 Lumbar puncture anticoagulation and antiplatelet considerations

- If the patient is being treated with prophylactic LWMH, the LP should not be performed until 12 hours after the last dose
- Post LP, prophylactic LWMH should not be given until at least 4 hours have elapsed
- For patients on warfarin, INR must be ≤1.4 before performing the LP. Patients on other anticoagulants should be discussed with a haematologist prior to performing an LP
- Aspirin and NSAIDs do not need to be held prior to the LP but clopidogrel should be held for 7 days prior to an LP unless a platelet transfusion or desmopressin has been administered following discussion with a haematologist. In the acute assessment of meningitis, the risk of a LP on clopidogrel must be weighed against the diagnostic benefits. This should be discussed with a senior clinician
- Platelet count should be ≥40 × 10^9/L.

Management

Call for help?

Meningitis and meningococcal septicaemia are medical emergencies and should be escalated to a senior clinician early.

Acute management

Pre-hospital

If meningitis is suspected in the community, antibiotics should be given urgently, e.g. IM/IV benzylpenicillin 1.2g, IM/IV ceftriaxone 2g, or IM/IV cefotaxime 2g. This should **not** delay transfer to hospital.

Emergency department

The mainstay of acute treatment is management of sepsis with:

Fluid resuscitation

Use crystalloids. A urinary catheter should be placed for accurate fluid balance measurements.

Antibiotics

Must be administered immediately after a LP and blood cultures, and at most within 1 hour of presentation, as per local guidance, e.g.:

- **Standard regimen:**
  - IV ceftriaxone 2g BD or IV cefotaxime 2g QDS
- **Penicillin/cephalosporin allergic:**
  - IV chloramphenicol 25mg/kg QDS
- **Immunocompromised or >60 years:**
  - As per **EITHER** standard **OR** penicillin/cephalosporin allergic regimen
    PLUS IV amoxicillin/ampicillin 2g, 4-hourly
- **If foreign travel within previous 6 months:**
  - Discuss with microbiology.

Steroids

- IV dexamethasone 10mg QDS within 12 hours of antibiotic administration. This should be continued for 4 days if pneumococcal disease is confirmed. For other causes, it should be stopped.

> Due to overlapping presentations, patients are often simultaneously tested and treated for meningitis and encephalitis (see Chapter 49).

Critical care admission

Escalation to critical care must be considered in all patients, particularly if they have:

- Rapidly evolving rash
- GCS score <12
- Organ support requirements
- Uncontrolled seizures.

> **Don't forget the 'Sepsis Six':** oxygen, fluid, and antibiotics **IN**; lactate, blood cultures, and urine output **OUT**.

Treatment after stabilization

Antibiotic therapy

- Liaise with local microbiology/infectious diseases teams and rationalize antibiotic therapy once an organism is confirmed
- Treatment is usually continued for 10–14 days unless a viral organism is found in which case antibiotics should be stopped.

Isolation

- All patients with suspected meningococcal meningitis should be isolated until they have received 24 hours of therapy or as per local policy.

Secondary prevention

- All cases must be notified to public health authorities
- Contact prophylaxis will be commenced by the consultant in the notified health protection team.

Screening for immunosuppression

- Test for HIV
- In any patient with more than one episode of meningitis or a family history of multiple episodes, further immunological investigations should be carried out.

Complications of meningitis

- Subdural empyema (suspect if persistent fever and new neurology develops)
- Seizures
- Hydrocephalus (suspect if ↓ consciousness)
- Cerebral venous sinus thrombosis (suspect if ↓ consciousness and new neurology develops)
- Cerebral ischaemia.

Complications of meningococcal sepsis

- Purpura fulminans (suspect if rapidly progressive rash)
- Septic shock.

Further reading

1. Wilkinson IB, Raine T, Wiles K, et al. (2017). Meningitis. In: *Oxford Handbook of Clinical Medicine*, 10th ed (pp. 822–3). Oxford: Oxford University Press. Available at: https://doi.org/10.1093/med/9780199689903.003.0019

Chapter 53

Metastatic spinal cord compression

Guideline:
NICE CG75 (Metastatic spinal cord compression in adults: risk assessment, diagnosis and management): https://www.nice.org.uk/guidance/cg75

OUP disclaimer: Oxford University Press makes no representation, express or implied, that the drug dosages are correct and that the recommendations are an exclusive or mandatory course of care. All health professionals reading this text have a responsibility to evaluate its appropriateness and take the individual needs of the patient into account.

Local trust guideline: please refer to your local guidelines as necessary.

Overview

Metastatic spinal cord compression (MSCC) is compression of the spinal cord due to tumour growth or pathological vertebral collapse. Pathology below L1 will produce cauda equina compression. MSCC is more common in lung, breast, prostate, renal, and thyroid malignancies, especially in patients with bone metastases. It can also occur in lymphoma and myeloma. MSCC should be considered in all patients with known cancer and it may be a presenting feature of a previously undiagnosed cancer.

Diagnosis is via MRI whole spine. The urgency of MRI is dependent on whether there are neurological symptoms or signs; the presence of these constitutes an emergency. All hospitals should have a point of contact available 24/7 to advise on MSCC (this is sometimes via the acute oncology team).

Diagnosis

History

Symptoms suggestive of spinal metastases:

- Pain in the cervical, thoracic, or lumbar spine
- Sudden onset, progressive, severe, or unremitting pain
- Spinal pain worsened by straining (e.g. with passing stool, coughing, sneezing)
- Nocturnal spinal pain preventing sleep
- Localized spinal tenderness.

Neurological symptoms or signs suggestive of MSCC:

- Limb weakness
- Difficulty walking
- Sensory loss
- Bladder or bowel dysfunction (e.g. retention of urine, incontinence, or constipation).

Other important information:

- Premorbid function (mobility, general fitness, performance status)
- Underlying cancer (when diagnosed, histology, previous treatments and response, extent of metastatic disease)
- Medication history: steroids, anticoagulants, and antiplatelets.

Examination

Perform a full neurological examination. Findings are shown in Table 53.1.

Table 53.1 Neurological examination findings in spinal cord compression

Tone	• Initial sign—tone ↓ below the lesion • Late sign—spasticity
Power	• Weakness below the lesion
Reflexes	• Initial sign—spinal shock phase—reflexes are ↓ • Late sign—reflexes are ↑ • In more gradual or incomplete compression, reflexes may be ↑ earlier • Extensor plantars
Sensation	• Look for a sensory level—pinprick, vibration, proprioception, and temperature • The absence of a sensory level does not exclude cord compression
Coordination	• Impaired, may be ataxic

Perform a rectal examination and specifically document anal tone (normal, reduced, or absent) and any sensory impairment.

Patients with MSCC may have autonomic dysreflexia. This tends to occur in the acute phase of paralysis or with high cord lesions (above T6). Signs include:

- Hypotension or hypertension
- Hypoventilation
- Bradycardia.

Investigations

Bloods

- FBC, U&E, LFT, INR
- Serum glucose/CBG may be raised secondary to steroid use
- Bone profile (check for hypercalcaemia)
- If unknown primary malignancy, perform myeloma screen (protein electrophoresis, immunoglobulins, Bence Jones protein) and PSA.

Imaging

- MRI whole spine:
    - Must be performed within 24 hours if neurological symptoms or signs are present, or sooner if pressing need for emergency surgery
    - Within 7 days if moderate clinical suspicion without neurological symptoms or signs
- If MRI is contraindicated (e.g. some types of pacemaker), discuss options with MSCC coordinator
- If MRI is urgently indicated but is unavailable, transfer the patient to another hospital that has MRI availability
- Do not perform plain radiographs of the spine to make or exclude the diagnosis of spinal metastases or MSCC.

Management

See Fig. 53.1.

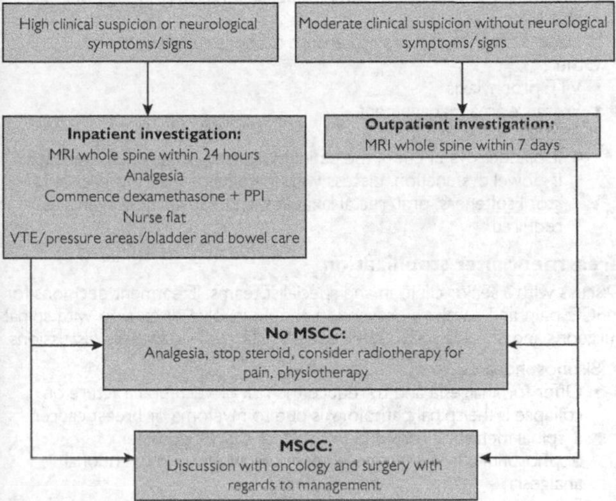

Fig. 53.1 Summary of investigation and management of suspected MSCC.

Acute management

- Analgesia:
    - Offer analgesia titrated to requirements
    - Laxatives should be given with opiate-based analgesia
    - If intractable pain, consider specialist pain team involvement
- Corticosteroids:
    - Consider on suspicion of MSCC, pending MRI result
    - Loading dose 16mg dexamethasone PO, followed by 16mg dexamethasone daily, e.g. 16mg OD (morning) or 8mg BD (morning and lunchtime):
        - Dexamethasone can also have an analgesic effect
        - Once definitive treatment is started (surgery or radiotherapy), taper the dose over 5–7 days to stop. If neurological function deteriorates, the dose should be ↑ again
    - May be contraindicated in suspected lymphoma (impairs histological diagnosis making biopsy difficult); discuss with MSCC coordinator prior to giving
    - Consider PPI cover, e.g. omeprazole 20mg OD
    - Monitor patients for hyperglycaemia, epigastric pain (particularly if on NSAIDs/aspirin), and steroid-induced psychosis

- Mobilization:
  - Nurse flat until bony and neurological stability are ensured
  - Turn using a log-rolling technique every 2–3 hours
  - Worsening neurology or severe mechanical back pain suggests spinal instability
  - Liaise with physiotherapy to ensure cautious remobilization
- Other:
  - VTE prophylaxis
  - Pressure area management
  - Bladder/bowel function:
    - If bladder dysfunction, the patient will need urinary catheterization
    - If bowel dysfunction, discuss with the patient their preference for stool softeners, oral/rectal laxatives, and constipating agents as required.

Treatment after stabilization

Discuss with a senior clinician and specialist teams. Treatment decisions for MSCC pain and paralysis prevention should involve discussion with spinal surgeons and oncologists, with the patient fully involved in these discussions.

- Bisphosphonates:
  - Offer for analgesia and to reduce the risk of vertebral fracture or collapse if the spinal pathology is due to myeloma or breast cancer
  - If spinal metastases are due to prostate cancer, consider bisphosphonates if the pain is not controlled with conventional analgesia
  - Do not use for tumours other than myeloma, breast, or prostate
- Surgery:
  - Aims to achieve spinal cord decompression and stability of the spinal column when instability is seen on imaging. If the patient has been paraplegic or tetraplegic for ≥24 hours, only offer surgery to provide pain relief
  - Consider vertebroplasty or kyphoplasty when pain is not controlled by analgesia or there is vertebral body collapse
- Radiotherapy:
  - Should be offered to all patients with MSCC who are not suitable for surgery, unless they have had tetra/paraplegia ≥24 hours and their pain is well controlled, or their overall prognosis is too poor
- Rehabilitation:
  - Consider admission to a specialist rehabilitation centre on discharge, dependent on prognosis, activity tolerance, and rehabilitation potential.

Special considerations

Patients with cancer, bone metastasis, or at risk of developing bone metastasis must be informed about the symptoms of MSCC.

Further reading

1. Al-Qurainy R, Collis E (2016). Metastatic spinal cord compression: diagnosis and management. *BMJ*. 353:i2539.

Chapter 54

Neuropathic pain

Guideline:
NICE CG173 (Neuropathic pain in adults: pharmacological management in non-specialist settings): https://www.nice.org.uk/guidance/cg173

OUP disclaimer: Oxford University Press makes no representation, express or implied, that the drug dosages are correct and that the recommendations are an exclusive or mandatory course of care. All health professionals reading this text have a responsibility to evaluate its appropriateness and take the individual needs of the patient into account.

Local trust guidelines: please refer to your local guidelines as necessary.

Overview

Neuropathic pain is caused by a lesion or disease of the neural tissue. Causes of neuropathic pain include:

- Diabetic neuropathy
- Post-herpetic neuralgia
- Trigeminal neuralgia
- Radicular pain
- Post-surgical chronic neuropathic pain
- Spinal cord injury
- Multiple sclerosis.

Diagnosis

- Neuropathic pain can be intermittent or constant, and spontaneous or provoked
- Patients describe the pain as shooting, stabbing, electric shock-like, burning, tingling, tight, numb, prickling, itching, or as a sensation of pins and needles.
- See Table 54.1

Table 54.1 Key characteristics for common causes of neuropathic pain

Diagnosis	Characteristic
Diabetic neuropathy	Patients with diabetes mellitus, tends to affect lower limbs before upper
Post-herpetic neuralgia	Pain that continues for months-years after the resolution of a VZV rash. Usually involves a specific nerve and localizes to one dermatome unilaterally
Trigeminal neuralgia	Often paroxysmal but can also be triggered by light touch. Lasts for seconds rather than minutes in the distribution of the trigeminal nerve. Usually unilateral. Often associated with autonomic symptoms such as lacrimation and rhinorrhea
Radicular pain	Due to inflammation of a spinal nerve root causing a dermatomal distribution of pain

Management

- Where possible, treat the cause of the pain
- When agreeing a treatment plan with a patient, consider the following:
  - The effect the pain has on the patient's lifestyle and activities of daily living, e.g. difficulties sleeping due to the pain
  - Whether the underlying condition that causes the pain has deteriorated
  - The importance of titrating medication dose to achieve adequate control but considering the benefits and adverse effects of pharmacological treatments
  - Non-pharmacological treatments such as psychological and physical therapies
- When introducing a new treatment, consider overlap with old treatments initially to avoid deterioration of pain control.

Pharmacological treatment

Trigeminal neuralgia

- Offer carbamazepine 100mg 1–2 times a day. Usual dose 200mg 3–4 times a day—titrate as needed. Maximum daily dose 1.6g daily.

Other causes of neuropathic pain

Options:

- Amitriptyline 10–25mg at night. Escalate if tolerated every 3–7 days. Usual daily dose 25–75mg **OR**
- Duloxetine 60mg OD (particularly helpful in diabetic neuropathy) **OR**
- Gabapentin 300mg OD on day 1, 300mg BD on day 2, 300mg TDS on day 3, with further titration as required (maximum 3.6mg/day, in three divided doses) **OR**
- Pregabalin 50mg TDS. Dose may be ↑ if needed after 3–7 days. Maximum 600mg OD in 2–3 divided doses.

Consider:

- Switching drug if the first is ineffective—all four can be trialled if necessary
- Tramadol 50–100mg QDS as a short-term rescue medication
- Capsaicin cream if the patient wishes to avoid oral analgesia and the pain is localized.

Follow up

- After initial treatment, review after 1–2 weeks
- Once established on treatment, review regularly to monitor effectiveness of treatment
- At each review, assess:
  - Pain control
  - Impact on lifestyle and daily activities
  - Physical and psychological well-being
  - Adverse effects of therapy, e.g. prolonged QTc and arrhythmias with amitriptyline use
  - Whether continued treatment is needed
- After 6 months of treatment consider gradual dose reduction
- When withdrawing or switching treatment, taper the drugs to reduce the risk of interval pain symptoms.

Special considerations

Specialist pain clinic referral

Refer to a specialist pain clinic if:

- The patient has severe pain **OR**
- The pain significantly impairs activities of daily living **OR**
- The underlying health condition that is causing the pain has deteriorated.

Elderly

Be cautious with the starting dose of amitriptyline due to ↑ risk of psychiatric and cardiac side effects.

Chapter 55

Parkinson's disease

Guideline:
NICE NG71 (Parkinson's disease in adults): https://www.nice.org.uk/guidance/ng71

OUP disclaimer: Oxford University Press makes no representation, express or implied, that the drug dosages are correct and that the recommendations are an exclusive or mandatory course of care. All health professionals reading this text have a responsibility to evaluate its appropriateness and take the individual needs of the patient into account.

Local trust guidelines: please refer to your local guidelines as necessary.

Overview

Parkinson's disease (PD) is a degenerative, incurable movement disorder resulting from the loss of dopamine-containing cells in the substantia nigra pars compacta.

Diagnosis

History and examination

The UK Parkinson's Disease Society Brain Bank Clinical Diagnostic Criteria must be met[1]:

Bradykinesia and at least one of:

- Muscular rigidity
- 4–6Hz resting tremor
- Postural instability not caused by primary visual, vestibular, cerebellar, or proprioceptive dysfunction.

Exclusion criteria

Symptoms suggestive of alternative neurological diagnoses that might also explain the presenting clinical symptoms, e.g. recurrent head injury or previous stroke.

Supportive criteria

≥3 must be present:

- Unilateral onset
- Resting tremor
- Progressive symptoms
- Persistent asymmetry affecting side of onset most
- Excellent response to levodopa
- Severe levodopa-induced chorea
- Levodopa response for ≥5 years
- Clinical course ≥10 years.

If PD is suspected, refer without starting medication for prompt specialist review.

Investigations

- Diagnosis is based on clinical findings
- MRI is only helpful in the differential diagnosis of other causes of parkinsonism
- Consider SPECT if unable to rule out essential tremor.

1 UK Parkinson's Disease Society Brain bank diagnostic criteria. Available at: https://www.ncbi.nlm.nih.gov/books/NBK379754/

Management

Lifestyle and simple interventions

- Involve physiotherapists and occupational therapists for balance, motor, and functional problems
- Liaise with a dietician as:
  - Some foods may interact with PD medications
  - Tremor, stiffness, and impaired swallow may mean patients need to change their diet
- Speech and language therapists can improve speech and swallow, aiding communication and reducing the risk of aspiration.

Pharmacological management

Main aim of drug therapy

- Improvement in motor symptoms and activities of daily living: levodopa, MAO-B inhibitors, COMT inhibitors. See Fig. 55.1
- Improving off time (when symptoms worsen in between doses due to 'wearing off' of the medication): dopamine agonists.

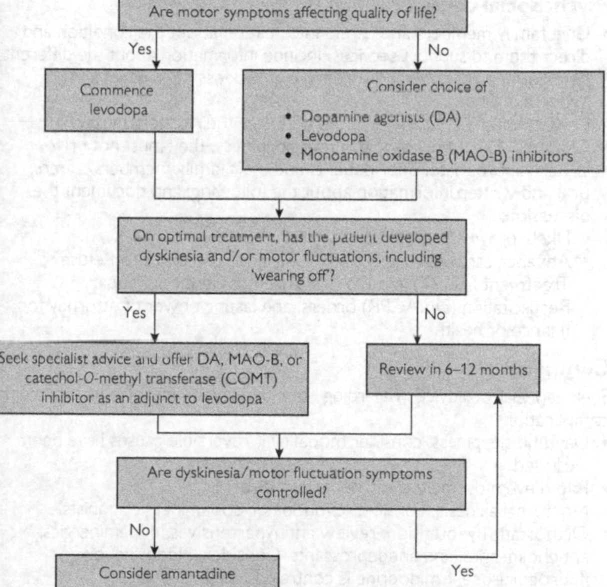

Fig. 55.1 Drug therapy options in Parkinson's disease.

Possible adverse effects

- Greater risk of motor complications: levodopa
- Greater risk of sleepiness, hallucinations, and impulse control disorders: dopamine agonists
- PD patients are prone to missing their medications when admitted to hospital, or receiving them at the wrong times, potentially leading to acute akinesia or neuroleptic malignant syndrome due to sudden withdrawal of therapy.
- Be vigilant for causes of poor treatment adherence e.g. gastroenteritis, missed prescriptions, being kept nil by mouth—and be proactive in removing barriers to treatment, e.g. use nasogastric tubes, self-administration
- Changes of formulation may be necessary, e.g. to a topical patch, with senior clinician assistance. A helpful resource for drug formulation conversion is available online (the OPTIMAL calculator[2]).

Surgical management

Deep brain stimulation may be considered in advanced PD where optimal medical therapy has failed to adequately control symptoms.

Psychosocial considerations

- Give family members and carers information about the condition and direct them to support services. Include information about the different types of impulse control disorders, e.g. reckless behaviours and hypersexuality
- Drivers with PD must inform the DVLA of their condition (see Chapter 115). If they have daytime sleepiness, they must not drive
- Where appropriate, offer patients and their family members/carers oral and written information about the following, and document the discussion:
  - Likely progression of PD
  - Advance care planning, including Advance Decisions to Refuse Treatment (ADRT) and Do Not Attempt Cardiopulmonary Resuscitation (DNACPR) orders, and lasting power of attorney for finance or health.

Complications

Seek specialist advice regarding the management of the following complications:

- Daytime sleepiness: consider modafinil if reversible causes have been excluded
- Rapid eye movement sleep behaviour disorder
- Nocturnal akinesia: consider levodopa or dopaminergic agonists
- Orthostatic hypotension: review antihypertensives, dopaminergics, anticholinergics, and antidepressants. Consider midodrine, or fludrocortisone if midodrine is contraindicated
- Depression (see Chapter 38)

2 OPTIMAL calculator—very useful for converting patients' medications to avoid missed doses, e.g. if they are nil by mouth during an acute admission. Available at: http://www.parkinsonscalculator.com/

- Psychotic symptoms (hallucinations and delusions): consider reducing the dosages of contributing PD drugs. Consider starting quetiapine or clozapine
- PD dementia: consider a cholinesterase inhibitor, or memantine if contraindicated
- Drooling of saliva: refer to speech and language therapy. If unsuccessful, consider glycopyrronium bromide
- Impulse control disorders.

Monitoring and follow-up

- Regular reviews every 6–12 months
- Consider alternative diagnoses if atypical features develop such as Parkinson's plus syndromes
- Assess for impulse control disorder development at each review
- Ensure the patient/family have access to a reliable source of information, e.g. specialist nurse
- Consider referring patients at any stage of PD to the palliative care team.

Chapter 56

Stroke and transient ischaemic attack

Guideline:
NICE NG128 (Stroke and transient ischaemic attack in over 16s: diagnosis and initial management): https://www.nice.org.uk/guidance/ng128

OUP disclaimer: Oxford University Press makes no representation, express or implied, that the drug dosages are correct and that the recommendations are an exclusive or mandatory course of care. All health professionals reading this text have a responsibility to evaluate its appropriateness and take the individual needs of the patient into account.

Local trust guidelines: please refer to your local guidelines as necessary.

Overview

A stroke is defined as a rapid-onset, focal neurological deficit due to a vascular lesion lasting >24 hours. If the deficit lasts <24 hours, this is termed a transient ischaemic attack (TIA). Patients with a stroke present with focal neurological deficit which can be classified into different syndromes (Table 56.1).

Table 56.1 Bamford/Oxford classification of stroke

Syndrome	Definitions
Total anterior circulation stroke (TACS)	All three of: • Unilateral weakness ± sensory deficit • Homonymous hemianopia • Higher cortical dysfunction, i.e. dysphasia, dyspraxia, or neglect
Partial anterior circulation stroke (PACS)	Two of three of TACS criteria
Lacunar syndrome (LACS)	Pure hemimotor or sensory loss, or both, or ataxic hemiparesis
Posterior circulation syndrome (POCS)	One of: • Cranial nerve palsy and a contralateral motor or sensory deficit • Bilateral motor or sensory deficit • Conjugate eye movement disorder • Cerebellar dysfunction (ataxia, nystagmus, vertigo, incoordination) • Isolated homonymous hemianopia or cortical blindness

Diagnosis

History

Take a focused history including the time of onset and type of neurological defect. Check if the patient takes anticoagulation or antiplatelet therapy and consider risk factors, i.e. smoking, diabetes, hypertension, hyperlipidaemia, AF, prosthetic valves, bleeding or thrombotic tendencies, and vasculitis.

Use a tool such as the Recognition of Stroke in the Emergency Room (ROSIER) scale. Stroke is likely if score >0 (Table 56.2).

Table 56.2 ROSIER[1] scale for recognition of stroke

Loss of consciousness or syncope	–1
Seizure activity	–1
New, acute onset (or new on waking) asymmetric facial weakness	+1
New, acute onset (or new on waking) asymmetric arm weakness	+1
New, acute onset (or new on waking) asymmetric leg weakness	+1
New, acute onset (or new on waking) speech disturbance	+1
New, acute onset (or new on waking) visual field defect	+1

Be aware of, and rule out, stroke mimics including hypoglycaemia, head injury, epilepsy (Todd's paresis), space-occupying lesion, drug overdose and central nervous system infection.

Examination

Systemically examine the patient using an ABCDE assessment (Table 56.3).

Table 56.3 Clinical signs in the ABCDE assessment of a patient with stroke or TIA

A	Airway may be compromised if GCS score is significantly ↓
B	↓ air entry due to aspiration pneumonia
C	Hypertension (may have caused, or be caused by stroke) AF Prosthetic heart valves Carotid bruit (carotid artery stenosis)
D	Reduced GCS score Hypoglycaemia (stroke mimic)
E	Papilloedema (↑ intracranial pressure) Bruising or bleeding (secondary to injury) Systematic neurological examination to help localize the area of infarct

1 Nor AM, Davis J, Sen B, Shipsey D, Louw SJ, Dyker AG, Davis M, Ford GA. The Recognition of Stroke in the Emergency Room (ROSIER) scale: development and validation of a stroke recognition instrument. *Lancet Neurology* 2005, 4(11): 727–34.

The National Institutes of Health Stroke Scale (NIHSS) should be used to assess neurological deficit and stroke severity. Full details can be accessed online.[2]

The deficits assessed for in the NIHSS are:

1. Level of consciousness
2. Eye gaze abnormality
3. Visual fields
4. Presence of facial palsy
5. Upper limb motor
6. Lower limb motor
7. Presence of ataxia
8. Sensory deficit
9. Language
10. Presence of dysarthria
11. Presence of inattention (neglect).

Investigations

Bedside

- Routine observations: including blood pressure and heart rate
- Electrocardiogram: AF or signs of ischaemic heart disease
- Point-of-care glucose.

Bloods

- FBC
- U&E
- LFT
- Glucose
- Lipid profile
- Coagulation profile
- Consider additional bloods in 'young stroke' patients (Box 56.1).

Box 56.1 'Young stroke' bloods

In young stroke patients, look for stroke risk factors on bloods such as polycythaemia, thrombocytopenia, ↑ CRP or ESR (vasculitis), HIV, syphilis, deranged coagulation profile (thrombophilia screen), and deranged renal function (vasculitis).

Imaging

CT head: to identify an intracranial haemorrhage or an established infarct. Should be done immediately if acute onset, persistent neurological symptoms, and:

- Thrombolysis or thrombectomy would potentially be indicated (see below)
- On anticoagulation or known bleeding tendency
- GCS score <13

2 NIHSS. Available at: https://www.stroke.nih.gov/resources/scale.htm

- Unexplained progressive or fluctuating symptoms
- Papilloedema, neck stiffness, or fever
- Severe headache at onset.

If the patient does not have one of the indications above, they should still have a CT head within 24 hours.

CT contrast angiography ± CT perfusion imaging: if thrombectomy is indicated (NIHSS >5, and the patient has a good premorbid function, i.e. a Modified Rankin Scale score <3).[3]

MRI brain: usually performed to assess the posterior fossa due to posterior stroke symptoms, in diagnostic uncertainty, or in TIAs after specialist assessment.

Other

- **Carotid imaging (Doppler ultrasound, CT angiography, or magnetic resonance angiography):** to identify carotid artery stenosis if the patient is considered a candidate for carotid endarterectomy
- **Holter monitoring/event recorder:** to investigate for paroxysmal AF
- **Echocardiogram:** to rule out an embolic cause of stroke.

3 van Swieten, J. C., Koudstaal, P. J., Visser, M. C., Schouten, H. J., & van Gijn, J. (1988). Interobserver agreement for the assessment of handicap in stroke patients. Stroke, 19(5), 604–607. https://doi.org/10.1161/01.str.19.5.604.

Management

Acute management

General measures

Use an ABCDE approach to ensure that there is a safe airway, adequate oxygenation and ventilation, effective circulation, and reversible disabilities are corrected.

Stroke

- Contact a senior member of staff and the **acute stroke team** and arrange for an **urgent CT head**
- **Thrombolysis** (Box 56.2) for acute ischaemic stroke is indicated if:
  - Within 4.5 hours of stroke onset **AND**
  - Intracranial haemorrhage has been excluded
- **Antiplatelet therapy:** aspirin 300mg (route: PO/nasogastric/rectal depending on swallow assessment) immediately once intracerebral haemorrhage has been excluded, unless thrombolysis has been given (withhold until a CT scan at 24 hours has excluded any haemorrhage). Aspirin is continued for 2 weeks after stroke onset and switched to long-term antithrombotic treatment after, e.g. clopidogrel 75mg OD
- **Prothrombin complex concentrate and vitamin K** if haemorrhagic stroke and the patient takes warfarin. Discuss with haematology if being treated with a DOAC
- Admit to a specialist acute stroke unit.

Suspected or confirmed transient ischaemic attack

- Offer aspirin (300mg daily) immediately unless contraindicated
- Refer any suspected TIA for specialist assessment and investigation to be seen within 24 hours of symptom onset
- Offer secondary prevention as soon as possible after the diagnosis is confirmed
- CT head is not required unless there is a clinical suspicion of an alternative diagnosis.

Box 56.2 Important considerations in thrombolysis

- Thrombolysis must only be administered by staff trained in delivering thrombolysis and monitoring for any complications
- The agent used for thrombolysis is tissue plasminogen activator (tPa), e.g. alteplase
- Suspect intracranial bleeding following thrombolysis if there is neurological deterioration, new headache, reduction in GCS score, acute hypertension, seizure, nausea, or vomiting. If haemorrhagic transformation is suspected during thrombolysis, stop the tPa infusion, arrange an urgent repeat CT scan, and contact a senior clinician immediately
- Follow local hospital protocols.

Blood pressure control in stroke

Acute ischaemic stroke

- Thrombolysis candidate: blood pressure reduction to ≤185/110mmHg should be considered

- Otherwise, antihypertensive medications in acute stroke are only recommended if there is:
  - Hypertensive encephalopathy, nephropathy, cardiac failure, or myocardial infarction
  - Aortic dissection
  - Pre-eclampsia or eclampsia.

Acute intracerebral haemorrhage

- Offer rapid blood pressure control to those who present within 6 hours of symptom onset **AND** have a systolic blood pressure of 150–220mmHg.
- Consider rapid blood pressure control in those who present beyond 6 hours of symptom onset **OR** have a systolic blood pressure >220mmHg
- Aim for a systolic blood pressure target of 130–140mmHg within 1 hour of starting treatment and maintain this blood pressure for at least 7 days
- Do not rapidly lower the blood pressure in people with an underlying structural cause, GCS score <6, awaiting early neurosurgical intervention to evacuate a haematoma, or who have a massive haematoma with poor expected prognosis.

Treatment after stabilization

Nutrition

- Assess swallow as soon as possible by trained staff. If swallow is impaired, refer to speech and language therapy and consider inserting a nasogastric tube for nutrition, fluids, and medications
- If a nasogastric tube is not tolerated, consider trying a nasal bridle tube or gastrostomy
- Screen the patient for malnutrition using the Malnutrition Universal Screening Tool (MUST).

> Remember to review the patient's medications and change the formulation or route if necessary.

Multidisciplinary team assessment

- This includes a specialist team of nurses, physiotherapists, occupational therapists, speech and language therapists, dieticians, and stroke physicians
- Patients should be assisted out of bed as soon as it is safe for them to do so.

Management of risk factors

- **Carotid stenosis:** consider carotid endarterectomy in people with acute non-disabling stroke or TIA who have symptomatic carotid stenosis of 50–99% according to the North American Symptomatic Carotid Endarterectomy Trial (NASCET) criteria, or 70–99% according to the European Carotid Surgery Trial (ECST) criteria

- **Cardiovascular risk factors[4]:**
  - Diet and lifestyle advice
  - Control of blood pressure—aim for blood pressure <130/80mmHg
  - Antiplatelet therapy, e.g. clopidogrel 75mg OD
  - Cholesterol-lowering drugs, e.g. atorvastatin 40–80mg at night
- **AF:** consider starting anticoagulation 2 weeks post stroke.

4 Royal College of Physicians. National clinical guideline for stroke, fifth edition. 2016. Available at: https://www.rcplondon.ac.uk/guidelines-policy/stroke-guidelines

Special considerations

Thrombectomy

This is offered in some centres alongside thrombolysis. If thrombectomy is indicated, a CT contrast angiography should follow the initial non-enhanced CT to confirm occlusion of the proximal anterior circulation or basilar artery. Patients with stroke symptoms who were last known to be well up to 24 hours previously can be considered for thrombectomy with appropriate specialist imaging.

Prosthetic heart valve

If the patient has a prosthetic heart valve and an acute disabling stroke which is at high risk of haemorrhagic transformation, they should stop their anticoagulation for a week, and be managed during this time with 300mg aspirin daily.

Cerebral venous sinus thrombosis (including those with secondary cerebral haemorrhage)

Full-dose anticoagulation treatment (initially with LMWH, then warfarin) should be offered.

Further reading

1. Royal College of Physicians (2016). National clinical guideline for stroke, fifth edition. Available at: https://www.rcplondon.ac.uk/guidelines-policy/stroke-guidelines

Part 9

Obstetrics and gynaecology

Chapter 57

Antenatal care

Guideline:
NICE NG201 (Antenatal care): https://www.nice.org.uk/guidance/ng201

OUP disclaimer: Oxford University Press makes no representation, express or implied, that the drug dosages are correct and that the recommendations are an exclusive or mandatory course of care. All health professionals reading this text have a responsibility to evaluate its appropriateness and take the individual needs of the patient into account.

Local trust guidelines: please refer to your local guidelines as necessary.

Overview

This chapter summarizes the antenatal care that should be received by women with uncomplicated (midwife-led) singleton pregnancies. Women with more complicated pregnancies should also receive this baseline of care and have additional scans and appointments as required.

Antenatal information

The following items should be discussed:

At the first contact with a healthcare professional

- Folic acid supplementation
- Reducing the risk of food-acquired infections
- Smoking cessation and avoiding drug and alcohol use
- Screening programmes including risks and benefits.

At booking

- Fetal development
- Nutritional information, including vitamin D supplementation
- Exercise, including pelvic floor exercises
- Place of birth
- Breastfeeding
- Antenatal classes
- Mental health issues.

Before or at 36 weeks

- Breastfeeding
- Preparation for labour and birth, including pain management
- Neonatal vitamin K prophylaxis
- Newborn screening tests
- Postnatal self-care
- Recognition of postpartum depression.

At 38 weeks

- Options if the pregnancy is likely to be overdue.

Antenatal appointments

In an uncomplicated pregnancy, nulliparous women should have ten appointments, and parous women should have seven. See Table 57.1.

At all appointments:

- Measure blood pressure and test urine for proteinuria
- Measure and plot symphysis–fundal height (after 25 weeks).

Table 57.1 Summary of antenatal appointments

Gestation	Content
Booking appointment (ideally by 10 weeks)	• Take past medical, obstetric and family history, including risk factors for pre-eclampsia (see Chapter 61) • Identify women who may need additional care • Check FBC, blood group, and rhesus D status • Offer screening • Arrange ultrasound scans for dating and anomalies • Measure height, weight, and BMI • Identify women who have had female genital mutilation (FGM) • Ask about mood and psychiatric history • Ask about occupation to identify potential risks
16 weeks	• Review results of screening tests • Start iron supplementation if anaemic
25 weeks*	• Routine • Discuss fetal movements and how to seek medical help if they notice reduced fetal movements
28 weeks	• Second screening for anaemia, blood group, and atypical red cell alloantibodies • Anti-D prophylaxis if rhesus negative
31 weeks*	• Review results of screening tests
34 weeks	• Second dose of anti-D if rhesus negative
36 weeks	• Offer external cephalic version (ECV) if suspected breech
38 weeks	• Routine
40 weeks*	• Routine
41 weeks	For women who have not given birth by 41 weeks: • Offer a membrane sweep • Offer induction of labour. If declined, offer ↑ monitoring

* Signifies extra appointments for nulliparous women.

Scanning

- **10+0–13+6 weeks:** dating scan to determine gestational age using crown–rump length measurement (and check for multiple pregnancies)
- **18+0–20+6 weeks:** structural anomaly scan to look for congenital abnormalities and placental position. If the placenta is low, then a re-scan should be booked for 32–36 weeks.

Lifestyle considerations

Nutritional supplements

- **Folic acid:** 400 micrograms per day. Ideally from 3 months prior to conception and throughout the first 12 weeks to reduce the risk of neural tube defects
- **Vitamin D:** 10 micrograms per day during pregnancy and breastfeeding. Higher-risk women include those with darker skin or limited exposure to sunlight (e.g. housebound or skin covered for cultural reasons)
- **Iron:** not routinely offered as there is no benefit if not anaemic and it may have side effects
- **Vitamin A:** avoid supplementation (liver/liver products also contain high levels) as it may be teratogenic.

Sleeping position

- Advise women not to sleep on their back after 28 weeks.

Reducing risk of infection

Listeria

- Drink only pasteurized or ultra-high temperature (UHT) milk
- Avoid eating ripened soft cheese, blue cheese, or any pate
- Avoid eating undercooked ready meals.

Salmonella

- Avoid raw or partially cooked eggs or food containing them (e.g. mayonnaise)
- Avoid raw or partially cooked meat, particularly poultry.

Toxoplasmosis

- Wash hands before handling food
- Wash all fruits and vegetables
- Ensure all food is thoroughly cooked for consumption
- Wear gloves and wash hands after gardening
- Avoid touching cat faeces in cat litter or soil.

Medication

- Few medicines have been established as safe for use in pregnancy
- Prescription should be limited to situations where benefit outweighs risk. Over-the-counter medicines and complementary therapies should be avoided.

Exercise in pregnancy

- Moderate-intensity exercise is safe in pregnancy
- Contact and high-impact sports with risk of abdominal trauma or falls should be avoided
- Scuba diving is unsafe.

Smoking in pregnancy

- There is an ↑ risk of adverse pregnancy outcomes in women who smoke or who are exposed to second-hand smoke. These include intrauterine growth restriction, pre-term birth, and stillbirth

- All women should have their smoking status explored and be offered smoking cessation advice and referral to local NHS Stop Smoking Services if required
- The risks and benefits of nicotine replacement therapy in pregnancy should also be explored.

Travel during pregnancy

Air travel

- Long-haul air travel is generally associated with an ↑ risk of DVT and PE. It is unclear whether pregnancy increases this risk
- Wearing compression stockings may reduce the risk.

Car travel

- Ensure the correct use of seatbelts, i.e. three-point seatbelt above and below the bump, not over it.

Travel abroad

- Discuss considerations such as flying (airline rules vary), travel insurance, and vaccinations (not all vaccinations are safe for the fetus).

Management of common pregnancy symptoms

Nausea and vomiting in early pregnancy

- See Chapter 63 for more details
- Most cases will resolve by 20 weeks without treatment. It does not affect pregnancy outcome. First-line treatment options include:
  - Ginger
  - Wrist acupressure
  - Antihistamines.

Heartburn

- Consider lifestyle and diet modification. Antacids can be trialled, e.g. ranitidine or omeprazole.

Constipation and haemorrhoids

- Give advice regarding dietary changes such as increasing fibre intake. Consider standard haemorrhoid creams if necessary.

Varicose veins

- Common, harmless pregnancy symptom. Compression stockings may improve symptoms but will not prevent varicose vein development.

Vaginal discharge

- ↑ discharge is a common physiological change. Consider an underlying infection if it is associated with itching, pain, offensive smell, or dysuria
- 7 days of topical imidazole should be given for vaginal candidiasis. An alternative is a clotrimazole pessary (500mg, once only) with clotrimazole topical cream. Oral treatments should not be used.

Vaginal bleeding

- Unexplained vaginal bleeding after 13 weeks:
  - Offer anti-D if rhesus D negative and at risk of isoimmunization
  - Refer to secondary care. The decision to admit depends on the risk of placental abruption and pre-term delivery, severity of bleeding, and the woman's ability to return to secondary care in an emergency
  - Check placental location if unknown (?placenta praevia).

Back pain

- Back pain is common in pregnancy and may be eased by water-based exercise and massage.

Screening

No screening is compulsory, so women should be given sufficient information to make an informed decision. Women should be monitored and screened for gestational diabetes (see Chapter 59) and pre-eclampsia (see Chapter 61) throughout pregnancy.

Anaemia

- A FBC should be taken at booking and at 28 weeks to screen for anaemia
- A haemoglobin concentration of <110g/L at booking or <105g/L at 28 weeks should be treated with a trial of oral iron.

Blood grouping

- A group and save and antibody screen should be performed at booking **and again** at 28 weeks, irrespective of previous status
- All women who are rhesus D negative should be given anti-D prophylaxis
- Women who have clinically significant red cell alloantibodies should be referred to fetal medicine for further investigation and management.

Haemoglobinopathies

- Preconception counselling and carrier testing should be available to those at high risk of haemoglobinopathies.

Hypertension

- Blood pressure should be measured at every antenatal appointment, as well as a urinalysis to check for proteinuria
- If >20+0 weeks with a first recording of hypertension (≥140/90mmHg), they should be seen in secondary care within 24 hours
- If blood pressure is ≥160/110mmHg, they should be seen urgently in secondary care on the same day
- See Chapter 61 for further details.

Screening for structural anomalies

- USS for fetal anomalies is performed between 18+0 and 20+6 weeks. Identifying fetal anomalies allows:
  - Termination of pregnancy
  - Preparation for any treatment, disabilities, or palliative care
  - Planning of birth in a specialist centre.

Screening for Down's syndrome

- Ideally, screening should be done using the 'combined test' (nuchal translucency plus βHCG plus pregnancy-associated plasma protein-A (PAPP-A)) by 13+6 weeks
- If a patient books later, or where nuchal translucency cannot be measured, offer serum screening (triple or quadruple test) between 15+0 and 20+0 weeks
- The routine anomaly scan should not be used for Down's syndrome screening; however, if there are suspicious findings the woman should be referred to fetal medicine.

Screening for infections

Early screening should be offered for:

- Asymptomatic bacteriuria, syphilis, HIV, and hepatitis B
- If <25 years, direct the woman to the national chlamydia screening programme
- Do not screen for the following: asymptomatic bacterial vaginosis, cytomegalovirus, hepatitis C virus, group B streptococci, rubella, or toxoplasmosis.

Further reading

1. NHS. The Healthy Start programme. Available at: https://www.healthystart.nhs.uk/
2. NICE (2014, updated 2020). Antenatal and postnatal mental health: clinical management and service guidance (CG192). Available at: https://www.nice.org.uk/guidance/cg192

Chapter 58

Antepartum haemorrhage

Guideline:
Royal College of Obstetricians and Gynaecologists (RCOG) GTG63 (Antepartum haemorrhage): https://www.rcog.org.uk/en/guidelines-research-services/guidelines/gtg63/

OUP disclaimer: Oxford University Press makes no representation, express or implied, that the drug dosages are correct and that the recommendations are an exclusive or mandatory course of care. All health professionals reading this text have a responsibility to evaluate its appropriateness and take the individual needs of the patient into account.

Local trust guidelines: please refer to your local guidelines as necessary

Overview

Antepartum haemorrhage (APH) is bleeding from the genital tract between 24+0 weeks' gestation and birth. It occurs in 3–5% of pregnancies and can affect the morbidity and mortality of both mother and baby.

Diagnosis

Causes

- Labour
- Local bleeding from the vulva, vagina, or cervix:
  - Cervical ectropion or polyp
  - Infection
  - Trauma
  - Malignancy
- Placental abruption
- Placenta praevia
- Ruptured vasa previa
- Unexplained.

Risk factors

- Domestic violence (ask if repeated presentations)
- Anticoagulant use or coagulopathies
- Previous APH
- Smoking and drug abuse
- For placental abruption: previous abruption, pre-eclampsia, fetal growth restriction, non-vertex presentations, advanced maternal age, premature rupture of membranes, intrauterine infection, abdominal trauma
- For placenta praevia: previous placenta praevia, previous caesarean section, previous termination, multiparity, advanced maternal age, multiple pregnancy, deficient endometrium due to past procedure or infection, assisted conception.

Preventing APH

The following interventions may reduce the risk of APH:
- Stopping smoking and the use of illicit drugs
- Avoiding vaginal and rectal examinations in women with placenta praevia
- Avoiding penetrative sexual intercourse in placenta praevia.

History

- Onset of bleeding
- Amount of bleeding (see Box 58.1 Quantifying blood loss)
- Associated pain—if continuous think **abruption,** if intermittent think labour
- Triggers—trauma, sexual intercourse, exercise
- Associated rupture of membranes
- Presence of fetal movements
- Cervical smear history
- Presence of risk factors for placenta previa or abruption
- Current medication (particularly LMWH or warfarin—patients taking these medications should withhold doses if they have any vaginal bleeding and attend hospital for urgent assessment with haematology input to advise about future doses)
- Obstetric history
- Known placenta or vasa praevia.

Box 58.1 Quantifying blood loss

- Spotting = spotting/staining/streaking noted on underwear
- Minor haemorrhage = self-limiting blood loss <50mL
- Major haemorrhage = blood loss 50–1000mL with no signs of shock
- Massive haemorrhage = blood loss >1000mL and/or signs of clinical shock (see Chapter 94)
- Remember, bleeding may be **occult** (e.g. concealed placental abruption).

Examination

Examine with senior support. Initial assessment should be with an ABCDE approach with ongoing resuscitation measures (see 'Management').

Abdominal palpation

- Assess for uterine contractions
- Tense or 'woody' uterus suggests abruption.

Speculum examination

- To assess for cervical dilatation or a lower genital tract cause of the bleeding
- If the cervix appears suspicious, refer the patient for colposcopy.

Digital vaginal examination

- Do **not** perform a digital vaginal examination if there is any suspicion of placenta praevia—an USS should be done first to exclude this.

Investigations

Maternal

Bloods

- **Minor haemorrhage:** FBC (coagulation profile only if platelets abnormal), group and save
- **Major haemorrhage:** FBC, coagulation profile, U&E, LFT, cross-match 4 units (+VBG)
- **If rhesus D negative:** Kleihauer test (to quantify degree of fetomaternal haemorrhage (FMH) and therefore gauge dose of anti-D Ig).

Ultrasound

- To confirm or exclude placenta praevia, if the site of the placenta is not yet known.

Fetal

Fetal investigations should be performed only once the mother is stable or resuscitation has been commenced.

- External auscultation of the fetal heart: <26 weeks
- Cardiotocograph (CTG): >26 weeks where knowledge of the fetal condition may influence the timing/mode of delivery
- If the fetal heart cannot be heard, perform USS to determine viability.

Management

Acute management

See Table 58.1 and Table 58.2.

Massive APH (blood loss >1000 mL ± signs of clinical shock)

> *The mother's life should always take priority, regardless of fetal gestation. She must be resuscitated and stabilized first, before any decisions are made regarding delivery of the baby.*

CALL FOR HELP

Put out a major obstetric haemorrhage crash call as per hospital protocol. This should alert:

- A senior midwife
- An obstetric registrar ± consultant
- An anaesthetic registrar ± consultant
- Porters to collect urgent specimens and deliver cross-matched blood
- Blood bank ± consultant haematologist on call
- A senior paediatrician/neonatologist in case of an emergency delivery.

Designate one member of the team to record events, fluids, drugs given, and vital signs.

Table 58.1 ABCDE approach in massive APH

	Typical ranges for vital signs are provided, but use local protocols/obstetric early warning scores if available
A + B	Assess **Airway** + **Breathing** • Respiratory rate—⚑ <10/min or >30/min • Saturations—⚑ <95% • Administer high-flow oxygen (10–15L/min) via a facemask
C	Evaluate **Circulation** • Heart rate—⚑ <40bpm or >120bpm • Systolic blood pressure—⚑ <90mmHg or >160mmHg • Diastolic blood pressure—⚑ >100mmHg • Insert 2× large bore (ideally 14G) IV lines to commence fluid resuscitation (Table 58.2) • Send bloods for FBC, assessment of FMH if rhesus D negative, coagulation profile, U&E, LFT, and cross-match 4 units of blood • Position left lateral tilt • Keep patient warm • Insert catheter for fluid balance monitoring • Transfuse blood as soon as available—until then up to 2L of warmed crystalloid solution • Give other blood products if required as per Table 58.2
D	Assess the fetus and decide on **Delivery**

If there is any concern that the patient has developed disseminated intravascular coagulation (DIC), urgent haematology advice should be sought.

APH up to 1000mL with no clinical shock

- Admit to hospital if APH is heavier than spotting or bleeding is ongoing:
  - Obtain IV access (1 large bore cannula)
  - Commence crystalloid infusion if required.

Treatment after stabilization

Antepartum

- If the patient has a significant APH between 24+0 and 34+6 weeks, consider giving a single course of steroids
- Following unexplained APH or APH due to placental abruption, the pregnancy should be reclassified as 'high risk', subsequent antenatal care should be consultant led, and serial growth scans performed
- Administer anti-D Ig if required to a non-sensitized rhesus D-negative woman after any presentation with APH (irrespective of whether they have received routine prophylaxis):
  - Administer at least 500IU (additional dose may be indicated following test for FMH)
  - If recurrent bleeding after 20+0 weeks, give at 6-weekly intervals.

Intrapartum

- If there is fetal compromise, a caesarean section should be performed, with simultaneous resuscitation of the mother
- Continuous fetal monitoring should be used in women with active bleeding, previous major or recurrent minor APH, or suspicion of abruption
- Patients with APH should receive active management of the third stage of labour due to the elevated risk of postpartum haemorrhage (PPH; see Chapter 65). This should be with ergometrine-oxytocin (Syntometrine®) unless contraindicated.

Postpartum

- Thromboprophylaxis should be commenced as soon as the immediate risk of haemorrhage is reduced, as both haemorrhage and blood transfusion are risk factors for VTE
- Debrief by a senior obstetrician both at the earliest opportunity after the event and at a follow-up appointment in 4–6 weeks
- Clinical incident reporting should be undertaken in major obstetric haemorrhage.

Table 58.2 Fluid therapy and blood product transfusion in APH

Crystalloid	Up to 2L crystalloid solution
Blood	Ideally cross-matched If cross-matched blood is unavailable and the clinical situation is urgent, give group-specific or O-negative blood Consider the use of cell salvage if available
FFP*	4 units of FFP (12–15mL/kg or total 1L) • For every 4 units of red cells **OR** • If PT and/or APTT are >1.5× normal
Pooled platelets	If platelet count <75 × 10^9/L
Cryoprecipitate*	If fibrinogen <2g/L

*With continuing massive haemorrhage and while awaiting coagulation studies, up to 4 units of FFP and 10 units of cryoprecipitate may be given empirically.

Source: data from Mavrides E, Allard S, Chandraharan E, Collins P, Green L, Hunt BJ, Riris S, Thomson AJ on behalf of the Royal College of Obstetricians and Gynaecologists. Prevention and management of postpartum haemorrhage. BJOG 2016;124:e106–e149; https://www.rcog.org.uk/en/guidelines-research-services/guidelines/gtg52/

Special considerations

Each woman must be assessed on an individual basis. For example, if a woman presents with spotting and has a past history of intrauterine fetal death resulting from placental abruption, then hospitalization would be appropriate.

Further reading

1. RCOG (2018). Placenta praevia and placenta accreta: diagnosis and management (GTG27a). Available at: https://www.rcog.org.uk/en/guidelines-research-services/guidelines/gtg27a/
2. RCOG (2018). Vasa praevia: diagnosis and management (GTG27b). Available at: https://www.rcog.org.uk/en/guidelines-research-services/guidelines/gtg27b/
3. British Committee for Standards in Haematology (BCSH) (2014). BCSH guideline for the use of anti-D immunoglobulin for the prevention of haemolytic disease of the fetus and newborn. Available at: https://onlinelibrary.wiley.com/doi/full/10.1111/tme.12091
4. RCOG (2015). Blood transfusions in obstetrics (GTG47). Available at: https://www.rcog.org.uk/en/guidelines-research-services/guidelines/gtg47/
5. RCOG (2019). Maternal collapse (GTG56). Available at: https://www.rcog.org.uk/en/guidelines-research-services/guidelines/gtg56/
6. NHS Cervical Screening Programmes (NHSCSP) (2010). *Colposcopy and Programme Management: Guidelines for the NHS Cervical Screening Programme*, 2nd ed. Sheffield: NHSCSP. Available at: http://www.cancerscreening.nhs.uk/cervical/publications/nhscsp20.html

Chapter 59

Diabetes in pregnancy

Guidelines:
NICE NG3 (Diabetes in pregnancy: management from preconception to the postnatal period): https://www.nice.org.uk/guidance/ng3

Joint British Diabetes Societies for Inpatient Care (Management of glycaemic control in pregnant women with diabetes on obstetric wards and delivery units): https://www.diabetes.org.uk/professionals/resources/shared-practice/inpatient-and-hospital-care/joint-british-diabetes-society-for-inpatient-care/management-of-glycaemic-control-in-pregnant-women-with-diabetes-on-obstetric-wards-and-delivery-units

OUP disclaimer: Oxford University Press makes no representation, express or implied, that the drug dosages are correct and that the recommendations are an exclusive or mandatory course of care. All health professionals reading this text have a responsibility to evaluate its appropriateness and take the individual needs of the patient into account.

Local trust guidelines: please refer to your local guidelines as necessary.

Overview

Approximately 5% of pregnancies are complicated by either pre-existing diabetes mellitus or gestational diabetes mellitus (GDM). Diabetes in pregnancy is associated with a number of risks to both women and their babies including miscarriage and stillbirth (Table 59.1).

Table 59.1 Complications of diabetes in pregnancy

Maternal	Fetal
Miscarriage	Congenital malformation
Pre-eclampsia	Macrosomia leading to shoulder dystocia
Pre-term labour	Polyhydramnios
Worsening complications of diabetes (e.g. retinopathy)	Birth injury
Stillbirth	Perinatal mortality
Perineal trauma	Postnatal adaptation problems (e.g. hypoglycaemia)

Preconception care for women with diabetes

- The most important part of preconception care is for the patient to achieve blood glucose levels within the target ranges (Box 59.1) and HbA1c <48mmol/mol, as this reduces many of the risks associated with diabetes in pregnancy (e.g. miscarriage, congenital defects, stillbirth)
- HbA1c:
  - Check monthly
  - Aim for <48mmol/mol (6.5%) if achievable without causing hypoglycaemia. Reassure women that any reduction towards this target will reduce the risk of congenital malformation
  - If >86mmol/mol (10%), strongly advise women not to get pregnant because of the risks
- Use metformin as an adjunct or alternative to insulin in the preconception period and during pregnancy (all other oral blood glucose-lowering agents should be discontinued before pregnancy)
- Perform retinal assessment if not done in last 6 months
- Perform renal assessments before contraception is discontinued. Refer to nephrology if creatinine ≥120μmol/litre, urinary ACR >30mg/mmol, or eGFR <45/min/1.73m².
- Stop ACE inhibitors, ARBs, and statins and find alternatives
- Advise women with a BMI >27kg/m² to lose weight
- Encourage appropriate use of contraception to avoid unplanned pregnancies to reduce the risk of problems during pregnancy, ideally until CBG measurements are well controlled
- Recommend folic acid (5mg OD) to reduce the risk of neural tube defects
- Provide the woman with a glucose meter for self-monitoring, and a ketone meter if T1DM.

Box 59.1 Preconception blood glucose targets

- Fasting (on waking): 5–7mmol/L
- Pre-meal: 4–7mmol/L.

Diagnosis

Who to test for gestational diabetes mellitus

- Women with any of the following risk factors:
  - Previous GDM
  - BMI >30kg/m^2
  - Previous macrosomic baby weighing >4.5kg
  - First-degree relative with diabetes
  - Minority ethnic family origin with a high prevalence of diabetes
- Glycosuria of 2+ on one occasion **OR** 1+ on ≥2 occasions, detected during routine antenatal care.

Investigations

HbA1c

- Measure in all women with pre-existing diabetes or those with newly diagnosed GDM.

Oral glucose tolerance test (OGTT)

- Previous GDM: Perform OGTT as soon as possible after booking and repeat at 24–28 weeks if the first test is normal
- Other risk factors for GDM (see 'Who to test for gestational diabetes mellitus'): Perform OGTT at 24–28 weeks
- Diagnose GDM if the woman has either:
  - A fasting plasma glucose level ≥5.6mmol/L **OR**
  - A 2-hour plasma glucose level ≥7.8mmol/L.

Antenatal management

Patient education

Explain to the patient that good blood glucose control during the pregnancy will reduce the risk to herself and her baby, including: birth trauma, need for caesarean section, fetal macrosomia, neonatal hypoglycaemia, and perinatal death.

Women should be taught to self-monitor blood glucose (Box 59.2).

Lifestyle and simple interventions

- Advise a healthy diet and refer to a dietician; emphasize that eating low glycaemic index (GI) foods should replace high GI ones
- Advise regular exercise (such as walking for 30 minutes).

Pharmacological management

Gestational diabetes

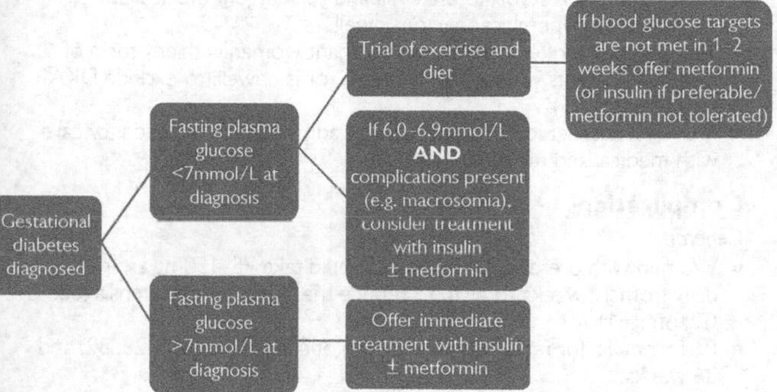

Fig. 59.1 Pharmacological management of gestational diabetes. Glibenclamide is a second-line option for patients who do not respond well to metformin and who decline insulin.

Risk of hypoglycaemia with insulin treatment

- Ensure awareness of the risks of hypoglycaemia and impaired awareness of hypoglycaemia in pregnancy, particularly in the first trimester
- Ensure constant availability of a fast-acting form of glucose (e.g. dextrose tablets)
- Provide glucagon if T1DM—instruct the woman and family members in its use
- Consider insulin pump if adequate control is not achieved despite multiple daily injections
- Consider continuous glucose monitoring for patients with severe hypoglycaemia or very unstable blood glucose levels, under the guidance of an expert joint diabetes and antenatal care team.

Box 59.2 Blood glucose monitoring

The following are targets for CBG if achievable without causing problematic hypoglycaemia. CBG should be kept at >4mmol/L:

- Fasting: <5.3mmol/L
- Post-meal: 1 hour after meal <7.8mmol/L or 2 hours after meal <6.4mmol/L
- If on insulin or glibenclamide: >4mmol/L.

When to monitor:

- T1DM/T2DM/GDM on multiple daily insulin regimen: fasting, pre meal, 1-hour post meal, and bedtime
- T2DM/GDM on diet/exercise, oral therapy, or single-dose insulin: fasting and 1-hour post meal.

Ketone monitoring

- Offer women with T1DM blood ketone testing strips and a meter—advise them to test for ketonaemia and seek urgent medical advice if they become hyperglycaemic or unwell
- Test urgently for ketonaemia if a pregnant woman with any form of diabetes presents with hyperglycaemia, or is unwell, to exclude DKA (see Chapter 15)
- If DKA is suspected during pregnancy, admit to high dependency care with medical and obstetric input.

Complications

General

- Women with pre-existing diabetes should take 75–150mg aspirin daily from 12 weeks to birth to reduce the risk of pre-eclampsia (see Chapter 61)
- Perform USS for fetal growth and amniotic fluid volume at 28, 32, and 36 weeks.

Retinopathy

Assessment:

- Offer at booking and again at 28 weeks
- If there is retinopathy at booking, assess again at 16–20 weeks.

If retinopathy is diagnosed at any point, refer for ophthalmological follow-up.

Nephropathy

Assessment:

- Arrange at booking if not done within the previous 3 months
- Refer to nephrology if creatinine ≥120μmol/L, urinary ACR >30mg/mmol or total urinary protein >0.5g/day.

Monitoring and follow-up

Offer women with a diagnosis of GDM a review with the joint diabetes and antenatal clinic within 1 week. Patients should be seen every 1–2 weeks.

Timing and mode of delivery

- **T1DM/T2DM with no complications:** elective birth by induction of labour or caesarean section between 37+0 and 38+6 weeks
- **T1DM/T2DM with complications:** consider delivery before 37+0 weeks
- **GDM:** advise delivery no later than 40+6 weeks; offer elective birth if not delivered by then (if complications, consider earlier elective birth)
- Explain to women with a macrosomic fetus about the risks and benefits of vaginal birth (e.g. ↑ risk of shoulder dystocia), induction of labour, and caesarean section
- Steroids can be used in preterm labour with careful glucose monitoring. As steroids can cause elevated blood glucose levels, patients requiring steroids will often need a VRII for 24 hours.

Intrapartum management

- Monitor CBG hourly during labour and half-hourly if caesarean section under general anaesthetic. Target = 4–7mmol/L
- All patients with T1DM and some with T2DM/GDM may require a VRII in established labour. If a VRII is used, reduce the rate by 50% (or change to lowest scale) once the placenta is delivered, and then follow the insulin plan made antenatally

Postpartum management

Pre-existing diabetes

- Women with insulin-treated pre-existing diabetes should reduce their insulin immediately after birth as they are at risk of hypoglycaemia
- Careful CBG monitoring (4× daily) will be needed to establish what the new dose will be
- Contact the diabetes team to review ongoing insulin requirement
- Women should have a meal or snack before or during breastfeeding to prevent hypoglycaemia
- Women with T2DM who are breastfeeding can continue metformin, glibenclamide, and insulin, but there are limited data on safety in breastfeeding with other blood glucose-lowering agents
- Remind the patient of the importance of contraception and preconception care when planning future pregnancies.

Gestational diabetes

- Discontinue all blood glucose-lowering therapy immediately after birth
- Continue to monitor CBG pre and 1 hour post meal for up to 24 hours to capture pre-existing diabetes, new-onset diabetes, and to avoid hypoglycaemia
- If blood glucose has returned to normal, perform a fasting test or HbA1c 6–13 weeks after birth. If postnatal test is negative, offer annual HbA1c testing
- Explain the risk of GDM in future pregnancies. The risk of developing T2DM is also significantly increased so emphasize the importance of preventative measures, e.g. healthy diet, weight control, and exercise.

Further reading

1. RCOG (2018). Care of women with obesity in pregnancy (GTG72). Available at: https://www.rcog.org.uk/en/guidelines-research-services/guidelines/gtg72/
2. RCOG (2012). Shoulder dystocia (GTG42). Available at: https://www.rcog.org.uk/en/guidelines-research-services/guidelines/gtg42/

Chapter 60

Ectopic pregnancy and miscarriage

Guideline:
NICE NG126 (Ectopic pregnancy and miscarriage: diagnosis and initial management): https://www.nice.org.uk/guidance/ng126

OUP disclaimer: Oxford University Press makes no representation, express or implied, that the drug dosages are correct and that the recommendations are an exclusive or mandatory course of care. All health professionals reading this text have a responsibility to evaluate its appropriateness and take the individual needs of the patient into account.

Local trust guidelines: please refer to your local guidelines as necessary.

Overview

Vaginal bleeding and/or abdominal pain are common presentations seen in early pregnancy. Around 20% of pregnancies miscarry in the first trimester and early pregnancy loss accounts for >50,000 admissions annually in the UK. Ectopic pregnancies occur in 11 per 1000 pregnancies, and their complications (e.g. rupture) can lead to significant morbidity and mortality.

Diagnosis

History

A miscarriage commonly presents with vaginal bleeding ± passage of tissue (after amenorrhoea) and/or abdominal/pelvic pain. A miscarriage may also be identified on USS when a non-viable pregnancy is found incidentally with no preceding symptoms.

Ectopic pregnancy can also present with vaginal bleeding and/or abdominal/pelvic pain, usually between 4–10 weeks gestation. Other reported symptoms may include:

- Breast tenderness, missed period (and other signs of early pregnancy)
- Diarrhoea, tenesmus, rectal pressure, or pain with defecation
- Dizziness or syncope
- Shoulder tip pain (due to peritoneal irritation)
- Urinary symptoms.

Risk factors for ectopic pregnancy

- History of tubal damage or surgery
- Pelvic inflammatory disease
- Smoking
- Previous infertility
- In vitro fertilization
- Intrauterine contraceptive device in situ
- Endometriosis.

A third of ectopic pregnancies occur in the absence of any risk factors.

Examination

Remember that any woman of reproductive age is pregnant until proven otherwise! A pregnancy test should always be performed if there is any doubt about the patient's reproductive status.

Possible signs are listed in Table 60.1. However, signs may be limited to abdominal/pelvic pain and/or vaginal bleeding. Call for help early. Remember that young women compensate well and may not show signs of cardiovascular compromise until they have lost significant amounts of blood.

Suspected ectopic pregnancy

- If ectopic pregnancy is suspected following history and examination, the patient should be referred to an early pregnancy unit (EPU)/ gynaecology
- If the patient is high risk for rupture (previous ectopic or pelvic infection) **OR** is haemodynamically unstable **OR** is in significant pain, they should be urgently referred to EPU/gynaecology, or directly to the emergency department as this is a gynaecological emergency
- Ectopic pregnancies can rupture at any time and may be life-threatening, so it is advisable that patients with a suspected ectopic pregnancy who are discharged from hospital, should remain with an adult who could call an ambulance at all times.

Table 60.1 Examination findings in ectopic pregnancy or miscarriage

C	**Tachycardia (heart rate >100bpm)** **Hypotension (blood pressure <100/60mmHg or orthostatic)** **Shock/collapse**
D	**Reduced conscious level**
E	Pallor Abdominal distension* Enlarged uterus Abdominal/pelvic tenderness ± **rebound tenderness/ peritonitis*** Cervical excitation (pain on palpation of the cervix)* Adnexal mass or tenderness*

Signs in bold may be suggestive of a major haemorrhage secondary to a ruptured ectopic pregnancy or miscarriage.

* indicates specific findings suggestive of ectopic pregnancy

Investigations

Bedside

- Urine pregnancy test (UPT)
- Urinalysis: look for blood, rule out other causes of abdominal pain such as a UTI.

Bloods

See Table 60.2.

Table 60.2 Bloods for the investigation of ectopic pregnancy and miscarriage

Test	Rationale
FBC	Haemoglobin value to quantify blood loss
βHCG	Usually performed only after USS to guide management in pregnancies of unknown location or after diagnosis to direct treatment options with methotrexate
U&E	Differential diagnosis of abdominal pain Baseline check prior to prescribing methotrexate in ectopic pregnancies
LFT	Differential diagnosis of abdominal pain Baseline check prior to prescribing methotrexate in ectopic pregnancies
Group and save	To assess rhesus D status and cross-match for blood if required

Imaging

Ultrasound

- If UPT is positive, a USS should be performed to identify the location and status of the pregnancy, and to assess if a fetal pole and/or heartbeat is present (Fig. 60.1)
- Patients should be made aware that it is not possible to diagnose miscarriage with 100% certainty on a USS, especially at early gestations
- Transvaginal ultrasound is preferable, but transabdominal ultrasound may be necessary if the patient has pelvic pathology, e.g. fibroids, or due to patient preference
- Patients may require two scans, a minimum of 7 days apart, and can be reassured that waiting for a repeat scan will not impact the outcome of their pregnancy
- The USS may show the following findings:
  - Viable intrauterine pregnancy: pregnancy seen within the uterine cavity with a fetal heartbeat
  - Missed or incomplete miscarriage: pregnancy tissue seen within the uterine cavity, but pregnancy is not viable or has partially miscarried
  - Ectopic pregnancy: pregnancy or a mass seen outside of the uterine cavity
  - Complete miscarriage: no pregnancy tissue seen within uterine cavity. This can only be diagnosed if the patient has had a previous scan showing an intrauterine pregnancy, otherwise it should be labelled as a pregnancy of unknown location
  - Pregnancy of unknown location: no intrauterine or extrauterine pregnancy seen on transvaginal USS (see 'Management' and Fig. 60.2)
  - Heterotopic pregnancy: concurrent viable intrauterine and ectopic pregnancies.

A full pelvic scan should always be done even if there is an obvious ectopic pregnancy to rule out a heterotopic pregnancy and to reliably examine the adnexae.

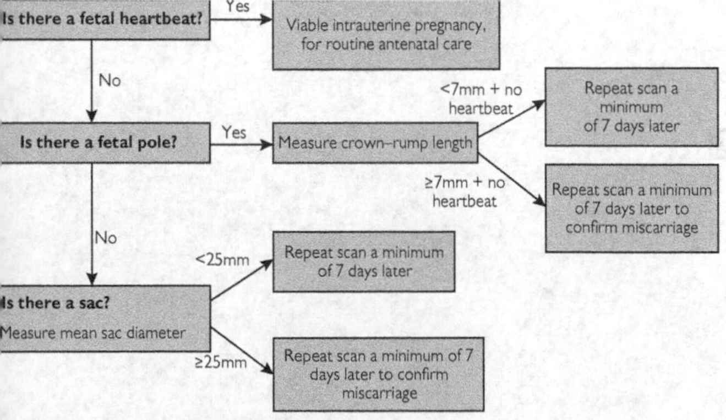

Fig. 60.1 Ultrasound investigation of viability.

Management

Acute management

- IV access and IV fluids for resuscitation (see Chapter 96) if haemodynamically unstable. Cross-match the patient urgently and activate the major haemorrhage protocol if necessary
- Make patient nil by mouth if awaiting surgery
- Give analgesia and antiemetics as required
- Provide the patient with appropriate information in a sensitive manner (Box 60.1).

Box 60.1 Providing information

Remember that pregnancy loss can cause significant distress and grief. Women and their partners should be given information in a sensitive manner. Information should be given on:

- Treatment options, including the risks and benefits
- What to expect during the course of the miscarriage, e.g. potential length of bleeding, advice regarding pain relief
- When and how to seek help if symptoms change or new symptoms develop
- What to expect during the recovery period, e.g. when it is possible to try to conceive again
- Signposting and support for bereavement.

Pregnancy of unknown location

Pregnancy of unknown location is diagnosed when the patient has a positive pregnancy test but no intrauterine or extrauterine pregnancy can be seen on a transvaginal USS. Eventual outcomes may include a healthy pregnancy (which was missed or too small to be detected on scan), a miscarriage that has already occurred (the pregnancy test may remain positive for another 2–3 weeks), or an ectopic pregnancy which is too early to be seen on scan or was missed. Management is summarized in Fig. 60.2.

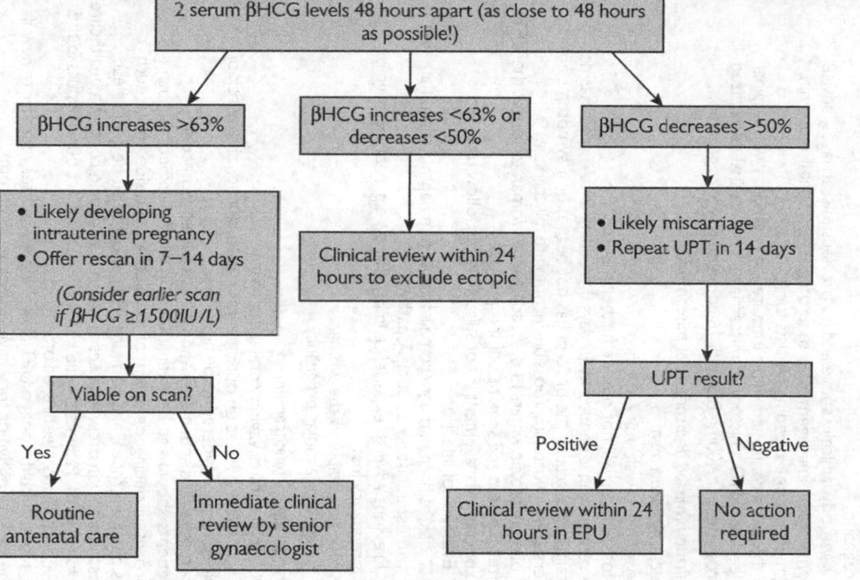
2 serum βHCG levels 48 hours apart (as close to 48 hours as possible!)
βHCG increases >63%
βHCG increases <63% or decreases <50%
βHCG decreases >50%
• Likely developing intrauterine pregnancy
• Offer rescan in 7–14 days
(Consider earlier scan if βHCG ≥1500IU/L)
Clinical review within 24 hours to exclude ectopic
• Likely miscarriage
• Repeat UPT in 14 days
Viable on scan?
Yes
No
Routine antenatal care
Immediate clinical review by senior gynaecologist
UPT result?
Positive
Negative
Clinical review within 24 hours in EPU
No action required

Fig. 60.2 Interpretation of serial βHCG levels in the management of pregnancy of unknown location.

Treatment after stabilization: miscarriage

Threatened miscarriage

- Any vaginal bleeding in early pregnancy should be considered a threatened miscarriage if the patient has a confirmed viable intrauterine pregnancy
- If haemodynamically stable and no previous miscarriages, advise conservative management with further assessment if worsening symptoms or if bleeding persists for >14 days
- If there is a confirmed viable intrauterine pregnancy with vaginal bleeding **AND** a history of miscarriage, offer vaginal micronized progesterone 400mg BD until 16 completed weeks gestation.

Confirmed (missed or incomplete) miscarriage

Expectant management

- 'Watch and wait' for 7–14 days
- Most women will not require further treatment
- A repeat scan is needed at 14 days if bleeding and/or pain has not started (suggesting the process has not begun) or if symptoms are persistent/worsening (possible incomplete miscarriage)
- If bleeding stops within 14 days, advise the woman to repeat the UPT after 3 weeks and seek help if it is positive
- Expectant management is not suitable in the following cases:
  - Evidence of infection
  - ↑ risk of haemorrhage/complications from haemorrhage (late first trimester, history of coagulopathy)
  - Previous adverse experience in pregnancy, e.g. haemorrhage or pregnancy loss
  - Not acceptable to the woman
  - Chance of a molar pregnancy.

Pharmacological management

- 800 micrograms vaginal/oral misoprostol
- This can be given as an outpatient, or as an inpatient if the risk of bleeding is considered to be high
- Pain relief and antiemetics should be provided as needed
- Patients should also be given advice on what to expect through the process including the extent of the bleeding and side effects such as pain, diarrhoea, and vomiting. They should also be given clear instructions on circumstances in which they should contact a healthcare professional. Patients should know who to contact out of hours in the event of heavy bleeding or other concerns
- Patients should repeat a UPT after 3 weeks and seek further review if the test is positive or they have worsening symptoms.

Surgical management

- Surgical management can be performed under local anaesthetic (manual vacuum aspiration) or general anaesthetic
- Pregnancy tissue should be analysed to exclude molar pregnancy.

Treatment after stabilization: ectopic pregnancy

Possible ectopic

Until an ectopic pregnancy or miscarriage is diagnosed, the patient should be treated as a pregnancy of unknown location. This will require follow-up in an EPU. Patients should be advised to attend the EPU at any time if they have pain or worsening bleeding.

Confirmed ectopic

Confirmed ectopic pregnancies should be managed on the EPU. Patients should be safety netted carefully and able to attend the EPU at any time if any complications develop. If not undergoing surgical management, patients should live with an adult who could call for help if required, due to the risk of rupture.

Expectant management

Offer if:

- Clinically stable and pain free
- Initial serum βHCG <1500IU/L
- Acceptable to the patient
- Able to return for follow-up:
  - Repeat βHCG at days 2, 4, and 7
  - If βHCG levels decrease >15% between tests, repeat weekly until negative result (<20IU/L), otherwise arrange urgent senior review
  - Be prepared to abandon expectant management if there are symptoms of pain or bleeding.

Medical management

- Should be offered if expectant management criteria fulfilled and no significant pain, and βHCG <1500IU/L
- Consider offering medical management if expectant management criteria fulfilled and no significant pain, and βHCG 1500–5000IU/L
- Treatment is IM methotrexate at a dose of 50mg/m^2. Estimated body area (m^2) can be calculated based on the patient's height and weight
- It must only be offered if there is a definitive diagnosis of ectopic pregnancy and a viable intrauterine pregnancy has been excluded
- Side effects include GI upset (flatulence and bloating), transient liver function abnormalities, stomatitis, and bone marrow suppression
- Follow up with repeat βHCG at days 4 and 7, with weekly levels until negative. A 15% decrease in βHCG should be expected by day 7. If levels plateau or rise, reassess clinically
- Patients with failed medical management are likely to require surgical management.

Surgical management

- Laparoscopic salpingectomy or salpingostomy
- Offer surgery as first line if significant pain, adnexal mass >35mm, fetal heartbeat present, or βHCG >5000IU/L
- Follow up with a repeat UPT in 3 weeks
- If risk factors for infertility (e.g. previous ectopic, contralateral tube damage, previous surgery or pelvic inflammatory disease), consider salpingostomy. One in five women will need further treatment (e.g. methotrexate and/or salpingectomy) and follow-up includes βHCG at day 7, and weekly until a negative result is obtained.

Anti-D prophylaxis (250IU or 50 micrograms) should only be given to women who undergo a surgical procedure to manage an ectopic pregnancy or miscarriage.

Further reading

1. RCOG (2016). Diagnosis and management of ectopic pregnancy (GTG21). Available at: https://www.rcog.org.uk/en/guidelines-research-services/guidelines/gtg21/
2. Miscarriage Association website. Available at: https://www.miscarriageassociation.org.uk/
3. The Ectopic Pregnancy Trust website. Available at: https://ectopic.org.uk

Chapter 61

Hypertension in pregnancy

Guideline:
NICE NG133 (Hypertension in pregnancy: diagnosis and management): https://www.nice.org.uk/guidance/ng133/

OUP disclaimer: Oxford University Press makes no representation, express or implied, that the drug dosages are correct and that the recommendations are an exclusive or mandatory course of care. All health professionals reading this text have a responsibility to evaluate its appropriateness and take the individual needs of the patient into account.

Local trust guidelines: please refer to your local guidelines as necessary.

Overview

Hypertension in pregnancy includes the following conditions:

- Chronic hypertension which requires ongoing management while the patient is pregnant
- Gestational hypertension
- Pre-eclampsia.

Careful blood pressure (BP) monitoring is critical for both maternal and fetal well-being, and antihypertensive treatment (AHT) may be required. Severe pre-eclampsia and eclampsia are life-threatening, and patients may require critical care support. See Fig. 61.1.

Diagnosis

History/diagnostic criteria

Hypertension in pregnancy is defined as systolic BP >140mmHg, or diastolic BP >90mmHg.

Chronic Hypertension	Gestational Hypertension	Pre-Eclampsia	Severe Pre-Eclampsia
• Hypertension present at booking visit **OR** • Already established on antihypertensive medications at booking **OR** • Hypertension which presents **before** 20 weeks	• New onset of hypertension presenting **after** 20 weeks gestation **without significant proteinuria or other features suggestive of pre-eclampsia**	• New onset of hypertension **after** 20 weeks gestation with ≥1 of (new onset): ◦ Proteinuria ◦ Renal insufficiency ◦ Liver involvement ◦ Neurological complications ◦ Haematological complications ◦ Uteroplacental dysfunction	• Pre-eclampsia with: ◦ Severe hypertension (systolic BP >160 mmHg or diastolic BP >110 mmHg) that is refractory to treatment ◦ Persistent symptoms ◦ Deteriorating blood tests ◦ Failure of fetal growth or abnormal Doppler finding

Fig. 61.1 Hypertensive disorders of pregnancy.

If the patient has chronic hypertension, determine which AHT they are using currently.

History in pre-eclampsia may include:

- Severe headache
- Visual disturbances (e.g. blurring, flashing lights)
- Severe upper abdominal pain (right upper quadrant and/or epigastric pain)
- Nausea and vomiting
- Sudden swelling of the face, hands, and feet
- Feeling generally unwell.

Risk factors for gestational hypertension and pre-eclampsia are listed in Box 61.1.

Box 61.1 Risk factors for gestational hypertension and pre-eclampsia

- Nulliparity
- Age >40 years
- Pregnancy interval >10 years
- Multiple pregnancy
- Family history pre-eclampsia
- BMI >35kg/m^2
- Renal disease
- Vascular disease
- History of pre-eclampsia or gestational hypertension.

Pre-eclampsia prophylaxis

- Patients with **any** of the following risk factors should take 75–150mg of aspirin daily from 12 weeks to birth as pre-eclampsia prophylaxis:
  - Autoimmune disease, e.g. systemic lupus erythematosus or antiphospholipid syndrome
  - Chronic hypertension
  - CKD
  - History of hypertension in a previous pregnancy
  - T1DM or T2DM
- Patients with **two or more** of the following risk factors should take 75–150mg of aspirin daily from 12 weeks to birth as pre-eclampsia prophylaxis:
  - Age >40 years
  - BMI ≥35kg/m^2 at first contact
  - Family history of pre-eclampsia
  - First pregnancy
  - Multiple pregnancy
  - Pregnancy interval >10 years.

Table 61.1 Examination findings in a hypertensive pregnant patient

B	Tachypnoea: possible pulmonary oedema Hypoxia: possible pulmonary oedema
C	Hypertension: systolic BP >160mmHg particularly concerning Tachycardia: possible pulmonary oedema Oliguria: possible renal insufficiency
E	Right upper quadrant or epigastric tenderness Swollen face, hands, or feet Clonus, hyperreflexia, or other signs of impending eclampsia Seizures (eclampsia) Visual scotomata Signs of fetal compromise

Examination

Possible examination findings in the hypertensive pregnant patient are listed in Table 61.1.

Investigations

Bedside

- **Urinalysis:** screen for proteinuria. Do not use first morning void:
  - If positive (>1+), send ACR or protein:creatinine ratio (PCR)
  - Significant proteinuria = ACR ≥8mg/mmol **OR** PCR ≥30mg/mmol.

Bloods

- **FBC:**
  - Thrombocytopenia—a concerning sign in pre-eclampsia
  - Haemolysis

- **LFT:**
  - ↑ transaminases (ALT or AST >40IU/L)—a concerning sign in pre-eclampsia
- **U&E:**
  - ↑ creatinine (>90μmol/L)—a concerning sign in pre-eclampsia
  - Note baseline creatinine is lower during pregnancy
- **Coagulation profile:**
  - Possible DIC

Imaging

- **Ultrasound:** may find fetal growth restriction, abnormal umbilical artery flow, or stillbirth.

Other

- **CTG:** assess fetal well-being
- **Placental growth factor testing:** used when pre-eclampsia is suspected in women between 20–35 weeks with chronic or gestational hypertension. Abnormally low plasma/serum levels suggest placental dysfunction and may indicate the development of pre-eclampsia.

Management

Acute management

Antenatal antihypertensive treatment options are listed in Fig. 61.2.

First line - labetalol

Second line - nifedipine

Third line - methyldopa

Fig. 61.2 Antenatal AHT choices.

Management of chronic hypertension

Table 61.2 summarizes the management of chronic hypertension in pregnancy.

Table 61.2 Management of chronic hypertension during pregnancy

Lifestyle advice	Weight management, exercise, healthy eating including salt reduction
AHT	**New diagnosis:** Start AHT as per Fig. 61.2 **If already using AHT:** • If medications are safe in pregnancy, continue unless systolic BP <110mmHg or diastolic BP <70mmHg • ACE inhibitors and angiotensin II receptor blockers (ARBs) are associated with ↑ risk of congenital abnormalities, therefore stop immediately and seek a safe alternative. Thiazides and thiazide-like diuretics may also increase the risk of congenital abnormalities
Aspirin	Give aspirin 75–150mg daily from 12 weeks until birth
BP target	≤135/85mmHg
BP measurement	Review every 2–4 weeks if BP is below target. If poor control, review weekly
Fetal assessment	Arrange ultrasound growth scans at 28, 32, and 36 weeks
	Perform a CTG only if clinically indicated

Management of gestational hypertension

Table 61.3 summarizes the management of gestational hypertension.

Management of pre-eclampsia

Table 61.4 summarizes the management of pre-eclampsia.

Management of severe pre-eclampsia

- Get senior help
- Consider labetalol PO/IV, nifedipine PO, or hydralazine IV
- Consider giving magnesium sulphate as prophylaxis to all patients with severe pre-eclampsia after discussion with a senior clinician

Table 61.3 Management of gestational hypertension

	Gestational hypertension BP 140/90mmHg - 159/109mmHg	Severe gestational hypertension BP >160/110mmHg
Admission	No	Yes
AHT	As per Fig. 61.2	
Target BP	≤135/85mmHg	
BP measurement	1–2 times/week until BP below target	Every 15–30 minutes until BP <160/110mmHg
Urinalysis	With BP measurements	Daily while admitted
Bloods	FBC, U&E, and LFT at presentation, then weekly	
Fetal assessment	Auscultate fetal heart at every appointment	
	Ultrasound assessment at diagnosis. If normal, repeat every 2–4 weeks as clinically indicated	Ultrasound assessment at diagnosis. If normal, repeat every 2 weeks if severe hypertension persists
	CTG only if clinically indicated	CTG at diagnosis. If normal, only repeat if clinically indicated

Table 61.4 Management of pre-eclampsia

	Pre-eclampsia BP 140/90mmHg - 159/109mmHg	Severe pre-eclampsia BP >160/110mmHg
Admission	Yes, if clinical concerns or high risk	Yes
AHT	As per Fig. 61.2	
Target BP	≤135/85mmHg	
BP measurement	At least every 48 hours, more often if admitted	Every 15–30 minutes until BP <160/110mmHg, then at least 4 times/day
Urinalysis	Repeat only if clinically indicated (e.g. new symptoms, uncertain diagnosis)	
Bloods	FBC, U&E, and LFT **twice** a week	FBC, U&E, and LFT **three times** a week
Fetal assessment	Auscultate fetal heart at every appointment	
	Ultrasound assessment at diagnosis. If normal, repeat every 2 weeks	
	CTG at diagnosis and if normal, only repeat if clinically indicated	

- Give a loading dose 4g IV over 5–15 minutes, followed by an infusion of 1g/hour maintained for 24 hours after delivery
- Patients who have had seizures should also be given a loading dose and maintenance dose to treat the seizure and prevent further seizures
- Recurrent fits can be treated with an additional dose of 2–4g IV over 5–15 minutes.

Blood pressure measurement and management in labour

- All women in labour should have their blood pressure measured hourly
- In severe hypertension, blood pressure should be checked every 15–30 minutes until <160/110mmHg
- Continue usual AHT during labour.

Treatment after stabilization

Patient education

- Inform the patient that their risk is approximately 1 in 5 of a hypertensive disorder occurring in a future pregnancy
- Inform the patient of an ↑ risk of hypertension and cardiovascular disease in later life.

Timing of birth

- Mode and timing of delivery should be decided by a senior obstetrician—consider whether the neonatal team should be present
- If an early birth is planned, consider whether to give antenatal steroids and magnesium sulphate.

Postnatal management and monitoring

The use of antihypertensive medications postnatally is summarized in Fig. 61.3. Table 61.5 summarizes the postnatal management of hypertensive disorders of pregnancy.

If well controlled on **labetalol** or **nifedipine** - continue

If on **methyldopa** - change to an alternative within 2 days of birth

If starting AHT - use **enalapril** but monitor renal function

If starting AHT for women of black African/Caribbean family origin - consider **nifedipine** (or **amlodipine** if previously used)

If BP not controlled with a single agent - consider combination therapy

If not breastfeeding - treat as per standard hypertension guidelines

Use once daily preparations where possible

Fig. 61.3 Postnatal AHT choices.

Table 61.5 Postnatal management and monitoring of hypertensive disorders of pregnancy

	Chronic hypertension	Gestational hypertension	Pre-eclampsia
Postnatal BP monitoring	• Check BP daily for first 2 days • Check BP at least once between days 3–5 • Check BP whenever AHT is modified		If patient didn't use AHT in pregnancy: • At least 4×/day while inpatient • At least once between days 3–5 postpartum • On alternate days until normal if abnormal at days 3–5 postpartum If patient used AHT in pregnancy: • At least 4×/day while inpatient • Every 1–2 days for up to 2 weeks until off AHT and normotensive Ask women about severe headache and epigastric pain at each BP measurement
Starting, stopping, and continuing postnatal AHT	Keep BP <140/90mmHg—continue AHT if necessary to achieve this	• Continue AHT if still needed • Reduce AHT if BP <130/80mmHg • Start AHT if BP >150/100mmHg	• Start AHT if BP ≥150/100mmHg • If already using AHT, continue after birth and consider reducing when BP <140/90mmHg

(Continued)

Table 61.5 *Continued*

	Chronic hypertension	Gestational hypertension	Pre-eclampsia
Outpatient review and follow-up	Review at 2 weeks, then again at 6–8 weeks	• Review at 2 weeks, then again at 6–8 weeks • Provide community staff with a clear plan for follow-up including frequency of monitoring and thresholds for stopping treatment	• Check platelets, creatinine, and transaminases 48–72 hours after birth—does not need repeating if normal • Transfer to community care when asymptomatic, BP (treated or untreated) <150/100mmHg, and bloods stable or improving • Review at 2 weeks, then again at 6–8 weeks • Do urinalysis at 6–8 weeks, if ≥1 proteinuria then reassess kidney function at 3 months. If abnormal, refer to specialist • Provide community staff with a clear plan for follow-up including frequency of monitoring and thresholds for stopping treatment

Special considerations

Breastfeeding

- Treatment options for breastfeeding patients include enalapril, nifedipine, amlodipine, atenolol, and labetalol.
- Many AHTs can pass into breastmilk at very low levels. They are unlikely to have any clinical effect
- Consider monitoring the BP of the baby (especially if pre-term) if they have symptoms of low BP in the first few weeks of life
- Parents should monitor babies for drowsiness, lethargy, pallor, cold peripheries, and poor feeding

Further reading

1. NICE (2016). PlGF-based testing to help diagnose suspected pre-eclampsia (Triage PlGF test, Elecsys immunoassay sFlt-1/PlGF ratio, DELFIA Xpress PlGF 1-2-3 test, and BRAHMS sFlt-1 Kryptor/BRAHMS PlGF plus Kryptor PE ratio) (DG23). Available at: https://www.nice.org.uk/guidance/dg23
2. Thangaratinam S, Allotey J, Marlin N, et al. (2019). PREP-S: risk of complications in early-onset pre-eclampsia. Available at: https://www.evidencio.com/models/show/1038

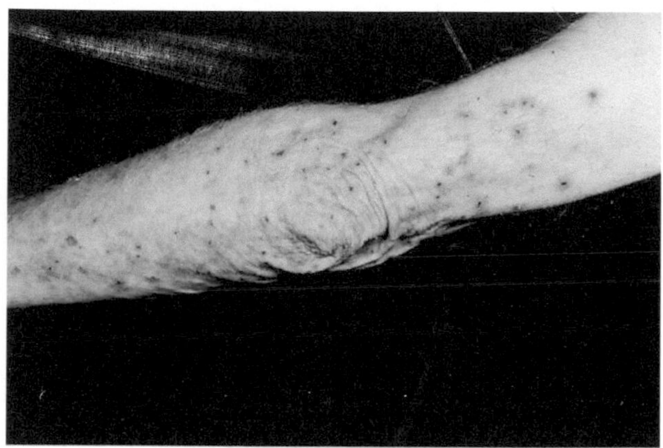

Plate 1 Dermatitis Herpetiformis. Reproduced from Bloom S et al (2011) 'Oxford Handbook of Gastroenterology and Hepatology 2e' Oxford University Press: Oxford, with permission from Oxford University Press.

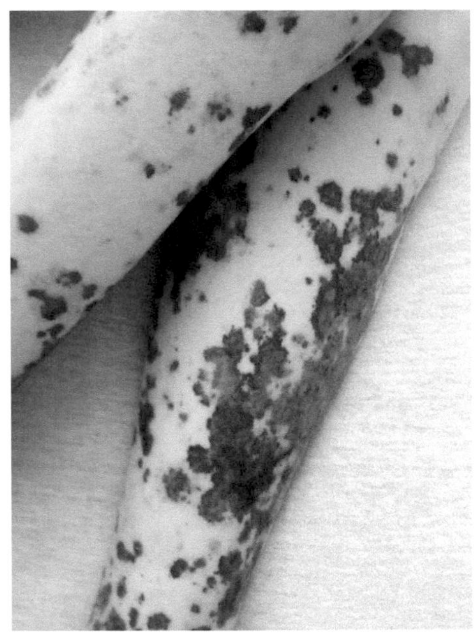

Plate 2 Non-blanching petechial rash. Reproduced from the original by Dr FO. Jr. Tn under the Creative Commons CC-BY-SA 3.0 license

(a)

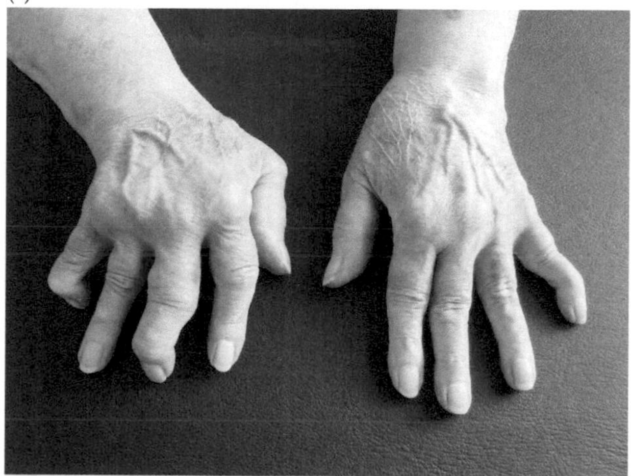

(b)

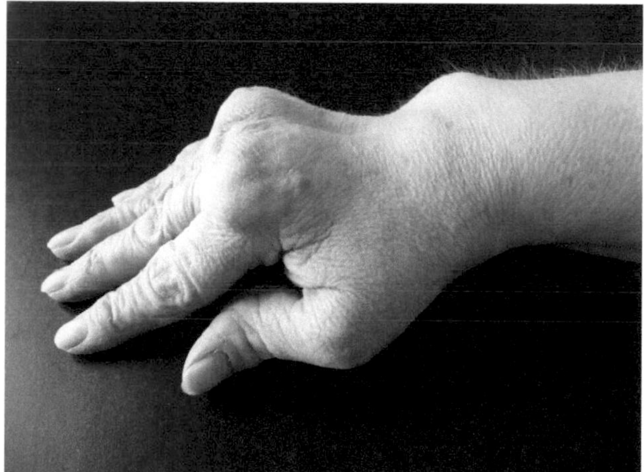

Plate 3 (a) Patient with RA presenting with a radial deviation (right wrist), swan-neck deformity with hyperextension of the proximal interphalangeal (PIP) and flexion of distal interphalangeal (DIP) joints (digits 3 right and 5 on both sides) and boutonnière deformity with flexion of the PIP and hyperextension of DIP joints (digit 2 right). (b) Patient with RA presenting with volar subluxation of the right hand with a visible sliding at the radiocarpal joint and Z-deformity (or 90–90 thumb) with flexion of the first metacarpophalangeal joint and hyperextension of the interphalangeal joint. Reprinted from Watts R et al (2013) 'Oxford Textbook of Rheumatology' 4th Edition Oxford University Press: Oxford, with permission from Oxford University Press.

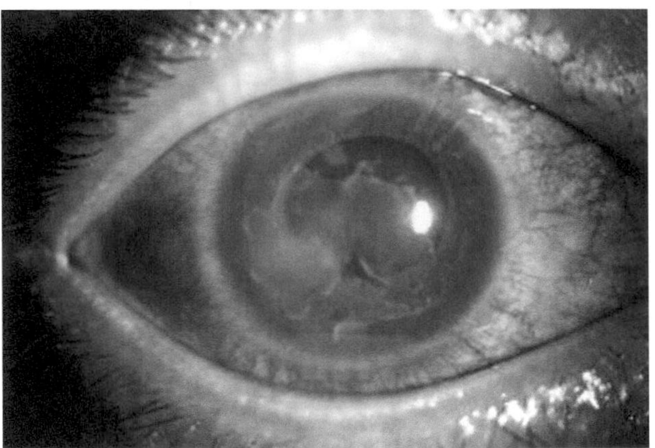

Plate 4 Anterior uveitis. A red eye with circumcorneal congestion, miosis and a hypopyon. Reprinted from Machemer R and Michelson G "Atlas of Ophthalmology: Online Multimedia Database" with kind permission from Prof. Dr. med. Georg Michelson

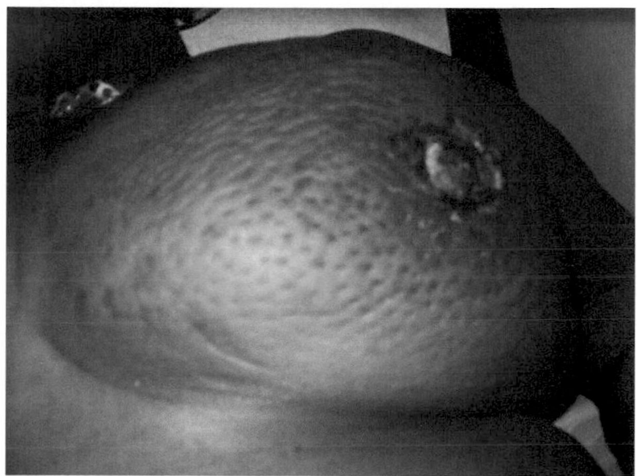

Plate 5 Peau d'orange skin changes which may be seen in breast cancer. Reproduced "Creative Commons Patient with inflammatory breast cancer" by Epidemiology and surgical management of breast cancer in gynecological department of Douala General Hospital (Scientific Figure on ResearchGate) is licensed under Creative Commons 2.0. Available from: https://www.researchgate.net/figure/Patient-with-inflammatory-breast-cancer_fig2_234162338

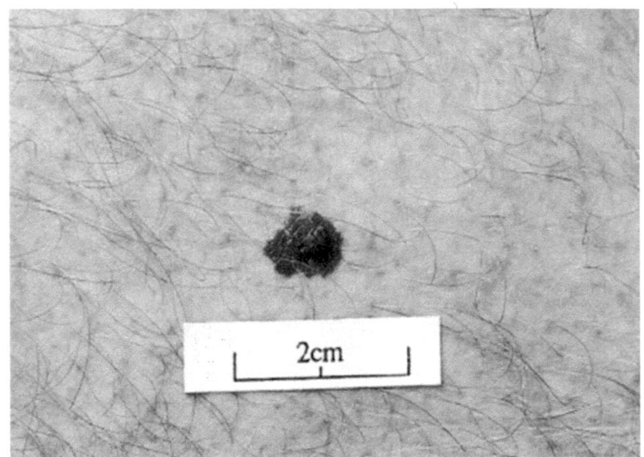

Plate 6 Superficial spreading melanoma. Reproduced from Firth J, Conlon C, and Cox T (2020) 'Oxford Textbook of Medicine 6th edition' Oxford University Press: Oxford, with permission from Oxford University Press.

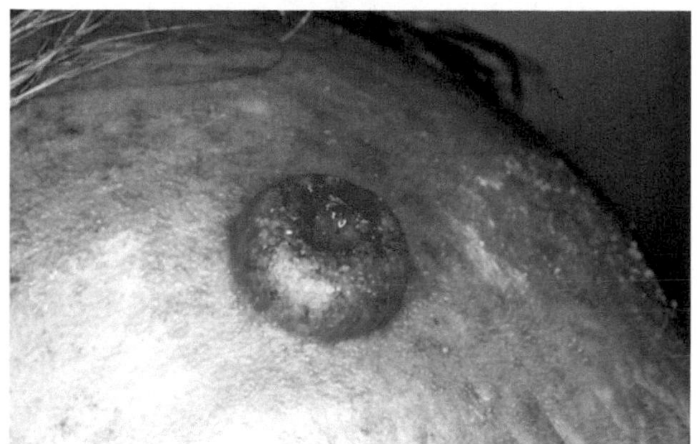

Plate 7 Squamous cell carcinoma presenting as a nodule. Reproduced from Firth J, Conlon C, and Cox T (2020) 'Oxford Textbook of Medicine 6th edition' Oxford University Press: Oxford, with permission from Oxford University Press.

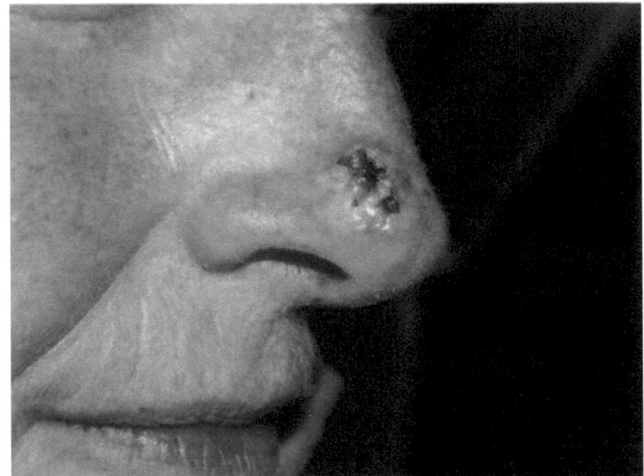

Plate 8 Morphoeic basal cell carcinoma. Reproduced from Gosney M and Harris T (2009) "Managing Older People in Primary Care: A Practical Guide' Oxford University Press, with permission from Oxford University Press

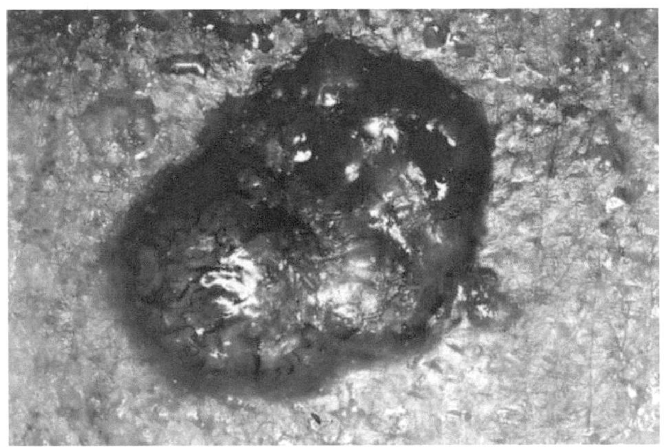

Plate 9 Basal cell carcinoma

Chapter 62

Intrapartum care

Guideline:
This chapter was based on: NICE CG190 (Intrapartum care for healthy women and babies): https://www.nice.org.uk/guidance/cg190/, updated 2017. Since the chapter was written, the guideline has been updated to NICE CG190 (Intrapartum care for healthy women and babies): www.nice.org.uk/guidance/cg190/, updated December 2022. NICE have updated the recommendations on monitoring during labour and transferred them to the new guideline NICE NG229 (Fetal monitoring in labour): https://www.nice.org.uk/guidance/ng229. NICE have also withdrawn content on fetal blood sampling.

OUP disclaimer: Oxford University Press makes no representation, express or implied, that the drug dosages are correct and that the recommendations are an exclusive or mandatory course of care. All health professionals reading this text have a responsibility to evaluate its appropriateness and take the individual needs of the patient into account.

Local trust guidelines: please refer to your local guidelines as necessary.

Overview

This chapter deals with standard care during labour for pregnancies where the birth is taking place at term (between 37 and 42 weeks).

Initial assessment of a woman in labour

Start by reviewing antenatal notes and relevant investigations such as bloods and screening results.

History

- Contractions: length, strength, and frequency
- Pain: full history, and discuss analgesia options (Table 62.1)
- Vaginal loss: bleeding, liquor, discharge
- Fetal movements over the past 24 hours: any change?

Examination

- Observations: pulse, blood pressure, and temperature
- Abdomen: fundal height, fetal lie, fetal presentation, fetal position, engagement of presenting part. Assess contractions if relevant
- Vaginal examination: perform if in established labour, or consider if the diagnosis is uncertain.

Investigations

- Urinalysis.

Fetal monitoring—should continue for the duration of labour

- Fetal heart auscultation (with Pinard stethoscope or Doppler ultrasound):
  - For 1 minute immediately after a contraction
  - Feel the woman's pulse simultaneously to differentiate
  - If abnormalities are suspected, use CTG
- CTG:
  - If the patient has any of the risk factors in Box 62.1 which mean they should have obstetric-led care, use continuous CTG
  - If fetal heart auscultation suggests abnormalities, use CTG for 20 minutes and then return to intermittent auscultation if normal
  - CTG can be offered to low-risk women if they are not yet in established labour but they should be aware of the risks and benefits and that it may require them to be transferred to obstetric-led care.

Box 62.1 Transfer to obstetric-led care

The patient should be transferred to obstetric-led care (if they are currently being cared for by a midwife) if any of the following are noted:

Signs of possible pre-eclampsia (see Chapter 61)

- Systolic blood pressure ≥160mmHg **OR** ≥140mmHg on two consecutive readings, 30 minutes apart
- Diastolic blood pressure ≥110mg **OR** ≥90mmHg on two consecutive readings, 30 minutes apart
- ≥2+ proteinuria **WITH EITHER** systolic blood pressure ≥140mmHg **OR** diastolic blood pressure ≥90mmHg
- Maternal collapse or seizure.

Signs of possible sepsis (see Chapter 66)

- Pulse >120bpm on two occasions, 30 minutes apart
- Temperature ≥38°C **OR** ≥37.5°C on two consecutive readings, 1 hour apart
- Suspected chorioamnionitis or sepsis.

Other concerns

- Pain that is not consistent with normal contractions
- Contractions >60 seconds
- >5 contractions in 10 minutes
- Use of oxytocin
- Wish for regional analgesia
- Antepartum haemorrhage (see Chapter 58)
- Rupture of membranes >24 hours before onset of established labour
- Significant meconium
- Reduced fetal movements in last 24 hours
- Cord prolapse
- Delayed first or second stage of labour
- Any abnormal presentation including transverse or oblique lie
- High or free-floating head in a nulliparous woman
- Suspected fetal growth restriction or macrosomia
- Anhydramnios or polyhydramnios
- Fetal heart rate <110bpm or >160bpm
- Decelerations on intermittent auscultation.

Postpartum complications

- Need for neonatal resuscitation
- Postpartum haemorrhage (see Chapter 65)
- Third- or fourth-degree tear (see 'Perineal trauma').

Table 62.1 Pain relief options in labour

Non-pharmacological	Breathing and relaxation techniques, massage, music, use of water or pool	
Pharmacological	**Advantages**	**Disadvantages**
Entonox (50:50 oxygen: nitrous oxide)	Inhaled route only Available in all birth settings	Nausea, vomiting, light-headedness
Opioids (pethidine or diamorphine)	Available in all birth settings IM single injection Lasts 2–4 hours Only takes 20 minutes to work	Requires concurrent administration of antiemetic *Maternal:* nausea and vomiting, drowsiness, interferes with breastfeeding *Fetal:* short-term respiratory depression and drowsiness
Regional anaesthesia (epidural or combined spinal epidural)	More effective analgesia Does not increase risk of caesarean section Does not increase risk of longer first stage of labour	Only available in obstetric units Requires IV access and continuous fetal monitoring so mobility may be reduced Associated with longer second stage of labour Associated with ↑ chance of instrumental birth

General points which apply throughout labour

- Encourage the woman to mobilize and use any position she finds comfortable
- Document if meconium is present at any point
- Encourage the woman to drink during labour, preferably isotonic drinks
- The woman may eat a light diet unless she has received opioids or is likely to require a general anaesthetic.

Fetal monitoring during labour

Low-risk women: intermittent auscultation

- Auscultate immediately after a contraction for 1 minute, at least every 15 minutes, and palpate maternal pulse hourly. Increase monitoring if concerned
- If there are definite concerns, summon help, transfer to obstetric care, and undertake continuous CTG.

High-risk women: CTG

- Assess and document the following features:
  - Contractions
  - Baseline fetal heart rate
  - Baseline fetal heart rate variability
  - Presence of accelerations (abrupt increase >15bpm in baseline fetal heart rate for >15 seconds)
  - Presence of decelerations (abrupt decrease >15bpm in baseline fetal heart rate for >15 seconds):
    - Early: start when uterine contraction begins, recover when uterine contraction stops—physiological
    - Variable: rapid fall in baseline fetal heartrate with variable recovery phase—may suggest pressure on the umbilical cord
    - Late: start at peak of uterine contraction, recover after uterine contraction stops—fetal hypoxia
    - Prolonged: >3 minutes
- Interpret the CTG according to Table 62.2.

Categorizing CTG traces (see Table 62.2)

- *Normal:* all features are reassuring
- *Suspicious:* one non-reassuring **AND** two reassuring features
- *Pathological:* one abnormal **OR** two non-reassuring features.

- If normal—continue usual care
- If suspicious:
  - Repeat maternal observations
  - Correct underlying cause, e.g. hypotension
  - Start conservative measures, e.g. mobilization, alternative positions, IV fluids, reduce or stop oxytocin, tocolysis to reduce contractions
  - Inform an obstetrician or senior midwife
- If pathological:
  - As per suspicious
  - Exclude acute events e.g. cord prolapse, placental abruption, uterine rupture
  - If no improvement, offer fetal scalp stimulation
  - If the CTG remains abnormal, consider fetal blood sampling and expediting the birth
- If acute bradycardia or deceleration lasting ≥3 minutes:
  - Urgent intervention is required
  - After correcting underlying cause and starting conservative measures, if bradycardia persists for >9 minutes or an acute event is confirmed, prepare for urgent delivery.

Table 62.2 Classification of CTG readings

	Baseline fetal heart rate	Baseline variability	Decelerations
Reassuring	110–160bpm	5–25bpm	None **OR** Early **OR** Variable <90 minutes
Non-reassuring	100–109bpm **OR** 161–180bpm	<5bpm for 30–50 minutes **OR** >25bpm for 15–25 minutes	Variable ≥90 minutes **OR** Variable with concerning features in up to 50% of contractions for ≥30 minutes **OR** Variable with concerning features in >50% contractions for <30 minutes **OR** Late in >50% contractions for <30 minutes with no significant clinical risk factors
Abnormal	<100bpm **OR** >180bpm	<5bpm for >50 minutes **OR** >25bpm for >25 minutes **OR** Sinusoidal	Variable with concerning features >50% contractions for >30 minutes **OR** Late for 30 minutes **OR** Acute bradycardia **OR** Deceleration lasting ≥3 minutes

Fetal blood sampling

Involves taking a small sample of blood from the baby's scalp during a vaginal speculum examination. Results are classified as per Table 62.3. Use **either** pH **or** lactate.

Table 62.3 Classification of fetal blood sampling results

	pH	Lactate	Action
Normal	≥7.25	≤4.1mmol/L	Repeat sample with 1 hour if CTG remains pathological
Borderline	7.21–7.24	4.2–4.8mmol/L	Repeat sample within 30 minutes if CTG remains pathological
Abnormal	≤7.20	≥4.9mmol/L	Expedite birth

First stage of labour

- Typically lasts 8–18 hours for primiparous woman and 5–12 hours for multiparous woman
- **Latent stage:** painful contractions and cervical effacement and dilatation **up to 4cm**
- **Established stage:** regular painful contractions and progressive cervical dilation **from 4cm until fully dilated (10cm)**
- Complete a partogram to monitor progression. Document:
  - Frequency of passing urine
  - Frequency of contractions every 30 minutes
  - Hourly pulse
  - 4-hourly temperature
  - 4-hourly blood pressure
  - 4-hourly vaginal examination (or if there is clinical concern)
- **Delay in the established first stage:** cervical dilation <2cm in 4 hours in any patient **OR** slowing of progress if multiparous. If membranes are intact, offer amniotomy and obstetric review to consider oxytocin augmentation.

Second stage of labour

- **Passive stage:** where the cervix is fully dilatated before the commencement of involuntary contractions or active maternal effort
- **Active stage:** baby visible **OR** expulsive contractions **OR** active maternal effort at full dilatation
- Document:
  - Frequency of passing urine
  - Frequency of contractions every 30 minutes
  - Hourly blood pressure
  - Hourly vaginal examination
  - 4-hourly temperature
- Fetal auscultation should be done after a contraction at least every 5 minutes
- **Delay in the second stage:** if active stage >2 hours (nulliparous) or >1 hour (multiparous). Arrange obstetric review to decide if oxytocin augmentation, instrumental birth, or caesarean section is necessary
- Encourage the woman to adopt any comfortable position that is not lying down or sitting in bed.

Third stage of labour

- **Definition:** time from the birth of the baby to the expulsion of placenta and membranes
- Management can be active or passive
- **Active management:** 10IU oxytocin IM after birth, deferred cord clamping (1–5 minutes), and controlled cord traction. There is a higher risk of nausea and vomiting compared to passive management
- **Passive (physiological) management:** waiting until the cord stops pulsing before clamping, and natural delivery of the placenta. There is a higher risk of haemorrhage and requiring a blood transfusion compared to active management
- Active management is recommended due to the significant reduction in the incidence of postpartum haemorrhage (see Chapter 65)
- **Prolonged third stage:** >30 minutes (active management) or >60 minutes (passive management). Secure IV access and consider if examination under anaesthetic is required in theatre for possible manual removal of retained placenta.

Postpartum

- Document pulse, temperature, blood pressure, uterine contraction, and lochia (vaginal discharge after birth)
- Assess that the placenta and membranes are complete
- The woman should have urinated within 6 hours of the birth.

Special considerations

Perineal trauma

- Classified into four degrees dependent on tissue involvement:
  - **First degree:** skin/vaginal mucosa only (does not require repair if the skin edges are well opposed)
  - **Second degree:** skin, vaginal mucosa, and perineal muscles but **not** the anal sphincter
  - **Third degree:** tear involving the anal sphincter complex
    - **3A:** <50% of external anal sphincter complex torn
    - **3B:** >50% of external anal sphincter complex torn
    - **3C:** internal anal sphincter torn
  - **Fourth degree:** tear involving anal epithelium ± anal sphincter complex (external and internal anal sphincter)
- An episiotomy is indicated for instrumental birth and/or suspected fetal compromise. This is an iatrogenic second-degree trauma originating from vaginal fourchette and is mediolateral at an axis of 45–60° (usually towards the right)
- Repair should be carried out as soon as possible after birth to minimize the risk of infection and blood loss. Use appropriate local or regional anaesthetic
- Third- and fourth-degree tears should be repaired in theatre and patients should receive a 7-day course of antibiotics. They should also be discharged with laxatives and should receive appropriate physiotherapy review and follow-up
- The patient should be given advice regarding hygiene and wound care and the wound should be reviewed prior to discharge. Patients should receive safety net advice to seek medical advice if they experience any signs of infection.

Further reading

1. Geeky Medics. How to read a CTG. Available at: https://geekymedics.com/how-to-read-a-ctg/
2. RCOG. Assessment of fetal wellbeing. Available at: https://elearning.rcog.org.uk/assessment-fetal-wellbeing/assessment-fetal-wellbeing

Chapter 63

Nausea and vomiting in pregnancy

Guideline:
RCOG GTG69 (The management of nausea and vomiting of pregnancy and hyperemesis gravidarum): https://www.rcog.org.uk/en/guidelines-research-services/guidelines/gtg69/

OUP disclaimer: Oxford University Press makes no representation, express or implied, that the drug dosages are correct and that the recommendations are an exclusive or mandatory course of care. All health professionals reading this text have a responsibility to evaluate its appropriateness and take the individual needs of the patient into account.

Local trust guidelines: please refer to your local guidelines as necessary.

Overview

Nausea and vomiting in pregnancy (NVP) is a common reason for hospital attendance and admission in the pregnant woman. About 80% of pregnant women will experience these symptoms although 90% of cases resolve by 20 weeks. When NVP is severe, it may satisfy the criteria to be termed hyperemesis gravidarum (HG) (see later in chapter). Women with multiple or trophoblastic pregnancies are at ↑ risk; however, the majority of patients will have a singleton pregnancy.

Diagnosis

Diagnosis is in the first trimester. Typical onset is at approximately 4–7 weeks with symptoms usually peaking at 9 weeks. Other causes of nausea and vomiting need to be excluded, particularly if presenting >10+6 weeks.

Differential diagnosis

- *Acute abdomen:* cholecystitis, pancreatitis, appendicitis, bowel obstruction
- *Gastrointestinal:* peptic ulcer, gastroenteritis, hepatitis
- *Endocrine:* diabetic ketoacidosis, hypothyroidism
- *Urinary:* UTI, pyelonephritis
- *Other:* drug induced.

History

- Protracted nausea and/or vomiting
- Inability to tolerate food/fluids
- Dehydration
- Hypersalivation
- Weight loss (>5% from pre-pregnancy)
- Haematemesis (secondary to Mallory–Weiss tears).

History to exclude other causes:

- Abdominal pain
- Fevers
- Urinary/bowel symptoms
- PV loss
- Drug history.

Severity of NVP can be quantified using the Pregnancy-Unique Quantification of Emesis (PUQE) index (Table 63.1).

Table 63.1 Total score is sum of replies to each of the three questions

In the last 24 hours, how long have you felt nauseated?	0 times (1)	1 hour or less (2)	2–3 hours (3)	4–6 hours (4)	More than 6 (5)
In the last 24 hours, how many times have you vomited?	0 times (1)	1–2 times (2)	3–4 times (3)	5–6 times (4)	7 or more times (5)
In the last 24 hours, how many times have you had retching/dry heaves without vomiting?	0 times (1)	1–2 times (2)	3–4 times (3)	5–6 times (4)	7 or more times (5)

PUQE-24 score: mild ≤6; moderate = 7–12; severe = 13–15.

Reprinted from Koren G, Boskvocic R, Hard M, Maltepe C, Navioz Y, Einarson A. Motherisk-PUQE (pregnancy-unique quantification of emesis and nausea) scoring system for nausea and vomiting of pregnancy. American journal of obstetrics and gynecology. 2002;186:S228–31 with permission from Mosby.

Hyperemesis gravidarum

This is a triad of:

- >5% pre-pregnancy weight loss
- Dehydration
- Electrolyte imbalance.

Examination

The main focus should be on performing an abdominal examination, and to look for any clinical signs of dehydration or wasting. Consider a thyroid examination if hypothyroidism/hyperthyroidism is a differential diagnosis.

Investigations

Bedside

- Basic observations
- Weight
- Urinalysis (ketonuria, and to exclude UTI)
- Midstream urine to be sent for MC&S
- Capillary blood glucose ± blood ketone level if diabetic.

Bloods

- FBC (infection, anaemia, haematocrit)
- U&E (hyponatraemia, hypokalaemia, renal disease)
- Amylase
- Consider checking TFT (although these may be transiently abnormal due to the biochemical structural similarity between HCG and TSH) and LFT in refractory cases

Imaging

- Pelvic USS to confirm viability and gestational age (check for trophoblastic/multiple pregnancy). This should be arranged as a routine scan unless the patient is not improving with treatment or there are other medical reasons for an earlier and more urgent scan
- Abdominal USS may also be required if the patient has severe abdominal pain
- OGD may also be required if pregnancy seems to be an unlikely cause of the symptoms.

Other

- Consider screening for *Helicobacter pylori* if the patient has severe abdominal pain.

Management

Initially NVP can be managed in the community with oral antiemetics. If this has failed, ambulatory/day care management may be suitable, particularly for patients with a PUQE <13.

Acute management

Inpatient admission is required if there is continued NVP with an inability to tolerate oral antiemetics, NVP associated with clinical dehydration, ketonuria, or weight loss, or NVP associated with a comorbidity such as a UTI.

Pharmacological management

Offer parenteral administration of medications until oral intake is tolerated. Use drugs from different classes if the first choice is ineffective. Combinations of antiemetics may also be required.

Antiemetics

- First line—antihistamines/phenothiazines. There is no evidence of teratogenicity:
  - Cyclizine:
    - 50mg PO, IM, or IV, TDS
  - Prochlorperazine:
    - 5–10mg PO, TDS–QDS
    - 12.5mg IM, TDS
    - 25mg rectally, OD
  - Promethazine:
    - 12.5–25mg PO, IM, IV, or rectally, 4–8-hourly
  - Chlorpromazine:
    - 10–25mg PO, IV, or IM, 4–6-hourly
    - 50–100mg rectally, 6–8-hourly.

Xonvea® (doxylamine with pyridoxine) is a newer antihistamine-based antiemetic which is increasingly being offered as an option for patients who do not respond to conservative management. Some prescribers and patients may prefer this medication as it is specifically licensed for NVP, whereas this is not the case for traditional first- and second-line treatments. Discuss with a senior obstetrician if Xonvea® may be an option locally.

- Second line—safe and effective, but second line due to either side effects or limited data:
  - Metoclopramide:
    - 5–10mg PO, IM, or IV, TDS
    - Maximum 5-day course due to possible maternal neurological side effects e.g. extrapyramidal side effects, tardive dyskinesia. Contraindicated in bowel obstruction
  - Domperidone:
    - 10mg PO, TDS
    - 30–60mg rectally, TDS
    - Maximum 7-day course, contraindicated in cardiac disease
  - Ondansetron:
    - 4–8mg PO, TDS–QDS
    - 8mg IV over 15 minutes, BD

- Third line, on senior obstetric advice—corticosteroids:
  - Hydrocortisone 100mg IV BD
  - Once there is clinical improvement, convert to prednisolone 50–60mg PO OD, with the dose gradually tapered until the lowest maintenance dose that controls the symptoms is reached.

IV rehydration

- Normal saline with added potassium, e.g. 1L 0.9% saline with 20mmol potassium over 2 hours. Multiple bags will be required
- Avoid dextrose due to the risk of precipitating Wernicke's encephalopathy if thiamine deficient
- Fluid status should be reassessed after 2L of fluid and then regularly thereafter. U&E should be tested daily.

Thiamine

- When oral intake is re-established
- If not tolerating any oral intake, discuss with a senior clinician if Pabrinex® should be used.

If symptoms of GORD/gastritis

- Start PPI/H_2 receptor antagonist, e.g. omeprazole 20mg OD.

VTE prophylaxis

Remember that pregnancy is a risk factor for VTE and that this risk is heightened by dehydration. Unless contraindicated, prescribe LMWH and antiembolic stockings for inpatients which may be stopped on discharge.

Treatment after stabilization

If symptoms continue into the second or third trimester, consider arranging serial scans to monitor growth from 28 weeks.

Special considerations

- NVP/hyperemesis gravidarum can be extremely isolating and can adversely affect quality of life. Consider mental health status in pregnancy and refer for psychological support if necessary. Direct patients to information online in order to feel less isolated with the condition
- A termination of pregnancy should not be considered for NVP alone until all other treatment options have been tried. This is a senior MDT decision
- Complementary therapies such as ginger and acupuncture can be effective in some cases of mild NVP.

Further reading

1. Collins S, Arulkumaran S, Hayes K, et al. (2013). Hyperemesis gravidarum. In: *Oxford Handbook of Obstetrics and Gynaecology*, 3rd ed (pp. 546–7). Oxford: Oxford University Press. Available at: https://doi.org/10.1093/med/9780199698400.003.0016
2. Pregnancy Sickness Support website. Available at: https://www.pregnancysicknesssupport.org.uk/

Chapter 64

Pelvic organ prolapse in women

Guideline:
NICE NG123 (Urinary incontinence and pelvic organ prolapse in women: management): https://www.nice.org.uk/guidance/ng123

OUP disclaimer: Oxford University Press makes no representation, express or implied, that the drug dosages are correct and that the recommendations are an exclusive or mandatory course of care. All health professionals reading this text have a responsibility to evaluate its appropriateness and take the individual needs of the patient into account.

Local trust guidelines: Please refer to your local guidelines as necessary.

Overview

Pelvic organ prolapse occurs when one of the pelvic organs (bladder or urethra, uterus or vaginal vault, or rectum or bowel) descends beyond the normal anatomical position. These conditions are common and can have a major psychological and social impact on the patient, leading to severely reduced quality of life. Bladder prolapse is commonly associated with urinary incontinence (see Chapter 68).

Diagnosis

History

Ask about onset, duration, and severity of the symptoms. Check coexisting medical conditions and medications. Consider using a validated pelvic floor symptoms questionnaire.

- Urinary symptoms:
  - Frequency (>4–7 voids/day)
  - Dysuria
  - Haematuria
  - Nocturia or nocturnal enuresis
  - Urgency
  - Voiding difficulties: hesitancy, straining, slow or intermittent stream, needing to change position or reduce prolapse manually to void completely
  - Postmicturition symptoms: feeling of incomplete emptying, terminal dribble
  - Bladder or urethral pain
  - Incontinence (see Chapter 68)
- Rectal symptoms:
  - Constipation, needing to strain or requiring digital evacuation to pass stool
  - Urgency or incontinence of flatus or stool
- Vaginal symptoms:
  - Dyspareunia
  - Sensation of pressure or heaviness
  - Difficulty using tampons.

Red flags

New-onset urinary incontinence or retention, or faecal incontinence along with acute neurological symptoms, or new or changed back pain, are ⚑ for cauda equina syndrome.

Examination

- Abdominal examination (exclude pelvic mass, retention).
- Pelvic examination:
  - Skin assessment (atrophy, erythema, oedema)
  - Assessment of urethral/bladder descent on straining
  - Presence and degree of prolapse (Table 64.1). If the examination findings do not match the symptoms, re-examine whilst standing, squatting, or at another time
  - Digital vaginal exam assessing pelvic floor muscle contraction
  - Digital rectal exam assessing tone/voluntary contraction if there are neurological symptoms.

Investigations

Bedside

- Weight and BMI.

Table 64.1 Grading of urogenital prolapse (Baden–Walker classification)

First degree	Lowest part of prolapse descends halfway down vaginal axis to the introitus
Second degree	Lowest part of prolapse extends to the level of the introitus and through the introitus on straining
Third degree	Lowest part of prolapse extends through the introitus and lies outside the vagina Procidentia describes a third-degree uterine prolapse

Chronic management

Management is dependent on patient preferences, comorbidities, and desire for childbearing.

Lifestyle and simple interventions

- Weight loss (if BMI >30kg/m^2)
- Preventing and/or treating constipation
- Minimizing heavy lifting.

Pelvic floor muscle training

- First-line treatment for stage 1 and 2 prolapse
- Offer a trial of supervised training for at least 3 months
- It should include eight contractions, sustained for 6–8 seconds, performed three times daily.

Pessaries

- Consider vaginal oestrogen if there are signs of vaginal atrophy before pessary insertion
- Explain that more than one fitting may be needed and that the pessary should be removed every 6 months to avoid complications which include bleeding, discharge, difficulty removing, and expulsion.

Surgical management

There are numerous surgical procedures available for the treatment of prolapse, e.g. vaginal repairs, colposuspension, vaginal sacrospinous fixation with sutures or sacrocolpopexy with mesh, hysteropexy, sacrospinous fixation, and colpocleisis. The procedure of choice depends on patient and surgeon preference, and the exact type and degree of prolapse. Careful counselling and senior decision-making are required for procedures involving synthetic mesh. An important consideration for some procedures is whether the patient wants to have more children.

Further reading

1. Collins S, Arulkumaran S, Hayes K, et al. (2013). Urogynaecology. In: *Oxford Handbook of Obstetrics and Gynaecology*, 3rd ed (pp. 653–84). Oxford: Oxford University Press. Available at: https://doi.org/10.1093/med/9780199698400.003.0022

Chapter 65

Postpartum haemorrhage

Guideline:
RCOG GTG52 (Prevention and management of postpartum haemorrhage): https://www.rcog.org.uk/en/guidelines-research-services/guidelines/gtg52/

OUP disclaimer: Oxford University Press makes no representation, express or implied, that the drug dosages are correct and that the recommendations are an exclusive or mandatory course of care. All health professionals reading this text have a responsibility to evaluate its appropriateness and take the individual needs of the patient into account.

Local trust guidelines: please refer to your local guidelines as necessary.

Overview

Primary postpartum haemorrhage (PPH) is defined as the loss of >500mL of blood from the genital tract within 24 hours of delivery. Secondary PPH is excessive bleeding occurring from 24 hours to 12 weeks postpartum. PPH is an obstetric emergency and a senior obstetrician should be informed at the earliest opportunity.

Diagnosis

History/diagnostic criteria

- **Minor PPH:** 500–1000mL
- **Major PPH:** >1000mL.

Risk factors

Antenatal

- Tone:
  - Previous PPH
  - BMI >35 kg/m^2
  - Uterine abnormalities, e.g. fibroids
  - Multiparity
  - Multiple pregnancy
  - Polyhydramnios
  - Macrosomia (>4kg)
- Tissue:
  - Placenta praevia
  - Placenta accreta
- Thrombin:
  - Pre-eclampsia/HELLP (**h**aemolysis, **e**levated **l**iver enzymes, **l**ow **p**latelets) syndrome
  - Hypertension
  - Anticoagulant use
  - Bleeding disorders
- Other:
  - Age >40 years
  - First pregnancy
  - APH (see Chapter 58).

Intrapartum and postpartum

- Tone:
  - Use of muscle relaxants including general anaesthetic, magnesium sulphate, and terbutaline
  - Infection
  - Rapid or prolonged labour
  - Bladder distension
- Tissue:
  - Retained placenta, part of placenta, or membranes
  - Retained blood clots
- Trauma:
  - Perineal tears or episiotomy
  - Assisted vaginal delivery
  - Caesarean section
  - Cervical tears
  - Uterine rupture or inversion

- Thrombin:
  - DIC
  - Intrauterine death
  - Amniotic fluid embolism
  - Sepsis
  - Placental abruption.

PPH prophylaxis and risk reduction

- Treat antenatal anaemia: aim for haemoglobin concentration >110g/L at booking, and >105g/L at 28 weeks. Give iron supplementation if needed
- In a patient with no risk factors, delivering vaginally, give oxytocin 10IU IM in the third stage of labour
- In a patient undergoing a caesarean section, give oxytocin 5IU via a slow IV infusion, and consider giving IV tranexamic acid 0.5–1g
- Ergometrine-oxytocin (Syntometrine®) may be used in patients at ↑ risk of haemorrhage, if there are no contraindications (e.g. hypertension and cardiac disease).

Management

Acute management

See Table 65.1.

Table 65.1 The acute management of primary PPH

<table>
<tr><td colspan="3">Call for help!
Put out a PPH call—this should alert the midwife in charge, obstetric and anaesthetic teams, porters, and haematology
One team member should scribe, including sequence of events and timings of interventions</td></tr>
<tr><td colspan="2">Minor PPH, with no clinical shock</td><td>Major PPH</td></tr>
<tr><td>B</td><td>• Check respiratory rate every 15 minutes</td><td>• Continuous respiratory rate and pulse oximetry recording
• Give high-flow oxygen irrespective of saturations</td></tr>
<tr><td>C</td><td>• Check pulse and blood pressure every 15 minutes
• Gain IV access (minimum 14G) and send bloods for: FBC, coagulation profile including fibrinogen, and group and save
• Give warmed crystalloids</td><td>• Continuous pulse and blood pressure recording
• Insert 2× large-bore cannulae and send bloods for: FBC, U&E, LFT, VBG, coagulation profile including fibrinogen, and cross-match a minimum of 4 units of blood
• Transfuse blood as soon as possible
• Give 2L of warmed isotonic crystalloid as fast as possible, then a further 1.5L of colloid if necessary, until blood is available. Do not give more than 3.5L to avoid dilutional coagulopathy
• If required use emergency group O, rhesus D-negative and K-negative blood, switch to group-specific red cells as soon as possible</td></tr>
<tr><td>D</td><td></td><td>• Check temperature every 15 minutes
• Keep the patient warm</td></tr>
<tr><td>E</td><td colspan="2">Examine for possible bleeding source:
Palpate uterus for uterine atony
Assess vagina and cervix for tears
Examine uterine cavity for retained placenta or membranes</td></tr>
<tr><td></td><td colspan="2">• Palpate and rub the uterine fundus to stimulate contractions
• Insert urinary catheter—emptying the bladder may help to increase uterine tone
• Lie the patient flat to minimize blood loss and maintain central perfusion
• External aortic compression may buy time (use fist to administer pressure just above the umbilicus)
• Consider intraoperative cell salvage at caesarean section
Medications:
• Oxytocin 5IU by slow IV injection (can repeat dose once)
• Ergometrine 0.5mg by slow IV/IM injection (not if hypertensive)
• Oxytocin IV infusion (40IU in 500mL isotonic crystalloid at 125mL/hour)
• Carboprost 0.25mg IM, every 15 minutes, max. 8 doses (not if asthmatic)
• Misoprostol 800 micrograms sublingually or rectally
• Tranexamic acid 1g IV</td></tr>
</table>

Examination and management pitfalls

- Estimating blood loss:
  - Patients with PPH are usually young and fit, and pregnancy causes an increase in circulating blood volume, therefore hypovolaemia is often not apparent initially. Clinicians often underestimate blood loss when visually estimating, it is therefore important to weigh all blood and swabs in order to accurately estimate blood loss
  - Approximate indicators of blood volume loss:
    - Blood pressure and heart rate in the normal range: loss of <1000mL blood
    - Blood pressure ↓ (but >80mmHg systolic), heart rate ↑, and tachypnoea: loss of 1000–1500mL blood
    - Blood pressure <80 mmHg systolic, worsening tachycardia and tachypnoea, and impaired mental state: loss of >1500mL blood
- Point-of-care haemoglobin tests:
  - These can be falsely reassuring and should not be relied upon if there is clinical concern of PPH.

If bleeding continues after initial fluid and blood resuscitation

- FFP:
  - Infuse 4 units at a dose of 12–15mL/kg if bleeding is continuing after 4 units of red cells and coagulation profile are still unavailable **OR**
  - If coagulation profile show prolonged PT or APTT, give 12–15mL/kg
- Platelets:
  - Give one pool if bleeding ongoing and platelets <75 × 10^9/L
- Cryoprecipitate:
  - Give two pools if bleeding ongoing and fibrinogen <2g/L
- Aim to maintain:
  - Haemoglobin >80g/L
  - Platelets >50 × 10^9/L
  - Fibrinogen >2g/L
  - PT and APTT <1.5× normal.

Treatment after stabilization

Surgical management

If basic measures do not stop bleeding, initiate surgical interventions promptly:

- Intrauterine balloon tamponade is first line if atony is considered to be the main cause
- Haemostatic sutures may be used, e.g. B-lynch
- Stepwise uterine devascularization (successive ligation of various uterine arteries) requires a senior gynaecologist or vascular surgeon due to a high risk of ureteric injury
- Internal iliac artery ligation, or arterial occlusion, or embolization by interventional radiology
- Early hysterectomy (usually subtotal) if indicated, especially if uterine rupture or placenta accreta. Ideally a second obstetric consultant should be involved with this decision.

Monitoring and debriefing

- Consider whether the patient should be transferred to intensive or high dependency care and if an arterial line would be appropriate
- Monitor observations closely including urine output
- Recheck haemoglobin 4–6 hours after onset of PPH
- Look for evidence of any further bleeding
- Debrief the woman and her partner, PPH can be a traumatic experience and can lead to post-traumatic stress disorder and tokophobia (fear of pregnancy and childbirth).

Special considerations

Secondary PPH

- Send infection markers (and blood cultures if pyrexial) with initial bloods
- Take vaginal and cervical swabs
- Give broad-spectrum antibiotics for suspected endometritis
- Consider arranging a USS to rule out retained placental tissue after discussion with a senior clinician
- Theatre may be required for evacuation of retained products of conception.

Further reading

1. MBRRACE-UK (2020). *Saving Lives, Improving Mothers' Care: Lessons Learned to Inform Maternity Care from the UK and Ireland Confidential Enquiries into Maternal Deaths and Morbidity 2016–18.* Oxford: National Perinatal Epidemiology Unit, University of Oxford. Available at: https://www.npeu.ox.ac.uk/assets/downloads/mbrrace-uk/reports/maternal-report-2020/MBRRACE-UK_Maternal_Report_Dec_2020_v10_ONLINE_VERSION_1404.pdf
2. Hofmeyr GJ, Abdel-Aleem H, Abdel-Aleem MA (2013). Uterine massage for preventing postpartum haemorrhage. *Cochrane Database Syst Rev.* 7:CD006431.
3. RCOG (2015). Blood transfusion in obstetrics (GTG47). Available at: https://www.rcog.org.uk/en/guidelines-research-services/guidelines/gtg47/

Chapter 66

Sepsis in and following pregnancy

Guidelines:

RCOG GTG64a (Sepsis in pregnancy, bacterial): https://www.rcog.org.uk/en/guidelines-research-services/guidelines/gtg64a/

RCOG GTG64b (Sepsis following pregnancy, bacterial): https://www.rcog.org.uk/en/guidelines-research-services/guidelines/gtg64b/

OUP disclaimer: Oxford University Press makes no representation, express or implied, that the drug dosages are correct and that the recommendations are an exclusive or mandatory course of care. All health professionals reading this text have a responsibility to evaluate its appropriateness and take the individual needs of the patient into account.

Local trust guidelines: please refer to your local guidelines as necessary.

Overview

Sepsis during and following pregnancy is a leading cause of maternal death in the UK. The 2016–2018 report on maternal mortality (MBRRACE-UK[1]) showed that 11% of women who died during, or in the 6 weeks after their pregnancy, died from sepsis.

1 Available at: https://www.npeu.ox.ac.uk/assets/downloads/mbrrace-uk/reports/maternal-report-2020/MBRRACE-UK_Maternal_Report_Dec_2020_v10_ONLINE_VERSION_1404.pdf

Diagnosis

Risk factors

See Table 66.1.

Table 66.1 Risk factors for antenatal and postnatal sepsis

<table>
<tr><th>Risk factors for antenatal sepsis</th><th>Risk factors for postnatal sepsis</th></tr>
<tr><td>History of group B streptococcal infection</td><td></td></tr>
<tr><td></td><td>Caesarean section</td></tr>
<tr><td></td><td>Retained products of conception</td></tr>
<tr><td></td><td>Vaginal trauma</td></tr>
<tr><td></td><td>Wound haematoma</td></tr>
<tr><td colspan="2">Anaemia</td></tr>
<tr><td colspan="2">Amniocentesis and other invasive procedures</td></tr>
<tr><td colspan="2">Ethnic minority group origin</td></tr>
<tr><td colspan="2">Group A streptococcal infection in close contacts or family members</td></tr>
<tr><td colspan="2">History of pelvic infection</td></tr>
<tr><td colspan="2">Impaired glucose tolerance or diabetes</td></tr>
<tr><td colspan="2">Impaired immunity or use of immunosuppressant medication</td></tr>
<tr><td colspan="2">Obesity</td></tr>
<tr><td colspan="2">Prolonged spontaneous rupture of membranes (>24 hours prior to the start of labour)</td></tr>
<tr><td colspan="2">Vaginal discharge</td></tr>
</table>

Common organisms causing sepsis in pregnancy and the postpartum period

- *Escherichia coli*
- *Staphylococcus aureus*
- *Streptococcus pneumoniae*
- Coliforms
- Group A *Streptococcus* (*Streptococcus pyogenes*)
- Methicillin-resistant *Staphylococcus aureus* MRSA).

History

Focused history taking is paramount in determining the potential source of sepsis. Remember that non-gynaecological foci of infection must also be considered during pregnancy and the postpartum period.

Note recent illnesses or exposure to unwell contacts.

Table 66.2 Common sources of antenatal and postnatal sepsis

Causes of antenatal sepsis	Causes of postnatal sepsis
Chorioamnionitis	
	Endometritis
	Mastitis
	Retained products of conception
	Skin and soft tissue infections—from IV cannula, caesarean section, and episiotomy wounds
	Spinal abscess (post-epidural)
Gastroenteritis	Gastroenteritis
Pharyngitis	Pharyngitis
Pneumonia	Pneumonia
UTI	UTI

The following features may be suggestive of sepsis:

- Systemic:
  - Fever or rigors
  - Vomiting or diarrhoea
  - Rash
  - Lethargy
  - Reduced appetite
- Gynaecological:
  - Antenatal and postnatal:
    - Abdominal or pelvic pain or tenderness
    - Offensive vaginal discharge (smelly suggests anaerobes, serosanguinous suggests streptococcal)
  - Antenatal:
    - Rupture of membranes or contractions (may suggest chorioamnionitis)
  - Postnatal:
    - Uterine tenderness
    - Offensive or excessively heavy lochia (vaginal discharge after birth)
    - Symptoms of infection in caesarean section wound, e.g. pain around site, discharge from wound
    - Breast engorgement or redness
- Non-gynaecological:
  - Urinary symptoms
  - Productive cough.

Examination

Consider possible sources of infection (Table 66.2). Examine using an ABCDE approach (Table 66.3).

Table 66.3 Findings which may be suggestive of sepsis during pregnancy or postnatally

B	Tachypnoea >20 breaths/min Hypoxia
C	Tachycardia >100bpm Systolic blood pressure <90mmHg, or decrease in systolic blood pressure from baseline >40mmHg, or mean arterial pressure <70mmHg Oliguria (urine output <0.5mL/kg/hour for ≥2 hours despite fluid resuscitation)
D	Impaired level of consciousness Temperature >38°C or <36°C

E	Head-to-toe examination including:
	• Antenatal:
	  • Palpating uterus for tenderness
	• Postnatal:
	  • Breast examination
	  • Caesarean section wounds, vulva and vagina for evidence of infection
	  • Palpate uterus for evidence of lack of involution
	• Cardiac, respiratory, abdominal, ENT, and skin examinations as appropriate to consider non-gynaecological sources of infection

Investigations

Bedside

- Record basic observations on an appropriate maternity chart ('MEOWS')
- Urinalysis and MC&S
- Swabs and cultures as appropriate, e.g. throat, high vaginal, wound, placental, sputum, epidural, episiotomy, caesarean section wound, expressed breast milk
- Antenatally, a CTG should be performed as the fetus may show signs of distress if chorioamnionitis is the source of sepsis.

Bloods

- FBC
- U&E
- CRP
- Lactate
- Blood cultures, ideally taken before antibiotics, as long as treatment is not delayed
- ABG.

Imaging

- Chest X-ray
- Any other imaging which may be appropriate to confirm a source of infection, e.g. pelvic USS
- CT if pelvic abscess is suspected.

Management

Acute management

General

There is a significant overlap between sepsis during pregnancy and the postpartum period and sepsis in the general adult population. Therefore, much of the management is the same (see Chapter 122) but there are a few extra considerations:

- IV immunoglobulin is recommended for severe invasive streptococcal or staphylococcal infections, if other therapies have failed
- Isolate the patient in a side room if possible and wear appropriate personal protective equipment.

Antibiotics

- Give broad-spectrum empirical antibiotics within 1 hour as per trust guidelines, e.g. Tazocin® (4.5g IV TDS) plus clindamycin (0.6–4.8g IV in 2–4 divided doses)
- An alternative may be carbapenem plus clindamycin
- If MRSA positive, add vancomycin or teicoplanin
- Take care if the patient is breastfeeding as some antibiotics will be unsuitable—consult with a microbiologist if there is any doubt.

Antenatally

- Delivery of the baby may be beneficial to the mother, the baby, or both. In the event of chorioamnionitis, urgent delivery is usually the only treatment option. However, in other circumstances, e.g. an uncomplicated pneumonia, the baby would not be delivered unless it would improve maternal outcomes
- The decision regarding timing and mode of delivery should be made by a senior obstetrician
- If preterm delivery is likely, steroids should be considered due to fetal lung immaturity, but they should be used cautiously as they can worsen maternal sepsis
- Continuous CTG is recommended. Significant changes in CTG should prompt clinical reassessment of the septic mother for possible urgent delivery
- Epidural and spinal anaesthesia should be avoided in septic patients. A general anaesthetic will usually be required for a caesarean section.

Postnatally

- Seek advice from a paediatrician for all deliveries involving maternal sepsis.

Group A streptococcal infections

- If the mother has had an invasive group A streptococcal infection, the baby should also receive antibiotics
- Discuss with a microbiologist whether household contacts require prophylaxis if the mother has had a group A streptococcal infection.

Treatment after stabilization

- Treatment after stabilization is as per sepsis in the general adult population (see Chapter 122).

Further reading

1. MBRRACE-UK (2020). *Saving Lives, Improving Mother's Care: Lessons Learned to Inform Maternity Care from the UK and Ireland Confidential Enquiries into Maternal Deaths and Morbidity 2016–18.* Oxford: National Perinatal Epidemiology Unit, University of Oxford. Available at: https://www.npeu.ox.ac.uk/assets/downloads/mbrrace-uk/reports/maternal-report-2020/MBRRACE-UK_Maternal_Report_Dec_2020_v10_ONLINE_VERSION_1404.pdf

Chapter 67

Thrombosis and embolism during pregnancy and the postnatal period

Guideline:
RCOG GTG37b (Thromboembolic disease in pregnancy and the puerperium: acute management): https://www.rcog.org.uk/en/guidelines-research-services/guidelines/gtg37b/

OUP disclaimer: Oxford University Press makes no representation, express or implied, that the drug dosages are correct and that the recommendations are an exclusive or mandatory course of care. All health professionals reading this text have a responsibility to evaluate its appropriateness and take the individual needs of the patient into account.

Local trust guidelines: please refer to your local guidelines as necessary.

Overview

Venous thromboembolism (VTE) includes deep vein thrombosis (DVT) and pulmonary embolism (PE) and is a major cause of maternal morbidity and mortality. The risk of thromboembolic events is ↑ in pregnancy as it is a hypercoagulable state. In addition to this, subjective clinical assessment of VTE can be difficult in pregnancy so there should be a high index of suspicion of VTE in those with symptoms and a low threshold for objective testing. The investigation and management of VTE in the non-pregnant general population is covered in Chapter 99.

Diagnosis

VTE in pregnancy presents in the same way as in non-pregnant patients. See Chapter 99 for typical history findings and other risk factors.

Investigations

Bedside

- ECG:
  - Possible findings:
    - Sinus tachycardia
    - Right axis deviation and right bundle branch block
    - Right heart strain (T wave inversion in V1–4 and sometimes II, III, and avF)
    - Deep S in lead I, Q wave and inverted T wave in lead III (S1Q3T3)
- ABG if saturations <94% (see Chapter 79):
  - Type 1 respiratory failure is suggestive of a ventilation/perfusion (V/Q) mismatch.

There is currently no evidence for the use of Well's score in pregnancy.

Bloods

- FBC
- U&E
- LFT
- Coagulation profile.

D-dimer should not be used in pregnancy, as pregnancy itself will cause it to be raised.

Imaging

- DVT:
  - Compression duplex ultrasound: if positive and PE is also suspected, no further investigations are required
- PE:
  - Echocardiogram if evidence of right heart strain on ECG
  - Chest X-ray to assess for changes resulting from a PE and also to rule out alternative pathologies (the radiation risk is negligible)
  - V/Q scanning or computed tomography pulmonary angiogram (CTPA) (Box 67.1). A CTPA is preferred if the chest X-ray is abnormal.

Box 67.1 V/Q scanning or CTPA in pregnancy

Seek senior advice as both CTPA and V/Q scanning expose the fetus to radiation. Patients should be counselled on the risks and benefits of both options and be allowed to make an informed decision.

- V/Q scanning may carry a slightly ↑ risk of childhood cancers. One extra case of fatal childhood cancer will be caused for every 34,000 V/Q scans that are performed
- CT scanning is associated with a lower radiation dose to the fetus (approximately 20% of the radiation dose used in V/Q scanning), but a slightly higher risk of maternal breast cancer
- CT scanning increases the mother's **background** risk of breast cancer by approximately 13%, e.g. if the patient's background risk of developing cancer over 10 years is 0.1% (1 in 1000), their new risk will be 0.013% extra, i.e. 0.113% in total (1.13 in 1000)
- CT scanning also has the advantage that other pathologies may be diagnosed, e.g. pneumonia
- The absolute risk of harm is very low for both scanning methods; however, the risk of not having either scan needs to be weighed against the risk of having an undiagnosed PE, or inappropriately treating a patient who does not have a PE
- The negative predictive values are comparable.

Management

Acute management

All venous thromboembolism

- Give treatment-dose LMWH, as per local guidelines, until thrombosis can be excluded

> Use **booking weight** to calculate the dose for LMWH.

Deep vein thrombosis

- If ultrasound is negative + low level of clinical suspicion → discontinue treatment
- If ultrasound is negative + high level of clinical suspicion → discontinue treatment and repeat the scan on day 3 and day 7
- Elevate the leg
- Compression stockings may help to reduce pain and swelling.

Pulmonary embolism

- Give oxygen to target saturations ≥94%
- Gain IV access
- Give analgesia as required
- If the patient is haemodynamically unstable (i.e. possibility of massive PE), give 100% oxygen and carry out urgent echocardiogram or CTPA within 1 hour. Patients may require IV unfractionated heparin (UFH), thrombolytic therapy, thoracotomy, or surgical embolectomy.

Treatment after stabilization

- Therapeutic anticoagulation should be continued for the duration of the pregnancy and for at least 6 weeks postnatally. A minimum of 3 months of treatment should be given in total
- Women should be taught to self-inject with LMWH
- Before stopping treatment, the ongoing risk of thrombosis should be reassessed
- Women should be offered a choice of LMWH or warfarin *postnatally*, after discussing the need for regular coagulation monitoring with warfarin

> Warfarin **MUST NOT** be used antenatally unless specifically being prescribed and monitored by an obstetric consultant, as it can cause birth defects, and placental, fetal and neonatal haemorrhage

- Postpartum warfarin should be avoided until at least the fifth day, and longer for women with an ↑ risk of PPH
- Both heparin/LMWH and warfarin can be used in breastfeeding
- The patient should be reviewed postnatally in a joint obstetric and haematology/medicine clinic
- Thrombophilia screening should be considered once anticoagulation has been stopped, only if it would affect the woman's future management.

Special considerations

Labour and delivery

- Women should stop LMWH when they think they are in labour
- If delivery is planned, hold treatment doses of LMWH for 24 hours prior to the planned delivery (whether induction or operative)
- LMWH should not be used for 4 hours after the removal of epidural catheters, or after spinal anaesthesia. Epidural catheters should not be removed within 12 hours of an injection
- It may be necessary to use wound drains during caesarean section if patients are anticoagulated to avoid the formation of haematomas.

Women at high risk of haemorrhage

- If women are at high risk of haemorrhage but still require anticoagulation, it is preferable to use UFH rather than LMWH.

Further reading

1. Wan T, Skeith L, Karovitch A, et al. (2017). Guidance for the diagnosis of pulmonary embolism during pregnancy: consensus and controversies. *Thromb Res*. 157:23–8.

Chapter 68

Urinary incontinence in women

Guideline:
NICE NG123 (Urinary incontinence and pelvic organ prolapse in women: management): https://www.nice.org.uk/guidance/ng123

OUP disclaimer: Oxford University Press makes no representation, express or implied, that the drug dosages are correct and that the recommendations are an exclusive or mandatory course of care. All health professionals reading this text have a responsibility to evaluate its appropriateness and take the individual needs of the patient into account.

Local trust guidelines: please refer to your local guidelines as necessary.

Overview

Urinary incontinence is the involuntary leakage of urine. Sometimes, it can be secondary to pelvic organ prolapse; the external protrusion of the vagina, uterus, bladder, or rectum (see Chapter 64). These conditions are common and can have a major psychological and social impact on the patient, leading to a severely reduced quality of life.

Diagnosis

Categories of urinary incontinence

- **Stress incontinence:** leakage of urine on physical effort or exertion, e.g. coughing. Usually occurs due to sphincter weakness
- **Urge incontinence/overactive bladder:** leakage of urine accompanied or preceded by a sudden strong desire to pass urine
- **Mixed incontinence:** leakage of urine associated with symptoms of both stress and urge incontinence. Usually one of these is predominant and treatment should be directed at the predominant symptom
- **Overflow incontinence:** occurs when the bladder becomes large and flaccid with little or no detrusor tone/function. This usually occurs due to injury, e.g. postoperatively or postpartum. It is diagnosed when the residual volume is >50% of bladder capacity.

History

Aim to establish the type of incontinence, e.g. when does incontinence occur, how frequently, etc. Ask about onset, duration, and the severity of symptoms. Check for coexisting medical conditions and medications. Take a full obstetric history.

> **Red flags**
>
> New-onset urinary incontinence or retention, or faecal incontinence along with acute neurological symptoms, or new or changed back pain, are ⚑ for cauda equina syndrome.

Examination

- Abdominal examination (exclude pelvic mass, retention)
- Assess pelvic floor digitally for tone and prolapses
- Consider checking for a post-void residual with a bladder scan if the patient complains of recurrent UTI.

Investigations

Bedside

- Weight and BMI
- Urinalysis (exclude UTI) ± pregnancy test ± send midstream urine sample for MC&S.

Other

Urodynamics is a combination of tests that looks at bladder function and consists of uroflowmetry, post-void residual measurement, and cystometry:

- Uroflowmetry: patient voids on a commode with urinary flow meter and flow rates are measured on a graph
- Cystometry: patient is catheterized and the bladder is filled with saline. Sensations of filling and voiding are recorded. Intra-abdominal and intravesical pressures can be recorded allowing detrusor pressures to be calculated. The patient is asked to cough/stand and incontinence is noted
- Video-urodynamics and ambulatory monitoring are also used.

Chronic management

Management is dependent on patient preferences, comorbidities, and desire for childbearing.

Lifestyle and simple interventions

- Bladder diaries: encourage patients to complete at least 3 days of the diary covering variations in their usual activities to correlate which activities are associated with worsening of symptoms
- Reduce caffeine intake
- Weight loss (if BMI >30 kg/m^2).

> **Overflow incontinence**
>
> Overflow incontinence can be difficult to treat, as it is often secondary to an irreversible neurological issue such as multiple sclerosis. Occasionally there is a physical obstruction which can be treated with surgery, but usually overflow incontinence is managed with the use of long-term, or intermittent self-catheterization.

Pelvic floor muscle training

- First-line treatment for stress or mixed urinary incontinence
- Offer a trial of supervised training for at least 3 months
- It should include eight contractions, sustained for 6–8 seconds, performed three times daily.

Bladder training

- First-line treatment for urge or mixed urinary incontinence
- Minimum of 6 weeks.

Absorbent containment products

- Offer as a coping strategy pending definitive treatment or if treatment options have already been explored.

Pharmacological management

Stress incontinence

- Duloxetine:
  - Second-line treatment, if surgery is not desired or appropriate
  - Side effects: nausea, dyspepsia, dry mouth, insomnia.

Overactive bladder

- Anticholinergics (oxybutynin, solifenacin, etc.):
  - Discuss side effects, e.g. dry mouth, constipation, exacerbation of glaucoma
  - Consider coexisting conditions such as dementia as adverse effects also include cognitive impairment. Oxybutynin should not be offered to older women as anticholinergic treatment may trigger or exacerbate deterioration in their physical or mental health
- Intravaginal oestrogens:
  - Can be used to treat overactive bladder symptoms in postmenopausal women with vaginal atrophy.

Surgical management

Stress incontinence

- Colposuspension
- Autologous rectus facial sling
- Intramural bulking agent
- Mid-urethral sling—however, any procedure using mesh requires very careful counselling and a specialist consultant decision within an MDT.

Overactive bladder

An MDT discussion is required and invasive treatment may be trialled if pharmacological management has not been successful and urodynamic studies have demonstrated overactive bladder symptoms secondary to detrusor overactivity:

- Botulinum toxin type A injection
- Percutaneous sacral nerve stimulation
- Augmentation cystoplasty
- Urinary diversion.

Some procedures may cause urinary retention and patients need to consider if they are willing to perform intermittent self-catheterization.

Further reading

1. Collins S, Arulkumaran S, Hayes K, et al. (2013). Urogynaecology. In: *Oxford Handbook of Obstetrics and Gynaecology*, 3rd ed (pp. 653–84). Oxford: Oxford University Press. Available at: https://doi.org/10.1093/med/9780199698400.003.0022
2. TeachMeObGyn (2017). Urinary incontinence. Available at: https://teachmeobgyn.com/gynaecology/vaginal-vulval/urinary-incontinence/

Part 10

Paediatrics

Chapter 69

Child maltreatment

Guideline:
NICE CG89 (Child maltreatment: when to suspect maltreatment in under 18s): https://www.nice.org.uk/guidance/cg89

OUP disclaimer: Oxford University Press makes no representation, express or implied, that the drug dosages are correct and that the recommendations are an exclusive or mandatory course of care. All health professionals reading this text have a responsibility to evaluate its appropriateness and take the individual needs of the patient into account.

Local trust guidelines: please refer to your local trust guidelines as necessary.

Overview

Safeguarding children and young people is a fundamental aspect of paediatric care. Child maltreatment encompasses neglect, physical (often described as non-accidental injury), sexual, and emotional abuse, and fabricated or induced illness. Whenever there are concerns about safeguarding, **ALWAYS** discuss with a senior clinician and follow local pathways.

Diagnosis

History

Approach to history taking

- Listen and observe
- Seek an explanation for findings
- Record—ensure that all findings gathered are documented
- **Consider**, **suspect**, or **exclude** maltreatment—after discussion with a senior clinician:
  - Consider: if maltreatment is unlikely but possible, gather more information and discuss with a senior clinician
  - Suspect: if maltreatment is suspected, see 'Management'
  - Exclude: if maltreatment is excluded after a review of the evidence and discussion with senior clinician
- Record the actions taken.

Key question: is the history appropriate and consistent with the findings?

An unsuitable explanation for a presentation is either implausible, does not adequately explain the findings, or is inconsistent. It may be out of keeping with the child's age, function, others' accounts, the presentation, or existing medical conditions—e.g. a child who is not mobile would not be expected to have accidental bruises from falling over.

The story may be **inconsistent** over time or between different people's accounts.

Seek information from several sources, which could include parents, other caregivers, other family members, staff at school, a GP, a practice nurse, a school nurse, a health visitor, or a social worker.

Presentations which may raise suspicion

- Unusual or frequent pattern of presentation to healthcare services
- Poisoning
- Fabricated or induced illness
- Repeated apparent life-threatening or brief resolved unexplained events which have only been witnessed by one parent/carer and do not have a medical explanation
- Inappropriately poor school attendance.

Examination

There are three main aspects to the examination in a situation where maltreatment is being considered:

1. **Physical examination**—look for injuries and signs of neglect
2. **Child's behaviour**
3. **Parent or caregiver's interaction** with the child.

Physical examination and observation

Injuries

Child maltreatment may be suspected in the presence of the physical features listed in Table 69.1, especially in the absence of an appropriate explanation or underlying medical condition (e.g. coagulation profile disorder).

Table 69.1 Examination findings which may be suggestive of maltreatment

Type of injury or finding	Factor which might increase suspicion of maltreatment
Bruises	• Bruise in the shape of a hand, stick, teeth, or other implement • Bruises on non-bony areas, e.g. ears, buttocks • Bruises that look like strangulation or ligature marks • Multiple bruises which are clustered or of similar size/shape • Bruising or petechiae with no suitable explanation and no underlying medical condition
Bites	• Any human bite inconsistent with being caused by another child
Lacerations, abrasions, and scars	• On areas of the body that are normally covered by clothes • Multiple or symmetrical • On eyes, ears, and face
Burns and cold injuries	• Any area which would be unlikely to touch a hot object in an accident, e.g. back, buttocks, backs of hands, soles of feet • The size and shape are consistent with an implement, e.g. cigarette or iron • Distribution suggestive of forced immersion, e.g. limb scalds in glove-and-stocking distribution, scald with sharp edges, buttock or perineal scalds • Swollen and inflamed hands or feet might be consistent with a cold injury
Fractures	• Several fractures of different ages
Intracranial injuries	• Any head injury without major confirmed accidental trauma • Child age <3 years with head injury • Associated retinal haemorrhages, rib/long bone fractures, or other injuries • Multiple subdural haemorrhages
Anogenital signs and symptoms	• Genital symptom, e.g. dysuria, bleeding, discharge or injury without medical explanation • Foreign bodies in vagina or anus
Pregnancy and sexually transmitted infections	• Child aged <13 years who is pregnant, or with any STI (unless caused by contaminated blood transfusion, non-sexual transmission, or vertical transmission) • Child aged 13–15 years with any of the above, unless certain that sexual transmission was from consensual activity with a peer • Child aged 16–17 years with any of the above if concerns over exploitation or differences in power/mental capacity between the young person and the sexual contact

Signs of neglect

Neglect is defined as a sustained failure to meet the basic needs of a child or young person, to the detriment of their health or development (Table 69.2).

Table 69.2 Examining for signs of neglect

Type of neglect	Examples
Lack of provision of basic needs	• Persistent infestation, e.g. head lice or scabies • Inappropriate clothing or footwear • Persistently unwashed body or hair • Malnutrition or poor growth • Injuries consistent with inadequate supervision
Failure to ensure access to medical care	• Delayed presentations • Failure to attend appointments • Failure to administer prescribed treatments • Failure to engage with health promotion, e.g. immunization and screening

Child's behaviour

A number of behaviours may be witnessed or described which could be a cause for concern (Table 69.3).

Table 69.3 Assessing a child's behaviour

Type of behavioural change	Examples
Significant changes in emotional and behavioural states (if not with social explanation such as recent bereavement or parental separation, or medical explanation such as delayed development)	• Nightmares, extreme distress, social withdrawal • Aggression • Rocking • Repeated, extreme or sustained emotional response out of keeping with the situation, e.g. temper tantrum in school-aged child, inconsolable crying • Dissociation episodes
Inappropriate interpersonal behaviour	• Inappropriate behaviour with strangers, e.g. over-friendly • Appears to show excessively good behaviour towards parent/carer to avoid angering them • Excessive clinginess • Unable to recognize or understand emotions
Inappropriate response to medical examination	• Unusual or developmentally inappropriate response, e.g. extreme passivity, refusal, or resistance
Other inappropriate or unusual behaviours	• Deliberate self-harm • Scavenging, stealing, or hoarding food • Secondary day or night enuresis or deliberate wetting • Defecation in inappropriate place or faecal smearing • Sexualized talk or behaviour • Running away from home

Parent or caregiver's interaction with the child

Consider emotional abuse if the behaviour of the carer towards the child appears inappropriate. For example:

- Negativity or hostility
- Rejecting or scapegoating
- Developmentally inappropriate expectations, including inappropriate methods of disciplining
- Emotional unavailability of the parent/carer
- Refusing to allow the child to speak to healthcare staff on their own.

Management

What action should be taken if child maltreatment is suspected?

- Involve a senior clinician and/or local safeguarding lead as soon as any suspicious features are identified
- Follow local child safeguarding protocols
- Perform a full history and comprehensive physical examination. This is usually done by a senior paediatrician
- Involve the MDT including social services.

Further reading

1. Tasker RC, Acerini CL, Holloway E (eds) (2021). Child safeguarding. In: *Oxford Handbook of Paediatrics* (pp. 911–24). Oxford: Oxford University Press. Available at: https://doi.org/10.1093/med/9780198789888.003.0026

Chapter 70

Fever in under 5s

Guideline:
NICE NG143 (Fever in under 5s: assessment and initial management): https://www.nice.org.uk/guidance/ng143/

OUP disclaimer: Oxford University Press makes no representation, express or implied, that the drug dosages are correct and that the recommendations are an exclusive or mandatory course of care. All health professionals reading this text have a responsibility to evaluate its appropriateness and take the individual needs of the patient into account.

Local trust guidelines: please refer to your local guidelines as necessary.

Overview

Fever is a common presentation in children <5 years of age in primary and secondary care. Identifying serious bacterial infection can be challenging in this age group and this guideline aims to aid healthcare professionals in clinical assessment and differentiation between non-serious and serious illnesses. Relevant chapters relating to more specific conditions are signposted within the chapter. If a more focused approach is required, please refer to the following chapters: Chapter 73, 'Paediatric bacterial meningitis and meningococcal septicaemia, Chapter 76, 'Paediatric gastroenteritis', and Chapter 78, 'Paediatric urinary tract infections'.

Diagnosis

History

A focused yet comprehensive history is required, including:

- Duration of fever and evolution of illness. Take parental report of fever into account even if the temperature was not measured at home
- Specific symptoms which may help to identify an underlying focus of infection (Table 70.1)
- Travel history
- Exposure to others with an infectious disease, including in childcare or educational settings
- History of previous infections and any concerns regarding immunodeficiency
- Vaccination history (vaccinations may cause transient fevers, especially in children aged <3 months).

Examination

Complete a physical examination using an ABCDE approach, and identify and treat any immediately life-threatening features. Assess for signs of dehydration (see Chapter 76). See Box 70.1 regarding measuring temperature in children.

Do not use forehead chemical thermometers as these are unreliable.

Look for signs and symptoms which could be predictive of a serious illness using Table 70.2 and carefully look for a fever source. If the child has developmental delay or disabilities take these into account when interpreting the table. Table 70.1 lists signs and symptoms suggestive of specific illnesses.

Investigations

Use Table 70.2 to ascertain which set of investigations are relevant.

Infants <3 months (red)

- Urine testing (see Chapter 78)
- Bloods:
  - FBC
  - CRP
  - Blood cultures
- Chest X-ray (if respiratory signs are present)
- LP (unless contraindicated) in:
  - Infants <1 month
  - Infant 1–3 months and appears unwell
  - Infant 1–3 months with a white cell count $<5 \times 10^9$/L or $>15 \times 10^9$/L
- Stool culture (if diarrhoea present).

Children >3 months with ≥1 high-risk feature (red)

- Urine testing (see Chapter 78)
- Bloods:
  - FBC
  - CRP
  - Blood cultures
- Additionally, consider the following based on clinical assessment:
  - U&E and blood gases
  - Chest X-ray
  - LP.

Table 70.1 Signs and symptoms suggestive of specific illnesses

Child with fever and following signs/ symptoms	Consider
• Non-blanching rash, especially with ≥1 of: • Unwell looking • Purpura (lesions >2mm diameter) • Capillary refill time >2 seconds • Neck stiffness	Meningococcal disease (see Chapter 73)
• Neck stiffness • Bulging fontanelle (<2 years) • Reduced level of consciousness • Status epilepticus	Bacterial meningitis (see Chapter 73)
• Focal neurology or focal seizures • Reduced level of consciousness	Herpes simplex encephalitis
• Crackles on auscultation • Signs of respiratory distress, e.g. nasal flaring, subcostal recession, cyanosis • Oxygen saturations ≤95% on room air • Tachypnoea: • **≤5 months:** >60 breaths/min • **6–12 months:** >50 breaths/min • **>12 months:** >40 breaths/min	Pneumonia
• Vomiting • Reduced feeding • Irritability or lethargy • Abdominal pain • Dysuria or urinary frequency (older children)	Urinary tract infection (see Chapter 78)
• Limb or joint swelling • Refusing to weight bear or use limb, or limping	Septic arthritis
• Fever of ≥5 days. Other features include: • Bilateral red eyes with no exudate • Cervical lymphadenopathy • Rash • Erythema of oral/pharyngeal mucosa and lips, or strawberry tongue • Erythema and swelling of hands and feet	Kawasaki disease

Box 70.1 Measurement of body temperature

Take into consideration whether the child has already received antipyretic medication.

Use:

- Age <1 month: axillary electronic thermometer
- Age >1 month: electronic or chemical dot thermometer in the axilla, or infrared tympanic thermometer.

Children >3 months with ≥1 moderate-risk feature (amber)

- Urine testing (see Chapter 78)
- Bloods (discuss necessity of bloods with a senior doctor):
  - FBC
  - CRP
  - Blood cultures
- Chest X-ray if fever >39°C and white cell count $>20 \times 10^9$/L
- LP—consider if aged <1 year.

Children >3 months with only low-risk features (green)

- Urine testing (see Chapter 78).

Table 70.2 Traffic light system for identifying risk of serious illness

	Green: low risk	Amber: intermediate risk	Red: high risk
Colour (of skin, lips, or tongue)	• Normal colour	• Pallor reported by parent/carer	• Pale/mottled/ashen/blue
Activity	• Responds normally to social cues • Content/smiles • Stays awake or awakens quickly • Strong normal cry/not crying	• Not responding normally to social cues • No smile • Wakes only with prolonged stimulation • ↓ activity	• No response to social cues • Appears ill to a healthcare professional • Does not wake or if roused does not stay awake • Weak, high-pitched or continuous cry

Respiratory		• Nasal flaring
		• Tachypnoea:
		  • RR >50 breaths/minute, age 6–12 months
		  • RR >40 breaths/minute, age >12 months
		• Oxygen saturation ≤95% in air
		• Crackles in the chest
			• Grunting
			• Tachypnoea: RR >60 breaths/minute
			• Moderate or severe chest indrawing

	Green: low risk	Amber: intermediate risk	Red: high risk

Circulation and hydration	• Normal skin and eyes
	• Moist mucous membranes
		• Tachycardia:
		  • >160bpm, age <12 months
		  • >150bpm, age 12–24 months
		  • >140bpm, age 2–5 years
		• CRT ≥3 seconds
		• Dry mucous membranes
		• Poor feeding in infants
		• Reduced urine output
			Reduced skin turgor

Other	• None of the amber or red symptoms or signs	• Age 3–6 months, temperature ≥39°C • Fever for ≥5 days • Rigors • Swelling of a limb or joint • Non-weight-bearing limb/not using an extremity	• Age <3 months, temperature ≥38°C* • Non-blanching rash • Bulging fontanelle • Neck stiffness • Status epilepticus • Focal neurological signs • Focal seizures

CRT, capillary refill time; RR, respiratory rate. * Some vaccinations have been found to induce fever in children aged <3 months.
This traffic light table should be used in conjunction with the recommendations in the NICE guideline on fever in under 5s

Management

Acute management

Management in the community or by non-paediatric services

- Life-threatening features (compromised airway, breathing, circulation, or reduced level of consciousness): immediate transfer to paediatric emergency care, usually by ambulance
- Any high-risk features (red): urgent referral to a paediatric specialist (within 2 hours)
- Any moderate-risk features (amber): referral to a healthcare professional for in-person assessment. If no diagnosis is reached, consider referral to a paediatric specialist or discharge with appropriate safety net advice (Box 70.2)
- Low-risk features only (green): care for at home with appropriate safety net advice (Box 70.2).

In hospital with paediatric specialty service

Decision to admit to hospital

When assessing the need for hospital admission, take the following factors into account:

- Social circumstances
- Illness in other family members
- Parental anxiety, especially if previous serious illness/death in another child
- Repeated presentations within same illness episode
- Duration of illness longer than expected
- Unwell contacts or recent travel.

Consider a period of observation in hospital for children aged <3 months with no obvious source of infection, even if no investigations are carried out.

Fluids

- If clinically shocked, give a 20mL/kg fluid bolus of 0.9% sodium chloride immediately
- Continue to monitor and give further fluid boluses as required
- If shocked, the child should be urgently reviewed by a senior paediatrician to consider the need for intensive care.

Antibiotics and antivirals

Always refer to local protocols and antibiotic guidelines when available. General principles of prescribing include:

- IV antibiotics should be given in the following circumstances:
  - <1 month with fever
  - 1–3 months and appears unwell
  - 1–3 months with a white cell count $<5 \times 10^9$/L or $>15 \times 10^9$/L (see Chapter 71).

Use an IV third-generation cephalosporin, e.g. ceftriaxone or cefotaxime, and give ampicillin or amoxicillin **as well** for cover against listeria:

- Give IV antibiotics **immediately** if the child is unrousable, shocked, or has signs of meningococcal disease (see Chapter 73) (or IM benzylpenicillin if pre-hospital transfer)

- Careful consideration should be given to immediate antibiotics if the child has a reduced level of consciousness. Give IV aciclovir if herpes simplex encephalitis is suspected.

Oxygen

- Give oxygen if signs of shock or SpO_2 <92% on room air.

Management of fever

- Consider giving either paracetamol or ibuprofen if the child is distressed due to their fever. The two medications can be alternated but should not be given together
- Antipyretics should not be used purely to reduce body temperature or prevent febrile convulsions.

Treatment after stabilization

Children with low-risk features only (green)

- Can be cared for at home
- Give safety net advice (Box 70.2) and advice regarding managing a feverish child at home (Box 70.3).

Children with any moderate or high-risk features but no clear diagnosis (amber or red)

- Consider arranging follow-up
- Give safety net advice (Box 70.2) and advice regarding managing a feverish child at home (Box 70.3).

Box 70.2 Safety net advice

Safety net advice should include:

- Written/verbal information regarding potential symptoms of concern
- Information regarding how to access healthcare services if needed
- Arranging specific follow-up or further assessment if appropriate.

Monitoring and follow-up

Give specific instructions on when to seek further medical review. Further review should occur if:

- The child fits
- The child develops a non-blanching rash
- The parents feel the child is less well/they are more worried than when they previously sought advice
- The fever lasts ≥5 days.

Box 70.3 Advice on how to manage a feverish child at home

- Dehydration (see Chapter 76):
  - Give/encourage regular fluids (breastmilk if the child is still being breastfed)
  - Assess for signs of dehydration, e.g. dry mouth, sunken eyes or fontanelle
- Rashes:
  - How to identify non-blanching rash
- Fever:
  - How to manage fever (see 'Management of fever')
- To check the child during the night
- Advice regarding return to school/nursery—child should stay away while feverish
- Safety net advice (Box 70.2).

Further reading

1. BMJ Learning. Fever in under 5s: putting NICE guidelines into practice. Available at: https://learning.bmj.com/learning/module-intro/feverish-illness-in-young-children--in-association-with-nice.html?moduleId=6052018

Neonatal infections

Guideline:
NICE NG195 (Neonatal infection: antibiotics for prevention and treatment): https://www.nice.org.uk/guidance/ng195

OUP disclaimer: Oxford University Press makes no representation, express or implied, that the drug dosages are correct and that the recommendations are an exclusive or mandatory course of care. All health professionals reading this text have a responsibility to evaluate its appropriateness and take the individual needs of the patient into account.

Local trust guidelines: please refer to your local guidelines as necessary.

Overview

Infection is a significant cause of neonatal morbidity and mortality. Neonatal sepsis may be early onset (<72 hours after birth) or late onset (>72 hours after birth). Group B *Streptococcus* (GBS) and *Escherichia coli* are the most common causative organisms in early-onset infection. Coagulase-negative staphylococci, *Staphylococcus aureus*, and Enterobacteriaceae are common pathogens in late-onset infection in babies on neonatal units. Reducing mortality and morbidity due to sepsis requires early recognition and prompt antibiotic treatment.

Diagnosis

History

Risk factors for early-onset neonatal infection

- Intrapartum fever >38°C (if suspected/confirmed bacterial infection)
- Invasive GBS infection in a previous baby
- Maternal GBS bacteriuria/colonization/infection during the current pregnancy
- Prelabour rupture of membranes (>24 hours before onset of labour) in term birth
- Confirmed rupture of membranes >18 hours before a pre-term birth
- Pre-term birth (<37 weeks) after a spontaneous labour
- Suspected/confirmed chorioamnionitis
- ⚑ In a multiple pregnancy: suspected/confirmed infection in another baby.

Risk factors for late-onset neonatal infection

- Prematurity
- Mechanical ventilation
- Presence of a central catheter
- History of surgery.

Examination

Examination may be unremarkable. Perform a thorough examination including vital signs and specifically look for the presence of indicators highlighted in Table 71.1 (early onset, before 72 hours) and Table 71.2 (late onset, after 72 hours).

Table 71.1 Clinical indicators of possible early-onset neonatal infection (<72 hours) during a structured assessment

Red flags	⚑ Apnoeic episodes ⚑ Signs of shock ⚑ Need for mechanical ventilation ⚑ Need for CPR ⚑ Seizure activity
Behaviour	Altered behaviour or responsiveness (e.g. inconsolable crying or listlessness) Difficulties with feeding (e.g. refusal, vomiting, feed intolerance)
Breathing	Signs of respiratory distress Hypoxia
Circulation	Tachycardia or bradycardia Persistent pulmonary hypertension of the newborn
Other	Hypo or hyperglycaemia Metabolic acidosis (base deficit ≥10mmol/L) Jaundice within 24 hours of birth Abdominal distension Unexplained excessive bleeding or coagulation profile abnormalities Altered muscle tone (e.g. floppiness) Signs of possible neonatal encephalopathy Temperature <36°C or >38°C

Table 71.2 Clinical indicators of possible late-onset neonatal infection (>72 hours) during a structured assessment

Behaviour	Does not wake, or unable to stay awake Weak, high-pitched or continuous cry Altered feeding pattern
Breathing	Respiratory rate >60 breaths/min Cyanosis of skin, lips, or tongue Grunting Apnoea Saturations <90% on room air, or ↑ oxygen requirement
Circulation	Tachycardia ≥160bpm Bradycardia <100bpm Pale, mottled, or ashen skin
Other	Appears unwell Seizures Bulging fontanelle Temperature <36°C or ≥38°C Non-blanching rash Abdominal distension Parental concern

Investigations

Risk assessment

Suspected early-onset neonatal infection

Based on Table 71.1 and section 'Risk factors for early onset neonatal infection':

- **With any ⚑ OR ≥2 'non-red flag' risk factors or clinical indicators:** send investigations and start antibiotics without waiting for investigation results
- **Without ⚑ OR only one 'non-red flag' risk factor or clinical indicator:** Use clinical judgement to decide regarding further monitoring and need for antibiotic treatment

Suspected late onset neonatal infection

- Use Table 71.2 and discuss further management with a senior doctor.

Bedside

- Urinalysis

Bloods

- CRP
- Blood cultures (before administering first dose of antibiotics).

Other

- LP: if strong clinical suspicion of infection or signs of meningitis
- Swabs for microbiology:
  - If purulent eye discharge (Box 71.1)
  - If signs of periumbilical infection.

Box 71.1 Eye discharge

Remember that eyelid crusting and minor conjunctivitis are common in neonates and usually benign, but purulent eye discharge may be indicative of a serious infection such as gonorrhoea or chlamydia. Liaise with your laboratory to ensure you send the correct swab type.

Management

Acute management of early-onset infection (<72 hours)

If antibiotics are indicated, give within 1 hour of the decision to treat.

In babies without ⚑, or only one risk factor/clinical indicator, use clinical judgement and discuss further management with a senior paediatrician. A period of clinical monitoring including vital signs may be required (usually at least 12 hours).

Ensure parents/carers are updated and involved with discussions regarding management. Provide information on treatment rationale, investigations required, and the likely treatment duration. Ensure every effort is being made to continue breastfeeding and/or support the mother to express breastmilk if unable to breastfeed.

Empirical treatment of suspected early-onset infection

- IV benzylpenicillin **AND**
- IV gentamicin (usually every 36 hours if still indicated). Subsequent doses/intervals should be guided by local protocols and serum levels—see Box 71.2
- Local resistance patterns may guide different antibiotic choices.

Umbilical infection or periumbilical cellulitis

- IV flucloxacillin and gentamicin (see previous bullet list).

Meningitis

This applies to babies in neonatal units. In older children, see Chapter 73.

Unknown causative pathogen

- IV amoxicillin and cefotaxime.

CSF Gram stain available

- Gram-positive bacteria in CSF: continue IV amoxicillin and cefotaxime
- Gram-negative bacteria in CSF: stop amoxicillin and continue IV cefotaxime.

Await CSF culture results and seek microbiological advice to decide on further antibiotic management and the length of treatment.

Box 71.2 Principles of gentamicin prescribing

- Consult local protocols where available
- Measure the trough dose immediately before the second dose is given
- Use the result to decide the dose and interval for the third dose
- If the result is unavailable, give the next dose unless there is evidence of renal dysfunction
- Measure levels at least every third dose, or more frequently if concerned about previous levels or renal function
- Adjust dose interval to achieve trough level <2mg/L or <1mg/L if gentamicin course >3 doses
- Review at every dose whether it continues to be clinically indicated.

Acute management of late-onset infection (>72 hours)

Empirical treatment of suspected late-onset infection

- Hospital acquired (babies already on the neonatal unit):

- Give a combination of narrow-spectrum antibiotics (e.g. IV flucloxacillin with gentamicin) according to local protocol, to cover both Gram-negative and Gram-positive pathogens
- Add an antibiotic against anaerobes (e.g. metronidazole) if necrotizing enterocolitis is suspected
- Community acquired (admitted from home):
  - Ceftriaxone 50mg/kg. If <40 weeks corrected gestational age, give cefotaxime 50mg/kg
- Antifungal:
  - Give prophylactic oral nystatin if the baby is receiving antibiotics and:
    - Has a birthweight of <1500g **OR**
    - Was born <30 weeks' gestation.
- Meningitis:
  - As per early-onset infection

Management after starting antibiotic therapy

Investigations during antibiotic therapy

- Repeat CRP 18–24 hours after the initial measurement
- Consider performing a LP (if not already done) and:
  - The baby has a positive blood culture (excluding coagulase-negative staphylococci) **OR**
  - The baby has a poor response to antibiotics **OR**
  - There is a strong suspicion of infection **OR**
  - The baby has signs/symptoms of meningitis.

Length of treatment (sepsis without meningitis)

Assess the baby clinically every 24 hours and review the ongoing need for antibiotics:

- If **early-onset infection**—at 36 hours
- If **late-onset infection**—at 48 hours:
- Consider stopping if:
  - Blood cultures are negative **AND**
  - The initial clinical suspicion was not strong **AND**
  - The clinical condition of the baby is reassuring without any clinical indicators of potential infection **AND**
  - CRP levels/trends are reassuring
- If blood cultures are positive: continue antibiotics for at least 7 days, or longer if advised by microbiology based on the causative pathogen or infection site. In late-onset infection, antibiotics may be stopped sooner if the baby recovered well or the pathogen is a common commensal
- If blood cultures are negative but there is still a strong clinical suspicion of sepsis:
  - Continue antibiotics (usually for 7 days)
  - Review the baby daily and consider stopping antibiotics taking into account clinical progress and CRP trend.

Discharge advice

Advise parents to seek medical advice if the baby:

- Becomes unusually floppy
- Has feeding difficulties or does not tolerate feeds
- Behaves abnormally, e.g. inconsolable crying
- Has breathing difficulties
- Has an unexplained temperature <36°C or >38°C
- Has a change in skin colour.

Special considerations

Intrapartum antibiotic prophylaxis

Intrapartum antibiotic prophylaxis to prevent early-onset neonatal infection should be given to women who are in preterm labour **OR** have had:

- A previous baby with invasive GBS infection
- GBS bacteriuria, colonization, or infection in the current pregnancy **OR** in a previous pregnancy without a negative GBS culture or PCR (taken between 35–37 weeks) in the current pregnancy
- Suspected or confirmed chorioamnionitis.

Give IV benzylpenicillin (cephalosporin if non-severe penicillin allergy, or vancomycin if severe allergy). Add gentamicin and metronidazole if treating chorioamnionitis.

Give the first dose as soon as labour is confirmed or chorioamnionitis is suspected. Stop antibiotics when the baby is born (unless treatment for chorioamnionitis is ongoing).

Group B streptococcal infection

In babies with GBS infection, give the following advice (applicable to future pregnancies) on discharge and inform the GP:

- The risk to a future baby of early-onset GBS is increased
- The maternity team in future pregnancies should be made aware of GBS infection in this baby
- Antibiotics during labour are recommended.

Further reading

1. RCOG (2017). Group B streptococcal disease, early-onset (GTG36). Available at: https://www.rcog.org.uk/en/guidelines-research-services/guidelines/gtg36/
2. Group B Strep Support. Group B Streptococcus (GBS) in pregnancy and newborn babies. Available at: https://gbss.org.uk/info-support/about-group-b-strep/what-is-group-b-strep/group-b-strep-in-pregnancy-and-newborn-babies-html/

Chapter 72

Paediatric asthma

Guideline:
British Thoracic Society, Scottish Intercollegiate Guidelines Network (British guideline on the management of asthma, 2019): https://www.brit-thoracic.org.uk/document-library/guidelines/asthma/btssign-guideline-for-the-management-of-asthma-2019/

OUP disclaimer: Oxford University Press makes no representation, express or implied, that the drug dosages are correct and that the recommendations are an exclusive or mandatory course of care. All health professionals reading this text have a responsibility to evaluate its appropriateness and take the individual needs of the patient into account.

Local trust guidelines: please refer to your local guidelines as necessary.

Overview

Paediatric asthma is a common condition encountered in both primary and secondary care. Asthma is a chronic disease characterized by variable airflow obstruction with airway hyper-responsiveness and inflammation in the presence of symptoms. There is no single diagnostic test for asthma and the diagnosis is based on clinical assessment supported by objective tests (depending on the age of the child). Acute exacerbations in children are often triggered by viral upper airway infections.

Assessing acute wheeze in children aged <5 years can be challenging (Box 72.1) as the pattern of wheezing is heterogeneous and the evidence is limited. There is a lack of objective diagnostic tests in this age group. This guideline should not be used for children aged <1 year.

Box 72.1 Viral-induced wheeze

Often, children who have had episodes of wheeze prior to age 2–3 years ('preschool wheeze' or 'viral-induced wheeze'), are no longer symptomatic by mid-childhood and do not go on to have chronic asthma. Wheezing is often triggered by viral upper respiratory tract infections and usually there are no symptoms between episodes. Risk factors for the development of chronic asthma or persistent wheeze are personal or family history of atopy, and frequent and severe episodes of wheezing.

History

A detailed history is **key**:

- Symptoms: >1 of the following—cough, chest tightness, shortness of breath, and wheeze (Box 72.2). See Box 72.3 for ⚑ symptoms which should prompt consideration of an alternative diagnosis
- Episodic pattern of symptoms: intervals with no or minimal symptoms
- Triggers: e.g. viral infections, pets, dust, passive smoking, exercise, emotion or laughter, and cold air
- Diurnal variability: symptoms are typically worse at night or early in the morning
- Personal or family history of other atopic illnesses, e.g. allergic rhinitis, eczema, allergies, or asthma
- Wheeze heard on auscultation and recorded by a healthcare professional.

Box 72.2 Never assume a parent knows what wheeze is!

- Parents often use the term wheeze to describe any abnormal respiratory sound they have heard such as stridor or rattly breathing and it is important to make the distinction
- Audio recordings and GP records may be helpful if the child is asymptomatic at presentation.

Box 72.3 Red flags which may indicate an alternative diagnosis

- ⚑ Symptoms from birth
- ⚑ Excessive vomiting or posseting (consider gastro-oesophageal reflux)
- ⚑ Persistent productive cough (consider cystic fibrosis or bronchiectasis)
- ⚑ Failure to thrive
- ⚑ Family history of lung disease
- ⚑ Nasal polyps
- ⚑ Dysphagia
- ⚑ Stridor or abnormal voice (consider laryngeal or tracheal disorders)
- ⚑ Signs not in keeping with asthma diagnosis, e.g. focal signs.

Existing diagnosis of asthma

Ask about asthma control and treatment compliance:

- How often does the child use their salbutamol inhaler each week? Does salbutamol help? What other preventer therapy is the child on? Does the child sometimes forget doses?
- Has the child had any admissions to hospital or intensive care with respiratory-related illnesses?

Examination

- May be normal between episodes
- Expiratory wheeze may be present on auscultation

- Growth and development: check height and weight
- Signs of an acute asthma exacerbation: see 'Acute asthma attack'.

Investigations

High probability of asthma

Criteria:

- Recurrent asthma symptoms (attacks) **AND**
- Wheeze heard by a healthcare professional **AND**
- Documented variable airflow obstruction **AND**
- History of atopy **AND**
- No ⚑ symptoms indicating an alternative diagnosis.

No further diagnostic investigations are required.

Start a trial of treatment and review after 6 weeks using a validated questionnaire. If there is a good response, diagnose as asthma. If there is a poor response, consider additional testing.

Intermediate probability of asthma

Criteria:

- Some of the features of asthma on clinical assessment, but not all (see 'High probability of asthma') **OR**
- Poor response to trial of treatment.

Age >5 years

- First line: spirometry with bronchodilator reversibility
- Second line (if spirometry normal): challenge tests (e.g. methacholine challenge) and/or fractional excretion of nitric oxide (FeNO) (Box 72.4).

Box 72.4 Fractional excretion of nitric oxide

High levels of nitric oxide are released when there is bronchial wall inflammation; therefore, higher levels are suggestive of eosinophilic inflammation.

Age <5 years (or unable to perform objective tests)

- If symptomatic, a trial of treatment may be commenced and monitored over 6–8 weeks. If there is clear evidence that symptoms have improved, the child should be considered to have a diagnosis of asthma
- If asymptomatic, consider watchful waiting. This usually applies to children with intermittent wheeze or who have respiratory symptoms during viral upper respiratory tract infections only.

Management

Patient education

Patient education is an important aspect of asthma management and every respiratory consultation should be used to review and improve knowledge and skills.

Compliance

- Check and reiterate the need for compliance with treatment
- Check inhaler technique.

Inhaler device

- Pressurized metered-dose inhaler (pMDI) and spacers are more appropriate in children and should always be used during acute exacerbations. A face mask is required until the child can form a seal and effectively breathe with a mouthpiece (usually >5 years)
- In older children, dry powder inhaler or breath-actuated inhaler devices can be used which are smaller and may be more practical. Their ability to use the device effectively should be assessed prior to using the device. This should be performed by a trained healthcare professional, e.g. asthma nurse
- Spacers should be washed with detergent monthly and allowed to air dry, and replaced every 6–12 months.

Personalized asthma management plan (asthma action plan)

- Provide written asthma management plan which includes regular treatment and stepwise management during an asthma exacerbation (see 'Further reading')
- Ensure the family and child understand the difference between 'preventer' and 'reliever' (salbutamol) inhalers.

Lifestyle and simple interventions

- Weight reduction if obese or overweight
- Discourage smoking within the household and signpost smoking cessation support
- Trigger avoidance.

Pharmacological management

Start treatment at the most appropriate step according to symptom burden. Use the lowest effective doses to maintain control. If well controlled (see Box 72.6), consider reducing the inhaled corticosteroid dose by 25–50% every 3 months.

Always check inhaler technique and review possible trigger factors before altering treatment or starting new therapies.

Intermittent reliever therapy

- SABA e.g. salbutamol, as required. For children with short-lived wheeze this may be the only treatment required.

Regular preventer therapy

- Very low dose ICS, e.g. beclomethasone dipropionate **OR**
- If age <5 years (and unable to take ICS): leukotriene receptor antagonist (e.g. oral montelukast).

Initial add on therapy

Very low-dose ICS **PLUS**:

- If age ≥5 years:
  - LABA, e.g. formoterol (ICS–LABA combination inhalers may improve adherence) **OR**
  - Leukotriene receptor antagonist, e.g. oral montelukast
- If age <5 years: add leukotriene receptor antagonist, e.g. oral montelukast.

Additional controller therapy

- Consider increasing ICS to low dose **OR**
- If age ≥5 years: add a leukotriene receptor antagonist or LABA
- If no response to LABA, consider stopping it.

Specialist therapies

- Refer to specialist care if asthma is still not controlled.

Monitoring and follow-up

Children with asthma should be reviewed at least annually in primary or secondary care.

Review the following:

- Current symptoms and control: current use of therapies and whether escalation or de-escalation is required, impact on life, e.g. time off school, exercise-induced asthma (Box 72.5)
- Future risk of attacks: past history of attacks, history of poor asthma control
- Management strategies: medication adherence and inhaler technique
- Supported self-management: provision or review of personal asthma management plan.

Box 72.5 Exercise-induced asthma

- Exercise-induced asthma frequently reflects poor asthma control
- Advise the child to use an inhaled short-acting beta-2 agonist immediately prior to exercise.

There are validated questionnaires which aid the assessment of symptom control (see 'Further reading'). Box 72.6 lists the key criteria that determine if asthma is controlled.

Box 72.6 When is asthma controlled?

Asthma may be considered controlled if there have **not** been:

- Attacks or symptoms during the day
- Restrictions on physical activity or exercise
- Symptoms at night that disturb sleep
- Any occasions where rescue medication was needed
- Side effects due to an asthma medication.

Reasons for secondary care referral

Most children with asthma can be managed in primary care. The following are reasons to refer to secondary care:

- Referral for tests not available in primary care
- Diagnosis unclear
- Poor response to initial asthma treatment
- Severe/life-threatening asthma attack
- ⚑ signs which may indicate an alternative diagnosis (Box 72.3).

Acute asthma attack

Exercise caution in younger children (especially if <2 years) without a confirmed diagnosis of asthma. An alternative diagnosis should be considered (e.g. pneumonia, bronchiolitis, recurrent wheezing due to prematurity, aspiration pneumonitis). The management described here applies to children with acute wheeze due to an underlying diagnosis of asthma. Similar management principles apply for younger children with suspected viral-induced wheeze but prednisolone is often not necessary (discuss with a senior paediatrician).

Severity of attack

Before giving treatment for an acute asthma attack, it is essential to assess severity (Table 72.1). The following clinical signs should be recorded:

- Pulse rate
- Respiratory rate, degree of breathlessness (are they able to speak in full sentences?) and oxygen saturations
- Use of accessory muscles of respiration (intercostal recession, subcostal recession, sternal recession, tracheal tug, head bobbing)
- Amount of wheezing—which might become biphasic or less apparent with increasing airway obstruction
- Degree of agitation and level of consciousness.

> Clinical signs correlate poorly with the severity of airways obstruction. Some children with acute severe asthma do not appear distressed and the absence of wheeze (silent chest) can be a sign of life-threatening asthma!

Investigations during an acute attack

Blood gas

Consider performing a venous or capillary blood gas if there are life-threatening features that do not respond to treatment.

Chest X-ray

Not routinely indicated. Perform if:

- Life-threatening asthma that is not responding to treatment
- Suspecting a pneumothorax or lobar consolidation/collapse (persisting unilateral signs).

Initial treatment

- Give oxygen if saturations <94%
- Salbutamol is the first-line treatment:
  - **Mild–moderate attack:** 100 micrograms per dose via pMDI inhaler with spacer, 2–10 puffs, repeat every 10–20 minutes or when needed
  - **Severe or life-threatening attack:** nebulizer every 20–30 minutes as needed:
    - Age <5 years: 2.5mg
    - Age ≥5 years: 5mg
- If symptoms are refractory to initial salbutamol: add ipratropium bromide (250 micrograms/dose) to nebulized salbutamol

Table 72.1 Acute asthma attack severity levels

Severity	PEF rate % of best/predicted	Oxygen saturation	Clinical features
Moderate	>50	≥92%	Able to talk in sentences *Respiratory rate:* **Age 1–5 years:** ≤40 breaths/min **Age >5 years:** ≤30 breaths/min *Heart rate:* **Age 1–5 years:** ≤140bpm **Age >5 years:** ≤125bpm
Severe	33–50	<92%	Unable to talk in sentences *Respiratory rate:* **Age 1–5 years:** >40 breaths/min **Age >5 years:** >30 breaths/min *Heart rate:* **Age 1–5 years:** >140bpm **Age >5 years:** >125bpm
Life-threatening	<33	<92%	Any of the following in a child with severe asthma: • Exhaustion • Hypotension • Cyanosis • Silent chest • Poor respiratory effort • Confusion

- Give oral prednisolone early. Remember to continue usual ICS inhaler while on oral steroid therapy:
  - Age <2 years: 10 mg
  - Age 2–5 years: 20 mg
  - Aged >5 years: 30–40 mg
  - Consider IV hydrocortisone 4mg/kg 4-hourly if unable to take orally
  - Treatment for 3 days is usually sufficient
  - In children with suspected viral-induced wheeze: discuss the need for prednisolone with a senior paediatrician.

Second-line treatment (with senior support)

Consider the following for children with severe symptoms or a poor initial response to treatment:

- Nebulized magnesium sulphate 150mg added to each nebulizer in the first hour
- Early administration of an IV salbutamol bolus (age >2 years: 15 micrograms/kg) over 10 minutes (often followed by a continuous IV infusion) with continuous ECG monitoring (Box 72.7)
- IV magnesium sulphate (40 mg/kg)
- Aminophylline for children with severe or life-threatening asthma unresponsive to maximal doses of bronchodilators and steroids.

Call for senior help urgently for any child with severe or life-threatening symptoms, children not responding to initial management, and/or requiring oxygen.

Box 72.7 Salbutamol side effects and toxicity

Salbutamol side effects include tachycardia (common), low potassium, and metabolic acidosis leading to tachypnoea. This is a particular concern if salbutamol is used IV. Consider replacing potassium and monitoring lactate especially if salbutamol is used IV.

Discharge

The child can be safely discharged once oxygen saturations are >94% (and PEF rate >75% of best predicted, if available), and stable on 3–4-hourly inhaled bronchodilators.

Prior to discharge:

- Provide patient education (see 'Patient education') including a written asthma action plan and check inhaler technique
- Arrange follow-up by primary care services within 48 hours
- Consider follow-up in a paediatric asthma clinic.

Further reading

1. NICE (2017, updated 2021). Asthma: diagnosis, monitoring and chronic asthma management (NG80). Available at: https://www.nice.org.uk/guidance/ng80
2. Asthma UK website: https://www.asthma.org.uk/
3. Generic children's asthma action plan. Available at: https://www.asthma.org.uk/971689d1/globalassets/health-advice/resources/children/myasthmaplan-trifold-interactive-041219.pdf
4. Childhood Asthma Control Test. Available at: https://www.asthma.com/understanding-asthma/severe-asthma/asthma-control-test/

Chapter 73

Paediatric bacterial meningitis and meningococcal septicaemia

Guideline:
NICE CG102 (Meningitis (bacterial) and meningococcal septicaemia in under 16s: recognition, diagnosis and management): https://www.nice.org.uk/guidance/cg102

OUP disclaimer: Oxford University Press makes no representation, express or implied, that the drug dosages are correct and that the recommendations are an exclusive or mandatory course of care. All health professionals reading this text have a responsibility to evaluate its appropriateness and take the individual needs of the patient into account.

Local trust guidelines: please refer to your local guidelines as necessary.

Overview

Meningococcal disease is an umbrella term for invasive infection caused by the bacteria *Neisseria meningitides*. It can present as bacterial meningitis (15% of cases), meningococcal septicaemia (25% of cases), or a patient can have both (60% of cases).

This chapter covers the diagnosis and management of children presenting with suspected or confirmed bacterial meningitis (secondary to *Neisseria* (meningococcal meningitis) or any other organism) and children presenting with suspected or confirmed meningococcal septicaemia.

Children commonly present with fever and a petechial rash. The majority of these children will not have meningococcal septicaemia, but identifying children at high risk of this life-threatening disease is paramount. Children with unexplained fever and petechial rash are treated as suspected meningococcal septicaemia.

All children with suspected or confirmed meningococcal septicaemia should be assessed for the presence of signs of meningitis and, if present, the management of bacterial meningitis should be followed.

Careful assessment and laboratory investigations will help to identify children who should be treated for suspected meningococcal septicaemia. This chapter should be used in conjunction with Chapter 70 and paediatric elements of the NICE sepsis guideline NG51 (see 'Further reading').

Diagnosis

History

Children often present with non-specific symptoms or signs which are challenging to distinguish from less serious viral infections. Over time, symptoms and signs may become more specific and/or severe making bacterial meningitis or meningococcal septicaemia more likely.

Symptoms and signs that present in bacterial meningitis (from any organism), meningococcal disease (any presentation caused by *Neisseria*), and meningococcal septicaemia include:

Common, non-specific:
- Fever (not always present in neonates)
- Nausea and vomiting
- Reduced appetite
- Lethargy
- Irritability
- Myalgia and/or arthralgia
- Respiratory symptoms/breathing difficulties
- Headache
- Unwell appearance.

Less common, non-specific:
- Chills/shivering
- GI symptoms (diarrhoea, abdominal pain/distension)
- ENT symptoms/coryza.

Other non-specific features:
- Degree of parental concern—how unwell the child is compared to previous illnesses
- Illness progression—how quickly the signs/symptoms are progressing
- Clinical concern—how worried the assessing doctors and nurses are about the child's condition.

More specific signs and symptoms are given in Table 73.1. Specific signs of meningitis (e.g. neck stiffness) are often absent in infants. Signs of shock and meningeal irritation are shown in Box 73.1 and Box 73.2, respectively.

> Consider a mechanical cause of symptoms, e.g. coughing or vomiting may cause petechiae limited to the head and neck, or localized petechiae due to local pressure.

Examination

Perform a careful examination following an ABCDE approach, especially in children with a petechial rash. Look for signs and symptoms previously detailed.

Investigations

All children with suspected septicaemia or meningitis

Bloods
- FBC
- U&E

Table 73.1 More specific signs and symptoms

Symptom/sign	Bacterial meningitis	Meningococcal disease	Meningococcal septicaemia
Non-blanching rash	✓	✓	✓
Shock (Box 73.1)/moribund state	✓	✓	✓
Unconscious/altered mental state	✓	✓	✓
Poor perfusion: • Hypotension • Capillary refill time >2 seconds • Cold extremities • Unusual skin colour	NK	✓	✓
Leg pain	NK	✓	✓
Bulging fontanelle (<2 years)	✓	✓	NK
Signs of meningeal irritation: • Photophobia • Kernig's/Brudzinski's sign (Box 73.2) • Stiff neck • Back rigidity	✓	✓	X (NK) (NK)
Neurological signs: • Focal neurological deficit • Paresis • Seizures	✓	✓	X

✓ = symptom/sign present; X = symptom/sign not present; NK= not known.

- CRP
- Coagulation profile
- Blood glucose
- Blood gas
- Blood cultures
- Sample for *Neisseria meningitidis* PCR (EDTA tube).

A normal FBC or CRP make meningococcal disease or meningitis less likely but do not exclude it.

Suspected bacterial meningitis

Imaging

- Perform a CT head in children with focal neurological signs or reduced/ fluctuating consciousness (GCS score <9 or decrease >3) to look for alternative intracranial pathology. Do not delay treatment and stabilization to undertake a CT scan.

Lumbar puncture

- Perform in suspected meningitis unless contraindicated (Box 73.3) *but without delaying administration of antibiotics*:
  - CSF samples may give useful results if taken up to 96 hours after admission
- In children with suspected meningococcal septicaemia who also have signs of meningitis or children with confirmed meningococcal septicaemia—discuss LP with a senior clinician
- Send CSF for microscopy including white cell count and Gram stain, total protein and glucose (measure corresponding blood glucose), and culture
- Consider sending additional samples for microbiological investigations to assess for alternative diagnoses (e.g. herpes simplex encephalitis, tuberculous meningitis).

Box 73.1 Signs of shock

- Prolonged capillary refill time >2 seconds
- Unusual skin colour (pale or mottled skin)
- Cold extremities
- Poor urine output
- Tachycardia and/or hypotension
- Respiratory symptoms or breathing difficulty
- Leg pain
- Toxic/moribund state
- Altered mental state/↓ conscious level.

Box 73.2 Kernig's and Brudzinski's signs

- Kernig's sign = pain on attempting to straighten the leg when the hip and knees are flexed to 90°
- Brudzinski's sign = passive flexion of the neck causes the hips and knees to flex due to extreme neck stiffness.

Box 73.3 Contraindications for lumbar puncture

- Signs suggestive of ↑ intracranial pressure:
  - Deteriorating or fluctuating consciousness—GCS score <9 or a decrease ≥3
  - Papilloedema
  - Unequal, dilated, or poorly responsive pupils
  - Abnormal 'doll's eye' movements
  - Focal neurological signs
  - Relative bradycardia and hypertension
  - Abnormal posture or posturing
- Shock
- Respiratory insufficiency (high risk of precipitating respiratory failure)
- Extensive or spreading purpura
- Post seizure (until stabilized)
- Coagulation profile abnormalities, platelet count $<100 \times 10^9$/L, or receiving anticoagulant therapy
- Superficial infection at the LP site.

Management

Acute management

Request prompt senior review to decide further management.
Monitor for clinical change and record at least hourly:

- Heart rate, blood pressure, and perfusion (capillary refill time)
- Respiratory rate and SpO_2
- Neurological assessment (e.g. AVPU scale/GCS score, signs of ↑ intracranial pressure)
- Skin changes (rash spreading or purpura developing).

Consider if disease notification to public health authorities is required (see 'Notification').

Management of suspected meningococcal septicaemia

Immediate stabilization of child with suspected meningococcal sepsis (including children with fever and petechial rash)

No signs of shock

- Reassess with blood results after a period of observation (usually after 4–6 hours, or sooner if clinical concern)
- If the risk of meningococcal disease is felt to be low (unremarkable bloods, well child, rash not spreading), consider discharge with advice to return if the child appears ill (see Box 70.2 in Chapter 70)
- Give IV antibiotics immediately (see 'Antibiotics') and treat as suspected meningococcal septicaemia if at any point during the observation period:
  - The rash starts to spread or becomes purpuric (>2mm)
  - The child appears ill or specific signs of shock or bacterial meningitis develop (Table 73.1),
  - CRP and/or WBC are raised.

Signs of shock

- Give high-flow (15L) oxygen via non-rebreathe mask
- IV fluids:
  - Give an IV/intraosseous bolus of sodium chloride 0.9% 20mL/kg over 5–10 minutes
  - Reassess, if there is no improvement give a second bolus of sodium chloride 0.9% or human albumin 4.5%
  - If signs of shock persist, seek paediatric critical care and senior support. Some children and young people may require large volumes of fluid over a short period of time and/or inotropic support
- Monitor for and correct:
  - Hypoglycaemia, hypokalaemia, hypocalcaemia, hypomagnesaemia
  - Acidosis
  - Anaemia
  - Coagulopathy
- Keep nil by mouth in case intubation is required.

Antibiotics

Primary care

- If a non-blanching rash is detected in a febrile, ill-appearing child in the community, give urgent IM or IV benzylpenicillin (unless there is a clear history of anaphylaxis) but do not delay hospital transfer.

Secondary care

- Give a third-generation cephalosporin such as ceftriaxone or cefotaxime IV for 7 days in total.

Management of suspected bacterial meningitis

- Monitor for seizures and ↑ ICP (in infants record and plot serial head circumference measurements).

Antibiotics

The majority of children with suspected bacterial meningitis will already have received antibiotics before the CSF microscopy results are available. If appropriate antibiotics have not already been given, start if:

- CSF white cell count in neonates: >20 cells/µL
- CSF white cell count in older children: >5 cells/microlitre **OR** >1 neutrophil/µL.

Examples of empiric antibiotic choices are given in the following sections. Treat as per local antimicrobial guidelines and seek microbiology advice where needed. Ensure a dose appropriate to meningitis is prescribed (usually a higher dose).

Age <3 months

- IV cefotaxime (see Box 73.4 regarding use of ceftriaxone as an alternative) plus either amoxicillin or ampicillin, for at least 14 days.

Box 73.4 Use of ceftriaxone

Ceftriaxone may be used instead of cefotaxime in children aged <3 months (with/without ampicillin/amoxicillin); however, note that ceftriaxone should be avoided in premature or jaundiced babies, or babies with acidosis or low albumin, as ceftriaxone may worsen hyperbilirubinaemia. Ceftriaxone should **NOT** be used in combination with calcium-containing infusions.

Age ≥3 months

- IV ceftriaxone for at least 10 days
- If recent travel outside the UK, or prolonged/multiple exposures to antibiotics in the last 3 months, add vancomycin (seek microbiology advice).

Specific antibiotic choices and durations

- Group B streptococci: IV cefotaxime for at least 14 days
- *Listeria monocytogenes*: IV amoxicillin or ampicillin for 21 days and gentamicin for at least the first 7 days
- Gram-negative bacilli: IV cefotaxime for at least 21 days
- *Haemophilus influenzae* type b: IV ceftriaxone for 10 days
- *Streptococcus pneumoniae*: IV ceftriaxone for 14 days
- If herpes simplex meningoencephalitis or tuberculous meningitis are part of the differential diagnosis, investigate accordingly and initiate specific empiric treatment.

Steroids

Give dexamethasone (0.15 mg/kg to a maximum dose of 10 mg, four times daily for 4 days) to children >3 months if:

- Frankly purulent CSF
- CSF white cell count >1000/μL
- ↑ CSF white cell count and protein concentration >1g/L
- Bacteria on Gram stain testing.

If dexamethasone is indicated, administer within 12 hours (ideally within 4 hours) of starting antibiotics.

> Discuss with a senior clinician if tuberculous meningitis is suspected, as starting steroids without also giving antituberculous drugs can be harmful.

IV fluids

Give full-volume maintenance fluid (use enteral feeds if tolerated):

- Consider IV fluids if oral intake is inadequate:
    - *Neonates*: use glucose 10% and add NaCl for maintenance fluids
    - *Infants/children*: use IV NaCl 0.9% with glucose 5%
- Monitor fluid balance, electrolytes, and blood glucose regularly
- Do not restrict fluids unless there is evidence of intracranial hypertension or ↑ antidiuretic hormone secretion
- If signs of shock present: treat as described previously for meningococcal disease.

Treatment after stabilization

Children with low risk of meningococcal disease (septicaemia and/or meningitis)

- Give appropriate safety net advice (see Box 76.2 in Chapter 70).

Children with confirmed meningitis or meningococcal sepsis

Before discharging

- Discuss potential long-term effects (depending on the diagnosis of sepsis or meningitis these include sensory, neurological, developmental, psychosocial, orthopaedic, dermatological, and renal problems) and the need for follow-up
- Offer contact details for peer support, charities, and counselling
- Offer an audiological assessment within 4 weeks
- Inform GP, health visitor, and school nurse.

Follow-up

- Follow-up with a paediatrician within 4–6 weeks.

Notification

- Meningitis is a notifiable disease and *Neisseria meningitidis* and other organisms that can cause meningitis or septicaemia are notifiable organisms. Urgent notification to the local public health authority is required (see 'Further reading'), who will assess the need for contact prophylaxis.

Special considerations

Immune testing

Discuss testing for complement deficiency with immunology or paediatric infectious disease teams if:

- More than one episode of meningococcal disease **OR**
- One episode of meningococcal disease caused by serogroups other than B **OR**
- One episode of meningococcal disease of any serogroup along with a history of other bacterial infections.

Further reading

1. GOV.UK. Meningococcal disease: guidance on public health management. Available at: https://www.gov.uk/government/publications/meningococcal-disease-guidance-on-public-health-management
2. GOV.UK. Notifiable diseases and causative organisms: how to report. Available at: https://www.gov.uk/guidance/notifiable-diseases-and-causative-organisms-how-to-report
3. Meningitis Research Foundation website. Available at: https://www.meningitis.org/
4. Meningitis Now website. Available at: https://www.meningitisnow.org/
5. NICE (2016). Sepsis (NG51). Available at: https://www.nice.org.uk/guidance/ng51

Chapter 74

Paediatric bronchiolitis

Guideline:
NICE NG9 (Bronchiolitis in children): https://www.nice.org.uk/guidance/ng9

OUP disclaimer: Oxford University Press makes no representation, express or implied, that the drug dosages are correct and that the recommendations are an exclusive or mandatory course of care. All health professionals reading this text have a responsibility to evaluate its appropriateness and take the individual needs of the patient into account.

Local trust guidelines: please refer to your local guidelines as necessary.

Overview

Bronchiolitis is a viral respiratory illness seen in children <2 years of age, most commonly in the first year of life with a peak between 3 and 6 months of age. The most common causes are respiratory syncytial virus (RSV) and rhinovirus, with the remainder caused by other respiratory viruses such as influenza, parainfluenza, adenovirus, or metapneumovirus.

Diagnosis

History/diagnostic criteria

Criteria

Coryzal prodrome for 1–3 days, followed by:

- Persistent cough **AND**
- Wheeze or crackles on auscultation **AND**
- Respiratory distress:
  - Tachypnoea **OR**
  - ↑ breathing effort (Table 74.2).

> Very young infants (typically <6 weeks) with bronchiolitis may present with apnoea without other clinical signs.

Other common symptoms

- Fever (usually <39°C)
- Reduced feeding.

When assessing severity and need for hospital admission, consider that symptoms often peak between days 3–5.

Common differential diagnoses are listed in Table 74.1.

Table 74.1 Common differential diagnoses in bronchiolitis

Diagnosis	Features
Pneumonia	Localized crackles on chest examination and/or fever (>39°C)
Viral-induced wheeze/early-onset asthma (unusual <1 year)	Persistent wheeze without crackles or recurrent episodic wheeze or personal/family history of atopy

Examination

Examine the patient using an ABCDE approach (Table 74.2).

Hospital admission criteria

Involve a senior paediatrician early, particularly if the child is in a high-risk group (Box 74.1). Admit to hospital if:

- Witnessed or reported apnoea
- Child looks seriously unwell
- Severe respiratory distress
- Respiratory rate >60 breaths/min
- Oxygen saturation <92% on air
- Central cyanosis
- Insufficient fluid intake (50–75% of usual volume).

Also consider factors that might affect a carer's ability to look after the child including social circumstances, distance to healthcare if the child deteriorates, and the carer's confidence in identifying ⚑ symptoms.

Table 74.2 ABCDE assessment in bronchiolitis

B	• ↓ oxygen saturations • Central cyanosis • Tachypnoea • Signs of respiratory distress (grunting, head bobbing, nasal flaring, subcostal/intercostal recession, use of accessory muscles) • Apnoea • Bilateral crackles and/or wheeze • Characteristic cough (dry, raspy)
C	• Tachycardia • Prolonged capillary refill • Pale or mottled skin • ↓ urine output
D	• Agitation or drowsiness
E	• Fever

Box 74.1 High-risk groups

The following children are at risk of more severe disease:
- Born prematurely (especially <32 weeks)
- Chronic lung disease
- Young infants (especially <3 months)
- Neuromuscular disease
- Haemodynamically significant congenital heart disease
- Immunodeficiency.

Triggers for consideration of higher dependency care
- Impending exhaustion with decreasing respiratory effort
- Recurrent apnoeic episodes
- Oxygen therapy insufficient to maintain target saturations.

Investigations

Bronchiolitis is usually a clinical diagnosis.

Bedside
- Rapid viral respiratory syncytial virus testing is sometimes performed to enable cohorting (admitting patients with the same virus to the same bay/clinical area).

Bloods
- Do not routinely perform bloods or blood gases
- Take a capillary blood gas in children with suspected imminent respiratory failure or severe, worsening respiratory distress.

Imaging
- Do not perform chest X-rays routinely. Consider performing if the child may require escalation to intensive care.

Management

Acute management

Management of bronchiolitis involves feeding support and oxygen supplementation if required. No medication is routinely indicated.

Feeding

- Nasogastric or orogastric feeding is often required due to ↑ work of breathing
- If nasogastric/orogastric feeding is not tolerated or there is impending respiratory failure, IV fluids can be used
- Refer to local guidelines for the volume of enteral or IV fluids (two-thirds of usual maintenance is commonly advised in infants with respiratory distress).

Respiratory support

- Oxygen supplementation to maintain oxygen saturations >90% (>92% if <6 weeks or underlying health condition)
- Upper airway suctioning if required, e.g. infant has respiratory distress or reduced feeding due to secretions or has comorbidities associated with additional difficulty in clearing secretions
- Higher-level respiratory support (high-flow nasal oxygen therapy, CPAP, or mechanical ventilation) may be required in infants not responding to supportive treatment.

Treatment after stabilization

Discharge criteria once clinically stable

- Maintaining oxygen saturations >90% (>92% if <6 weeks or underlying health condition) on room air for >4 hours, including a period of sleep
- Adequate oral fluid intake (usually >75% of usual amount).

Discharge advice

Explain ⚑ symptoms and when to seek medical care:

⚑ Worsening work of breathing (grunting, nasal flaring, chest recessions)
⚑ Cyanosis
⚑ Apnoea
⚑ Exhaustion (not responding to social cues, difficult to wake)
⚑ Taking <50–75% feeds or no wet nappies in 12 hours.

Give advice on the usual course of illness:

- Expect worsening symptoms on days 3–5
- Resolution of cough and wheeze usually within 3 weeks.

Signpost to smoking cessation resources where there is smoking in the home.

Further reading

1. Cunningham S (2015). Oxygen saturations target in infants with bronchiolitis (BIDS): a double-blind, randomised equivalence trial. *Lancet*. 386:1041–8.

Chapter 75

Paediatric diabetic ketoacidosis

Guideline:
NICE NG18 (Diabetes (type 1 and type 2) in children and young people: diagnosis and management): https://www.nice.org.uk/guidance/NG18

OUP disclaimer: Oxford University Press makes no representation, express or implied, that the drug dosages are correct and that the recommendations are an exclusive or mandatory course of care. All health professionals reading this text have a responsibility to evaluate its appropriateness and take the individual needs of the patient into account.

Local trust guidelines: please refer to your local guidelines as necessary.

Overview

T1DM is characterized by deficient insulin production and some children present with DKA. Patients with an established T1DM diagnosis can also develop DKA if they are unwell or have received insufficient insulin. Suspected DKA in a child should be managed in a hospital with acute paediatric facilities. Other aspects of the diagnosis and management of T1DM in children, including the management of hypoglycaemia are covered in Chapter 77.

Diagnosis

History

DKA should be suspected in the context of hyperglycaemia (plasma glucose >11.1mmol/L) **OR** known diabetes in the presence of the following symptoms:

Excessive fatigue, polyuria, polydipsia, or unexplained weight loss
AND any of:

- Abdominal pain
- Dehydration
- Hyperventilation
- Nausea
- Vomiting
- Reduced level of consciousness.

Sepsis should be considered if there is concurrent fever, hypothermia, hypotension, lactic acidosis, or refractory acidosis.

Examination

- Perform an ABCDE assessment in all unwell children
- A drowsy child may require early anaesthetic involvement for airway support
- Check observations including heart rate, blood pressure, respiratory rate, and temperature
- Measure weight
- Examine for the following:
  - Kussmaul breathing
  - Evidence of dehydration or shock
  - Level of consciousness
  - Signs of ↑ intracranial pressure (cerebral oedema)
  - Focus of infection or signs of sepsis.

Investigations

- CBG
- Ketones—near-patient blood ketones (beta-hydroxybutyrate) testing should be used
- Blood gases (typically venous or capillary in patients who are not requiring intensive care)
- FBC
- U&E, plasma bicarbonate, plasma glucose
- CRP
- If a first presentation of T1DM, consider sending 'new diagnosis' investigations, e.g. HbA1c, TFT, coeliac screen
- Consider sending other investigations as clinically indicated, e.g. blood cultures, throat swabs, urine MC&S.

Diagnostic criteria

- Acidaemia (pH <7.3 or plasma bicarbonate <15mmol/L) **AND**
- Ketonaemia (blood beta-hydroxybutyrate >3mmol/L or ketonuria greater than ++).

> Plasma glucose is usually high (>11mmol/L), but some patients may have DKA with a **normal** blood glucose level (if already on insulin).

DKA severity should be determined as it may influence the decision to treat the child in a higher dependency environment:

- Mild: pH <7.3 **OR** bicarbonate <15mmol/L
- Moderate: pH <7.2 **OR** bicarbonate <10mmol/L
- Severe: pH <7.1 **OR** bicarbonate <5mmol/L.

Management

Management of paediatric DKA is complex. Request senior paediatric help urgently and consult local guidelines, especially for guidance on fluid management. Paediatric critical care and anaesthetic review may be required if the child with DKA cannot protect their airway due to a reduced level of consciousness.

The aim of DKA management is to reverse dehydration, reduce glucose levels, reverse ketosis, and avoid hypokalaemia and rapid changes in serum osmolarity or electrolyte imbalances.

Fluids

If alert, not nauseous or vomiting, and not dehydrated, consider treating with oral fluids (discuss specific management with a senior paediatrician). Otherwise, use IV fluids, giving a fluid bolus first, followed by rehydration fluids.

Initial fluid bolus

- All **non-shocked** children:
  - Give an initial IV bolus of 10mL/kg 0.9% sodium chloride, over 30 minutes
  - Rarely, a second bolus of 10mL/kg is required but this should always be discussed with a senior paediatrician
  - Remember: any fluid bolus given at this stage should be deducted when calculating fluid deficit (see step 2 of calculations)
- If **shocked** (Box 75.1):
  - Give an IV bolus of 20mL/kg 0.9% sodium chloride, over 15 minutes
  - This bolus volume should **NOT** be subtracted when calculating fluid deficit.

Box 75.1 Shock

Shock is relatively rare in DKA. A weak thready pulse and hypotension should be considered as signs of shock. Tachycardia, tachypnoea, or prolonged capillary refill time are signs of vasoconstriction and do not signify shock in this scenario.

IV rehydration fluids

IV rehydration fluid requirement for first 48 hours = deficit + maintenance, given over 48 hours.

How to calculate fluids

The British Society for Paediatric Endocrinology and Diabetes (BSPED) provides a useful calculator which helps with fluid calculations and creates a protocol to follow for DKA management (see 'Further reading').

Examples are based on a child weighing 30kg with mild DKA (5% dehydration), who did not have shock and received a single initial 10mL/kg bolus.

NOTE: *in rare instances, a second initial bolus may be given to a non-shocked child (10mL/kg + 10mL/kg), and the volume for the initial bolus in the calculations would need to be adjusted to 20mL/kg (see step 2).*

Step 1. Calculate fluid deficit

The degree of dehydration cannot be accurately clinically assessed. Estimation of fluid deficit in DKA is based on the **initial blood pH**:

- 5% fluid deficit in mild–moderate DKA (blood pH ≥7.1)
- 10% fluid deficit in severe DKA (blood pH <7.1).

> **Calculation:**
>
> Fluid deficit (mL) = weight (kg) × % dehydration × 10
>
> e.g. 30 (kg) × 5 (% dehydration) × 10 = 1500mL

Step 2. Deduct initial 10mL/kg fluid bolus from total fluid deficit

This does **not** apply to a 20mL/kg bolus given to a *shocked* child.

> **Calculation:**
>
> Fluid deficit less initial bolus volume (mL) =
> fluid deficit (mL) − 10mL/kg bolus volume (mL)
>
> e.g. 1500mL − 300mL bolus = 1200mL

Step 3. Calculate deficit replacement rate over **48 hours**

> **Calculation:**
>
> Deficit replacement rate (mL/hour) =
> fluid deficit less initial bolus [if not initially shocked] (mL) ÷ 48 hours
>
> e.g. 1200mL ÷ 48 hours = 25mL/hour

Step 4. Calculate **daily** maintenance requirement

> **Calculation:**
>
> Up to a maximum weight of 75kg
>
> - 100mL/kg/day for the first 10kg of body weight
> - 50mL/kg/day for the second 10kg of body weight
> - 20mL/kg/day for each additional kilogram above 20kg.
>
> E.g. in a 30kg child:
> Kilograms 0–10 = 100mL × 10 = 1000mL
> Kilograms 11–20 = 50mL × 10 = 500mL
> Kilograms 21–30 = 20mL × 10 = 200mL
> Total daily maintenance for 30kg child = 1700mL

Step 5. Calculate **daily** maintenance rate

> **Calculation:**
>
> Maintenance rate (mL/hour) = daily fluid requirement (mL) ÷ 24 hours
>
> E.g. 1700mL ÷ 24 = 70.83mL/hour

Step 6. Calculate starting fluid rate

> **Calculation:**
> Starting fluid rate (mL/hour) = maintenance rate (mL/hour) + deficit replacement rate (mL/hour)
> E.g. 70.83mL/hour + 25mL/hour = 95.83mL/hour
> **Therefore, 4600mL of fluid (1700mL maintenance for day 1 + 1700mL maintenance for day 2 + 1200mL deficit spread over days 1 and 2) should be given at a rate of 95.83mL/hour, over 48 hours.**
> Do not give additional IV fluids to replace urinary losses.

Type of fluid

- Use 0.9% sodium chloride with added potassium (20mmol/500mL), unless the patient is anuric or potassium is >5.5mmol/L, until plasma glucose concentration falls to 14mmol/L
- Once the plasma glucose concentration is <14mmol/L, switch to 0.9% sodium chloride with 5% glucose plus potassium (20mmol/500mL)
- If glucose decreases to <6mmol/L, increase the glucose concentration of the fluid under senior guidance, and continue to give at least 0.05 units/kg/hour of insulin if ketosis persists.

Insulin

- **WAIT** for 1–2 hours after fluids have commenced before starting an insulin infusion
- Administer insulin at a rate of 0.05–0.1 units/kg/hour
- If the blood beta-hydroxybutyrate levels are not falling within 6–8 hours, discuss with a senior paediatrician regarding increasing the insulin dosage
- If the child is already using SC basal insulin, discuss the management with a senior paediatrician
- If the child has an insulin pump *in situ*, disconnect it prior to commencing the insulin infusion.

Other

- Consider nasogastric tube insertion (if vomiting or reduced GCS score)
- Consider urinary catheterisation.

Monitoring

Children in DKA need frequent medical reviews and monitoring:

- Connect to a cardiac monitor (observe for signs of hyper/ hypokalaemia)
- Vital signs and GCS score
- Strict fluid balance
- Capillary glucose and ketones (usually hourly)
- Blood gases (pH and PCO_2) and plasma U&E and laboratory glucose (usually 4-hourly).

Monitor for complications and seek urgent senior support if the any of the following are suspected:

- Cerebral oedema (changes in conscious level or behaviour, headaches, oculomotor palsies, pupil inequality or dilatation, bradycardia, or hypertension)
- Cardiac dysrhythmias (secondary to electrolyte imbalances, especially potassium)
- Electrolyte abnormalities: monitor plasma sodium and potassium levels. Calculate corrected sodium level to identify hyponatraemia (see 'Further reading'). Corrected sodium levels should rise with falling blood glucose. If either the corrected sodium is falling or there is a rapid and ongoing rise, inform a senior paediatrician as these can precipitate cerebral oedema
- VTE, especially if there is a central venous catheter.

Resolution of DKA

It may be appropriate to stop the fluid infusion when all of the following apply:

- The child is alert and drinking
- The child does not have nausea and vomiting
- Ketone levels are falling
- pH is ≥7.3.

Do not give oral fluids to a child who is receiving IV fluids for DKA until ketosis is resolving and there is no nausea or vomiting.

SC insulin should be given at least 30 minutes before the insulin infusion is stopped.

If the child has an insulin pump, this should be restarted 60 minutes before the insulin infusion is stopped.

Avoiding future episodes of DKA

Following recovery, discuss with the child and their family what may have led to the episode and the management of intercurrent illness. Consider the possibility of non-adherence (in patients with an established diagnosis of T1DM) and ensure that the specialist paediatric diabetes team is happy that the child is ready for discharge and has appropriate follow-up in place. See Chapter 77.

Further reading

1. British Society for Paediatric Endocrinology and Diabetes. Paediatric DKA Calculator. Available at: https://www.dka-calculator.co.uk/
2. MDCalc. Sodium correction for hyperglycemia. Available at: https://www.mdcalc.com/sodium-correction-hyperglycemia
3. British Society for Paediatric Endocrinology and Diabetes. (2020). BSPED interim guideline for the management of children and young people under the age of 18 years with diabetic ketoacidosis. Available at: https://www.sort.nhs.uk/Media/Guidelines/BSPED-DKA-guideline-2020-update.pdf

Chapter 76

Paediatric gastroenteritis

Guidelines:
NICE CG84 (Diarrhoea and vomiting caused by gastroenteritis in under 5s: diagnosis and management): https://www.nice.org.uk/guidance/cg84

European Society for Paediatric Gastroenterology Hepatology and Nutrition (Guidelines for the management of acute gastroenteritis in children in Europe, ESPGHAN): https://www.espghan.org/knowledge-center/publications/Gastroenterology/2014_Guidelines_for_the_Management_of_Acute_Gastroenteritis_in_children_in_Europe

OUP disclaimer: Oxford University Press makes no representation, express or implied, that the drug dosages are correct and that the recommendations are an exclusive or mandatory course of care. All health professionals reading this text have a responsibility to evaluate its appropriateness and take the individual needs of the patient into account.

Local trust guidelines: please refer to your local guidelines as necessary.

Overview

Acute gastroenteritis commonly occurs in children, mostly due to a viral infection, although sometimes due to a bacterial or protozoal infection. Symptoms can often be managed at home, but are non-specific and children can develop dehydration and shock.

Diagnosis

History

Gastroenteritis

Suspect acute gastroenteritis if there is acute-onset diarrhoea and/or vomiting with or without fever. Typical symptom duration is outlined in Box 76.1.

Box 76.1 Duration of symptoms

- Diarrhoea: typically 5–7 days, usually no more than 14 days
- Vomiting: typically 1–2 days, usually no more than 3 days.

Ask about:

- Recent travel
- Recent exposure to a potential source (e.g. contaminated water or food)
- Recent contact with someone with diarrhoea and/or vomiting.

Alternative diagnoses

Key differential diagnoses include UTI (see Chapter 78), other non-gastroenteritis infections, acute appendicitis, and other causes of an acute abdomen. A careful review for alternative diagnoses is particularly important in children with isolated vomiting without diarrhoea.

Consider an alternative diagnosis and request a senior review in the presence of:

- Fever: ≥38°C if age <3 months or ≥39°C if age ≥3 months
- Respiratory symptoms, e.g. tachypnoea or respiratory distress
- Neurological symptoms, e.g. altered consciousness, neck stiffness, or bulging fontanelle
- Non-blanching rash
- Blood and/or mucus in stool
- Bilious vomit
- Severe or localized abdominal pain or tenderness, or abdominal distension.

Box 76.2 summarizes categories of children at ↑ risk of dehydration.

Box 76.2 Children at increased risk of dehydration

- Infants (<1 year old), especially if <6 months and/or low birth weight
- Diarrhoea >5 times and/or vomiting >2 times in the previous 24 hours
- Not tolerating replacement fluids or stopped breastfeeding
- Signs of malnutrition.

Examination

Assess dehydration and shock as per Table 76.1. Dehydration exists on a spectrum. Children with ⚑ signs are more likely to deteriorate to clinical shock.

Table 76.1 Assessing severity of dehydration

	Clinical dehydration	Clinical shock
Symptoms	⚑ Looks unwell	
	⚑ Altered responsiveness, e.g. irritable, fatigued	Reduced consciousness
	History of ↓ urine output	
Signs	⚑ Tachycardia	
	⚑ Tachypnoea	
	⚑ Sunken eyes	
	⚑ Reduced skin turgor	
	Dry mucous membranes (caution if 'mouth breather')	
	Warm extremities	Cold extremities
	Normal skin appearance	Pale or mottled skin
	Normal peripheral pulses	Weak peripheral pulses
	Normal capillary refill time	Prolonged capillary refill time
	Normal blood pressure	Hypotension

Suspect **hypernatraemic dehydration** if there are neurological signs, e.g. jittery movements, hypertonia, hyperreflexia, convulsions, drowsiness, or coma.

Investigations

Bloods

- Do not perform routine bloods
- If IV fluids are required or hypernatraemia is suspected, check sodium, potassium, urea, creatinine, and glucose
- If shock is suspected, perform a VBG
- If giving antibiotic therapy, send blood cultures
- Consider the possibility of haemolytic uraemic syndrome, especially in children with bloody diarrhoea, and discuss investigations with a senior paediatrician.

Microbiology

Perform stool microbiological investigations if:

- Septicaemia is suspected (see Chapter 73) (in addition to blood cultures and urgent antibiotic treatment)
- There is blood and/or mucus in the stool
- The child is immunocompromised.

Consider performing stool microbiological investigations if the child has been abroad, diarrhoea has lasted >7 days, or there is uncertainty over the diagnosis.

> If stool culture is positive for Shiga toxin-producing *Escherichia coli* (STEC), seek specialist advice on monitoring for haemolytic uraemic syndrome.

Management

Acute management

Enteral fluid management

No signs of dehydration

Continue usual fluid intake (including breastmilk and other milk feeds) and encourage additional oral fluids. Offer oral rehydration salts (ORS) solutions and discourage fruit juices and carbonated drinks.

Clinical dehydration

Enteral rehydration is associated with fewer adverse events and should be used as first line, including in children with hypernatraemia. Continue breastfeeding during rehydration but do not give solid food.

- Give 50mL/kg ORS for fluid deficit replacement over 4 hours as well as maintenance fluid
- Use ORS solution often and in small quantities
- If not tolerating oral ORS, give via a nasogastric tube
- Monitor with regular clinical assessment.

Antiemetics

Discuss with a senior clinician a single dose of ondansetron in children >6 months with persistent vomiting who are not tolerating oral rehydration (can cause diarrhoea as a side effect).

IV fluids

- Give IV fluids with senior guidance in:
  - Suspected/confirmed shock
  - Children with ⚑ signs who are deteriorating clinically, despite oral rehydration therapy
  - Children who persistently vomit ORS solution during oral or nasogastric rehydration
- Use 0.9% sodium chloride, or 0.9% sodium chloride with 5% glucose for fluid deficit replacement and maintenance.

> Start ORS orally/via nasogastric tube as early as possible during IV rehydration. Stop IV fluids as soon as oral/nasogastric fluids are tolerated, and continue rehydration with oral fluids.

No hypernatraemia

- Calculate maintenance fluid requirements over 24 hours and add a further 50mL/kg for fluid deficit replacement for those who were not shocked at presentation
- Measure plasma sodium, potassium, urea, creatinine, and glucose regularly and adjust fluids as needed.

Hypernatraemia present

- Calculate fluids as previously described but administer the fluids more slowly, e.g. over 48 hours, aiming to reduce the serum sodium by 0.5mmol/L per hour
- Monitor serum sodium levels closely.

Suspected or confirmed shock

- Call for senior help urgently
- Give a rapid IV fluid bolus of 20mL/kg of 0.9% sodium chloride over 10 minutes
- Give a second bolus if no response to initial bolus. If no improvement with the second bolus, consider an alternative diagnosis, e.g. sepsis.

Antibiotic therapy

- Antibiotics are not usually required
- Discuss with a senior paediatrician and/or microbiology if suspected sepsis, positive stool cultures, or significant travel history.

Treatment after stabilization

- After rehydration, encourage usual fluids (including breastmilk and other milk feeds) and solid food intake
- Avoid giving fruit juices and carbonated drinks until the diarrhoea has stopped
- Consider giving 5mL/kg ORS after each large watery stool in children at ↑ risk of dehydration (Box 76.2).

Discharge advice

Advise parents and carers:

- On signs of dehydration and ask them to contact a healthcare professional if their child appears dehydrated or symptoms do not resolve within the expected time frame (Box 76.1), particularly if the child is at ↑ risk of dehydration (Box 76.2)
- To encourage plenty of fluids ± additional ORS for large watery stools in at-risk children
- To wash their hands with soap frequently and thoroughly, particularly after changing nappies and before contact with food
- Infected children should not share towels with others
- Children should not return to their school or childcare facility until at **least 48 hours after the last episode** of diarrhoea or vomiting
- Children should not swim for **2 weeks** following resolution of diarrhoea.

Special considerations

Children with the following conditions are at risk of more severe or persistent disease:

- Underlying immune deficiency
- Inflammatory bowel disease
- Oncology patients.

Discuss with a senior clinician early as these children may need additional investigations and/or management.

Chapter 77

Paediatric type 1 diabetes

Guideline:
NICE NG18 (Diabetes (type 1 and type 2) in children and young people: diagnosis and management): https://www.nice.org.uk/guidance/NG18

OUP disclaimer: Oxford University Press makes no representation, express or implied, that the drug dosages are correct and that the recommendations are an exclusive or mandatory course of care. All health professionals reading this text have a responsibility to evaluate its appropriateness and take the individual needs of the patient into account.

Local trust guidelines: please refer to your local guidelines as necessary.

Overview

Type 1 diabetes mellitus (T1DM) (previously known as insulin-dependent, juvenile or childhood-onset diabetes) is characterized by deficient insulin production and often children are first diagnosed having presented with DKA (Fig. 77.1). Treatment of T1DM requires long-term insulin therapy. Type 2 diabetes mellitus (T2DM) is rare in children, although the prevalence is increasing. It should be considered as a differential diagnosis especially in overweight or obese children, those with a strong family history of T2DM, children of black or Asian family origin, those with insulin resistance, and/or sustained low insulin requirements. The management of T2DM in children is beyond the scope of this chapter.

Diagnosis

History/diagnostic criteria

See Fig. 77.1.

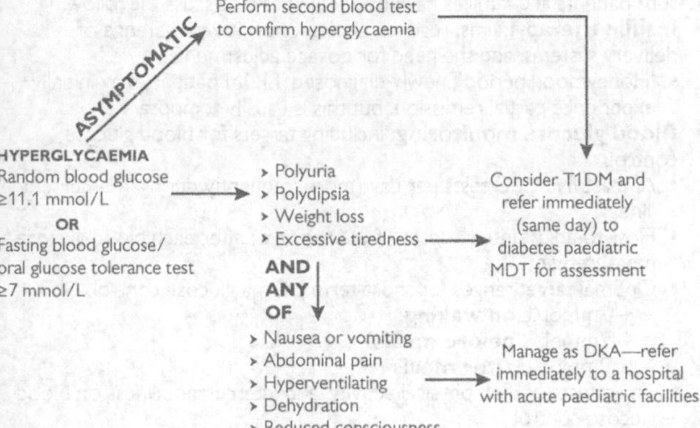

Fig. 77.1 Symptoms of T1DM and the diagnostic process.

Examination

- Check weight and height and plot on a growth chart. Significant changes in weight or growth may indicate a change in blood glucose control
- Assess hydration status
- Look for acute issues, e.g. a concomitant infection, which can worsen glucose control or trigger DKA
- Examine injection sites for signs of infection or lipodystrophy in children on SC insulin
- Look for signs of insulin resistance such as acanthosis nigricans (associated with T2DM)
- Look for signs of other autoimmune pathology such as coeliac disease, adrenal insufficiency, vitiligo, and hypothyroidism.

Investigations

- Blood glucose
- Blood ketones (to identify DKA if suspected)
- HbA1c (four times per year, or more frequently if challenging blood glucose management)
- Annual screening investigations (see 'Monitoring and follow-up').

Management

Chronic management of T1DM in children is primarily led by the local paediatric diabetes team.

Patient education

Ensure patients and families have opportunities to discuss the following:

- **Insulin therapy:** aims, regimen choices, how it works, range of delivery systems, and the need for dosage adjustments:
    - 'Honeymoon period': newly diagnosed T1DM patients may initially experience partial remission, but this is usually temporary
- **Blood glucose monitoring:** including targets for blood glucose control:
    - At least five CBG tests per day (more frequently during intercurrent illness)
    - How to adjust insulin doses (if appropriate) after each blood glucose measurement
    - Optimal target ranges for short-term plasma glucose control:
        - 4–7mmol/L **on waking**
        - 4–7mmol/L **before meals**
        - 5–9mmol/L **after meals**
    - The effects of diet, physical activity, and intercurrent illness on blood glucose control
    - Detecting and managing hypoglycaemia (see Chapter 21), hyperglycaemia, and ketosis
- **Managing intercurrent illness and 'sick-day rules':** including monitoring of blood ketones (see Chapter 17):
- **Diet:** carbohydrate-counting education and the benefits of low glycaemic index diets to help improve blood glucose control
- **Local/national support groups:** e.g. Diabetes UK
- **Medical alert identifiers:** encourage the wearing of, e.g. a medic alert bracelet.

Lifestyle and simple interventions

- **Smoking:** explain the risk of smoking and prevent uptake of smoking. Offer smoking cessation support to those who smoke
- **Additional immunizations:** pneumococcal and annual influenza immunization
- **Dietary:** healthy eating (low glycaemic index, fruit and vegetables, and appropriate fats)
- **Exercise:**
    - Children can participate in all forms of exercise, provided that insulin and diet are appropriately managed
    - Children should monitor blood glucose before **AND** after exercise to learn how their body responds and to avoid hypo- or hyperglycaemia
    - Additional carbohydrates should be consumed if plasma glucose levels are <7mmol/L before exercise
    - Exercise-induced hypoglycaemia may occur several hours after prolonged exercise.

Pharmacological management

Most children are on one of the following SC insulin regimens:

- Basal-bolus: short/rapid-acting insulin injections before meals plus ≥1 separate injection of intermediate/long-acting insulin
- Continuous SC insulin infusion or insulin pump.

Provide needles appropriate for the patient's size and a means of safely disposing of sharps.

Sick day rules

Apply to periods of intercurrent illness:

- Normal insulin doses **should be continued** and fluids encouraged
- Monitor blood glucose (2-hourly), as well as blood ketone levels, and food and fluid intake, and adjust insulin accordingly
- If DKA develops or sufficient oral intake is not possible, refer to hospital urgently.

Psychosocial considerations

Children and adolescents with T1DM are at a greater risk of emotional and behavioural difficulties and have an ↑ risk of mental health problems such as anxiety, depression, or eating disorders. Assess emotional well-being and support structures and consider whether specialist input (e.g. CAMHS) is needed, particularly if patients have frequent episodes of DKA or persistently suboptimal blood glucose control.

Monitoring and follow-up

Follow-up should take place in a paediatric diabetes clinic (usually four times a year).

Check/monitor for:

- Injection site problems
- Height, weight, and BMI on appropriate growth charts
- HbA1c (target level of 48mmol/mol)
- Diabetic retinopathy and hypertension (annually from 12 years)
- Diabetic kidney disease
- Diabetic foot problems
- Coeliac disease
- Thyroid disease (annually)
- Adherence to routine dental and eye examinations (every 2 years).

Be aware of rare complications: juvenile cataracts, necrobiosis lipoidica, and Addison's disease.

Hypoglycaemia

Hypoglycaemia is defined as a glucose level <4mmol/L and requires urgent treatment (Fig. 77.2). Symptoms are the same as in adults (see Chapter 21). Adolescents should be aware that alcohol use increases the risk of hypoglycaemia.

Hypoglycaemia (<4mmol/L)

Non-severe (patient able to self-treat)

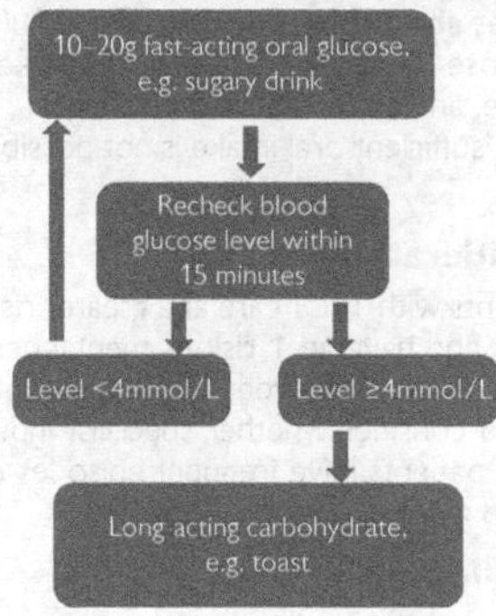

Severe (patient unable to self-treat) with IV access

10% IV glucose
maximum 5mL/kg body weight

Severe (patient unable to self-treat) without IV access

IM glucagon:
Age >8 years **OR** weight ≥25kg: 1mg
Age ≤8 years **OR** weight <25kg: 500 micrograms

OR

Oral glucose solution e.g. glucogel
(not if reduced GCS score)

Seek medical assistance if glucose levels or symptoms do not respond within 10 mins

Fig. 77.2 Hypoglycaemia management.

Further reading

1. British Society for Paediatric Endocrinology and Diabetes. Guidelines. Available at: https://www.BSPED.org.uk/clinical-resources/guidelines/
2. Diabetes UK. type 1 diabetes. Available at: https://www.diabetes.org.uk/type-1-diabetes

Chapter 78

Paediatric urinary tract infections

Guideline:
This chapter was based on: NICE CG54 (Urinary tract infection in under 16s: diagnosis and management): http://www.nice.org.uk/guidance/cg54. Since the chapter was written, the guideline has been updated with minor changes and renamed: NICE NG224 (Urinary tract infection in under 16s: diagnosis and management): https://www.nice.org.uk/guidance/ng224.

OUP disclaimer: Oxford University Press makes no representation, express or implied, that the drug dosages are correct and that the recommendations are an exclusive or mandatory course of care. All health professionals reading this text have a responsibility to evaluate its appropriateness and take the individual needs of the patient into account.

Local trust guidelines: please refer to your local guidelines as necessary.

Overview

Urinary tract infections (UTIs) are a common type of bacterial infection in children and are typically caused by *Escherichia coli*. Especially in young children, signs and symptoms may be non-specific and often overlap with common viral illnesses, which may cause diagnostic challenges. Clinical distinction between cystitis (lower UTI) and pyelonephritis (upper UTI) can be difficult in clinical practice (Box 78.1).

Diagnosis

History

Presenting signs and symptoms of UTIs differ depending on age (Fig. 78.1).

<3 months

Fever
Vomiting
Lethargy
Irritability
Poor feeding
Failure to thrive
Abdominal pain
Jaundice
Haematuria
Offensive urine

>3 months and pre-verbal

Fever
Abdominal pain
Loin tenderness
Vomiting
Poor feeding
Lethargy
Irritability
Haematuria
Offensive urine
Failure to thrive

Verbal

Frequency
Dysuria
Dysfunctional voiding
Changes to continence
Abdominal pain
Loin tenderness
Fever
Malaise
Vomiting
Haematuria
Offensive urine
Cloudy urine

Fig. 78.1 Presenting signs and symptoms of UTIs according to age group. Features are ordered by decreasing prevalence, with the most common feature at the top of the list. **Bold**: most common; normal font: moderately common; *italics*: least common.

Based on Table 1 from NICE CG54

Examination

Physical examination may be normal except for the presence of fever. Check vital signs including temperature and blood pressure. On examination, check for:

- Abdominal or loin pain
- Non-specific signs, e.g. lethargy, dehydration
- Signs of sepsis (see Chapter 77).

Box 78.1 Cystitis (lower UTI) versus pyelonephritis (upper UTI)

- Clinical distinction between cystitis (lower UTI) and pyelonephritis (upper UTI) can be difficult, especially in young children
- Pyelonephritis tends to include systemic features such as fever >38°C, lethargy, vomiting, and loin tenderness.

In children with confirmed or recurrent UTIs ask about and/or assess:

- Previous UTIs
- Poor urinary flow or dysfunctional voiding
- Recurrent pyrexia of unknown origin
- Congenital renal abnormality or family history of renal disease or vesicoureteric reflux
- Constipation
- Enlarged bladder or abdominal mass
- Spinal lesions
- Failure to thrive
- Hypertension.

Investigations

Collect urine for testing in all children with suspected UTI. Collection of urine to exclude UTI is not required if the child is well and there is a clear alternative focus of fever.

How to collect urine for testing

- Collect a clean catch urine sample
- If not possible, consider in/out catheterization or suprapubic aspiration (infants only after ultrasound confirmation of urine in bladder) under senior supervision.

Collect urine **before** starting antibiotics unless the child is seriously unwell and at risk of serious bacterial infection.

Use of urinalysis

Age <3 months

- Do not use a dipstick to diagnose a UTI
- Send urine for urgent microscopy and culture.

Age >3 months

- Test urine with a dipstick within 24 hours in children presenting with an unexplained fever >38°C
- If there is an alternative focus of infection, test urine only if the child remains unwell.

Interpretation of urinalysis results

A small number of false negatives may occur. Use clinical judgement when the test results are not in keeping with the clinical picture.

Age 3 months–3 years

- If leucocyte esterase **AND/OR** nitrites *positive*: send sample for culture and treat as a UTI
- If leucocyte esterase **AND** nitrites *negative*: do not treat as a UTI and only send urine for culture if specific criteria are met (see indications for urine culture given later).

Age >3 years

Interpret urinalysis in children >3 years of age as per Fig. 78.2.

Urine microscopy, culture, and sensitivity

Indications for sending urine for MC&S include:

- Suspected acute pyelonephritis/upper UTI (Box 78.1)
- Intermediate to high risk of serious illness
- Age <3 months
- Positive result for leucocyte esterase or nitrites
- Recurrent UTIs
- An infection that does not respond to treatment within 24–48 hours
- Clinical symptoms and dipstick results do not correlate.

Urine should be cultured within 4 hours of collection. If this is not possible it should be refrigerated or preserved with boric acid.

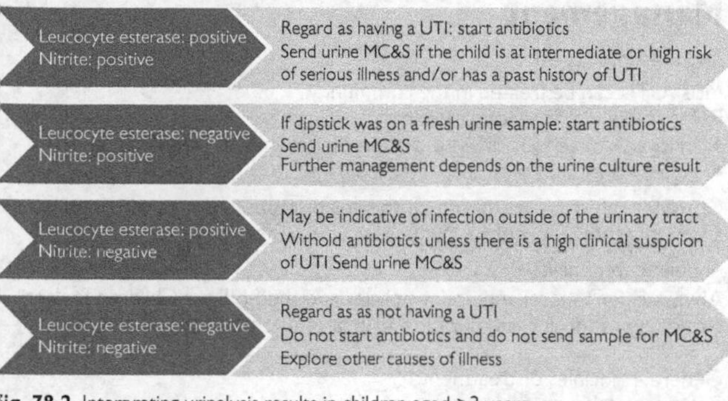

Leucocyte esterase: positive
Nitrite: positive
Regard as having a UTI: start antibiotics
Send urine MC&S if the child is at intermediate or high risk of serious illness and/or has a past history of UTI
Leucocyte esterase: negative
Nitrite: positive
If dipstick was on a fresh urine sample: start antibiotics
Send urine MC&S
Further management depends on the urine culture result
Leucocyte esterase: positive
Nitrite: negative
May be indicative of infection outside of the urinary tract
Withold antibiotics unless there is a high clinical suspicion of UTI Send urine MC&S
Leucocyte esterase: negative
Nitrite: negative
Regard as as not having a UTI
Do not start antibiotics and do not send sample for MC&S
Explore other causes of illness

Fig. 78.2 Interpreting urinalysis results in children aged >3 years.
Based on Table 2 from NICE CG54.

Interpretation of microscopy results while awaiting culture results

Bacteriuria present

- Symptomatic: consider as having a UTI and start antibiotics
- No symptoms (asymptomatic bacteriuria): do not treat.

Bacteriuria not present

- Pyuria (white cells) present: if symptomatic, consider as having UTI and start antibiotics
- No pyuria: regard as not having UTI.

Urine results pitfalls

- Epithelial cells suggest skin contamination and a poorly collected sample. Consider recollection
- Growth of a single organism at >100,000 colony-forming units (CFUs)/mL suggests infection. Lower CFUs and samples with mixed growth need to be correlated to clinical symptoms and the sample collection method and may need to be repeated.

Management

Acute management

Most UTIs can be treated in the community.

Refer to paediatric secondary care if:

- High risk of serious illness based on clinical findings (see Chapter 70)
- Aged <3 months with suspected UTI.

Consider referral if >3 months with signs of acute pyelonephritis, and have a low threshold for referral in infants aged <6 months.

Antibiotic treatment

Always refer to local antibiotics policies and the BNF for Children for antibiotic choice, dosing and duration as local resistance patterns vary.

General principles of treatment:

- Doses and durations are the same for boys and girls
- Seek specialist advice if aged <3 months
- In children aged >3 months, oral antibiotics are usually appropriate
- Oral antibiotic regimens include:
  - Cystitis: 3 days of trimethoprim, nitrofurantoin, amoxicillin, or cefalexin
  - Pyelonephritis: 7–10 days of cefalexin or co-amoxiclav
- IV antibiotics (sometimes in combination) may be required in seriously unwell children or when oral antibiotics are not tolerated. IV regimens include ceftriaxone, cefuroxime, gentamicin, amikacin, and co-amoxiclav
- Discuss children with recurrent UTIs and/or pre-existing uropathies with a senior paediatrician ± microbiology as antibiotic choices may be different and depend on previous urine cultures
- Children who do not clinically improve within 48 hours need reassessment.

Treatment after stabilization

Imaging tests

Children ≥6 months with a first time UTI responding to treatment do not need any imaging tests unless their UTI is atypical (Table 78.1).

Follow-up

- Follow-up is not routinely indicated after a UTI that does not require imaging
- Children with abnormalities on imaging tests will need appropriate follow-up with a paediatrician or nephrologist
- Give parents information and advice on:
  - Planned urinary tract investigation (if required)
  - Treatment and prognosis, including expected improvement within 48 hours
  - The possibility of the UTI recurring and prompt recognition of symptoms
  - Prevention:
    - Ensure adequate hydration
    - Treat constipation if present
    - Reduce delayed voiding with prompting and access to clean toilets
    - Antibiotic prophylaxis is not routinely recommended following a first UTI.

Table 78.1 Imaging schedule for children with UTIs

Type of scan	Age group	UTI feature		
		Clinical improvement within 48 hours	Atypical UTI	Recurrent UTI
Ultrasound in acute infection	<6 months	No	Yes[a]	Yes
	6 months – 3 years	No	Yes[a]	No
	≥3 years	No	Yes[a]	No
Ultrasound within 6 weeks	<6 months	Yes	No	No
	6 months– 3 years	No	No	Yes
	≥3 years	No	No	Yes
DMSA 4–6 months after infection (radionuclide scan to assess parenchyma)	<6 months	No	Yes	Yes
	6 months– 3 years	No	Yes	Yes
	≥3 years	No	No	Yes
Micturating cystoure throgram (MCUG)	<6 months	No	Yes	Yes
	6 months– 3 years	No	No[b]	No[b]
	≥3 years	No	No	No

An atypical UTIs is defined as:

- Seriously ill patient
- Poor urine flow
- Abdominal or bladder mass
- Raised creatinine
- Septicaemia
- Failure to respond to appropriate antibiotics within 48 hours
- Infection with non-*E. coli* organisms

A recurrent UTIs is defined as either:

- ≥2 episodes of upper UTI/pyelonephritis
- ≥3 episodes of lower UTI
- 1 episode of upper UTI/pyelonephritis plus ≥1 episodes of lower UTI

[a] In non-*E. coli*-UTIs, responding well to antibiotics and with no other features of atypical infection, the USS can be requested to take place within 6 weeks

[b] Consider performing MCUG if:

- Dilatation seen on ultrasound
- Poor flow of urine
- Non-*E. coli* infection
- Family history of vesicoureteric reflux

Further reading

1. NICE (2018). Urinary tract infection (lower): antimicrobial prescribing (NG109). Available at: http://www.nice.org.uk/guidance/ng109
2. NICE (2018). Pyelonephritis (acute): antimicrobial prescribing (NG11). Available at: http://www.nice.org.uk/guidance/ng111

Part 11

Respiratory

Chapter 79

Acute oxygen therapy

Guideline:
British Thoracic Society (British Thoracic Society Guideline for oxygen use in adults in healthcare and emergency settings): https://www.brit-thoracic.org.uk/document-library/guidelines/emergency-oxygen/bts-guideline-for-oxygen-use-in-healthcare-and-emergency-settings-summary-of-recommendations/

OUP disclaimer: Oxford University Press makes no representation, express or implied, that the drug dosages are correct and that the recommendations are an exclusive or mandatory course of care. All health professionals reading this text have a responsibility to evaluate its appropriateness and take the individual needs of the patient into account.

Local trust guidelines: please refer to your local guidelines as necessary.

Overview

Oxygen treats hypoxia but does not treat the underlying cause or the sensation of breathlessness. It should not be started in patients prophylactically, e.g. in stroke or myocardial infarction. Over- and under-oxygenation can be dangerous, which is why target saturations should be prescribed on admission.

Definitions

Hypoxia

Inadequate oxygenation at the tissue level which may be caused by hypoxaemia, or by a failure in the oxygen transport to the tissues, e.g. anaemia or cardiac failure.

Hypoxaemia

Arterial oxygen concentration (PaO_2) <10.7kPa.

Respiratory failure

Severe hypoxaemia where PaO_2 <8kPa. See Table 79.1 for differentiating between type 1 and type 2 respiratory failure.

Table 79.1 Types of respiratory failure

	Type 1 respiratory failure	Type 2 respiratory failure
$PaCO_2$	4.7–6kPa	>6kPa
Causes	Usually a problem with the diffusion of oxygen from alveoli into the blood: • Ventilation/perfusion mismatch e.g. PE • ↑ diffusion distance e.g. fibrosis, fluid	Usually a problem with ventilation, e.g. COPD, obesity, neuromuscular disease

Diagnosis

Signs of hypoxia

- Cyanosis:
  - Peripherally: blue skin colour and prolonged capillary refill time (>2 seconds)
  - Centrally: blue discolouration over the lips or under the tongue
- Respiratory distress:
  - Dyspnoea
  - Accessory muscle use
- Signs of carbon dioxide retention (see following section).

Carbon dioxide retention

Patients who retain carbon dioxide require lower target saturations, typically 88–92%, because they are reliant on their relative hypoxia for their respiratory drive (Fig. 79.2).

Presumed target saturations should be 94–98% *unless* you suspect carbon dioxide retention (Fig. 79.2).

Spotting the likely carbon dioxide retainers

History

- Drowsiness and confusion
- Headache (especially early morning).

Past medical history

- COPD
- Undiagnosed COPD (long-term smoker, aged >50 years, shortness of breath on exertion)
- Chest wall, spinal, or neuromuscular disease
- Morbid obesity: BMI >40
- Cystic fibrosis or severe bronchiectasis
- Previously required non-invasive ventilation (NIV).

Examination

- Flushed face
- Bounding pulse
- Carbon dioxide retention flap (asterixis)
- ↓ respiratory rate.

Bloods

- Raised HCO_3
- Polycythaemia.

Management

Emergency oxygen

Hypoxia kills before hypercapnia.

In all critically ill patients with acute hypoxia (initial saturations <85%), a 15L/min reservoir bag mask should be used.

Quickly decide on target saturations based on the patient's background, and adjust the device as saturations respond.

In patients who require a prolonged high rate of oxygen delivery, humidified nasal high flow should be used instead of a reservoir bag as it is more comfortable for the patient. Nasal high flow has the added advantage of being able to independently adjust the flow rate and percentage fraction of inspired oxygen (FiO_2) delivered. The flow rate can be increased up to 60L/min which can provide added pressure support to splint open alveoli (positive end-expiratory pressure). However, weaning nasal high flow can be more difficult in unwell patients and therefore only a senior clinician should consider commencing this.

Choosing the oxygen device

- Maintain the patient in an upright position to aid oxygenation
- Commence oxygen therapy using an appropriate device (Fig. 79.1 and Fig. 79.2) and perform a blood gas as soon as possible to measure carbon dioxide and decide on target saturations
- Venturi masks are useful to deliver specific oxygen concentrations and are colour coded accordingly (Fig. 79.1). Each venturi mask can only deliver up to its specified oxygen concentration and further increasing oxygen flow above the level required (printed on the mask) does **not** increase the oxygen concentration delivered to the patient.

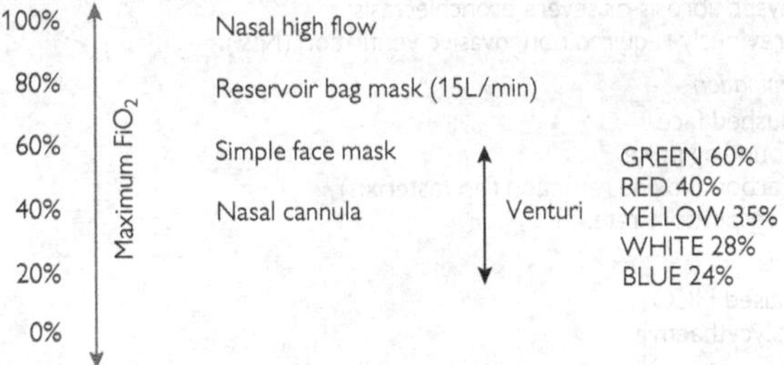

Fig. 79.1 Oxygen devices. FiO_2 (%) = (number of litres × 4) + 20.

> For non-carbon dioxide retainers who do not require high oxygen flow rates, nasal cannulae are often preferable to venturi masks. However, beware of predominant 'mouth breathers', who may not saturate well with nasal cannulae. For these patients it may be more appropriate to use a mask instead.

Monitoring oxygen

- Pulse oximetry:
  - Used to monitor oxygen saturation
  - Can be affected by peripheral perfusion—ensure that there is a good trace (even waveform seen on monitor)
- Blood gases:
  - ABG (consider using local anaesthetic):
    - Gold standard for assessment of hypoxaemia
    - Often painful for the patient
    - When interpreting the ABG, consider if the patient is on oxygen therapy. As a rule of thumb, the expected PaO_2 should be 10kPa lower than the FiO_2 received by the patient, e.g. a patient on 52% oxygen (8L/min) would be expected to have a PaO_2 of approximately 42kPa

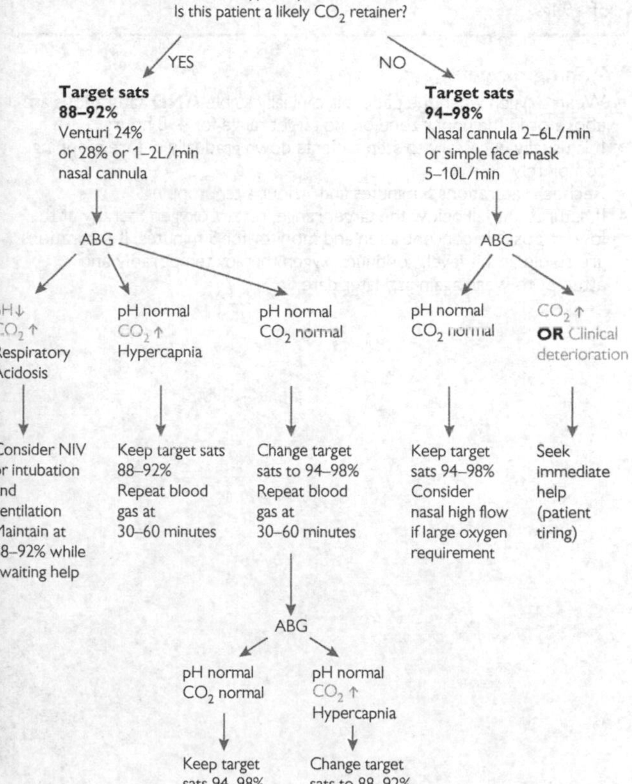

Fig. 79.2 Flow chart demonstrating the choice of target saturations and subsequent monitoring requirements.

- Capillary blood gas from the earlobe:
  - Less painful than ABG
  - Accurate for the measurement of pH, $PaCO_2$, and HCO_3 but less so for PaO_2
  - Useful where multiple samples are required for patient monitoring, e.g. during treatment with NIV.

Blood gases should be checked:
- In all critically unwell patients
- In all patients at risk of carbon dioxide retention
- If saturations drop <94% or deteriorate ≥3% from baseline
- If the patient has increasing oxygen requirements to maintain saturations
- New or worsening breathlessness.

> ABGs are not usually required for patients with no risk factors for hypercapnic respiratory failure and an oxygen saturation on air of ≥94%.

Weaning oxygen

- Wean oxygen when the patient is clinically stable **AND** saturations are above or in the upper zone of the target range for 4–8 hours
- It is usually necessary to step patients down gradually before stopping completely
- Recheck saturations 5 minutes and 1 hour after stopping
- If saturations fall below the target range, restart oxygen therapy at the lowest possible concentration and monitor for 5 minutes. If saturations are stable at this level, continue oxygen therapy temporarily and attempt to wean again at a later date.

Chapter 80

Asthma

Guideline:
British Thoracic Society, Scottish Intercollegiate Guidelines Network (British guideline on the management of asthma): https://www.brit-thoracic.org.uk/document-library/guidelines/asthma/btssign-guideline-for-the-management-of-asthma-2019/

OUP disclaimer: Oxford University Press makes no representation, express or implied, that the drug dosages are correct and that the recommendations are an exclusive or mandatory course of care. All health professionals reading this text have a responsibility to evaluate its appropriateness and take the individual needs of the patient into account.

Local trust guidelines: please refer to your local guidelines as necessary

Overview

Asthma is a very common condition associated with variable airflow obstruction, airway inflammation, and airway hyper-responsiveness. It tends to occur in atopic individuals. Symptoms can be triggered by environmental exposures and resolve spontaneously or with treatment. Exacerbations are often caused by infections (usually viral).

Diagnosis

Based on clinical assessment, supported by objective tests to demonstrate variable airflow obstruction or airway inflammation.

History

- Recurrent episodes of wheeze/cough/shortness of breath/chest tightness with no/minimal symptoms in between episodes. Symptoms may be worse at night/early morning or exhibit a seasonal pattern
- Symptoms triggered by various exposures, e.g. allergen exposure, viral infection, exercise, cold air, emotion, NSAIDs, beta-blockers
- Symptoms that improve outside of the workplace suggests an occupational cause or trigger
- Past history or family history of atopy, e.g. eczema or allergic rhinitis.

Examination

- Wheeze (may not be audible due to variable airflow obstruction).

Investigations

A single negative test does not rule out asthma due to the variable nature of the disease.

Investigations should include:

- Peak expiratory flow (PEF) rate monitoring over at least 2 weeks to identify diurnal variability (positive if >20% variability) or at least four times a day if occupational asthma is suspected
- Spirometry. Identifies airflow obstruction (forced expiratory volume in 1 second (FEV_1)/forced vital capacity (FVC) <70%). Perform pre and post bronchodilator to identify reversibility of obstruction (positive if >12% improvement in FEV_1). Normal spirometry does not rule out asthma.

Additional tests in selected patients:

- FBC—identifies eosinophilic inflammation
- Chest X-ray (if atypical symptoms, older patient, smoking history)
- FeNO (exhaled nitric oxide)—identifies airway inflammation (see Chapter 72)
- Total and specific IgE or skin prick tests to identify atopy and potential allergic triggers
- Challenge tests (histamine or methacholine)—to assess airway hyper-responsiveness.

'Suspected asthma' probability

Assess the probability of asthma diagnosis based on initial structured clinical assessment.

High probability of asthma (with a classical history and examination)

- Proceed to treatment. A good response to treatment after 6 weeks confirms the diagnosis. A poor response should prompt further testing and consideration of alternative diagnoses.

Intermediate probability of asthma (some features of asthma but diagnosis not clear)

- Perform further investigations to confirm diagnosis.

Low probability of asthma

- Consider alternative diagnoses (Box 80.1).

Box 80.1 Asthma mimics in adults

- COPD/smoking (fixed airway obstruction can be seen in chronic asthma)
- Obesity
- Dysfunctional breathing and vocal cord dysfunction
- GORD
- Rhinitis
- Heart failure
- Lung fibrosis
- Bronchiectasis
- Lung cancer

Management

Lifestyle and simple interventions

- Smoking cessation
- Weight loss
- Breathing exercise programmes—for quality of life and symptom improvement
- Patient education and personalized self-management plan
- Workplace adjustment when occupational asthma is diagnosed.

Pharmacological management

- Aim to achieve early control
- **Before** initiating a new medication or changing the dose; check adherence, inhaler technique, and triggers
- Discuss whether to provide the patient with a spacer device.

Reliever therapy: short-acting beta-2 agonist (SABA)

- E.g. salbutamol inhaler, 100–200 micrograms PRN, maximum QDS
- Requiring a SABA inhaler more often than once a month is an indication of poorly controlled asthma and should prompt an urgent review.

Regular preventer: low-dose inhaled corticosteroid (ICS)

Start a preventer therapy if:

- Symptomatic or using reliever ≥3 times per week **OR**
- Waking ≥1 night per week due to asthma **OR**
- Asthma exacerbation within last 2 years.

E.g. beclometasone dipropionate, 200 micrograms, BD.

> Consider encouraging the patient to quadruple their ICS dose when an asthma attack begins. This dose may be continued for up to 14 days to reduce the probability of needing oral steroids.

Initial add-on therapy

Long-acting beta-2 agonist (LABA): usually as a combined ICS/LABA inhaler

- E.g. beclometasone dipropionate/formoterol 100/6, 1 puff, BD.

If no response to adding LABA

Stop LABA and move to medium-dose ICS, or consider a leukotriene receptor antagonist (see below)

- E.g. beclometasone dipropionate, 400 micrograms, BD.

If limited response to adding LABA

Continue LABA and move to medium-dose ICS (or combination inhaler), or consider a leukotriene receptor antagonist (see below)

- E.g. beclometasone dipropionate/formoterol 100/6, 2 puffs, BD.

Leukotriene receptor antagonists

- E.g. montelukast, 10mg (oral), OD (evening)
- Leukotriene receptor antagonists are also useful in treating allergic rhinitis.

Additional controller therapies

If asthma is still poorly controlled, refer for specialist care where the following drugs will be considered:

Long-acting muscarinic antagonists

- E.g. tiotropium bromide, 5 micrograms, OD.

Theophylline

- E.g. theophylline, 250–500 micrograms (oral), BD. See Box 80.2.

Box 80.2 Prescribing theophylline

- It is important to prescribe by brand name due to variability in bioavailability between different products and the narrow drug therapeutic index of theophylline
- Theophylline many possible side effects including nausea, headaches, and arrhythmias
- Requires drug level monitoring.

High-dose ICS

- Provide the patient with a spacer device if not already done so
- E.g. beclometasone dipropionate, 800 micrograms, BD
- Refer for specialist care and consider bone protection to reduce the likelihood of side effects (Box 80.3).

Specialist therapies

Oral steroids

Used if the above-listed therapies have been unable to maintain adequate control of asthma. The lowest possible dose to maintain asthma control should be prescribed to reduce the likelihood of side effects (Box 80.3).

Box 80.3 Long-term steroid side effects monitoring

Monitor:

- Blood pressure
- Blood glucose
- Cholesterol
- Bone mineral density
- Eyes for cataract and glaucoma screening.

Monoclonal antibody therapy

- Considered in regional specialist asthma centres for patients with frequent exacerbations (≥4/year) or on continuous oral steroids.

Anti-IgE therapy (omalizumab)

- Subcutaneous injection every 2-4 weeks for patients with evidence of atopy.

Anti-IL-5 therapy (mepolizumab, reslizumab, benralizumab)
- SC or IV therapy
- Targets eosinophils—considered if the blood eosinophil count is raised (≥0.3 × 10^9/L).

Bronchial thermoplasty
- Heating of the airways to reduce smooth muscle mass
- Performed in selected specialist centres for patients with severe asthma despite maximum medical therapy.

Monitoring of asthma

- Use specific questions to review asthma control such as the Royal College of Physicians 'three questions' (Box 80.4) or asthma control test (ACT—five questions)
- Check inhaler use and technique and check how much they use their PRN inhaler.

Box 80.4 Royal College of Physicians 'three questions'
1. Impact of asthma symptoms on sleep
2. Any daytime symptoms
3. Impact of asthma symptoms on activities.

Medication reduction

Patients should step down treatment once stable for ≥3 months with regular review as treatment is being reduced. Patients should be maintained on the lowest possible dose of ICS, with a reduction of 25–50% every 3 months.

Acute asthma attack

Severity of attack

See Table 80.1.

Table 80.1 Acute asthma attack severity levels

Severity	PEF % of best/ predicted	Oxygen saturation %	Clinical features
Moderate	>50–75	≥92	
Severe	33–50	≥92	Respiratory rate ≥25/min Heart rate ≥110bpm Cannot speak in full sentences
Life-threatening	<33	<92	PaO_2 <8kPa $PaCO_2$ 4.6–6.0kPa Altered conscious level Exhaustion Arrhythmia Hypotension Cyanosis Silent chest Poor respiratory effort
Near fatal			Raised $PaCO_2$ **AND/OR** Requiring mechanical ventilation with raised inflation pressures

Admit patients with any feature of life-threatening or near fatal asthma, or any feature of severe asthma persisting after initial treatment.

Patients with PEF >75% best/predicted 1 hour after initial treatment may be discharged from the emergency department unless:

- Still have significant symptoms
- Social isolation
- Treatment adherence concerns
- Previous near-fatal asthma attacks
- Presentation despite oral steroids prior to presentation
- Presentation at night
- Patient is pregnant
- Psychological problems
- Physical disability or learning difficulties.

Investigations during an acute attack

Peak expiratory flow

- Measure on arrival to hospital, 15–30 minutes after starting treatment, and thereafter according to response.

Arterial blood gas

- Patients with oxygen saturation (SpO_2) <92% or features of life-threatening asthma require ABG measurement
- See Table 80.1 for interpretation
- If the ABG result suggests near fatal asthma, discuss with intensive care and a senior clinician urgently as the patient may need mechanical ventilation.

Chest X-ray

Perform if:

- Life-threatening asthma
- Suspecting a pneumothorax or consolidation
- The patient is not responding to treatment or is requiring mechanical ventilation.

Initial treatment

- Oxygen to target saturations 94–98%
- Salbutamol 5mg nebulised every 15–30 minutes as needed or continuous nebulizer (10mg/hour)
- Ipratropium 0.5mg nebulised QDS
- Prednisolone 40–50mg (IV hydrocortisone 100mg 6-hourly if unable to take orally)—continue for 5 days if improving

> - Use oxygen to drive the nebulizers
> - Give parenteral corticosteroids within 1 hour of arrival in hospital
> - Continue ICS while having oral steroid therapy.

Treatment escalation

- Continue nebulized bronchodilators
- Discuss with intensive care and with a senior clinician
- Consider IV magnesium sulphate 1.2–2g infusion over 20 minutes for patients with severe asthma or worse
- Consider an aminophylline infusion (5mg/kg loading dose over 20 minutes (omit if on oral theophylline normally) and then infusion of 0.5–0.7mg/kg/hour) for patients with life-threatening asthma or worse.

Monitoring

Severe asthma/life-threatening/near fatal

- PEF: repeat 15–30 minutes after starting treatment. Record PEF before and after nebulized therapy during the hospital stay
- ABG: repeat if the previous ABG was abnormal or if the patient is deteriorating, within 1 hour after starting treatment
- Bloods: monitor for hypokalaemia and check daily aminophylline levels if the patient is receiving an infusion (target is 10–20 mg/L)
- Refer all asthmatic patients to the respiratory team for review during their hospital stay and prior to discharge.

Discharge from hospital

When to discharge after medical admission

- Clinically improving and off oxygen and nebulizers
- PEF >75% best/predicated and <25% diurnal variability
- Established on medical therapy that they will continue at home—this should include ICS and oral steroids (unless the course was completed in hospital).

If the patient has taken oral steroids for >3 weeks, they will require a tapering regimen.

Discharge checklist and patient education

Check the following prior to discharge:

- Medication reviewed and optimized
- Medication adherence
- Inhaler technique assessed and advice given
- Asthma triggers addressed
- Smoking cessation advice/referral where appropriate
- Provision of self-management education including asthma action plan and PEF monitoring.

Follow-up

- GP or practice nurse review within 2 working days (discharge letter to contain patient's best/predicted PEF and PEF on discharge)
- Respiratory clinic in 2–4 weeks.

Chapter 81

Chronic obstructive pulmonary disease

Guideline:
NICE NG115 (Chronic obstructive pulmonary disease in over 16s: diagnosis and management): https://www.nice.org.uk/guidance/ng115

OUP disclaimer: Oxford University Press makes no representation, express or implied, that the drug dosages are correct and that the recommendations are an exclusive or mandatory course of care. All health professionals reading this text have a responsibility to evaluate its appropriateness and take the individual needs of the patient into account.

Local trust guidelines: please refer to your local guidelines as necessary.

Overview

Chronic obstructive pulmonary disorder (COPD) is a common condition, affecting over 1.2 million people each year in the United Kingdom. It is essential to know when it is appropriate to suspect COPD in order to initiate chronic management and to avoid potentially life-threatening acute exacerbations.

Diagnosis

COPD is diagnosed clinically, and the diagnosis should be supported by spirometry.

Suspect COPD in patients >35 years with a history of smoking and one of the following:

- Exertional shortness of breath (graded by the Medical Research Council (MRC) dyspnoea scale, see Box 81.1)
- Chronic cough and/or excessive sputum production
- Worsening of symptoms in winter
- Wheeze.

Consider if there is an occupational trigger which might be worsening symptoms, e.g. working in a dusty environment.

Ask about symptoms of commonly associated conditions including heart failure (see Chapter 5) (e.g. reduced exercise tolerance, paroxysmal nocturnal dyspnoea, and ankle swelling) and lung cancer (see Chapter 107) (e.g. weight loss, fatigue, chest pain, and haemoptysis) and provide focused management of these conditions as this improves prognosis.

Box 81.1 MRC dyspnoea scale

1. Breathless only with strenuous exercise
2. Breathless when hurrying, or walking up a slight incline
3. Breathless on flat terrain, walking slower than contemporaries
4. Breathless after walking about 100m or after a few minutes on level terrain
5. Impaired activities of daily living due to breathlessness, e.g. when getting dressed.

Investigations

Spirometry

See Table 81.1.

Table 81.1 Severity of airflow obstruction in patients with COPD

FEV_1/FVC	FEV_1 % predicted	Severity of airflow obstruction
<0.7	≥80%	Stage 1: mild
<0.7	50–79%	Stage 2: moderate
<0.7	30–49%	Stage 3: severe
<0.7	<30%	Stage 4: very severe

- To confirm diagnosis and monitor disease progression
- Perform post bronchodilator. Routine bronchodilator reversibility testing is not required
- If spirometry is suggestive of stage 1 disease, the patient must also have at least one COPD symptom to receive a diagnosis of COPD.

Further investigations at diagnosis

- FBC (check for anaemia or secondary polycythaemia).
- Chest X-ray (hyperinflated lung fields, flattened diaphragm, and bullae)

Additional tests (to identify additional or alternative diagnoses)

- Serial home peak flow diary if asthma is suspected
- Sputum culture if persistent purulent sputum is present
- Alpha-1 antitrypsin if early onset or there is a family history of COPD
- ECG, BNP, echocardiogram if cardiac disease or pulmonary hypertension are suspected
- CT thorax if symptom severity is disproportionate to the spirometry results or if the chest X-ray findings suggest possible fibrosis or bronchiectasis
- Full lung function testing if the symptom severity is disproportionate to the spirometry results.

Stable COPD

- At each clinical review (at least annually), ensure that there is understanding about COPD, exacerbation triggers, and the importance of **smoking cessation**
- Patients should be offered a pneumococcal and annual influenza vaccination
- Ensure that the patient is taught the correct inhaler and, if appropriate, spacer technique and observe their technique prior to prescribing inhalers. The choice of device is based on a number of factors including the patient's preference and their ability to use it correctly.

> Spacers should be cleaned using warm water and washing up liquid not more than once a month. The spacer should air dry.

Management

Pulmonary rehabilitation

- Offer if MRC breathlessness grade 3 and above and the patient is able to walk and does not have unstable angina or a recent myocardial infarction.

Initial pharmacological therapy

- SABAs or short-acting muscarinic antagonists (SAMAs) for acute breathlessness, e.g. salbutamol 100 micrograms, 1–2 puffs, as needed
- If still breathless or having exacerbations and there are no features suggesting steroid responsiveness (see Box 81.2): combination long-acting muscarinic antagonists (LAMAs) and LABAs, e.g. Spiolto® Respimat or Ultibro® Breezhaler
- If still breathless or having exacerbations and there are features suggestive of steroid responsiveness (see Box 81.2): combination LABA and ICS, e.g. Symbicort® Turbohaler, Flutiform® MDI, Seretide® Accuhaler, Seretide® Evohaler, Sirdupla® MDI, Symbicort® MDI.

Box 81.2 *Features suggestive of steroid responsiveness*

- Previous secure diagnosis of asthma or atopy
- High blood eosinophil count (>0.3)
- FEV_1 variation over time (≥400mL)
- Diurnal peak flow variability (≥20%).

Escalation (worsening symptoms OR if they have had a severe exacerbation requiring hospitalization OR two moderate exacerbations requiring prednisolone ± antibiotics in a year)

- Combination LAMA and LABA and ICS, e.g. Trelegy® Ellipta
- If treatment escalation was due to worsening symptoms and the patient was previously not using an ICS, review this therapy after a 3-month trial.

Additional therapies

- Oral modified-release theophylline for persistent breathlessness despite inhaled therapy or if the patient is unable to use inhaled therapy. Plasma levels must be monitored and clinicians should be aware that there are many potential drug interactions

- Mucolytic therapy (carbocisteine) for patients with a chronic productive cough
- Long-term oral corticosteroid therapy is not recommended but some patients with advanced COPD are unable to wean from oral steroids following an exacerbation
- Physiotherapy if excessive sputum production
- Dietetic advice ± nutritional support for abnormal BMI
- Management of anxiety and depression.

Further treatment escalation—with specialist COPD team guidance

- Oxygen—long-term oxygen therapy (LTOT) (see 'Criteria for assessment for long-term oxygen therapy') and ambulatory oxygen therapy (AOT) (see below)
- Home nebulizers for disabling breathlessness despite maximal inhaled therapy
- Prophylactic antibiotics if frequent, prolonged, or severe exacerbations, e.g. azithromycin 250mg three times a week (see Box 81.3)
- Lung volume reduction procedures and transplantation
- End-stage COPD with unresponsive breathlessness may require palliative opioids and sedatives.

Box 81.3 Azithromycin

- Prior to starting, the patient must have an ECG (to check QT interval), baseline LFT, and sputum culture to identify resistant organisms and atypical mycobacteria
- They must be warned about the small risk of hearing loss and tinnitus with this therapy
- Azithromycin does not need to be stopped during an acute exacerbation.

Criteria for referral to specialist COPD team

- Diagnostic uncertainty
- Alpha-1 antitrypsin deficiency is suspected
- Severe COPD, sudden worsening of condition, or difficulty managing symptoms
- Frequent infections/exacerbations
- The patient requires assessment for oxygen, home nebulizers, or continuous oral steroid therapy
- Onset of cor pulmonale
- Assessment for lung volume reduction procedures and transplantation.

Criteria for assessment for long-term oxygen therapy

Patients should have **stable COPD on optimal medical therapy**, with one of the following:

- Very severe COPD (FEV_1 <30%)
- Cyanosis
- Polycythaemia
- Peripheral oedema
- A raised JVP
- Oxygen saturations of ≤92% on room air.

The assessment process for LTOT is described in Box 81.4.

Box 81.4. Assessment process for long-term oxygen therapy

- Assessment comprises two ABGs at least 3 weeks apart
- LTOT may be supplied via a concentrator if:
  - PaO_2 is ≤7.3 kPa
  - PaO_2 7.3–8.0 kPa along with one of: secondary polycythaemia, peripheral oedema, or pulmonary hypertension
- LTOT should be used for ≥15 hours a day
- LTOT should not be offered to patients who continue to smoke after referral to specialist stop smoking services.

Ambulatory oxygen therapy

- AOT can be delivered via small lightweight cylinders or portable liquid oxygen systems along with oxygen-conserving devices
- AOT is suitable for motivated patients with resting hypoxaemia who on formal assessment are shown to have exercise desaturation and an improvement in exercise capacity with oxygen
- It can also be given to patients on LTOT who wish to continue oxygen therapy outside their home.

Exacerbations of COPD

An exacerbation of COPD is when there is an acute worsening of symptoms, beyond normal day-to-day variations.

- Mild: ↑ need of existing medication which the patient can manage in their own environment
- Moderate: requires prednisolone and/or antibiotics
- Severe: requires hospitalization.

Investigations

Primary care

Patients should be referred for urgent secondary care if oxygen saturations are <90% or if they are already on LTOT, have significant comorbidities or frailty, are unable to cope at home, or it would be clinically inappropriate to treat them in the community, e.g. severe breathlessness, impaired consciousness, etc.

Secondary care

Bedside

- Sputum MC&S if sputum is purulent
- ECG.

Bloods

- ABG—to assess for respiratory failure. **Record inspired oxygen concentration**
- FBC
- U&E
- CRP
- Theophylline levels (if taking orally)
- Blood cultures if pyrexic.

Imaging

- Chest X-ray.

Management

Pharmacological

- Nebulized bronchodilators, e.g. salbutamol 2.5mg QDS plus PRN, ipratropium bromide 500 micrograms QDS
- Nebulizers should be driven by **room air** with supplemental oxygen delivered by nasal cannula if needed
- Corticosteroids—in an emergency or if the patient is unable to swallow, an IV preparation may be given, e.g. hydrocortisone 100mg QDS. If able to have orally, prednisolone 30mg should be prescribed for 5 days
- Oxygen therapy targeted to achieve pulse oximetry saturation 88–92% for hypercapnic patients and >94% for other patients
- Antibiotics if bacterial infection is suspected. A broad-spectrum agent should be used initially, guided by local protocol, and reviewed following sputum or blood culture results. Oral regimens are typically given for

5 days. IV antibiotics are reserved for patients who are unable to take oral antibiotics or are severely unwell:

- Examples of broad-spectrum oral regimens: amoxicillin 500mg TDS, co-amoxiclav 500/125mg TDS, doxycycline 200mg initially and then 100mg OD, and clarithromycin 500mg BD

- IV theophylline can be used if steroids and inhaled bronchodilators do not lead to clinical improvement. Check theophylline level within 24 hours of starting.

Non-invasive ventilation

- Indicated if the patient has hypercapnic (type 2) ventilatory failure with acidosis (pH <7.35), despite maximal medical treatment
- Patients on NIV require high-level monitoring including regular arterial or capillary blood gas measurement. NIV should be delivered in a dedicated setting with appropriately trained staff
- All patients started on NIV should have a clearly documented escalation plan including agreed ceilings of therapy. Functional status and comorbidities are important determinants of suitability for intubation and ventilation on the intensive care unit, in addition to age and FEV_1.

> Oxygen therapy must be prescribed including target saturations. An arterial blood sample should be analyzed for pH, PaO_2, and $PaCO_2$ 30 minutes after oxygen therapy or NIV has been initiated, or after a change in the flow rate or NIV settings, or at any time if there is a change in clinical condition.

Recovery and discharge

- Daily measurement of peak flow or spirometry is not required but spirometry should be performed prior to discharge
- Physiotherapy can be helpful for selected patients to aid sputum clearance
- Patients with respiratory failure should have satisfactory oximetry and ABG results before discharge
- Establish patient on optimal inhaled therapy.
- Patients with COPD should be referred to the hospital respiratory clinical nurse specialist team who will assess medication including inhaler education and provide a written self-management plan, emergency drug pack, oxygen alert card, referral for smoking cessation, and pulmonary rehabilitation as applicable. They will also facilitate prescription or assessment for home oxygen if needed and liaise with the community respiratory service to arrange community follow-up after discharge.

Further reading

1. NICE (2018). Chronic obstructive pulmonary disease (acute exacerbation): antimicrobial prescribing (NG114). Available at: https://www.nice.org.uk/guidance/ng114

Chapter 82

Pleural effusion

Guideline:
British Thoracic Society (Investigation of a unilateral pleural effusion in adults: British Thoracic Society pleural disease guideline 2010): https://www.brit-thoracic.org.uk/document-library/guidelines/pleural-disease/bts-pleural-disease-guideline/

OUP disclaimer: Oxford University Press makes no representation, express or implied, that the drug dosages are correct and that the recommendations are an exclusive or mandatory course of care. All health professionals reading this text have a responsibility to evaluate its appropriateness and take the individual needs of the patient into account.

Local trust guidelines: please refer to your local guidelines as necessary.

Overview

A pleural effusion occurs when fluid builds up in the pleural space between the visceral and parietal pleura. A transudative (typically protein <30g/L) pleural effusion occurs when a change in hydrostatic or oncotic pressure forces fluid across the pleural membranes, whereas an exudative pleural effusion (typically protein >30g/L) occurs when there is ↑ permeability of the pleural membrane or capillaries.

This chapter covers the investigation and management of unilateral pleural effusion.

Box 82.1 Causes of pleural effusions

Transudate causes

Common

- Left ventricular failure
- Liver cirrhosis.

Uncommon

- Hypoalbuminaemia
- Peritoneal dialysis
- Hypothyroidism
- Nephrotic syndrome.

Rare

- Constrictive pericarditis
- Urinothorax
- Meigs' syndrome (underlying ovarian tumour).

Exudate causes

Common

- Malignancy
- Parapneumonic effusions (simple—sterile, complicated—colonized with bacteria, empyema—purulent)
- PE (most are small)
- TB.

Uncommon

- Rheumatoid arthritis and other autoimmune pleuritic diseases
- Benign asbestos effusion
- Pancreatitis
- Post myocardial infarction
- Post CABG.

Rare

- Yellow nail syndrome (and other lymphatic disorders, e.g. lymphangioleiomyomatosis)
- Drugs, e.g. nitrofurantoin, amiodarone, methotrexate
- Fungal infections.

Diagnosis

History

Patients may be asymptomatic or may report any of the following symptoms:

- Dyspnoea
- Chest pain
- Cough
- Night sweats
- Fever
- Haemoptysis
- Weight loss.

Examination

- Stony dullness on percussion on the affected side
- ↓ breath sounds on the affected side
- ↓ tactile fremitus on the affected side
- Asymmetrical chest expansion
- Aegophony (↑ vocal resonance (sounds like a bleating goat) over the superior part of the effusion)
- Mediastinal shift (rare).

Clinical findings may also suggest the underlying pathophysiology; e.g. peripheral oedema, distended neck veins and S_3 gallop, suggest congestive heart failure (see Chapter 5). Oedema may also be due to non-heart failure causes, such as nephrotic syndrome, pericardial disease (see Chapter 7), and yellow nail syndrome. Ascites suggests liver disease, and lymphadenopathy with a palpable mass suggests malignancy.

Investigations

See Fig. 82.1.

Bloods

- FBC—looks for anaemia which may be a sign of chronic disease, e.g. malignancy
- U&E, LFT (including albumin), CRP, and BNP can all provide information on aetiology
- Coagulation profile is necessary prior to aspiration (INR should be <1.5); platelets should also be >50 × 10^9/L
- Lactate dehydrogenase (LDH) should be measured for comparison with pleural LDH.

Imaging

Chest X-ray

The posteroanterior view will show effusions >200mL. See Fig. 82.2.

Ultrasound

Ultrasound is highly sensitive, provides clues to the aetiology and informs management of the effusion. It should be used in all pleural procedures to improve the success rate and reduce the risk of complications.

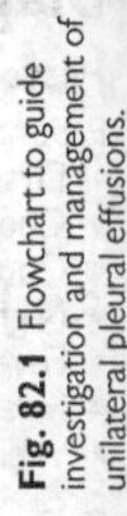

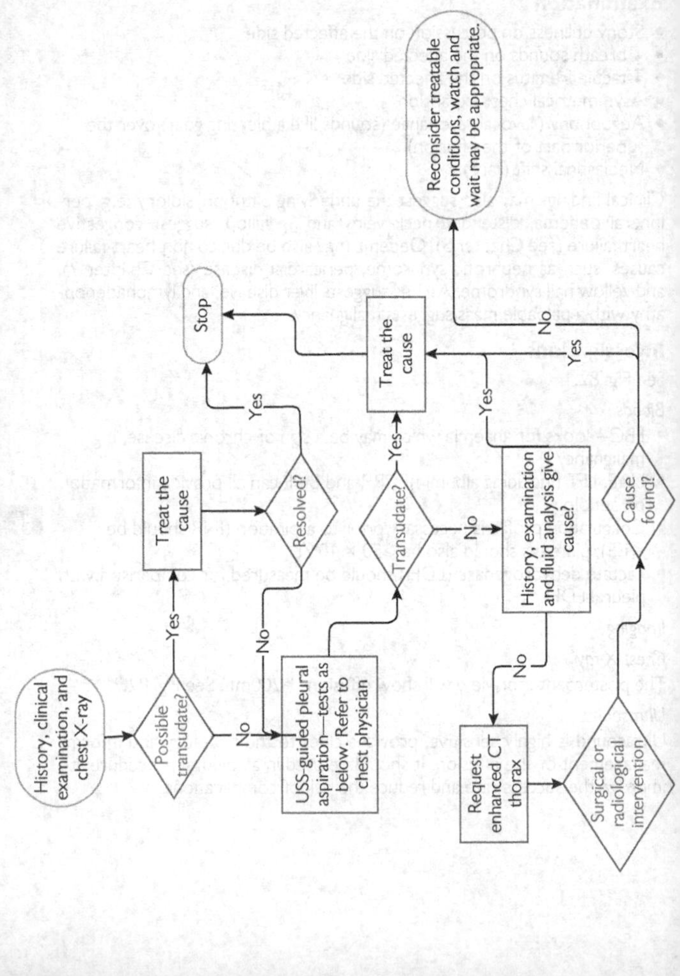

Fig. 82.1 Flowchart to guide investigation and management of unilateral pleural effusions.

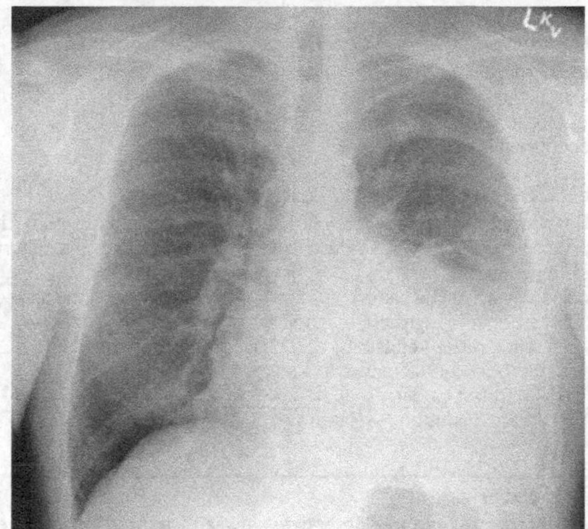

Fig. 82.2 Chest X-ray showing a moderately large left-sided pleural effusion with a meniscus-shaped upper border.

Reprinted from Desai S R et al (2012) 'Thoracic Imaging' Oxford University Press: Oxford, with permission from Oxford University Press.

CT thorax

CT scans should be performed in the investigation of all **exudative** pleural effusions. They are useful in differentiating malignant from benign causes and are important in planning the management of complex malignant and infective effusions. A CTPA should be performed if PE is suspected.

Pleural aspiration (thoracocentesis)

Assessment of pleural fluid allows the effusion to be distinguished as either an exudate or transudate. Additional investigations are sometimes indicative of the underlying cause of the effusion. Pleural aspiration should be performed under ultrasound guidance. Informed consent should be taken prior to the procedure.

Indications:

- Diagnostic—remove 50mL of fluid and record the appearance of the fluid (straw coloured is normal). Send samples for analysis as per Box 82.2. Perform:
  - For all effusions unless clinical features and other investigations provide a likely diagnosis
  - Urgently if empyema is suspected
- Therapeutic—up to 1.5L can be aspirated:
  - For the symptomatic relief of dyspnoea.

Risks:

- Pain
- Haemorrhage
- Visceral injury
- Pneumothorax
- Procedure failure.

Box 82.2 Pleural sample investigations

- All aspirates: protein, LDH, pH (if infection is suspected, unless fluid is obviously purulent, <7.2 suggests empyema), microscopy and culture, cytology
- Additional tests can be performed in certain clinical situations. If suspected:
  - Chylothorax → triglycerides, cholesterol
  - Pancreatic-related effusions, oesophageal rupture → amylase
  - Haemothorax → haematocrit
  - TB → acid-fast bacillus
  - Rheumatoid effusions → glucose.

Light's criteria

Light's criteria are used to differentiate between a transudate and an exudate when pleural fluid protein is >25g/L and <35g/L, or if serum protein is abnormal.

Pleural fluid is an exudate if one or more of the following criteria are met:

- Pleural fluid protein/serum protein is >0.5
- Pleural fluid LDH/serum LDH is >0.6
- Pleural fluid LDH >⅔ the upper limits of laboratory normal value for serum LDH.

Pleural biopsy

- Pleural fluid cytology confirms malignancy in around 60% of patients. Where this diagnosis is still suspected, a pleural biopsy should be performed
- Can be done percutaneously under ultrasound or CT guidance
- Alternatively, it may be performed using thoracoscopy, either under local or general anaesthetic. This is performed when there is insufficient pleural thickening for percutaneous biopsy and also when treatment of the pleural effusion is complex, e.g. in a multiloculated effusion.

Management

Acute management

- If the effusion is causing respiratory distress, drainage of the fluid should be done for symptom relief. This can be achieved in most cases by therapeutic aspiration
- Empyemas and low pH parapneumonic effusions should be drained by a senior clinician, as should significant haemothorax. Post-procedure requirements are summarised in Box 82.3.
- Empyemas that do not respond to chest drainage should be treated with surgical thoracoscopy
- Malignant effusions are usually drained to palliate symptoms and may require pleurodesis to prevent recurrence; this is done using sterile talc to adhere the two pleural layers
- Insertion of an indwelling pleural catheter is an alternative to talc pleurodesis and should be performed if pleurodesis is unsuccessful or as primary management of loculated malignant effusions.

Box 82.3 Post-procedure requirements for the insertion of a chest drain

Direct observation for 15 minutes

Chest X-ray to confirm the position and check for a pneumothorax

Observations following the chest X-ray:
- Repeat observations every 15 minutes for the first hour
- Hourly for the following 3 hours
- 4-hourly thereafter

Prescribe:
- Intrapleural saline flushes (20mL, at least QDS)
- Regular and PRN analgesia
- Oxygen if necessary
- VTE prophylaxis if necessary

Monitoring of drainage:
- Record cumulative output
- To reduce the risk of re-expansion pulmonary oedema:
  - First hour: drain max. 1L. Once 1L has drained, turn off three-way tap for 1 hour rest period
  - Note: large effusions can drain very quickly, so monitor the volume drained carefully
  - After 1 hour rest period, open three-way tap and drain fluid at a rate of 500mL/hour
  - Turn tap off for another 1-hour rest period between each drainage
  - Once draining <500mL/hour, leave on free drainage
- If during drainage the patient develops worsening breathlessness, chest pain, cough or vasovagal symptoms, or National Early Warning Score (NEWS) deteriorates, turn off the three-way tap and request an urgent senior review

Treatment after stabilization

Drains must be reviewed daily, including the site of the drain insertion, to check for wound infection, the volume that has drained, and whether the drain continues to be swinging (indicating that the drain remains within the intrapleural space and is patent, although swinging may cease as the lung re-expands and will be reduced if suction is used), and/or bubbling (which would suggest an air leak).

Drains can be removed when the output is <200mL/24 hours.

Chapter 83

Pneumonia

Guidelines:
British Thoracic Society (BTS guidelines for the management of community acquired pneumonia in adults): https://www.brit-thoracic.org.uk/quality-improvement/guidelines/pneumonia-adults/

NICE NG138 (Pneumonia (community-acquired): antimicrobial prescribing): https://www.nice.org.uk/guidance/ng138/chapter/Recommendations

NICE NG139 (Pneumonia (hospital-acquired): antimicrobial prescribing): https://www.nice.org.uk/guidance/ng139/chapter/Recommendations

OUP disclaimer: Oxford University Press makes no representation, express or implied, that the drug dosages are correct and that the recommendations are an exclusive or mandatory course of care. All health professionals reading this text have a responsibility to evaluate its appropriateness and take the individual needs of the patient into account.

Local trust guidelines: please refer to your local guidelines as necessary

Overview

Pneumonia is an acute lower respiratory tract infection where there is consolidation on a chest X-ray. If the patient developed the infection in the community, it is referred to as community-acquired pneumonia (CAP). If the patient is found to have pneumonia after they have been in hospital for at least 48 hours, their condition is referred to as hospital-acquired pneumonia (HAP).

Diagnosis

History

Pneumonia usually presents with cough as the main symptom. Other symptoms include:

- Fever
- Sputum production
- Breathlessness
- Wheeze
- Chest discomfort or pain.

Risk factors for CAP

- **Age:** especially infants, young children, and the elderly, in particular care home residents
- **Aspiration:** aspiration pneumonia is typically caused by anaerobes and Gram-negative organisms; commonly multiple pathogenic organisms are involved. It is seen more in patients who are elderly, those who have had a stroke, or who have myasthenia gravis, bulbar palsy, reduced consciousness, oesophageal disease, or poor dental hygiene
- **Comorbidities:** diabetes, chronic heart disease, chronic lung disease including COPD and bronchiectasis
- **Immunosuppression:** greater risk of presenting with an atypical or opportunistic infection, e.g. *Mycobacterium*, fungi, viruses, and parasites
- **Long-term prescribed opioid use:** due to impaired immune response to bacterial infections and supressed cough and mucus secretion
- **Lifestyle**: smoking; alcohol and drug misuse.

Examination

General

- Fever
- Tachypnoea
- Tachycardia
- Hypotension
- Hypoxaemia.

Respiratory (on the affected side)

- Crackles
- ↓ breath sounds
- Bronchial breathing
- ↑ vocal resonance
- Reduced chest expansion
- Reduced percussion note.

Box 83.1 CURB-65 and CRB-65 scoring

CURB-65 for severity scoring of CAP in hospital

CURB-65 is a scoring system for CAP that predicts mortality. It is calculated by giving 1 point for each of the following:

- **C**onfusion (AMTS ≤8, or new disorientation in person, place, or time)
- Raised **U**rea (>7mmol/L)
- Raised **R**espiratory rate (≥30 breaths per minute)
- Low **B**lood pressure (diastolic ≤60mmHg, or systolic <90mmHg)
- Age ≥**65** years.

Continued

Box 83.1 *Continued*

The score allows patient stratification as follows:

- 0–1: low risk (<3% mortality risk)
- 2: intermediate risk (3–15% mortality risk)
- 3–5: high risk (>15% mortality risk).

CRB-65 for severity scoring of CAP in the community

In the community, a CRB-65 score may be used, taking the CURB-65 criteria but excluding the urea value.

The score allows patient stratification as follows:

- 0: low risk (<1% mortality risk)
- 1–2: intermediate risk (1–10% mortality risk)
- 3–4: high risk (>10% mortality risk).

Investigations

Patients managed in the community

- Sputum culture and sensitivity if poor response to empirical antibiotic treatment
- Serological tests for *Legionella* or *Mycoplasma* if there is a current outbreak
- Sputum for *Mycobacterium tuberculosis* testing: consider if persistent productive cough with malaise, weight loss or night sweats or risk factors for TB, e.g. ethnic origin, social deprivation, elderly.

Patients managed in hospital

- Sputum culture and sensitivity if intermediate or high risk and antibiotics not yet received, or later in the admission if poor response to treatment
- Pneumococcal urinary antigen tests if intermediate to high risk
- Legionella urinary antigen tests if high risk. If positive, send sputum for *Legionella* culture
- Throat swab for *Mycoplasma pneumoniae* if clinically suspected (during epidemic years)
- Sputum for *Mycobacterium tuberculosis* testing: as in 'Patients managed in the community'.

Bloods

- FBC
- U&E
- LFT
- CRP
- Blood cultures: if intermediate to high risk, ideally before antibiotics are started. About 10% of patients with CAP will have positive blood cultures
- ABG if acutely unwell.

When performing an ABG, the inspired oxygen concentration must be documented.

Imaging

Chest X-ray

Should be done in all hospitalized patients with suspected pneumonia within 4 hours of hospital admission. A repeat film during the admission is not required unless there is clinical deterioration or a lack of improvement after 3 days of antibiotic therapy.

Findings which may be suggestive of pneumonia on chest X-ray (see Figure 83.1):

- Consolidation (dense shadowing that obscures blood vessels), often with air bronchograms (visible airways within the shadowing). Lower lobes are most commonly affected
- Pleural effusion is common
- A more diffuse interstitial and infiltrative pattern without focal consolidation
- Multifocal consolidation
- Cavitation.

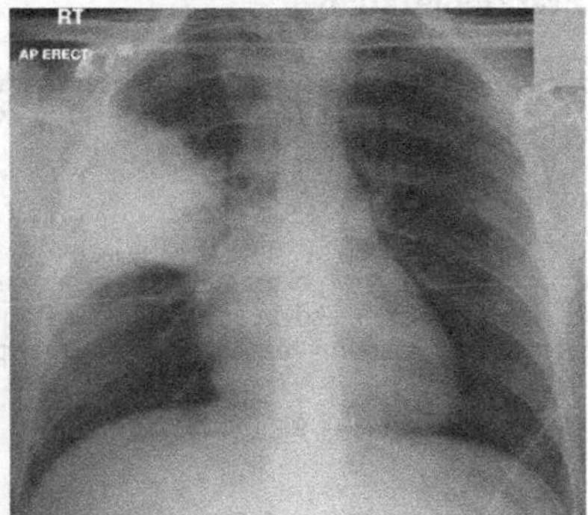

Fig. 83.1 Chest X-ray showing right upper lobe pneumonia.

Ultrasound

Consider if there is evidence of pleural effusion on chest X-ray. Can help to distinguish between simple and complex parapneumonic effusions and empyema. Pleural fluid can be aspirated under ultrasound guidance (see Chapter 82) and sent for MC&S; also pH to exclude empyema.

CT chest

Not required routinely but perform if the diagnosis is unclear or if the patient is critically ill and/or failing to respond to treatment. Also consider in the presence of cavitation, multifocal consolidation, significant or multiloculated pleural effusion, suspicion of malignant disease, or fibrosis on chest X-ray. CT pulmonary angiogram should be performed if there is a clinical suspicion of pulmonary embolism.

Management

Acute management

The management of CAP is dependent on the CURB-65 or CRB-65 score (see Box 83.1).

The duration of the antibiotic course is typically 5 days unless there is microbiological evidence or clinical indication that the patient needs a prolonged course (e.g. continued fever, haemodynamic instability, tachypnoea, or hypoxia). Patients with an empyema may require antibiotics for up to 6 weeks.

The prescription should be reviewed if microbiology sensitivities become available. IV antibiotics should be reviewed after 48 hours, and a switch to an oral formulation should be considered. In the community, patients should be reviewed after 48 hours (sooner if clinically needed) and if they have not improved or if they have deteriorated, a chest X-ray might be indicated and hospital admission should be considered.

Examples of typical antibiotic therapies are detailed in Table 83.1, but local protocols should be followed.

Treatment after stabilization

Lifestyle

Patients should be advised to rest, stay well hydrated and not to smoke.

In hospitalized patients with uncomplicated CAP, ideally they should sit out of bed for ≥20 minutes within the first day of admission if they are able to.

Pharmacological

Hypoxia

If required, and not contraindicated, oxygen therapy should be provided to achieve a target saturation ≥94% and arterial PaO_2 ≥8 kPa. If the patient is at risk of carbon dioxide retention, repeat ABGs should be performed.

Analgesia

Treat pleuritic pain initially with paracetamol.

Fluids

Patients should be assessed for volume depletion and may require IV fluids.

Thromboprophylaxis

Conduct a risk assessment for VTE prophylaxis (see Chapter 99) with LMWH.

Smoking cessation

Smoking cessation advice should be given to all patients who are current smokers.

Discharge

Consider discharge, if in the past 24 hours at least six out of seven criteria are met (exclude an abnormal feature if it reflects the patient's baseline state):

1. Temperature ≤37.8°C
2. Respiratory rate ≤23 breaths per minute
3. Heart rate ≤100bpm
4. Systolic blood pressure ≥90mmHg
5. Oxygen saturation ≥90% on room air
6. Baseline mental status
7. Able to maintain oral intake.

Table 83.1 Examples of antibiotic therapies that may be used in pneumonia

Community-acquired pneumonia			
Pneumonia severity (CURB65/CRB65 severity score)	Treatment site	Preferred treatment	Alternative treatment
Low severity CURB-65: 0–1 or CRB-65: 0	Home (hospital if other social factors or medical comorbidities that complicate management)	Amoxicillin 500mg TDS PO	Doxycycline 200mg loading dose then 100mg OD PO
Moderate severity CURB-65: 2 or CRB-65: 1–2	Hospital	Amoxicillin 500mg–1g TDS PO **plus** clarithromycin 500mg BD PO	Doxycycline 200mg loading dose then 100mg OD PO
High severity CURB-65: 3–5 or CRB-65: 3–4	Hospital (consider critical care review)	Co-amoxiclav 1.2g TDS IV **plus** clarithromycin 500mg BD PO or IV	Levofloxacin 500mg BD PO or IV
Hospital-acquired pneumonia			
Pneumonia severity (based on clinical judgement)		**Preferred treatment**	**Alternative treatment**
Non-severe		Co-amoxiclav 625mg TDS PO	Doxycycline 200mg loading dose then 100mg OD PO
Severe		Tazocin 4.5g TDS IV	Meropenem 0.5–1g TDS IV
		If suspected or confirmed MRSA, add vancomycin 15–20mg/kg BD–TDS IV (max dose 2g) **or** teicoplanin 6mg/kg BD IV for 3 doses, then OD	

Post discharge

After starting treatment, most patients can expect that by:

- 1 week: fever should have resolved
- 4 weeks: chest pain and sputum production should have substantially reduced
- 6 weeks: cough and breathlessness should have substantially reduced
- 3 months: most symptoms should have resolved but fatigue may still be present
- 6 months: most people will feel back to normal.

Post-discharge care:

- Patients should be reviewed 6 weeks following discharge either in a hospital clinic or by their GP.
- A follow-up chest X-ray should be arranged in patients 6 weeks post discharge if they have persistent symptoms or signs, or if they are at ↑ risk of a respiratory malignancy (age >50 years, smokers).
- If the pneumonia has not resolved after 6 weeks, a CT scan may be necessary to investigate further.
- Patients aged >65 years or at high risk for pneumococcal disease should receive a 23-valent pneumococcal vaccine if they have not already received one.

Part 12

Rheumatology and musculoskeletal

Chapter 84

Giant cell arteritis

Guideline:
British Society for Rheumatology (British Society for Rheumatology guideline on diagnosis and treatment of giant cell arteritis): https://academic.oup.com/rheumatology/article/59/3/e1/5714024

OUP disclaimer: Oxford University Press makes no representation, express or implied, that the drug dosages are correct and that the recommendations are an exclusive or mandatory course of care. All health professionals reading this text have a responsibility to evaluate its appropriateness and take the individual needs of the patient into account.

Local trust guidelines: please refer to your local guidelines as necessary.

Overview

Giant cell arteritis (GCA, also known as temporal arteritis) is a large vessel vasculitis, which untreated can cause ischaemic damage in the temporal arteries and branches of the aorta, potentially leading to serious complications including irreversible visual loss and stroke. It is considered to be a medical emergency because of the risk of irreversible blindness, but it is easily missed so a high index of suspicion is important. It is commonly associated with polymyalgia rheumatica (PMR; see Chapter 89).

Diagnosis

The diagnosis is most common between the ages of 70–79 years. GCA is unlikely under the age of 50 years[1] and women are affected more often than men.

History

Symptoms may include:

- Headache (classically temporal and severe)
- ↑ sensitivity or tenderness of the scalp—the patient may complain that they are unable to brush their hair due to the pain
- Claudication of the tongue, jaw (usually pronounced when chewing or talking) or limbs
- Tenderness or nodularity of the temporal artery
- Reduced or absent pulses in the temporal artery
- Visual loss or diplopia
- Symptoms suggestive of PMR including stiffness and pain in the shoulders or pelvic girdle
- Systemic symptoms including weight loss, fever, sweats, and malaise.

A detailed past medical history should also be taken. Ask specifically about symptoms which may be suggestive of previous PMR. It is also worth noting whether the patient has any pre-existing conditions such as diabetes, osteoporosis, or peptic ulcer disease, which may put them at higher risk of steroid-related toxicity.

Examination

- Height and weight
- Temperature
- Palpate the temporal arteries bilaterally to assess for tenderness, nodularity, or reduced pulsation
- Bruits of the carotid, axillary, or brachial arteries, or differing blood pressure between the two arms, may suggest the involvement of extracranial arteries
- Perform an ophthalmological assessment, looking for any abnormalities which may be suggestive of ischaemic changes, e.g. cotton wool spots, oedema of the optic nerve head.

Investigations

Bloods

- FBC, CRP, and ESR are essential, preferably before starting steroids, but do not wait for results to start treatment if suspicion is high. ESR is ≥50mm/hour in the majority of cases, but a normal ESR does not exclude the diagnosis. Consider a myeloma screen (serum protein electrophoresis and urinary Bence-Jones protein or serum free light chains) if ESR is disproportionately elevated compared to CRP
- U&E, calcium, glucose, HbA1c, and LFT including ALP should be measured as a baseline check.

1 Hunder G, Bloch A, Michel B, et al. The American College of Rheumatology 1990 criteria for the classification of giant cell arteritis. *Arthritis Rheum*. 1990; 33:1122–8.

Other

- PET-CT may be considered if there is suspicion of aortic involvement
- **All patients** should have **at least one of the following tests:**
  - USS of temporal ± axillary arteries is first line if available (Fig. 84.1). A 'non-compressible halo sign' is highly suggestive of GCA. It is more sensitive, but less specific, than temporal artery biopsy
  - Temporal artery biopsy used to be recommended in all cases, but usage now depends on the level of clinical suspicion and ultrasound availability. If both ultrasound and biopsy are available, the test should be chosen by the specialist according to the level of clinical suspicion, and the results should be interpreted as per Fig. 84.1.

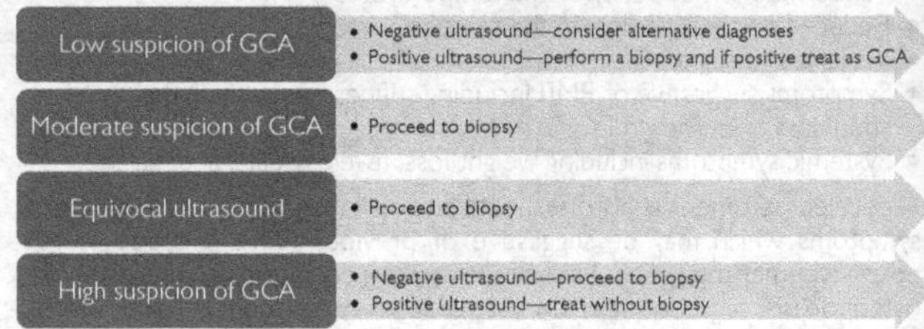

Low suspicion of GCA
• Negative ultrasound—consider alternative diagnoses
• Positive ultrasound—perform a biopsy and if positive treat as GCA
Moderate suspicion of GCA
• Proceed to biopsy
Equivocal ultrasound
• Proceed to biopsy
High suspicion of GCA
• Negative ultrasound—proceed to biopsy
• Positive ultrasound—treat without biopsy

Fig. 84.1 Choice and interpretation of specialist testing.

Management

Acute management

- Treat immediately with high-dose steroids, e.g. 40–60mg oral prednisolone, given as a single daily dose, if there is a strong suspicion of GCA (i.e. GCA is thought to be the best explanation for the patient's presentation). **Do not** wait for lab results if there is a high suspicion
- Patients with visual loss may be given 500mg to 1g IV methylprednisolone for 3 days before starting oral steroid. If IV treatment is not available this should not delay giving oral steroid
- Ideally co-prescribe a PPI, e.g. omeprazole 20mg OD for gastroprotection
- Bone protection as per osteoporosis guidelines, see Chapter 24
- Arrange same-day rheumatology review
- If the patient has new visual loss or diplopia, arrange same-day ophthalmology review.

Treatment after stabilization

Patient education

- Provide information about the diagnosis and treatment
- Encourage patients to stop smoking
- Encourage exercise and a healthy diet due to the ↑ risk of osteoporosis and diabetes with long-term steroid treatment
- Once asymptomatic, patients should be aware to seek urgent rheumatology review if any musculoskeletal symptoms return and urgent ophthalmology review if there is a recurrence of their visual disturbance.

Follow-up

- If the patient has not responded symptomatically to the steroid within 1 week, the diagnosis should be reconsidered
- Patients should be followed up by a rheumatologist every 2–8 weeks for the first 6 months, then every 3 months for the next 6 months, then every 3–6 months during the second year
- Follow-up should include a history, examination, and checking of FBC, ESR, and CRP
- There is no specific schedule for steroid weaning. Tapering should be done based on the patient's response. The dose is usually reduced to approximately 20mg of prednisolone once the patient has been asymptomatic for 1–2 months, and the dose should carry on being reduced cautiously over 1.5–2 years
- The dose of steroid may need to be ↑ again if any symptoms of GCA return
- Methotrexate and tocilizumab are sometimes given in combination with steroid to patients at high risk of steroid toxicity, so that the dose of steroid can be lowered more quickly.

Live vaccines are contraindicated in patients who have had >20mg prednisolone daily for ≥2 weeks.

Further reading

1. Vodopivec I, Rizzo J (2018). Ophthalmic manifestations of giant cell arteritis. *Rheumatology*. 57:ii63–72.

Chapter 85

Gout

Guideline:
British Society for Rheumatology (The British Society for Rheumatology guideline for the management of gout): https://academic.oup.com/rheumatology/article/56/7/e1/3855179

OUP disclaimer: Oxford University Press makes no representation, express or implied, that the drug dosages are correct and that the recommendations are an exclusive or mandatory course of care. All health professionals reading this text have a responsibility to evaluate its appropriateness and take the individual needs of the patient into account.

Local trust guidelines: please refer to your local guidelines as necessary.

Overview

Gout is a crystal arthropathy causing painful swollen joints. Worldwide, it is the most common cause of inflammatory arthritis. It tends to cause monoarthritis, typically affecting the first metatarsophalangeal joint. It can also affect the knees, ankles, hands, and wrists. In chronic gout, multiple joints can be affected. Risk factors are shown in Table 85.1.

Table 85.1 Risk factors for gout

Non-modifiable	Lifestyle	Medications	Conditions
Age	Obesity	Diuretics	Renal impairment
Male	Alcohol	Antihypertensives	Hypertension
Menopause	Excessive red meat	Aspirin	Diabetes
	Excessive seafood	Ciclosporin	Hyperlipidaemia
	Sugary drinks	Cytotoxic drugs	Lympho-/ myeloproliferative disorders
	Lack of, or excessive exercise	Vitamin B_{12}	Genetic, e.g. glycogen storage disorders

Diagnosis

History

- Sudden-onset painful, swollen, hot joint (see Chapter 86)
- Symptom onset often in the middle of the night
- Usually one joint affected.

Examination

- Erythematous, swollen joint
- Hot to touch
- Exquisitely tender on palpation
- Reduced range of movement
- Gouty tophi
- Fever.

> Gouty tophi are a late feature of untreated hyperuricaemia.

Investigations

Bloods

- FBC
- U&E
- CRP
- Blood cultures if pyrexial or if septic arthritis is a differential
- Serum urate level.

> A normal serum urate level does not exclude an acute gout flare.

Imaging

- X-ray the affected joint—the most common feature seen is joint effusion. Juxta-articular erosions may also be seen.

Joint aspiration

- This will obtain a definitive diagnosis
- Samples must be sent for both culture and crystal examination
- Negatively birefringent crystals of monosodium urate are seen in the joint fluid
- Positively birefringent crystals suggest crystal arthritis due to calcium pyrophosphate.

> Joint aspiration is not usually necessary in a patient with a previous history of gout and if their current presentation is suggestive of gout. If you are uncertain, discuss the case with a senior clinician.

Management

Acute management

- General:
  - Commence treatment as early as possible
  - Educate patient on the condition
  - Ice packs
  - Rest and elevate joints
  - Encourage good hydration
  - Encourage patient to reduce alcohol consumption and modify diet
- Pharmacological:
  - NSAID/cyclooxygenase (COX)-2 inhibitor (coxib), at maximum dose, e.g. naproxen 750mg initially, then 250mg TDS until the attack settles plus PPI, e.g. omeprazole 20mg OD **OR**
  - Colchicine 500 micrograms BD–QDS **OR**
  - Intra-articular corticosteroid injection or oral prednisolone 20mg/day, reducing by 5mg each week.
  - IL-1 inhibitors e.g. anakinra, canakinumab, rilonacept may be prescribed by a rheumatologist in refractory disease

Prescribing notes

- Choice of NSAID/coxib versus colchicine depends on comorbidities and patient preference
- Caution with NSAID use in those with renal impairment, heart failure, peptic ulcer disease, or previous GI bleed/perforation
- Colchicine is often associated with GI side effects, most commonly diarrhoea. The higher the dose, the higher the risk of side effects. Colchicine should be used cautiously in patients with eGFR <50mL/min/1.73m^2, those using statins, and those using cytochrome P450 inhibitors
- Intra-articular corticosteroid injection (± therapeutic joint aspiration) is an acute treatment option for those with comorbidities preventing NSAID or colchicine use. Alternatively, a single IM dose or a short oral course of corticosteroids can be used when joint injection is not feasible.

Treatment after stabilization

Review at 4–6 weeks, and then annually

- Assess lifestyle and cardiovascular factors (Table 85.1)
- Review medications, e.g. if a diuretic is being used for blood pressure management only, consider changing to a different antihypertensive
- Measure serum urate and assess renal function.

Urate-lowering therapy (ULT)

- ULT should be discussed and offered to all patients with a diagnosis of gout
- ULT is especially recommended for the following groups:
  - ≥2 attacks/year
  - Tophi
  - Chronic gouty arthritis
  - Joint damage
  - eGFR <60mL/min/1.73m^2

    - Previous urolithiasis
    - Diuretic use
    - Young age
- Starting ULT should be delayed until after an acute attack has settled, as it can trigger flares
- As commencing ULT may precipitate acute gout, prophylaxis with either an NSAID or colchicine (500 micrograms BD–TDS) is required.
- Allopurinol is first-line ULT—commence at low dose (50–100mg daily) and up-titrate as required every 4 weeks depending on serum urate level. Maximum dose 900mg daily (if renal function permits)
- Aim for serum urate <300μmol/L
- Febuxostat is second-line ULT if allopurinol is not tolerated or contraindicated
- Once started, do not stop ULT during acute attacks
- Continue ULT lifelong, unless modifiable risk factors are addressed.

Special considerations

Renal impairment

- CKD is common in patients with gout
- Colchicine can be used at lower doses if eGFR is 10–50mL/min/1.73m^2, but is contraindicated if eGFR <10mL/min/1.73m^2
- High-dose NSAIDs are contraindicated in moderate to severe renal impairment
- Steroids are generally considered safe to use.

Severe refractory tophaceous gout

- These patients require referral to a rheumatologist.

Further reading

1. NICE Clinical Knowledge Summaries (2018). Gout. Available at: https://cks.nice.org.uk/gout

Chapter 86

Hot swollen joint

Guidelines: British Society for Rheumatology (BSR & BHPR, BOA, RCGP and BSAC guidelines for management of the hot swollen joint in adults): https://doi.org/10.1093/rheumatology/kel163a

European League Against Rheumatism (EULAR recommendations for calcium pyrophosphate deposition. Part II: management): https://ard.bmj.com/content/70/4/571.long

OUP disclaimer: Oxford University Press makes no representation, express or implied, that the drug dosages are correct and that the recommendations are an exclusive or mandatory course of care. All health professionals reading this text have a responsibility to evaluate its appropriateness and take the individual needs of the patient into account.

Local trust guidelines: please refer to your local guidelines as necessary.

Overview

A hot swollen joint is a common presentation, with key differential diagnoses including septic arthritis, crystal arthropathies, and the inflammatory arthritides. Prompt management is important to avoid joint damage and loss of function.

Diagnosis

Possible aetiologies of a hot swollen joint

- Septic arthritis
- Crystal arthropathies:
  - Gout (see Chapter 85)
  - Pseudogout
- Autoimmune arthritides:
  - Rheumatoid arthritis (see Chapter 90)
  - Psoriatic arthritis
  - Connective tissue diseases
- Reactive arthritis
- Trauma
- Haemarthrosis
- Osteomyelitis
- Cellulitis
- Bursitis.

History

Ask about:

- Painful joint with a reduced range of movement or pain on weight bearing
- Visible changes noted such as obvious redness and swelling
- Number of joints affected and pattern:
  - Monoarthritis versus polyarthritis (see below)
  - Large versus small joints
  - Symmetrical versus asymmetrical
- Duration of symptoms
- Sudden versus gradual onset
- Recent trauma
- Fever and systemic symptoms
- Skin features and rashes
- Risk factors:
  - Past medical history: inflammatory arthritis, diabetes mellitus, immunosuppression, recurrent urinary tract infections, or recent intra-abdominal surgery
  - IV drug user
  - Elderly or frail.

Monoarthritis versus polyarthritis

Septic arthritis more commonly presents as a monoarthritis. However, polyarthritic disease does **NOT** rule out septic arthritis. Up to 22% of cases affect multiple joints. Septic arthritis can also occur in pre-existing polyarticular disease.

Red flags

If the joint affected is a prosthetic joint, seek senior orthopaedic input as soon as possible. Do **NOT** try to aspirate or inject a prosthetic joint.

Call for help?

If the patient is acutely septic, escalate early and seek senior advice.

Examination

- All joints must be examined, not only the affected joint
- Inspect for:
  - Erythema
  - Swelling
  - Deformity
  - Reduced range of active and passive movement
- Palpate for:
  - Warmth
  - Effusion
  - Tenderness
- Also perform a general systems examination considering the possibility of other infectious sources and systemic joint disease.

Investigations

Bedside

- Basic observations, e.g. pyrexia, tachycardia, and hypotension may be suggestive of sepsis
- Consider cultures and swabs (e.g. genital) if the history and examination are suggestive of reactive arthritis.

Bloods

See Table 86.1.

Table 86.1 Summary of bloods for investigation of the hot swollen joint

Bloods	Rationale
FBC, CRP, ESR	Monitor inflammatory markers
U&E, LFT	May affect antibiotic choice and dosing, e.g. flucloxacillin, the common first-line drug, will require dose reduction in renal impairment
Rheumatoid factor (RF), anti-cyclic citrullinated peptide (CCP), ANAs	Consider sending if autoimmune disease is suspected
Blood cultures	To guide antibiotic choices

Imaging

- Plain joint X-rays must be performed. X-rays tend to be normal in acute septic arthritis but will help to diagnose other arthritides
- If osteomyelitis is suspected, a MRI scan may be useful
- Ultrasound and CT may be considered if recommended by a specialist.

Other

- Synovial fluid aspiration:
  - Send for Gram stain, culture, and crystal analysis. This must be done prior to commencing antibiotics but antibiotic therapy should not be delayed if indicated

- Anticoagulation with warfarin is not a contraindication to immediate aspiration, but the INR should be checked first to ensure it is within the patient's target therapeutic range
- DOACs are safe to use during joint aspiration/injections and it is not necessary to hold treatment[1]
- Do not refrigerate samples if they cannot be transported to the laboratory immediately as this may affect processing. Store at room temperature
- Common pathogens found in aspirated fluid are shown in Table 86.2.

Table 86.2 Common pathogens found in the infected joint

Diagnosis	Common pathogens
Septic arthritis	*Staphylococcus* spp. *Streptococcus* spp. *Brucella* spp. *Mycobacterium* spp.
Osteomyelitis	*Staphylococcus* spp. *Streptococcus* spp.
Reactive arthritis	*Neisseria* spp. *Chlamydia* spp.
Septic arthritis in immunosuppressed patients	*Mycobacterium avium* complex *Mycobacterium malmoense*

Differential diagnosis

See Table 86.3.

1 Yui JC, Preskill C, Greenlund LS. Arthrocentesis and joint injection in patients receiving direct oral anticoagulants. *Mayo Clin Proc*. 2017; 92:1223–6.

Table 86.3 Clinical features of key differential diagnoses for the hot swollen joint

Clinical feature	Differential diagnosis				
	Septic arthritis	Gout	Pseudogout	Rheumatoid arthritis	Reactive arthritis
Typical number and pattern of joints affected	Most commonly monoarticular (~80%), affecting large joints. ~50% involve the knee	Most commonly monoarticular, classically affecting first metatarsophalangeal joint	Usually a monoarthritis of the wrists or knees	Symmetrical polyarthritis of the small joints	Typically asymmetrical, oligoarticular disease of the large joints, with preference for the lower limbs
Aspiration fluid findings	Yellow-green and opaque in gross appearance. High white cell count, glucose level lower than serum levels. Positive cultures	Needle-shaped crystals, blue in polarized light with negative birefringence. Moderate white cell count, glucose level lower than serum levels. Negative cultures. Urate crystals present	Rhombus-shaped crystals, yellow in polarized light with positive birefringence. Moderate white cell count, glucose level lower than serum levels. Negative cultures	Negative polarized light microscopy. Negative cultures	High white cell count. Glucose level equal to serum. Negative cultures

Acute management

See Fig. 86.1.

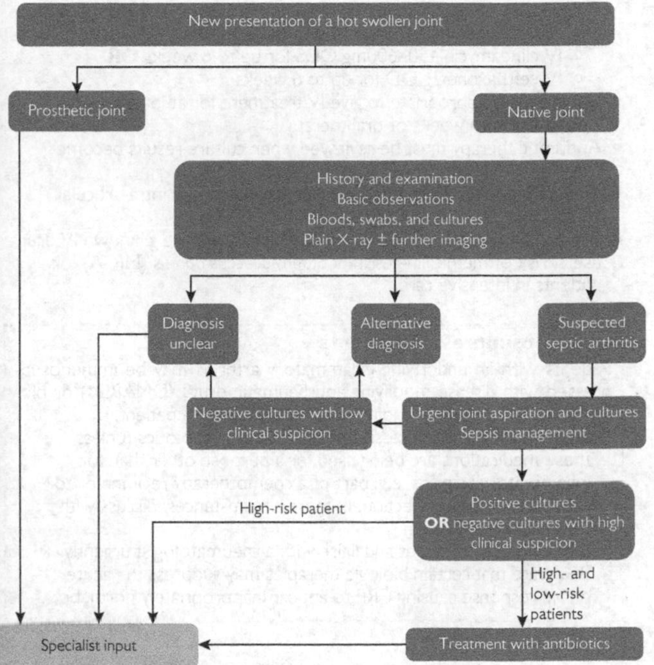

Fig. 86.1 Algorithm for management of the hot swollen joint.

- If clinical suspicion is high, treat as septic arthritis even in the absence of positive fluid cultures or Gram stains
- If only the great toe metatarsophalangeal joint is affected, a clinical diagnosis of gout may be considered without joint aspiration. The management of gout is covered in Chapter 85
- The management of rheumatoid arthritis is covered in Chapter 90.

Lifestyle and simple interventions

Septic arthritis

- There is no clear evidence regarding whether it is more beneficial to mobilize or immobilize the joint. Consider local policy and seek the advice of a physiotherapist.

Pseudogout

- Apply ice and rest the joint.

Pharmacological management

Septic arthritis

- Follow local antibiotic guidelines for the management of a septic joint:
  - Examples of typical antibiotic regimens include one of the following:
    - IV flucloxacillin 2g QDS for up to 6 weeks **OR**
    - IV clindamycin 450–600mg QDS for up to 6 weeks **OR**
    - IV ceftriaxone 2g OD for up to 6 weeks
  - It is usually appropriate to give IV treatment for at least 2 weeks, followed by 4 weeks of oral therapy
- Antibiotic therapy must be reviewed when culture results become available
- If there is any suspicion of sepsis (see Chapter 122), intra-articular steroid injections must not be used
- Always discuss high-risk patients with microbiology, e.g. known IV drug users, risk of methicillin-resistant *Staphylococcus aureus* (MRSA), or patients in intensive care.

Immunosuppressed patients

Patients with an underlying inflammatory arthritis may be immunosuppressed with disease-modifying antirheumatic drugs (DMARDs) or biologic therapies. If a septic joint is suspected in such a patient:

- Stop the immunosuppressive agent while on antibiotics (unless these medications are being used for a purpose other than for inflammatory arthritis, e.g. part of a chemotherapy regimen or to prevent transplant rejection. In these circumstances, discuss with the patient's specialist)
- Hold biologic therapies and liaise with a rheumatologist urgently
- Be aware that certain biologic therapies may suppress the acute-phase response causing CRP to appear inappropriately normal.

Pseudogout

- Options include oral NSAIDs with gastroprotection, e.g. ibuprofen 400mg TDS with omeprazole 20mg OD, or colchicine 0.5mg TDS/QDS (± loading dose of 1mg)
- Both are effective but caution should be applied in the older population due to comorbidities and toxicity
- A short course of oral steroid may also be used
- Therapeutic aspiration and intra-articular steroid injections may be appropriate.

Surgical management

Septic arthritis

- Needle aspiration, arthroscopic aspiration, and joint washouts must be discussed with the local rheumatology and/or orthopaedic teams. Joints may require multiple aspirations.

Complications

- Delayed treatment may lead to permanent joint destruction and loss of function.

Special considerations

Pregnancy and breastfeeding

Many drugs may not be suitable for use in pregnancy or breastfeeding, while others require dose adjustment. See Table 86.4.

Table 86.4 Summary of safety of antibiotics in pregnancy and breastfeeding (information from the BNF)

Drug	Safe in pregnancy?	Safe in breastfeeding?
Flucloxacillin	Not known to be harmful	Trace amounts in milk, but appropriate to use
Clindamycin	Not known to be harmful	Amount probably too small to be harmful but bloody diarrhoea was reported in one infant
Ceftriaxone	Manufacturer advises use only if benefit outweighs risk—limited data available. Specialist sources indicate suitable for use	Compatible with breastfeeding. Present in milk in low concentration but limited effects to infant

X-rays

- The use of X-rays risks exposing the fetus to radiation.

Hepatic and renal impairment

Be aware that most drugs will need dose adjustment in accordance with the severity of impairment. See Table 86.5.

Table 86.5 Summary of safety of antibiotics in hepatic and renal impairment (information from the BNF)

Drug	Safe in hepatic impairment?	Safe in renal impairment?
Flucloxacillin	Use with caution	Reduce dose if eGFR <10mL/min/1.73m^2
Clindamycin	No information	No information
Ceftriaxone	No information	Reduce dose if eGFR <10mL/min/1.73m^2

Further reading

1. Raine T, Collins G, Hall C, et al. (2018). Joint aspiration. In: *Oxford Handbook for the Foundation Programme*, 5th ed (pp. 570–1). Oxford: Oxford University Press. Available at: https://doi.org/10.1093/med/9780198813538.003.0017
2. Clunie GPR, Wilkinson N, Nikiphorou E, et al. (2018). Septic arthritis. In: *Oxford Handbook of Rheumatology*, 4th ed (pp. 708–11). Oxford: Oxford University Press. Available at: https://doi.org/10.1093/med/9780198728252.003.0025

Chapter 87

Low back pain and sciatica

Guideline:
NICE NG59 (Assessment and management of low back pain and sciatica in adults): https://www.nice.org.uk/guidance/ng59

OUP disclaimer: Oxford University Press makes no representation, express or implied, that the drug dosages are correct and that the recommendations are an exclusive or mandatory course of care. All health professionals reading this text have a responsibility to evaluate its appropriateness and take the individual needs of the patient into account.

Local trust guidelines: please refer to your local guidelines as necessary.

Overview

Low back pain is incredibly common and the majority of adults will be affected by it at some stage in their life. Although usually self-limiting, it is important to remain vigilant for sinister causes, especially if symptoms are new or progressive.

Diagnosis

Differential diagnosis

Low back pain is often mechanical and due to strain or degenerative disease. For specific causes see Table 87.1.

Table 87.1 Typical causes of back pain by age at first presentation

15–30 years	30–50 years	>50 years
Prolapsed disc	Prolapsed disc	Degenerative spinal disease
Trauma	Degenerative spinal disease	Osteoporotic vertebral collapse
Fractures	Malignancy (primary or secondary to lung, breast, prostate, thyroid, or kidney)	Malignancy
Ankylosing spondylitis (see Chapter 91)		Paget's disease
Spondylolisthesis		Myeloma
Pregnancy		Spinal stenosis
Rarer causes: discitis, psoas abscess, cauda equina tumours		

If a serious underlying pathology is suspected, then see the relevant chapter to initiate appropriate management e.g. metastatic spinal cord compression (see Chapter 53), spondyloarthritis (see Chapter 91), or spinal injury (see Chapter 120).

History

- **S**ite
- **O**nset
- **C**haracter
- **R**adiation
- **A**ssociated symptoms (possible ⚑)—see Table 87.2
- **T**iming
- **E**xacerbating/relieving factors
- **S**everity.

Examination

- Assess the **range of movement** in the lumbar spine—forward and lateral flexion and extension
- Palpate the sacroiliac joint (check for **sacroiliitis**)
- **Neurological deficits**—examine tone, power, sensation, and reflexes in the lower limbs. DRE for perianal tone and sensation if cord compression/cauda equina suspected
- **Nerve root pain**—positive straight leg and femoral stretch tests suggest disc injury
- Further examination will be guided by the suspected cause.

Table 87.2 Red flags for sinister causes of back pain

⚑ Age <20 years or >55 years	⚑ Thoracic
⚑ Acute onset in the elderly	⚑ Morning stiffness
⚑ Constant or progressive pain	⚑ Bilateral/alternating leg pain
⚑ Nocturnal pain, or pain worse on being supine	⚑ Neurological or sphincter disturbance
⚑ Weight loss, night sweats	⚑ Major trauma
⚑ Current or previous neoplasia	⚑ Immunosuppression, e.g. steroids/ HIV
⚑ Current or recent infection/ systemically unwell/raised inflammatory markers (is there a history of IV drug abuse?)	⚑ Leg claudication, or exercise-related leg weakness or numbness (spinal stenosis)

Acute low back pain seen in primary care will not usually require further investigation unless there are sinister features (⚑), or the pain persists for >4 weeks.

Investigations

Bloods

Perform focused testing as per clinical suspicion:

- FBC and CRP (infection or inflammatory cause)
- U&E, ALP (Paget's)
- Calcium, serum electrophoresis, serum free light chains, and urinary Bence Jones protein (myeloma)
- CRP or ESR (inflammation, e.g. ankylosing spondylitis)
- PSA (metastases from prostate primary).

Imaging

Emergency

- If a sinister cause such as acute cauda equina or cord compression is suspected, refer for an urgent MRI spine.

Routine

- Consider further imaging only in a specialist setting, e.g. musculoskeletal or rheumatology clinic, and only if the result is likely to change management.

Management

Risk assessment

Tools such as STarT Back (see 'Further reading') provide a prognostic guide for patients who present with acute back pain ± sciatica which can help to guide management.

Patient education

Empowering patients to self-manage their symptoms is key. Tailored advice should include:

1. Information on the causes of low back pain and sciatica
2. Encouragement to continue with normal activities of daily living
3. Facilitated return to work.

Lifestyle and simple interventions

- **Group exercise programmes**—particularly for patients at high risk of persistent disabling symptoms
- **Manual therapy**—spinal manipulation, mobilization or massage, in combination with an exercise programme.

Psychological interventions

- Consider **CBT** in addition to an exercise programme if symptoms are not relieved by treatment or there are significant psychosocial obstacles to recovery, e.g. avoiding normal activities due to a belief that they will worsen symptoms.

Pharmacological management

- **NSAIDs**, e.g. ibuprofen 400mg TDS if no contraindications:
  - Use the shortest possible course of the lowest effective dose
  - Consider co-prescribing a PPI for gastroprotection
  - Caution in the elderly and those with renal and hepatic impairment
- **Paracetamol**—use for low back pain in combination with other analgesics
- **Weak opioids**, e.g. codeine 30mg QDS only if NSAIDs are contraindicated, not tolerated, or ineffective for acute back pain. Do not use for chronic pain
- Do not use gabapentinoids, other anticonvulsants or antidepressants for low back pain
- Do not use gabapentinoids, other anticonvulsants, oral steroids, or benzodiazepines for sciatica.

Invasive non-surgical management

Radiofrequency denervation

Consider referring for chronic, moderate to severe pain if non-surgical treatments are ineffective and the pain is related to structures supplied by the medial branch nerve.

Epidural injections

Using local anaesthetic and steroid. This is an option for acute, severe sciatica.

Surgical management

Spinal decompression

Consider if radiological findings suggest sciatica, but non-surgical treatments have been ineffective.

> **Management options which are not recommended**
>
> A number of management options which patients often request are **not** recommended, as there is no evidence base for them. These include:
> - Belts, corsets, or foot orthotics
> - Traction therapy
> - Acupuncture
> - Electrotherapy (includes ultrasound, interferential therapy, percutaneous and transcutaneous electrical nerve stimulation)
> - Spinal injections
> - Spinal fusion
> - Disc replacement.

Further reading

1. Wilkinson IB, Raine T, Wiles K, et al. (2017). Back pain. In: *Oxford Handbook of Clinical Medicine*, 10th ed (pp. 542–3). Oxford: Oxford University Press. Available at: https://doi.org/10.1093/med/9780199689903.003.0012
2. Clutton J (2020). Orthopaedics [topics on back pain]. In: Baldwin A (ed) *Oxford Handbook of Clinical Specialties*, 11th ed (pp. 462–519). Oxford: Oxford University Press. Available at: https://doi.org/10.1093/med/9780198827191.003.0007
3. STarT Back Screening Tool. Available at: https://startback.hfac.keele.ac.uk/training/resources/startback-online/

Chapter 88

Osteoarthritis

Guideline:
This chapter was based on: NICE CG177 (Osteoarthritis: care and management): https://www.nice.org.uk/guidance/cg177. Since the chapter was written, the guideline has been updated and replaced with NICE NG226 (Osteoarthritis in over 16s: diagnosis and management): https://www.nice.org.uk/guidance/ng226. Please see the management section of NG226.

OUP disclaimer: Oxford University Press makes no representation, express or implied, that the drug dosages are correct and that the recommendations are an exclusive or mandatory course of care. All health professionals reading this text have a responsibility to evaluate its appropriateness and take the individual needs of the patient into account.

Local trust guidelines: please refer to your local trust guidelines as necessary.

Overview

Osteoarthritis is the most common type of arthritis and is a very common cause of joint pain. It occurs due to the loss of joint cartilage and remodelling of bone, leading to painful, stiff, and swollen joints, which may lead to reduced functional ability.

Diagnosis

History

- Common symptoms include:
  - Gradual onset of joint pain with movement
  - Reduced range of movement of the joint
  - Intermittent swelling of the joint
- It most commonly affects the hands, knees, and hips, but can affect any joint (see Box 88.1)
- History should take a holistic approach and include assessment of the following:
  - Social impact, e.g. activities of daily living, family duties, and hobbies
  - Occupational impact, e.g. ability to perform job, adjustments required
  - Mood, e.g. depression and stress
  - Sleep
  - Support network
  - Pain including analgesics used, and psychological approach to pain
  - Concerns, expectations, and understanding of treatment options.

Box 88.1 Diagnosing osteoarthritis

Diagnose clinically (without investigations) if:
- Age ≥45 years **AND**
- Activity-related joint pain **AND**
- No morning stiffness **OR** morning stiffness lasting <30 minutes.

Red flags for alternative diagnosis:
- Hot swollen joint
- Trauma
- Rapid worsening of symptoms
- Prolonged morning stiffness >30 minutes.

Examination

Findings in keeping with a diagnosis of osteoarthritis include:
- Pain on movement of the joint, especially at the extremes of range of motion
- Joint line tenderness
- Joint crepitus
- Bony swelling, e.g. Heberden's or Bouchard's nodes in hands (Fig. 88.1)
- Reduced range of movement.

Investigations

If the history is not typical of osteoarthritis, consider investigations to exclude common differential diagnoses such as septic arthritis (see Chapter 86), rheumatoid arthritis (RA; see Chapter 90), and gout (see Chapter 85).

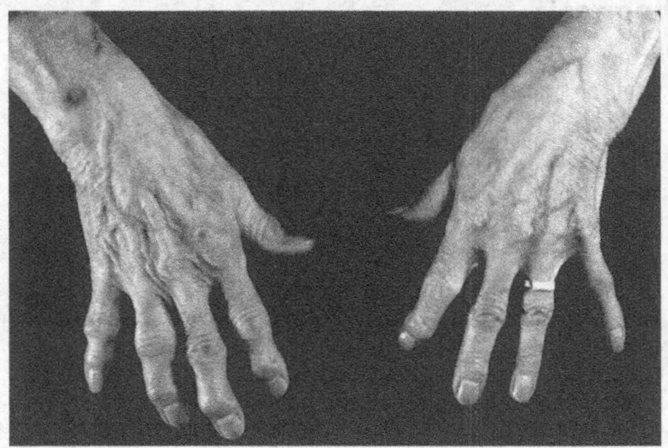

Fig. 88.1 Generalized osteoarthritis. Of note, prominent bony hypertrophy is seen at the proximal (Bouchard's nodes) and distal (Heberden's nodes) interphalangeal joints. The metacarpophalangeal joints are spared. Early hypertrophic changes are seen on profile at the first carpometacarpal joint, giving a slight squaring of the hand deformity, appreciated best in this patient's left hand.

Reproduced from Wittich C M (2019) 'Mayo Clinic Internal Medicine Board Review' 12th edition Oxford University Press: Oxford, with permission from Oxford University Press.

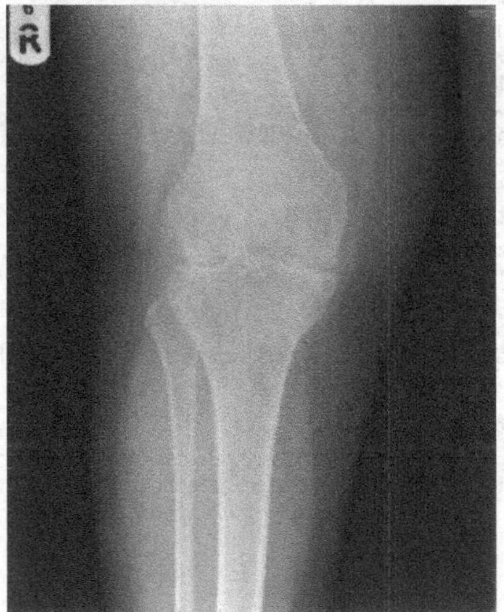

Fig. 88.2 Knee X-ray in a young woman showing severe loss of cartilage and secondary osteoarthritis due to RA.

Reproduced from Luqmani R, Pincus T, and Boers M (2010) 'Rheumatoid Arthritis: Oxford Rheumatology Library' Oxford University Press: Oxford, with permission from Oxford University Press.

There is a poor correlation between radiographic changes and symptom severity, i.e. minor X-ray changes can be associated with significant pain, or the reverse.

Imaging

X-ray changes consistent with osteoarthritis include:

- Narrowing of joint space (Fig. 88.2)
- Osteophytes
- Subchondral sclerosis and cysts.

Management

Psychosocial considerations

Osteoarthritis can have a significant impact on all areas of a person's life. This can be highlighted if a holistic history is taken.

Patient education

Formulate a management plan in conjunction with the patient, and empower the patient to manage their condition through access to appropriate education and information.

Lifestyle and simple interventions

Exercise and physical therapy

All patients should be encouraged to undertake regular exercise appropriate to their level of function, including aerobic activity and strengthening exercises. Exercise is considered a core treatment irrespective of the level of disability, severity of pain, and other comorbidities.

Weight loss

Patients should be supported with weight loss techniques if overweight or obese.

Other interventions

- Supportive footwear, joint supports, and braces
- Occupational therapy referral for walking sticks and other assistive devices
- Use of local heat and cold therapy
- Manipulation and stretching therapies
- Transcutaneous electrical nerve stimulation (TENS) for pain relief.

Pharmacological management

Pharmacological interventions should be used in conjunction with non-pharmacological treatments:

- First line: paracetamol and/or topical NSAIDs
- If ineffective, consider adding:
  - Topical capsaicin
  - Oral NSAIDs (see Box 88.2)/COX-2 inhibitors
  - Opioids (avoid chronic use)
- For moderate to severe pain, consider intra-articular steroid injections.

Box 88.2 Precautions when using NSAIDs

- Use NSAIDs at the lowest effective dose for the shortest possible time
- Co-prescribe a PPI, especially if there is any history of GI bleeding or ulceration
- Avoid if also taking aspirin
- Caution in the elderly and in patients with reduced renal function.

Surgical management

Consider referral for surgery if joint symptoms are having a significant impact on the patient's quality of life, and the patient's symptoms are refractory to simple interventions and pharmacological therapies.

Complications

Osteoarthritis may be a major factor contributing to frailty and falls in the elderly.

Monitoring and follow-up

- Follow up at least annually if the patient:
    - Has severe joint pain
    - Has symptoms in more than one joint
    - Has more than one comorbidity
    - Is using regular medication for osteoarthritis
- During the review:
    - Monitor symptoms and impact on daily life
    - Review treatments
    - Discuss self-management and provide information.

Further reading

1. Clunie G, Wilkinson N, Nikiphorou E, et al. (2018). Osteoarthritis. In: *Oxford Handbook of Rheumatology*, 4th ed (pp. 265–76). Oxford: Oxford University Press. Available at: https://doi.org/10.1093/med/9780198728252.003.0006

Chapter 89

Polymyalgia rheumatica

Guideline:
British Society for Rheumatology, British Health Professionals in Rheumatology (BSR and BHPR guidelines for the management of polymyalgia rheumatica): https://academic.oup.com/rheumatology/article/49/1/186/1789113

OUP disclaimer: Oxford University Press makes no representation, express or implied, that the drug dosages are correct and that the recommendations are an exclusive or mandatory course of care. All health professionals reading this text have a responsibility to evaluate its appropriateness and take the individual needs of the patient into account.

Local trust guidelines: please refer to your local guidelines as necessary.

Overview

Polymyalgia rheumatica (PMR) is the commonest inflammatory rheumatic disease of the elderly, typically affecting the shoulders and/or thighs. The most important diagnosis to exclude is GCA (see Chapter 84), which affects patients of a similar age group and occurs in around 10% of patients with PMR.

Diagnosis

History/diagnostic criteria

The diagnostic work-up should include three steps (Fig. 89.1):

Step 1: Identify the typical clinical features of PMR

- ➤ Patient aged >50 years
- ➤ Symptoms lasting >2 weeks
- ➤ Bilateral aching of shoulders and/or thighs
- ➤ Morning stiffness >45 minutes
- ➤ Acute phase response, e.g. raised inflammatory markers

Step 2: Consider and try to exclude potential differential diagnoses

Core exclusion criteria:

- ➤ **GCA: requires urgent high-dose steroids to prevent blindness**
- ➤ Active infection or cancer

Other exclusion criteria:

- o Other inflammatory rheumatic diseases, e.g. rheumatoid arthritis
- o Drug-induced myalgia
- o Chronic pain syndromes, e.g. fibromyalgia
- o Endocrine disorders
- o Neurological disorders, e.g. Parkinson's disease

Step 3: Assess steroid responsiveness

Standard starting dose for PMR = 15mg prednisolone, once daily

A successful response to steroids is defined as:

- ➤ Patient-reported global improvement of >70% within 1 week
- ➤ Normalization of inflammatory markers within 4 weeks

The combination of typical clinical features and a successful response to steroids are suggestive of an underlying diagnosis of PMR.

Fig. 89.1 Three-step diagnostic work-up for polymyalgia rheumatica.

Consider alternative diagnoses and early specialist referral in the presence of any of the following red flag features:

- Age <60 years
- Chronic onset (>2 months)
- No shoulder involvement
- No inflammatory stiffness
- Weight loss
- Focal neurology
- Pain that causes awakening from sleep
- Features of other rheumatic disease
- Normal inflammatory markers
- Extremely high inflammatory markers.

Examination

At diagnosis, the patient should be fully examined, focusing particularly on the musculoskeletal and neurological systems—to both confirm the classical features of PMR and to exclude possible alternative diagnoses, especially GCA (see 'Further reading').

Investigations

Although PMR can be diagnosed without raised inflammatory markers, they are typically raised.

Investigations to exclude differential diagnoses and ensure the safety of steroid treatment should be considered in the work-up of a PMR diagnosis, as shown in Table 89.1.

Table 89.1 Investigations to consider in the work-up of PMR

Bedside	Bloods	Imaging
Urinalysis	Haematology (FBC, ESR, and plasma viscosity)	Chest X-ray
Fracture assessment tool, e.g. FRAX (see 'Further reading')	Biochemistry (CRP, U&E, LFT, TFT, creatine kinase, bone profile, and HbA1c)	Joint X-rays (if rheumatoid arthritis in the differential)
	Immunology (serum electrophoresis, Bence Jones proteins, RF, and consider ANA and anti-CCP)	

Management

Acute management

- Oral steroids are the first-line treatment
- The starting dose of steroids is usually **15mg of prednisolone OD**, which is gradually tapered (Table 89.2)
- However, it is important to note that there is currently no evidence for a standardized steroid starting or tapering regimen, therefore treatment should be tailored to the individual patient.

Table 89.2 Sample steroid tapering regimen in PMR

Time since diagnosis	Prednisolone dose
0–3 weeks	15mg OD
4–6 weeks	12.5mg OD
7–12 weeks	10mg OD
13 weeks–up to 2 years	Alternate-day reductions, or reduce by 1mg every 4–8 weeks

NB: guidance only, doses should be tailored to the needs of the individual patient.

- In some cases, it may be preferable to give steroids IM using methylprednisolone.
- Bone protection is recommended on initiation of steroids for patients with PMR
- All patients should be given calcium and vitamin D supplementation
- If the patient is >65 years, has previously had a fragility fracture or requires a high initial steroid dose, they should be offered a bisphosphonate unless contraindicated
- Other patients should have a DXA scan to determine the need for bisphosphonates.

Treatment after stabilization

- Follow-up at: 1–3 weeks, 6 weeks, and then every 3 months for the first year
- At follow-up, re-examine for steroid responsiveness, e.g. improvement in pain proximally, fatigue, and morning stiffness. As GCA can complicate PMR, patients should be checked for features of this during follow-up, as well as other possible differential diagnoses (Fig. 89.1)
- Once on steroid therapy, review for side effects (see Chapter 80), e.g. hypertension, osteoporosis, glucose intolerance
- Consider routine follow-up bloods: FBC, ESR/CRP, U&E and glucose
- Given the heterogeneous nature of PMR, flexibility and clinical judgement is required in the tapering of steroids, which typically takes 1–2 years
- **Consider tapering steroids when the patient's inflammatory symptoms are no longer present.**

Specialist referral

If there are any difficulties with steroid management, consider referral for a specialist opinion.

Difficulties may include:

- Partial, inconsistent, or no response to steroids
- Difficulties in weaning a patient from steroids
- Contraindications to steroid treatment
- A chronic need for steroid treatment (>2 years).

In relapsing cases, specialists may consider higher doses of steroids or commence DMARDs.

Further reading

1. NICE Clinical Knowledge Summaries (2020). Giant cell arteritis. Available at: https://cks.nice.org.uk/giant-cell-arteritis
2. University of Sheffield. Fracture Risk Assessment Tool (FRAX). Available at: https://www.sheffield.ac.uk/FRAX/tool.aspx?country=9

Chapter 90

Rheumatoid arthritis

Guideline:
NICE NG100 (Rheumatoid arthritis in adults: management): https://www.nice.org.uk/guidance/ng100/

OUP disclaimer: Oxford University Press makes no representation, express or implied, that the drug dosages are correct and that the recommendations are an exclusive or mandatory course of care. All health professionals reading this text have a responsibility to evaluate its appropriateness and take the individual needs of the patient into account.

Local trust guidelines: please refer to your local guidelines as necessary.

Overview

Rheumatoid arthritis (RA) is the most common inflammatory arthritis in adults, usually presenting between the ages of 45–65 years. It is a chronic, multisystem illness which can have a profound impact on the patient's functional abilities. The exact cause is unknown although some risk factors have been identified.

Diagnosis

History/diagnostic criteria

- RA classically presents as a symmetrical polyarthritis of the small joints of the hands or feet, with morning stiffness lasting >30 minutes (Fig. 90.1)
- However, more rarely it can affect the larger joints, such as the knees, elbows, and shoulders
- It can also manifest in the hands in atypical patterns, e.g. asymmetrically, or as a monoarthritis.

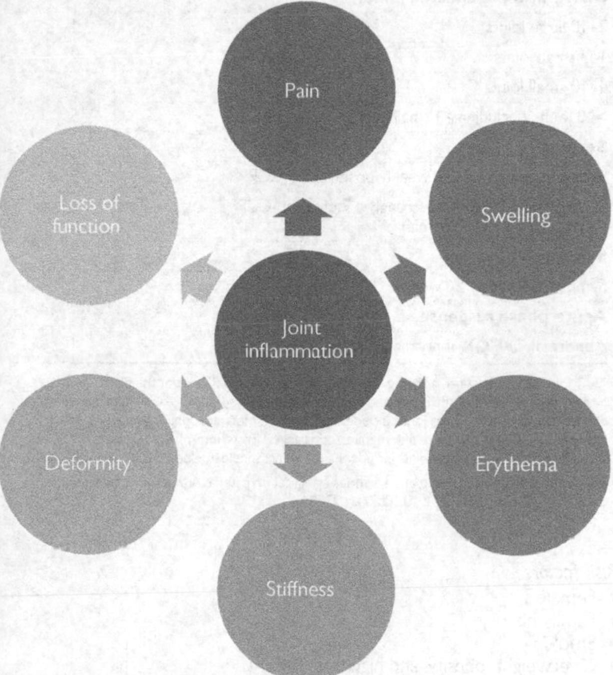

Fig. 90.1 Possible manifestations of joint inflammation.

- If patients present late, they may have already developed significant joint deformities (see 'Examination')
- Patients may also present with vague non-specific constitutional symptoms such as fever and fatigue
- RA may have extra-articular manifestations, affecting virtually any part of the body. Common manifestations include rheumatoid nodules, dry eyes (secondary Sjögren's syndrome), pulmonary fibrosis, and splenomegaly

- The 2010 American College of Rheumatology/European League Against Rheumatism criteria (Table 90.1) can be used to make a diagnosis in patients who have evidence of swelling in at least one joint, which is not better explained by an alternative condition. However, it should not be used to exclude a diagnosis of RA if there is still strong clinical suspicion.

Table 90.1 Classification criteria for rheumatoid arthritis

Scores for each category should be totalled. A score of ≥6/10 suggests definite RA	
Distribution of affected joints	
2–10 large joints*	1
1–3 small joints	2
4–10 small joints	3
>10 joints (including >1 small joint)	5
Serology	
Weakly positive RF **OR** weakly positive anti-CCP	2
Strongly positive RF **OR** strongly positive anti-CCP (>3× upper limit of normal)	3
Symptom duration	
Symptom duration ≥6 weeks	1
Acute phase response	
Abnormal CRP **OR** abnormal ESR	1

*Any joint can be classified as being 'affected' (swollen or tender) except the distal interphalangeal joints of the hands and feet, the first metatarsophalangeal joint, and the first carpometacarpal joint. Small joints include the following: metacarpophalangeal joints, proximal interphalangeal joints, second–fifth metatarsophalangeal joints, interphalangeal joint of the thumb, and the wrist. Large joints include the following: shoulder, elbow, hip, knee, ankles.

Source: data from 2010 rheumatoid arthritis classification criteria. *Arthritis & Rheumatism*. 62;9: 2010. 2569–2581. DOI: 10.1002/art.27584

Risk factors

- Female
- Family history
- Smoking
- Overweight, obesity, and high birth weight
- Various genetic factors including HLA-DR4 and -DR1.

Examination

- Perform a detailed examination of the hands, looking for erythema, swelling, or deformity
- Palpate each joint of the hand individually and monitor for tenderness and swelling (signs of synovitis)
- Test the patient functionally to establish which movements elicit pain
- Examine any other joints which the patient is concerned about
- Perform a general systems examination to look for extra-articular manifestations
- See Fig. 90.2 for two presentations of RA.

(a)

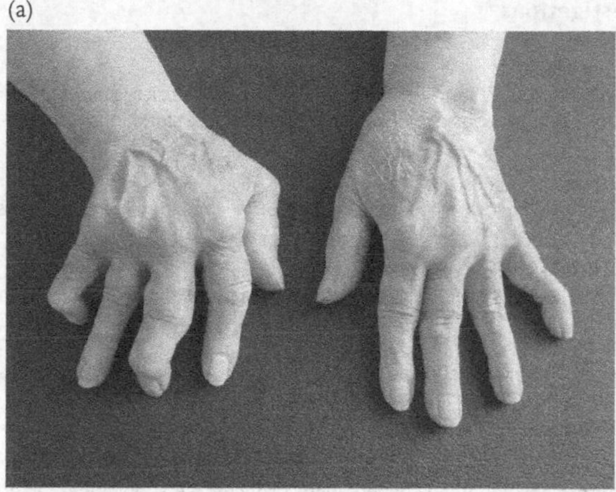

(b)

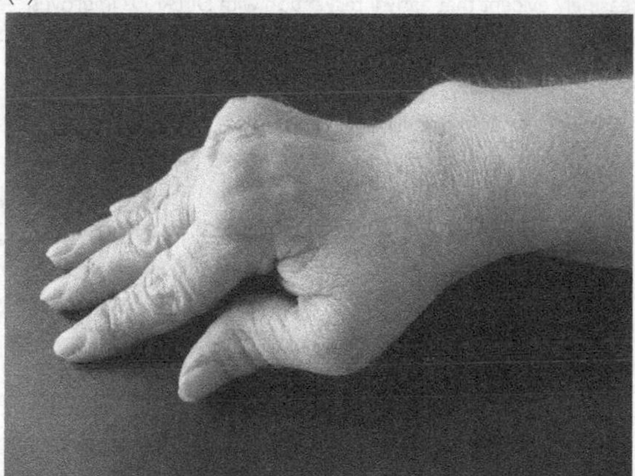

Fig. 90.2 (a) Patient with RA presenting with a radial deviation (right wrist), swan-neck deformity with hyperextension of the proximal interphalangeal (PIP) and flexion of distal interphalangeal (DIP) joints (digits 3 right and 5 on both sides) and boutonnière deformity with flexion of the PIP and hyperextension of DIP joints (digit 2 right). (b) Patient with RA presenting with volar subluxation of the right hand with a visible sliding at the radiocarpal joint and Z-deformity (or 90–90 thumb) with flexion of the first metacarpophalangeal joint and hyperextension of the interphalangeal joint.

Reprinted from Watts R et al (2013) 'Oxford Textbook of Rheumatology' 4th Edition Oxford University Press: Oxford, with permission from Oxford University Press. See colour plate 3.

Investigations

Bloods

See Table 90.2.[1,2]

Positive anti-CCP and erosions on X-ray both predict radiological progression, but this does not necessarily correlate with functional ability.

Imaging

- X-ray of the hands and feet
- USS of the hands to look for evidence of inflammation/early erosions.

Rheumatology referral

Refer to a rheumatologist if any patient has persistent synovitis with no obvious cause.

Refer **urgently** to a rheumatologist if:

- >1 joint affected
- >3 months between symptom onset and seeking medical advice
- Small joint of the hands or feet are involved.

Refer even if ESR, CRP, RF, and anti-CCP are within the normal range. If there is any doubt, any patient with suspected RA should be referred for a rheumatology opinion in case DMARDs are required, as it is increasingly evident that early intervention with DMARDs improves outcomes.[3]

1 Sauerland U, Becker H, Seidel M, et al. Clinical utility of the anti-CCP assay: experiences with 700 patients. *Ann N Y Acad Sci*. 2005; 1050:314–8.

2 Lee DM, Schur PH. Clinical utility of the anti-CCP assay in patients with rheumatic diseases. *Ann Rheum Dis*. 2003; 62:870–4.

3 Raza K, Buckley CE, Salmon M, et al. Treating very early rheumatoid arthritis. *Best Pract Res Clin Rheumatol*. 2006; 20:849–63.

Table 90.2 Bloods used in the diagnosis of rheumatoid arthritis

	Test	Rationale	May demonstrate
Baseline bloods	FBC	May be affected by DMARDs May show evidence of inflammatory response	Microcytic anaemia Thrombocytosis Raised white cell count
	U&E	DMARDs may cause renal impairment	Usually normal at baseline
	LFT	DMARDs are usually metabolized by liver	
Inflammatory markers	CRP	May show evidence of inflammatory response	Raised, but if normal does not rule out RA
	ESR	May show evidence of inflammatory response	
Autoantibodies	Rheumatoid factor	Sensitivity in RA ~70% Specificity in RA ~80%	Raised, but if normal does not rule out RA
	Anti-CCP	Sensitivity in RA ~65–75% Specificity in RA ~90–95%	
	ANA	Differential diagnosis	Positive ANA may suggest connective tissue disease

Management

Patient education

- Provide information regarding RA, and the risks and benefits of any treatments offered
- Patients should have a point of contact, e.g. a specialist nurse, who they can speak to in the event of a flare or issues with their medications.

Lifestyle and simple interventions

- Patients should be referred for specialist physiotherapy and occupational therapy
- If relevant, patients should be referred to hand exercise programmes and podiatry
- Patients should also be offered education on pain management options, e.g. TENS.

Psychological interventions

- Offer psychological support, e.g. relaxation, stress management, to help with the adjustment to living with a chronic disease.

Pharmacological management

- Functional ability should be assessed prior to starting treatment, e.g. using a questionnaire, in order to ascertain a baseline so that the response to treatment can be evaluated
- Disease activity is usually measured using a score such as the DAS28 score
- Treatment aims to either achieve complete remission or a low disease activity—the target must be decided on a case-by-case basis.

DMARDs

- First-line treatment is with conventional DMARDs (cDMARDs), e.g. oral methotrexate, leflunomide, or sulfasalazine. Hydroxychloroquine may be used in mild disease
- Treatment should be started as early as possible and the dose ↑ as necessary under specialist guidance
- Perform baseline bloods prior to starting any DMARD (see 'Further reading')
- If one cDMARD is not sufficient, two may be used in combination
- Some patients with severe disease may be eligible for biological treatments such as infliximab, rituximab, and tocilizumab. Patients are not usually eligible until they have failed two DMARD treatments
- See Fig. 90.3.

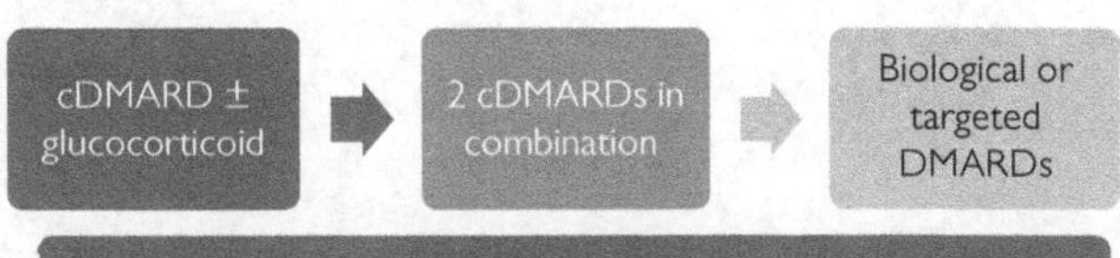

Fig. 90.3 Flowchart of pharmacological management steps in RA.

Symptomatic treatments

- Glucocorticoids are often used as a short-term bridging therapy to help with symptom control until the DMARD has reached an effective treatment dose (this can take up to 3 months)
- Glucocorticoids can also be used at any point to treat disease flares, but should not be used long-term unless there are no other options
- NSAIDs, e.g. naproxen, may also be used for short-term symptom control. Consider whether gastroprotection should be co-prescribed
- Simple analgesia. e.g. paracetamol or codeine, and drugs for neuropathic pain, e.g. amitriptyline, should also be considered.

Surgical management

- Consider referring for a surgical opinion if symptoms have not responded to optimal non-surgical management, e.g. persistent pain or synovitis, worsening deformity or function
- Refer early if there are issues such as stress fractures, nerve compression, or potential tendon rupture.

Psychosocial considerations

- Possible need to stop working, especially if the patient has significant hand deformities.

Complications

- ↑ risk of septic arthritis, osteoporosis, cardiovascular, and cerebrovascular events.

Monitoring and follow-up

- If the disease is active—review monthly in rheumatology clinic until the treatment target is reached:
  - Measure CRP and disease activity at every visit
- Once treatment target has been reached—review after 6 months and then annually. Assess/monitor for:
  - Disease activity
  - Functional ability
  - The development of comorbidities such as depression, hypertension, osteoporosis, ischaemic heart disease
  - The development of complications such as vasculitis
- Consider tapering down DMARDs if patients have been at their treatment target for 1 year without needing glucocorticoids.

Special considerations

Many medications used in rheumatology are not appropriate for use during peri-conception (both maternally and paternally), pregnancy, and breastfeeding. Detailed guidelines are available from the British Society for Rheumatology (see 'Further reading').

Further reading

1. BSR and BHPR Standards, Guidelines and Audit Working Group (2017). BSR and BHPR guideline for the prescription and monitoring of non-biologic disease-modifying anti-rheumatic drugs. *Rheumatology*. 56:865–8. Available at: https://doi.org/10.1093/rheumatology/kew479
2. BSR and BHPR Standards, Guidelines and Audit Working Group (2016). BSR and BHPR guideline on prescribing drugs in pregnancy and breastfeeding—Part I: standard and biologic disease modifying anti-rheumatic drugs and corticosteroids. *Rheumatology*.55:1693–7. Available at: https://doi.org/10.1093/rheumatology/kev404
3. BSR and BHPR Standards, Guidelines and Audit Working Group (2016). BSR and BHPR guideline on prescribing drugs in pregnancy and breastfeeding—Part II: analgesics and other drugs used in rheumatology practice. *Rheumatology*. 55:1698–702. Available at: https://doi.org/10.1093/rheumatology/kev405

Chapter 91

Spondyloarthritis

Guideline:
NICE NG65 (Spondyloarthritis in over 16s: diagnosis and management): https://www.nice.org.uk/guidance/ng65

OUP disclaimer: Oxford University Press makes no representation, express or implied, that the drug dosages are correct and that the recommendations are an exclusive or mandatory course of care. All health professionals reading this text have a responsibility to evaluate its appropriateness and take the individual needs of the patient into account.

Local trust guidelines: please refer to your local guidelines as necessary.

Overview

Spondyloarthritides (also known as spondyloarthropathies) are a group of progressive inflammatory rheumatological conditions that primarily involve the joints and entheses. Spondyloarthritis may be:

- **Axial spondyloarthritis (axSpA):** e.g. ankylosing spondylitis
- **Peripheral spondyloarthritis (pSpA):** e.g. psoriatic arthritis, reactive arthritis, or enteropathic spondyloarthritis.

Diagnosis

History

- Spondyloarthritides may present with axial or peripheral symptoms, a combination, or an extra-articular manifestation (see 'Examination')
- Pain is atraumatic and onset is often insidious.

Axial spondyloarthritis

axSpA should be considered if a patient presents with lower back pain before age 45 years, that has lasted >3 months. They should be referred to rheumatology if four or more of the following are present, **OR** if three are positive and a HLA-B27 test is positive:

- Age of onset <35 years
- Pain and stiffness improve with movement and exercise
- Waking during the second half of the night due to pain
- Improvement with NSAIDs within 48 hours
- Buttock pain
- Family history in a first-degree relative
- Current or previous arthritis, enthesitis, or psoriasis.

Peripheral spondyloarthritis

pSpA should be considered and an urgent referral to rheumatology made if:

- A patient presents with new-onset inflammatory arthritis (unless there is a high suspicion or evidence of rheumatoid arthritis (see Chapter 90), gout (see Chapter 85), or pseudogout (see Chapter 86))
- First presentation of dactylitis (Fig. 91.1)
- Enthesitis without an obvious cause that is persistent, in multiple locations or associated with any other suspicious features (such as family history in a first-degree relative, unexplained back pain, current or previous uveitis (see Box 91.1), current or previous psoriasis, GI or genitourinary infection or history of inflammatory bowel disease).

Box 91.1 Anterior uveitis

Patients with any symptoms of anterior uveitis, e.g. light sensitivity, eye pain, eye redness, or blurring of vision, should be referred for a same-day ophthalmology assessment.

Examination

Axial spondyloarthritis

- Reduced spinal range of movement
- Schober's test of lumbar spine flexibility may be performed. The test is considered positive if there is an increase of <5cm in the distance between lines marked 5cm above and 10cm below the posterior superior iliac spines when the patient flexes forwards as if trying to touch their toes (keeping their knees straight)
- Clinical tests for sacroiliitis: direct pressure, lateral compression, sacroiliac stretch test.

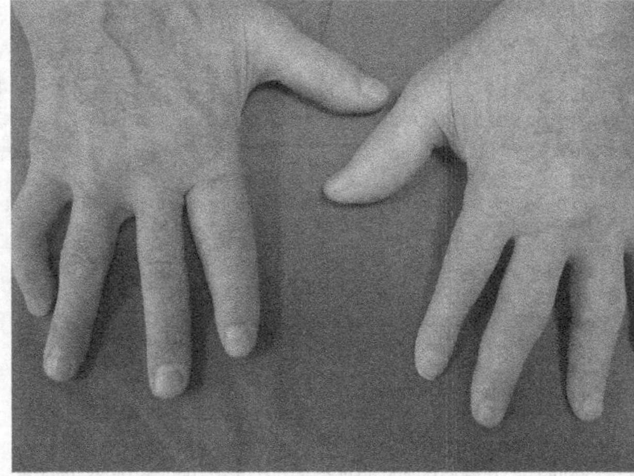

Fig. 91.1 Dactylitis of the right index finger and left thumb.

Reprinted from FitzGerald O and Gladman D (2018) 'Oxford Textbook of Psoriatic Arthritis' Oxford University Press: Oxford, with permission from Oxford University Press.

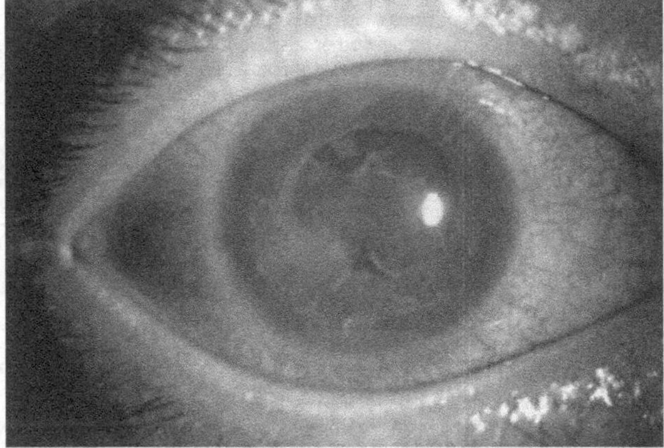

Fig. 91.2 Anterior uveitis. A red eye with circumcorneal congestion, miosis, and a hypopyon.

Reprinted from Machemer R and Michelson G 'Atlas of Ophthalmology: Online Multimedia Database' with kind permission from Prof. Dr. med. Georg Michelson. See colour plate 4.

Peripheral spondyloarthritis

- Most commonly present as asymmetrical oligoarthritis/polyarthritis
- Enthesitis e.g. plantar fasciitis, Achilles tendonitis, costochondritis
- Dactylitis (Fig. 91.1)

- Evidence of psoriasis/psoriatic nail changes, e.g. onycholysis
- Signs of extra-articular manifestations such as anterior uveitis—red, painful eye, blurred vision, and sensitivity to light (See Box 91.1 and Fig. 91.2).

Investigations

Bloods

- A diagnosis can be made even with a normal CRP and ESR.

Imaging

Axial spondyloarthritis

- Plain film radiograph of sacroiliac joints (Fig. 91.3). Spondyloarthritis can still be diagnosed even in the absence of clear X-ray evidence
- MRI whole spine and sacroiliac joints (Fig. 91.4). Some centres preferentially perform MRI first line without performing a prior X-ray.

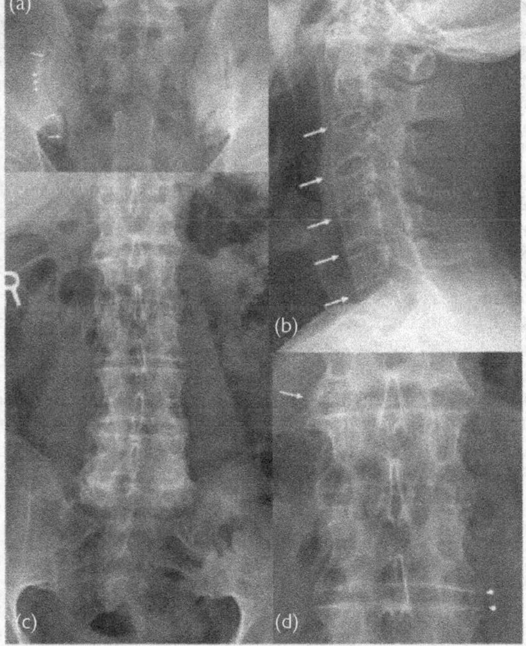

Fig. 91.3 Radiographic findings in ankylosing spondylitis. (a) Sacroiliitis and loss of subchondral bone causing apparent joint space widening. (b) Extensive syndesmophytes along the cervical spine and facet joint fusion at C2/3. (c) Syndesmophytes in the lumbar spine causing a characteristic 'bamboo spine' (further enlarged in (d)).

Reprinted from Østergaard M and Bianchi G (2012) 'Imaging in ankylosing spondylitis' Ther Adv Musculoskeletal Dis. 4(4):301–311 with permission from SAGE.

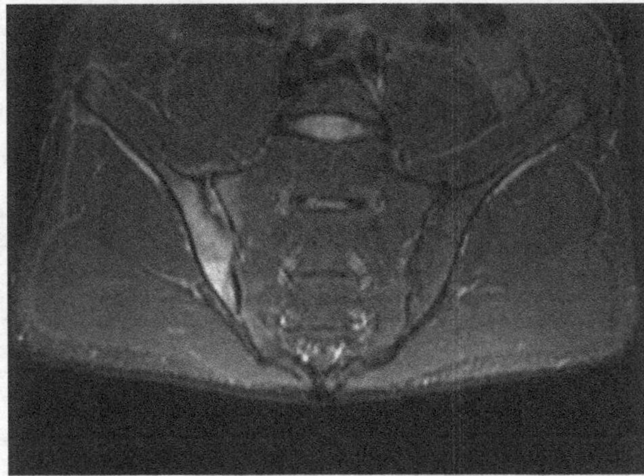

Fig. 91.4 Bright white (hyperintense) signal on MRI (STIR sequence) demonstrating inflammatory changes in the ileum and right sacroiliac joint.

Reprinted from Watts R et al (2013) 'Oxford Textbook of Rheumatology' 4th edition Oxford University Press: Oxford, with permission from Oxford University Press.

Peripheral spondyloarthritis

- Plain film radiograph of the symptomatic joint
- USS of hands and feet, and anywhere enthesitis is suspected
- If peripheral spondyloarthritis is confirmed, offer a plain film radiograph of the sacroiliac joints to assess for axial involvement even in the absence of symptoms. Some centres preferentially perform MRI first line without performing a prior X-ray.

Other

- HLA-B27 gene positivity raises the suspicion of spondyloarthritis, but if negative it does not exclude the diagnosis.

Management

Patient education

- Educate patients in how they can reduce the risk of complications and slow progression
- Provide information regarding the symptoms and management options, including how to manage flares
- Provide a named contact for patients to access during flares, e.g. a rheumatology specialist nurse.

Lifestyle and simple interventions

- Specialist physiotherapist referral for advice on stretching, strengthening, and postural exercises to improve pain and stiffness. Deep breathing and aerobic exercise may be beneficial
- Occupational therapy may also be required to assist with functional difficulties with activities of daily living
- Reduce cardiovascular and pulmonary complication risks (see 'Complications') by stopping smoking and maintaining a healthy, balanced diet
- Hydrotherapy may aid pain management.

Psychological interventions

- Recognise that there is a raised risk of depression and treat accordingly (see Chapter 38)
- Identify, support and normalize elements such as fatigue, ↑ need for sleep and demotivation
- Ensure access to local support, exercise groups, and places to develop coping strategies.

Pharmacological management

Axial spondyloarthritis

- NSAIDs, e.g. naproxen 250–500mg BD ± gastroprotection, e.g. omeprazole 20mg OD
- Switch to another NSAID if inadequate pain relief at maximum dose for 2–4 weeks
- Under specialist supervision, biological DMARDs (TNF-alpha inhibitors) are used in patients who have not responded to, or cannot tolerate NSAIDs, e.g. adalimumab, golimumab, and infliximab
- Switch to another TNF-alpha inhibitor if the first is ineffective or not tolerated
- Secukinumab (alternative biological DMARD) should be used if all other management is inadequate.

Peripheral spondyloarthritis

- Local steroid injections can be used for monoarthritis, or as an adjunct to systemic treatments
- Standard DMARDs (e.g. methotrexate/sulfasalazine) for oligo/polyarthritis
- After 3 months, switch to another standard DMARD, add a second DMARD, or consider a biological DMARD if the first treatment is inadequate

- NSAIDs may be used in addition to DMARDs to help with symptom control.

Reactive arthritis

- Treat the initial infection with an appropriate course of antibiotics. Long-term antibiotics (>4 weeks) are not part of the management of reactive arthritis.

Surgical management

- Surgical consultation should only be sought if a patient presents with acute unstable fractures or if severe or progressive spinal deformity is significantly affecting their quality of life.

Psychosocial considerations

- Daily activities such as getting dressed, transferring, and mobilizing can be affected which may have a significant impact on work and social activities.

Complications

- Most common extra-articular manifestation: anterior uveitis (requires same-day ophthalmological assessment, see Box 91.1)
- Osteoporosis (see Chapter 24)
- Bony fusion
- ↑ fracture risk:
  - A low threshold of suspicion should be adopted for acute pathological spinal fractures which may occur from low-energy mechanisms
  - They most commonly occur in the cervical spine and may present with pain and/or neurological deficit
  - They should be investigated using MRI or CT imaging and management should be led by an orthopaedic specialist
- Cardiovascular diseases such as ischaemic heart disease, aortitis, aortic valve disease, conduction disturbances, and cardiomyopathy
- Kyphosis which may contribute to ↓ vital capacity
- Apical pulmonary fibrosis
- Adverse effects of long-term NSAIDs, e.g. GI bleeds
- ↑ risk of skin cancer in those using long-term TNF-alpha inhibitors.

Monitoring and follow-up

- Tailored flare management plan
- Monitor cardiopulmonary risk factors
- 2-yearly osteoporosis assessment for patients with axSpA.

Further reading

1. Yu TD, van Tubergen A (2020). Clinical manifestations and diagnosis of peripheral spondyloarthritis in adults. UpToDate®. Available at: https://www.uptodate.com/contents/clinical-manifestations-and-diagnosis-of-peripheral-spondyloarthritis-in-adults
2. NICE Clinical Knowledge Summaries (2021). DMARDs. Available at: https://cks.nice.org.uk/dmards

Part 13

Surgery

Chapter 92

Preoperative care

Guidelines:
NICE NG45 (Routine preoperative tests for elective surgery): https://www.nice.org.uk/guidance/ng45

Royal College of Nursing (Perioperative fasting in adults and children, pp. 24–33): https://media.gosh.nhs.uk/documents/RCN_Perioperative_Fasting_Adults_and_Children.pdf

Joint British Diabetes Societies (Guideline for perioperative care for people with diabetes mellitus undergoing elective and emergency surgery): https://abcd.care/sites/abcd.care/files/site_uploads/CPOC_Diabetes_Surgery_Guideline_March_2021.pdf

ESA/European Society of Anaesthesiology (2014 ESC/ESA Guidelines on non-cardiac surgery: cardiovascular assessment and management, pp. 2401–3): https://academic.oup.com/eurheartj/article/35/35/2383/425095

NICE NG180 (Perioperative care in adults): https://www.nice.org.uk/guidance/ng180

OUP disclaimer: Oxford University Press makes no representation, express or implied, that the drug dosages are correct and that the recommendations are an exclusive or mandatory course of care. All health professionals reading this text have a responsibility to evaluate its appropriateness and take the individual needs of the patient into account.

Local trust guidelines: please refer to your local guidelines as necessary.

Overview

In all surgical specialities, high-quality preoperative and postoperative care is critical to ensure positive patient outcomes. This chapter covers the management of patients pre-operatively including preparations for surgery and the management of comorbidities. The use of blood products pre-operatively is covered in Chapter 94.

Preoperative testing for elective surgery

Prior to any preoperative test, it is necessary to consider the patient's medical and surgical history, in addition to medications being taken.

The patient's American Society of Anesthesiologists (ASA) grade (Table 92.1) and type of surgery (Table 92.2) that is planned will affect the tests chosen.

ASA grades V and VI have not been included as such patients should be assessed in conjunction with other specialities (anaesthetist, geriatrician, etc.) before considering any procedure on an elective basis.

Table 92.1 ASA physical status classification system

ASA grade	Patient description
ASA I	Healthy
ASA II	Mild systemic disease
ASA III	Severe systemic disease
ASA IV	Severe, life-threatening systemic disease

Table 92.2 Types of surgery

Type	Examples
Minor	Skin lesion excision, abscess incision and drainage
Intermediate	Inguinal hernia repair, tonsillectomy, knee arthroscopy
Major or complex	Organ removal, joint replacement, bowel resection

Tests under specific circumstances

- See Table 92.3
- Urine dipstick and microscopy and culture: only if a UTI would prevent surgery proceeding
- Pregnancy test: if a female patient is of childbearing age, ask sensitively about the possibility of pregnancy on the day of the procedure. Ensure women who may be pregnant understand the potential risks of the surgery and the anaesthetic, including the risks to the fetus, and gain the patient's consent to carry out a test if there is any possibility of pregnancy
- HbA1c test: offer to any diabetic patient not tested in the last 3 months
- Echocardiography:
  - If there is:
    - A heart murmur and a cardiac symptom (e.g. breathlessness, syncope, chest pain) **OR**
    - Clinical suspicion of heart failure
  - If considering this, perform an ECG and discuss with the anaesthetic team prior to requesting the echocardiogram.

Table 92.3 Preoperative investigations based on ASA grade of patient and type of planned surgery

	FBC	U&E	Coagulation profile	ECG	Lung function testing or ABG
ASA I	If undergoing major/ complex surgery	If at risk of AKI		If aged >65 years and no ECG from past year	
ASA II		If undergoing major/ complex surgery If undergoing intermediate surgery and at risk of AKI		If undergoing major surgery If undergoing intermediate surgery with cardiovascular disease, renal disease, or diabetes	
ASA III or IV	If undergoing major/ complex surgery If undergoing intermediate surgery with cardiovascular disease or renal disease, with symptoms that have not been investigated recently	As standard, unless minor surgery with low AKI risk	If the patient has chronic liver disease, unless minor surgery	Perform if undergoing intermediate or major/ complex surgery Consider performing if undergoing minor surgery and the patient has not had an ECG within the last year	After discussion with anaesthetist if known or suspected respiratory disease, unless minor surgery

Preoperative fasting in healthy adults

- Fluids: water and other clear fluids (e.g. clear tea and black coffee) may be consumed until 2 hours prior to anaesthesia induction. Tea and coffee with milk may be consumed until 6 hours prior to surgery
- Food: food including solids and milk should not be consumed within 6 hours of surgery
- Medication: continue preoperatively unless advised otherwise. May take with up to 30mL water.

Chewing gum is not permitted on the day of a surgical procedure.

Management of diabetes preoperatively

All diabetic patients for elective surgery should have a preoperative assessment. This should include:

- Review of glycaemic control and arrangement of a preoperative diabetic plan if needed:
  - HbA1c should ideally be <69mmol/mol prior to elective surgery
  - Refer to the diabetes specialist team if the HbA1c is ≥69mmol/mol as it may be possible to delay surgery if it is felt that further glycaemic improvement is possible and that it is safe to delay the procedure. Also refer if the patient has hypoglycaemic unawareness
- Optimization of comorbidities
- Medication review, with written instructions given to the patient with any changes that they need to make to their medications preoperatively clearly marked
- Pre-prescription of diabetes medications prior to admission and rescue treatment for hypoglycaemia and hyperglycaemia
- SGLT2 inhibitors should be held during admission and blood ketone levels should be checked daily regardless of glucose levels (risk of euglycaemic DKA)
- Recognition of high-risk patients who will require higher dependency care postoperatively.

Diabetic patients should be prioritized on the surgical list.

Glucose control

- CBG measurements should be taken hourly on the day of surgery
- Target glucose concentration: 6–10mmol/L (4-12mmol/L may be acceptable if the patient does not take a hypoglycaemic agent, e.g. insulin, sulphonylurea)
- If blood glucose >12mmol/L and blood ketones >3mmol/L, cancel the surgery and follow DKA guidance (see Chapter 15).

Preoperative fasting

- If a patient takes any diabetes medications (i.e. not just diet controlled) and it is planned that the patient will miss more than one meal, a VRII should be prescribed.

Feet

- In those at high risk of foot ulcers (previous/current ulceration, amputation, or dialysis) pressure-relieving footwear should be used, and antiembolism stockings avoided.

Drug chart

- VRIIs will vary based on local guidelines but an example is 50 units of a rapid-acting insulin, made up to a volume of 50ml with 0.9% sodium chloride. In addition, give 5% dextrose in 0.45% sodium chloride (with 0.15-0.3% potassium) as maintenance fluids:
  - If a VRII is started, the patient's usual long-acting insulin preparations **should** be given **but** reduced by 20%
- Prescribe 'as required' Glucogel®, glucagon, and SC rapid-acting insulin analogue (e.g. Actrapid®) to allow prompt hypo- or hyperglycaemia management:
  - In hyperglycaemia (without raised ketones or evidence of HHS):

- Type 1 diabetics: give 1 unit of a rapid-acting insulin analogue to reduce glucose by approximately 3mmol/L, to a target of <12mmol/L
- Type 2 diabetics: give 0.1 units/kg of a rapid-acting insulin analogue to reduce glucose by approximately 3mmol/L, to a target of <12mmol/L
- If the glucose level is not falling after 1 hour, commence a VRII if the surgery cannot be postponed

- In hypoglycaemia (only relevant to patients who are taking diabetic medications and who are **not** on a VRII):
  - Blood glucose 4–6mmol/L: give 50mL of 20% IV glucose as a stat IV bolus and recheck the glucose level after 10 minutes
  - Blood glucose <4mmol/L: give 75–100mL of 20% IV glucose over 15 minutes and recheck the glucose level after 10 minutes
  - If given, blood glucose should be rechecked 1 hour later. If surgery cannot be delayed or the response is inadequate, start a VRII
- In hypoglycaemia (only relevant to patients who are taking diabetic medications and who are on a VRII):
  - Blood glucose 4–6mmol/L: give 50mL of 20% IV glucose as a stat IV bolus and recheck the glucose level hourly
  - Blood glucose <4mmol/L: give 100mL of 20% IV glucose over 15 minutes and recheck the glucose level every 15 minutes until >6.0mmol/L, and then check hourly.

Management of anticoagulation preoperatively

Anticoagulants cause an ↑ surgical bleeding risk. A risk versus benefit analysis for medication continuation must be performed for all patients. Advice varies depending on the type of anticoagulation and the indication.

The patient is taking a vitamin K antagonist (e.g. warfarin)

Elective surgery

If INR <1.5, surgery can be performed safely.

If the patient is at high risk of thromboembolism (e.g. AF with a CHA_2DS_2-VASc score ≥4 or mechanical mitral valve):

- Stop vitamin K antagonist 3–5 days preoperatively
- Measure INR daily until ≤1.5 and also on the day of the procedure
- Start LMWH or unfractionated heparin (UFH) when the INR is <2.0, and at least 24 hours has elapsed since the last dose of vitamin K antagonist
- The final preoperative LMWH dose must be given at least 12 hours before the surgery.

Emergency surgery

Give 2.5–5mg of IV or oral vitamin K. This will take 6–12 hours to have an effect. If more immediate reversal is needed, prescribe prothrombin complex concentrate (PCC) or FFP as well with guidance from haematology.

The patient is taking UFH or a LMWH (e.g. dalteparin)

- If a patient is receiving IV UFH, stopping the therapy normalizes coagulation profile within 4 hours. If they are being given SC UFH, coagulation profile takes longer to normalize
- If the effects of UFH need to be reversed urgently, protamine sulphate may be given with haematology guidance
- If a patient is administered LMWH, coagulation profile will normalize within 8 hours after the last dose
- If the effects of LMWH need to be reversed urgently, protamine sulphate may be given with haematology guidance but the maximum efficacy of the reversal in this situation is 50%.

The patient is taking a direct oral anticoagulant (DOAC e.g. rivaroxaban, dabigatran)

Unless a patient is at high risk of thromboembolism, the medication can be stopped without starting LMWH or UFH. The timing of stopping the medication is medication specific and depends on the surgical bleeding risk and kidney function. Seek haematology guidance for precise timing.

In an emergency setting, seek haematology guidance.

Further reading

1. Jibawi A, Baguneid M, Bhowmick A (2018). Preoperative assessment. In: *Current Surgical Guidelines*, 2nd ed (pp. 55–78). Oxford: Oxford University Press. Available at: https://doi.org/10.1093/med/9780198794769.003.0007

Chapter 93

Postoperative care

Guidelines: Joint British Diabetes Societies (Guideline for peri-operative care for people with diabetes mellitus undergoing elective and emergency surgery): https://abcd.care/sites/abcd.care/files/site_uploads/CPOC_Diabetes_Surgery_Guideline_March_2021.pdf

ESA/European Society of Anaesthesiology (2014 ESC/ESA Guidelines on non-cardiac surgery: cardiovascular assessment and management, pp. 2401–3): https://academic.oup.com/eurheartj/article/35/35/2383/425095

NICE NG180 (Perioperative care in adults): https://www.nice.org.uk/guidance/ng180

Association of Anaesthetists, Royal College of Physicians, Society for Endocrinology UK (Guidelines for the management of glucocorticoids during the peri-operative period for patients with adrenal insufficiency): https://associationofanaesthetists-publications.onlinelibrary.wiley.com/doi/10.1111/anae.14963

NICE NG125 (Surgical site infections: prevention and treatment): https://www.nice.org.uk/guidance/ng125

OUP disclaimer: Oxford University Press makes no representation, express or implied, that the drug dosages are correct and that the recommendations are an exclusive or mandatory course of care. All health professionals reading this text have a responsibility to evaluate its appropriateness and take the individual needs of the patient into account.

Local trust guidelines: please refer to your local guidelines as necessary.

Overview

In all surgical specialities, high-quality preoperative and postoperative care is critical to ensure a favourable patient outcome. Postoperative management of surgical patients varies depending on the nature of the surgical procedure and any complications that may occur. It is important to adhere to the postoperative plan in the operation note written by the operating surgeon.

Postoperative pain management

A tailored postoperative pain management protocol may have been made preoperatively.

All postoperative patients must be assessed regularly to ensure analgesia is adequate, with few side effects. Such assessments include asking the patient about the location, quality, and intensity of the pain as well as carrying out a thorough examination.

A multimodal approach should be adopted whereby pain should be treated by a variety of medications and techniques, not all of which are pharmacological. For example, a patient may benefit from a TENS device in addition to pharmacological therapy or from cognitive behavioural modalities.

Pharmacological therapy

- Paracetamol is a typical starting point for non-opioid therapy and this can be accompanied by ibuprofen unless contraindicated
- If the pain is expected to be moderate or severe, give oral opioids as soon as the patient is able to safely eat and drink. If the patient cannot take oral therapy, a continuous epidural or IV patient-controlled analgesia should be considered. A continuous epidural may be preferable if the patient has cognitive impairment, is expected to have severe pain, or has had major laparotomy surgery
- If the pain is expected to be moderate or severe and it is thought that opioid therapy will not be sufficient, or if the patient has an opioid sensitivity, consider giving a single dose of ketamine during surgery or postoperatively, under specialist guidance
- Other pain adjuncts that may be considered include gabapentin and local anaesthetic injections.

The response to analgesia should be assessed using a validated pain assessment tool so that the patient may be regularly reassessed, e.g. a numeric rating scale of 0–10.

If pain relief is inadequate, a local hospital pain specialist should be consulted.

Management of long-term steroid therapy postoperatively

Surgical stress increases the bodily demand for cortisol, which, in patients who do not produce a sufficient quantity of cortisol, can lead to an adrenal crisis (see Chapter 14). Therefore, any patient who takes long-term steroid therapy (≥5mg a day of prednisolone or equivalent for 1 month or more) should be given hydrocortisone at anaesthesia induction (usually 100mg), followed by a continuous infusion (200mg every 24 hours) until the patient is able to take a double dose of their normal oral steroid. There may be some variation depending on the surgical procedure.

The ↑ oral dose should ideally be reduced back to their normal oral maintenance dose within 48 hours, but clinical judgement must be used as this could take up to a week with larger doses.

Management of diabetes postoperatively

- High-risk patients with poor glycaemic control should have a diabetes plan that should be followed postoperatively and any concerns should be escalated to the diabetes specialist team
- In all diabetic patients, early mobilization should be encouraged with resumption of normal diet and usual diabetes management. This may be supported by the use of antiemetics where needed
- Optimal blood glucose control should be maintained, aiming for a range of 6–12mmol/L
- Fluid balance should be assessed regularly and electrolyte levels monitored
- Foot and pressure areas should be reviewed regularly due to the risk of ulceration
- If the patient becomes unwell or has persistent hyperglycaemia (two or more CBG measurements >13mmol/L), measure capillary blood ketones
- If the patient normally takes an SGLT2 inhibitor, check capillary blood ketone levels daily regardless of glucose levels (risk of euglycaemic DKA)

Reducing the risk of infection postoperatively

- Postoperatively, if required, the wound should be dressed or changed using an aseptic non-touch technique. Sterile saline should be used for wound cleansing for 48 hours post procedure and tap water can be used thereafter, even if the wound has separated or been opened to drain pus
- A shower is generally permissible from 48 hours post procedure
- Topical antibiotics should not be used for wounds that are healing by primary intention. However, if a surgical site infection is suspected by the presence of cellulitis, give antibiotics as per local microbiology guidance
- Wounds healing by secondary intention should only use moist cotton gauze or mercuric antiseptic solutions for dressings. Appropriate dressings can be discussed with the tissue viability team
- On discharge, patients and carers should be given advice on how to care for and manage their wound, including how infection can be identified and where to seek medical advice should one occur.

Restarting anticoagulation postoperatively

- If required, LMWH or UFH is resumed at the preprocedural dose at least 12 hours after surgery if haemostasis has been achieved
- Vitamin K antagonists should be resumed on day 1 or 2 after surgery, depending on haemostasis, at 1.5× preoperative levels for the first 2 days. Prior to this, LMWH/UFH can be used for bridging and stopped once the INR is at a therapeutic level
- DOACs can be restarted 1–2 days after adequate haemostasis has been achieved. If LMWH/UFH are used postoperatively, they should be stopped immediately when the DOAC is restarted.

Further reading

1. Jibawi A, Baguneid M, Bhowmick A (2018). Chapters 7–9. In: *Current Surgical Guidelines*, 2nd ed. Oxford: Oxford University Press. Available at: https://doi.org/10.1093/med/9780198794769.003.0007

Part 14

Miscellaneous

Chapter 94

Blood transfusion

Guideline:
NICE NG24 (Blood transfusion): https://www.nice.org.uk/guidance/ng24

OUP disclaimer: Oxford University Press makes no representation, express or implied, that the drug dosages are correct and that the recommendations are an exclusive or mandatory course of care. All health professionals reading this text have a responsibility to evaluate its appropriateness and take the individual needs of the patient into account.

Local trust guidelines: please refer to your local guidelines as necessary.

Overview

This guideline highlights the scenarios where blood products and blood product alternatives may be required.

Unless a delay would be life-threatening, in all circumstances where a transfusion is offered, it is important to obtain informed consent (see Chapter 112).

In the UK, a patient who has received a blood transfusion cannot donate blood in future.

Transfusion due to anaemia or bleeding

Red cells

Unless a patient is actively bleeding, consider single-unit transfusions and clinically reassess the need for further transfusions afterwards. Assume an increment in haemoglobin levels of 10g/L per unit transfused for an average 70kg adult.

Consider a transfusion if the haemoglobin falls below 70g/L in a stable patient. Aim for a post-transfusion haemoglobin level of 70–90g/L, unless the patient has one of the following:

- Major haemorrhage:
  - Use frequent measurements of haemoglobin, including the use of point of care, to guide the use of red cell transfusion
- ACS:
  - Consider using a haemoglobin threshold of 80g/L and aim for a level of 80–100g/L
- Chronic anaemia requiring regular transfusions:
  - Consider setting individual thresholds; if uncertain consider transfusing to a haemoglobin level which alleviates symptoms.

Follow local protocols for specific indications such as post cardiac surgery, traumatic brain injury, acute cerebral ischaemia, or elderly patients.

Alternatives to blood transfusion

The cause of anaemia should be investigated and managed. Transfusion may be avoided if the patient is clinically well and the underlying cause can be addressed, e.g. use of oral or IV iron.

Platelets

Thresholds for platelet transfusion vary depending on the scenario. Do not routinely give more than a single pool of platelets unless a patient has severe thrombocytopenia and is bleeding in a critical site, e.g. eyes.

Thrombocytopenia without bleeding

Offer prophylactic platelet transfusions to most patients with a platelet count <10 × 10^9/L. If the patient has sepsis and thrombocytopenia, aim for a platelet count of 10–20 × 10^9/L.

Do not offer prophylactic platelet transfusions to patients with the following conditions:

- Chronic bone marrow failure
- Autoimmune thrombocytopenia
- Heparin-induced thrombocytopenia
- Thrombotic thrombocytopenic purpura.

Thrombocytopenia with bleeding

- Offer platelet transfusions in patients with clinically significant bleeding and a platelet count <30 × 10^9/L
- Consider thresholds up to 100 × 10^9/L in more severe bleeding (associated with haemodynamic instability) or bleeding in critical sites, e.g. traumatic brain injury.

Fresh frozen plasma

- Use in the management of major haemorrhage (refer to local trust guidelines)
- Use FFP if there is significant bleeding and abnormal coagulation profile, e.g. PT ratio/INR or APTT ratio >1.5
- Do not use in the absence of bleeding or if the coagulation profile derangement is due to a vitamin K antagonist which may be reversed using vitamin K
- The dose is usually 15mL/kg body weight, often equivalent to 4 units in adults.

Cryoprecipitate

- Cryoprecipitate is usually used with FFP
- Offer in patients with clinically significant bleeding, without major haemorrhage, and a fibrinogen level <1.5g/L
- The dose is usually 2 pooled units in adults and will increase fibrinogen by approximately 1g/L.

Prothrombin complex concentrate

- Used for emergency reversal of warfarin in patients with clinically significant bleeding or head injury with suspected intracerebral haemorrhage
- Consider using to reverse warfarin in patients due to undergo emergency surgery, depending on the level of anticoagulation and the surgical bleeding risk
- Monitor the INR to confirm that the anticoagulation has been adequately reversed
- Refer to local trust guidelines for dosing.

> NHS Blood and Transplant have created a smartphone app called 'Blood Components' which helpfully summarizes available blood products and circumstances for their use.

Surgery

Blood transfusion alternatives in surgery

If a patient requires surgery, there are a number of blood transfusion alternatives that may be considered.

Erythropoietin (EPO)

- Do not offer EPO unless a patient declines transfusion due to religious beliefs or the appropriate blood type is not available due to the patient's red cell antibodies.

Iron

- Oral iron can be offered to patients with iron deficiency anaemia before and after surgery
- IV iron may be considered in patients who cannot tolerate, absorb, or are not compliant with oral iron.

> IV iron has a faster response time than oral iron so may also be considered in patients where surgery is needed relatively soon.

Cell salvage and tranexamic acid

- Cell salvage with tranexamic acid should be considered for patients undergoing operations where large-volume blood loss is anticipated
- Tranexamic acid should be offered to adults undergoing surgery if at least moderate blood loss is expected (>500mL in adults).

Management of presurgical coagulation profile abnormalities

Platelets

- Consider prophylactic platelet transfusions aiming for a platelet count $>50 \times 10^9$/L
- Higher thresholds may be considered (seek senior advice) for procedures with a high risk of bleeding or for surgery at critical sites.

Fresh frozen plasma

- Consider prophylactic FFP transfusion in patients with abnormal coagulation profile tests (e.g. INR >1.5).

Cryoprecipitate

- Consider if fibrinogen level <1g/L.

Prothrombin complex concentrate

- Consider using to reverse warfarin in patients due to undergo emergency surgery, depending on the level of anticoagulation and surgical bleeding risk.

Special considerations

Jehovah's witness

- Be open, clear, and non-judgemental in discussions with patients whose religious beliefs may preclude transfusions
- Explain the blood products being offered as people may have individual beliefs that may allow certain blood products to be used, e.g. cryoprecipitate
- Make use of alternatives to transfusion
- Seek senior advice early.

Further reading

1. Provan D, Baglin T, Dokal I, et al. (2015). Blood transfusion. In: *Oxford Handbook of Clinical Haematology*, 4th ed (pp. 759–83). Oxford: Oxford University Press. Available at: https://doi.org/10.1093/med/9780199683307.003.0017_update_001

Chapter 95

Care of dying adults in the last days of life

Guideline:
NICE NG31 (Care of dying adults in the last days of life): https://www.nice.org.uk/guidance/ng31

OUP disclaimer: Oxford University Press makes no representation, express or implied, that the drug dosages are correct and that the recommendations are an exclusive or mandatory course of care. All health professionals reading this text have a responsibility to evaluate its appropriateness and take the individual needs of the patient into account.

Local trust guidelines: please refer to your local guidelines as necessary.

Overview

Recognizing when a patient is entering the final days of their life is crucial to ensure that their needs are met and their wishes are respected. However, this can be a challenging task. This guideline aims to highlight potential pitfalls and help with this process. See Box 95.1.

Box 95.1 Recognition of dying

Recognition of dying has two key aspects:

- Recognizing that a patient is 'approaching the end of life', i.e. that they have entered a terminally ill period with limited reversibility, and that they are likely to die within the next 6–12 months. Therefore, the nature of care should be predominantly palliative in nature
- Recognizing that a patient is actively and/or imminently dying within hours or days.

Recognizing that a patient may die within the next 6–12 months often happens in the community. The Gold Standards Framework and SPICT tools are used in this context to help support earlier recognition of these patients (see 'Further reading').

Some patients deteriorate more quickly than expected, which is why advance care planning for those thought to be in the last year of life is so important. Hospice UK and Marie Curie offer helpful resources to assist with this (see 'Further reading').

Recognition

What does the process of dying commonly look like?

Dying is an individual affair; however, the similarities outweigh the differences. Most commonly, it is a gradual process, and it is rarer that a sudden event occurs. The common natural course is that a patient gets increasingly tired, spending an increasing amount of time in bed resting and sleeping. There will usually be periods when the patient is 'themself', chatting and talking, but remains very weak and unable to leave the bed safely. These periods are often called 'windows of wakefulness', and get progressively shorter over time with sleep predominating. There appear to be two kinds of sleep; a 'shallow' sleep, whereby the patient is able to hear and may respond with their facial expressions, and a 'deeper' sleep. Families are encouraged to be by the patient's bedside and talk, listen to music, and interact with the patient during this time. Over time, the deeper sleep becomes more predominant. In the deep sleep periods, the patient is likely unaware of their surroundings and the patient may develop noisy breathing ('gurgly') as they breathe through their respiratory secretions (i.e. they are too weak and deeply asleep to clear them properly). The patient's level of consciousness may continue to fluctuate through to shallow sleep and even have brief windows of wakefulness. However, families must understand that this is the fluctuating nature of dying, that this is a normal pattern and that the patient is not getting better. Eventually, the periods of deep sleep become deeper still and the pattern of breathing begins to change, with pauses starting to appear. These are normally relatively short to begin with, but over time the pauses in the breathing lengthen. Eventually a pause starts, but doesn't stop, and the patient has died.

If it is thought that a patient is entering the last few days of their life, it is important to:

- Document:
  - Signs, symptoms, and physiological needs
  - Medical history and underlying diagnoses
  - Wishes of the patient and those important to them
  - Whether the patient has capacity. If they do not, whether there is a legal lasting power of attorney for health and welfare (legislation around this varies across the UK; see Chapter 112)
  - If the patient has expressed preferences about their care, e.g. refusal of certain treatments
  - If they have made a formal advance decision or have a 'do not attempt cardiopulmonary resuscitation' (DNACPR) order (see Chapter 114)
  - If the patient has specific psychological, social, or spiritual needs
  - Any multidisciplinary discussions
- Assess for changes such as:
  - Increasing fatigue
  - Agitation (terminal agitation is always a retrospective diagnosis and should never be assumed, i.e. exploration of reversible causes should always be considered)

  - Cheyne–Stokes breathing
  - Deteriorating level of consciousness
  - Skin mottling and cool peripheries
  - Noisy respiratory secretions
  - Weight or appetite loss
  - Change in communication or social withdrawal
- Reassessment:
  - It is important to regularly review and monitor symptoms. A patient's condition can stabilize or improve unexpectedly, particularly in non-malignant disease. If there is significant improvement, careful consideration should be given to whether the patient is still likely to be in the last days of their life. However, it is also important to appreciate that the dying process rarely follows a linear trajectory downwards.

Communication

Communication is the most important aspect of caring for patients as they approach the end of life. Poor communication, or lack of communication, is where most issues and complaints arise from. Including the patient and their family in these discussions and decisions is vitally important. Remember that communication needs may change at any point and should be reassessed regularly

- Establish communication expectations early including:
  - The patient's cognitive status, level of understanding, and how much information they would like to receive
  - Whether the patient would like someone with them during conversations
  - If the patient has any cultural, religious, social, or spiritual needs
- Decision-making and discussing prognosis:
  - Prognosis should be explained by a competent, confident healthcare professional who has a good rapport with the patient and those important to them
  - Provide accurate information and explain uncertainties, while avoiding false optimism
  - Provide opportunities for the patient and those important to them to discuss fears and anxieties and to ask questions
  - Explain how to contact the healthcare team, including out-of-hours services
  - Ensure that the patient and those important to them understand any changes to the plan.

Investigations

- Perform only appropriate investigations. It is important to consider the burden versus benefit of any investigations that are carried out.

Individualized care

- Organize required resources early, e.g. equipment, carers, meal deliveries
- Create an individualized care plan, involving the entire MDT, to include:
  - Individual goals and wishes
  - The preferred care setting and place of death
  - Patient preferences
  - Any advanced or legal decisions
  - Current and anticipated care and resource needs, including preferences for symptom management and needs for care after death
- Share this plan with the patient, those important to them, and the healthcare team
- **Update the plan as needed, at least every 24 hours**
- If it is not possible to meet the patient's wishes, explain why.

Hydration

- Support the patient to drink if they wish to
- Assess for swallowing problems and aspiration risk. If the patient has capacity, consider whether the patient can continue drinking 'at risk' of aspiration if they wish
- If the patient is unable to swallow, discuss the advantages and disadvantages of clinically assisted hydration, with the patient and those important to them:
    - Clinically assisted hydration may relieve signs and symptoms of dehydration such as dry mouth and thirst
    - It is uncertain if clinically assisted hydration will prolong life, hasten death, or extend the dying process
    - Clinically assisted hydration has risks including pulmonary oedema
- Provide mouth and lip care, including:
    - Help with cleaning teeth, mouth, and/or dentures
    - Regular sips of fluid
- Monitor the patient's hydration status regularly and assess if clinically assisted hydration may be appropriate. A trial may be useful
- If clinically assisted hydration is started:
    - Monitor every 12 hours for changes in signs or symptoms and evidence of benefit or harm
    - Continue if there are signs of benefit and consider stopping if there are signs of harm such as fluid overload, or if the patient no longer wants the intervention
- If the patient is already dependent on clinically assisted hydration:
    - Review the risks and benefits
    - Consider whether to continue, reduce, or stop as the patient nears death.

Pharmacological management

Review current medications and consider stopping any medications which are no longer providing benefit or may be causing harm.

Symptom control

- Ensure that the patient and those important to them are involved with decisions
- Explore possible causes of the patient's symptoms and treat any reversible causes
- Consider non-pharmacological management in all cases
- Discuss the benefits and harms of any medications offered
- Start with the lowest appropriate dose and titrate upwards (Table 95.1)
- Always consider side effects, compatibility, and drug interactions
- Consider the most effective route for administering medications based on the patient's ability to swallow and their preferences:
  - Avoid IM injections; SC or IV are preferable
  - Consider using a syringe pump to provide a continuous subcutaneous infusion (CSCI) over 24 hours if the patient requires regular SC injections (as a rough guide, more than 2–3 doses in 24 hours). CSCI advantages include:
    - It provides a continuous level of medications
    - It offers a mode of administration which avoids the oral route and GI absorption
    - It can be titrated on a daily basis in response to clinical need
- Seek palliative care advice if the patient's symptoms do not improve quickly or if there are unwanted side effects.

Anticipatory prescribing

- If using anticipatory prescribing, specify indications for use and dosages of any medications prescribed
- Ensure that anticipatory prescribing is done early
- Consider the:
  - Likelihood of specific symptoms occurring
  - Risks and benefits of giving or not giving medications
  - Risk of sudden deterioration which may require urgent symptom control
  - Place of care and time needed to obtain medications
- **Monitor benefits and side effects daily and adjust as needed. Seek specialist advice if symptoms remain poorly controlled.**

Pain management

- Treat any reversible causes, e.g. urinary retention
- Follow the WHO analgesic ladder and local guidance.

Managing breathlessness

- Treat any reversible causes, e.g. pulmonary oedema or pleural effusion
- Do not routinely start oxygen unless there is a clinical suspicion of hypoxaemia
- With senior/palliative input, consider using:
  - An opioid:
    - E.g. morphine sulphate 1–2mg, PO, every 6 hours and PRN
    - E.g. morphine sulphate 1–2mg, SC, PRN 2–4-hourly
  - A benzodiazepine:
    - E.g. lorazepam 0.5mg, PO, every 12 hours and PRN
    - E.g. midazolam 2mg, SC, PRN 2–4-hourly
  - Or a combination of these.

Managing nausea and vomiting

- Consider possible causes, including other medications, chemotherapy, radiotherapy, psychological causes, biochemical causes such as hypercalcaemia, raised intracranial pressure, GI dysmotility, or obstruction
- Consider using:
  - For central nausea:
    - Haloperidol 0.5mg, PO, BD–TDS **OR**
    - Haloperidol 0.5mg, SC, PRN 4-hourly
      —*Do not use in Parkinson's disease and be aware of potential extrapyramidal side effects*
  - For GI nausea:
    - Metoclopramide 10mg, PO, TDS **OR**
    - Metoclopramide 10mg, SC, PRN 4-hourly
      —*Do not use in Parkinson's disease and be aware of potential extrapyramidal side effects*
    - Domperidone 10mg, PO, TDS
      —*Can be used in Parkinson's diseases but should not be used in bowel obstruction*
  - For central nausea, intracranial pathology or vertigo:
    - Cyclizine 50mg, PO, TDS
      —*Be aware of anticholinergic side effects*
  - For chemotherapy- or radiotherapy-induced nausea:
    - Ondansetron 4mg, PO, BD–TDS **OR**
    - Ondansetron 4mg, SC, PRN 6-hourly
      —*Graniestron is another type of 5-HT_3 antagonist and is available as a patch (3.1mg/24 hours). It is currently the only transdermal antiemetic option*
  - For end of life nausea or vomiting of any cause:
    - Levomepromazine 6mg, PO, at bedtime **OR**
    - Levomepromazine 2–5mg, SC, PRN 4–6-hourly.

Managing anxiety, delirium, and agitation

- Isolated agitation may be associated with other unrelieved symptoms, e.g. unrelieved pain, urinary retention, or constipation
- Consider treating any reversible causes such as infections, or metabolic disorders such as renal failure or hyponatraemia
- In delirium, target non-pharmacological measures initially such as providing appropriate lighting, reducing loud noises, and encouraging family interaction (see Chapter 10)
- Provide appropriate psychological, spiritual, and social support
- For anxiety or agitation, consider a trial of a benzodiazepine, e.g. midazolam 2mg, SC, PRN 2–4-hourly **OR** lorazepam 0.5mg, PO, PRN 2–4-hourly
- For delirium or agitation, consider a trial of an antipsychotic medication, e.g. haloperidol 0.5mg, PO or SC, PRN 2–4-hourly
- Seek specialist advice if there is unwanted sedation or a poor response to treatment.

Managing noisy respiratory secretions

- Reassure patients and those important to them that although the noise can be distressing to those around the patient, it is unlikely to cause discomfort to the patient themselves
- Readjusting the patient's position may be helpful
- Consider a trial of medication if the respiratory secretions are causing distress
- Consider one of the following:
  - Glycopyrronium bromide, 200–400 micrograms, SC, PRN 2–4-hourly (maximum 1.2mg in 24 hours)
  - Hyoscine butylbromide 20–40mg, SC, PRN 2–4-hourly (maximum 120mg in 24 hours)
  - Hyoscine hydrobromide 0.4mg, SC, PRN 2–4-hourly (maximum 2.4mg in 24 hours). May cause drowsiness
- Monitor for improvement and side effects every 4–12 hours
- Consider stopping or changing medications if there is no improvement after 12 hours.

Table 95.1 Summary table of options for pharmacological management in anticipatory prescribing

Symptom	Pharmacological options
Agitation	**Midazolam 2mg,** SC, PRN 2–4-hourly **Lorazepam 0.5mg,** PO, PRN 2–4-hourly **Haloperidol 0.5mg,** PO or SC, PRN 2–4 hourly
Anxiety	**Midazolam 2mg,** SC, PRN 2–4-hourly
Breathlessness	**Morphine sulphate 1–2mg,** SC, PRN 2–4-hourly **Morphine sulphate 1–2mg,** PO, every 6 hours and PRN **Lorazepam 0.5mg,** PO, every 12 hours and PRN **Midazolam 2mg,** SC, PRN 2–4-hourly
Delirium	**Haloperidol 0.5mg,** PO or SC, PRN 2-hourly
Nausea and vomiting	**Haloperidol 0.5mg,** PO, BD–TDS **Haloperidol 0.5mg,** SC., PRN 4-hourly **Metoclopramide 10mg,** PO, TDS **Metoclopramide 10mg,** SC, PRN 4-hourly **Domperidone 10mg,** PO, TDS **Cyclizine 50mg,** PO, TDS **Ondansetron 4mg,** PO, BD–TDS **Ondansetron 4mg,** SC, PRN 6-hourly **Levomepromazine 6mg,** PO at bedtime **Levomepromazine 2–5mg,** SC, PRN 4–6-hourly
Noisy respiratory secretions	**Glycopyrronium bromide,** 200–400 micrograms, SC, PRN 2–4-hourly (maximum 1.2mg in 24 hours) **Hyoscine butylbromide 20–40mg,** SC, PRN 2–4-hourly (maximum 120mg in 24 hours) **Hyoscine hydrobromide 0.4mg,** SC, PRN 2–4-hourly (maximum 2.4mg in 24 hours)

Special considerations

Renal and liver impairment

Be aware that some drugs, in particular, opioid-based medications, may require dose adjustment in patients with severe renal and/or liver impairment. In this situation you should seek the advice of your palliative care team or pharmacist.

Further reading

1. Watson M, Ward S, Vallath N, et al. (2019). *Oxford Handbook of Palliative Care*, 3rd ed. Oxford: Oxford University Press. Available at: https://doi.org/10.1093/med/9780198745655.001.0001
2. Palliative Care Adult Network Guidelines. Available at: https://book.pallcare.info/
3. Wilkinson IB, Raine T, Wiles K, et al. (2017). Palliative care. In: *Oxford Handbook of Clinical Medicine*, 10th ed. (pp. 532–7). Oxford: Oxford University Press. Available at: https://doi.org/10.1093/med/9780199689903.003.0011
4. Simon C, Everitt H, von Dorp F, et al. (2020). Palliative care in general practice. In: *Oxford Handbook of General Practice*, 5th ed (pp. 1012–3). Oxford: Oxford University Press. Available at: https://doi.org/10.1093/med/9780198808183.003.0028
5. Simon C, Everitt H, von Dorp F, et al. (2020). The last 48 hours. In: *Oxford Handbook of General Practice*, 5th ed (pp. 1026–7). Oxford: Oxford University Press. Available at: https://doi.org/10.1093/med/9780198808183.003.0028
6. Simon C, Everitt H, von Dorp F, et al. (2020). Syringe drivers. In: *Oxford Handbook of General Practice*, 5th ed (pp. 1028–9). Oxford: Oxford University Press. Available at: https://doi.org/10.1093/med/9780198808183.003.0028
7. Wiffen P, Mitchell M, Snelling, et al. (2017). Syringe drivers and compatibility of medicines. In: *Oxford Handbook of Clinical Pharmacy*, 3rd ed. (p. 637). Oxford: Oxford University Press. Available at: https://doi.org/10.1093/med/9780198735823.003.0026
8. Gold Standards Framework. Available at: https://www.goldstandardsframework.org.uk/
9. SPICT Tool. Available at: https://www.spict.org.uk/
10. Hospice UK. What happens when someone is dying. Available at:https://www.hospiceuk.org/what-we-offer/clinical-and-care-support/what-to-expect/what-happens-when-someone-is-dying
11. Marie Curie. Palliative care knowledge zone. Available at: https://www.mariecurie.org.uk/professionals/palliative-care-knowledge-zone
12. Mannix K (2019). *With the End in Mind: How to Live and Die Well*. London: HarperCollins.

Chapter 96

Intravenous fluid therapy

Guideline:
NICE CG174 (Intravenous fluid therapy in adults in hospital): https://www.nice.org.uk/guidance/CG174

OUP disclaimer: Oxford University Press makes no representation, express or implied, that the drug dosages are correct and that the recommendations are an exclusive or mandatory course of care. All health professionals reading this text have a responsibility to evaluate its appropriateness and take the individual needs of the patient into account.

Local trust guidelines: please refer to your local guidelines as necessary.

Overview

IV fluid therapy should only be used if the patient's needs cannot be met orally or enterally. IV fluid therapy should be stopped when no longer needed. IV fluid therapy can be used for:

- Resuscitation
- Replacement
- Routine maintenance.

The advice here does not apply to patients aged <16 years, pregnant women, and those with severe liver or renal disease, diabetes, burns, or other groups with more specialized fluid prescribing needs.

Assessment and monitoring

Patients receiving IV fluids should receive frequent fluid balance assessments. Assess using an ABCDE assessment. Findings suggestive of hypovolaemia or hypervolaemia should prompt a fluid prescription review (Table 96.1).

Table 96.1 Summary of key findings in hypovolaemia and hypervolaemia

	Hypovolaemia	Hypervolaemia
History		
Input	↓ due to fasting ('nil by mouth'), reduced consciousness, or altered mental state	↑—usually iatrogenic (rarely psychogenic)
Output	↑ due to polyuria, diarrhoea, vomiting or ↑ insensible losses	↓
Examination		
JVP	Not visible	May be ↑
Pulse	↑ (>90bpm)	May be ↑
Systolic blood pressure	↓ (<100mmHg)	May be ↑
Capillary refill	↑ (>2 seconds) Cool peripheries	Normal
Respiratory rate	↑ (>20 breaths/minute)	↑ (>20 breaths/minute)
Other	Postural hypotension (early sign) National Early Warning Score (NEWS) ≥5 Positive passive leg raise (raising legs leads to a temporary improvement in blood pressure or heart rate after 30–90 seconds)	Pulmonary oedema Peripheral oedema
Bedside charts		
Fluid balance charts	Negative balance	Positive balance
Weight		Weight increasing
Investigations		
FBC, U&E, electrolytes	↑ urea and creatinine	Dilutional picture, e.g. ↓ haemoglobin, sodium, potassium

Acute management

Resuscitation

- Use crystalloids (0.9% sodium chloride, Hartmann's)
- Give 500mL over 15 minutes and reassess
- Give further boluses if still in need of resuscitation, up to a maximum of 2000mL, unless contraindicated
- Use 250mL boluses if elderly, patients with congestive cardiac failure, or at risk of fluid overload
- Human albumin solution 4–5% should be considered in severe sepsis only
- If the patient's ABCDE assessment is not improving during fluid resuscitation then seek senior advice.

Routine maintenance and replacement

An IV fluid regimen may be prescribed for up to 24 hours unless more frequent monitoring is required.

Average daily requirements

- 25–30mL/kg/day water
- 1mmol/kg/day of sodium, potassium, and chloride
- 50–100g/day of glucose (this limits starvation ketosis but does not meet patients' nutritional needs).

Adjust your prescription and seek senior advice if:

- Existing fluid/electrolyte deficits, e.g. hypo/hypernatraemia
- Ongoing losses
- Abnormal fluid distribution, e.g. postoperative fluid retention, severe oedema, ascites.

Important caveats

- In obese patients (BMI >25kg/m^2), use adjusted body weight (ABW), calculated from ideal body weight (IBW):
  - IBW (men) = 50kg + 2.3kg for each inch of height over 5 feet
  - IBW (women) = 45.5kg + 2.3kg for each inch of height over 5 feet
  - ABW = IBW + 0.4(actual weight – IBW)
- Seek senior advice and consider reducing fluid volume in high-risk patients:
  - Elderly or frail
  - Cardiac or renal failure
  - Malnourished or at risk of refeeding syndrome
- Don't forget to consider whether patients may be losing additional fluid that has not been accounted for, e.g. surgical drains, stomas, nasogastric tubes.

Reassessment

Reassess daily:

- Clinical fluid status
- Fluid balance charts
- Laboratory values (urea, creatinine, and electrolytes—beware of hyperchloraemic acidosis if giving 0.9% sodium chloride. Monitor by checking serum chloride levels).

Weights should be checked twice weekly. Stable patients on long-term IV therapy may be monitored less frequently.

Situations requiring more frequent or additional monitoring

Fluid resuscitation

- ABCDE approach
- Regular reassessment of vital signs (aim for a mean arterial pressure >65mmHg, normalization of heart rate and respiratory rate)
- Measure venous or arterial lactate/pH/base excess (these should normalize with resuscitation)
- Catheterize to measure urine output (aim for >0.5mL/kg/hour).

Consider the need for an arterial line and higher dependency care to allow more frequent assessment.

High-volume gastrointestinal losses

Check urinary sodium levels. Levels <30mmol/L may indicate total body sodium depletion, even if plasma sodium is normal. However, this may be unreliable in the presence of renal failure or diuretic use.

Chapter 97

Lower urinary tract symptoms in men

Guidelines:
NICE CG97 (Lower urinary tract symptoms in men: management): https://www.nice.org.uk/guidance/cg97

NICE NG109 (Urinary tract infection (lower): antimicrobial prescribing): https://www.nice.org.uk/guidance/ng109

NICE NG110 (Prostatitis (acute): antimicrobial prescribing): https://www.nice.org.uk/guidance/ng110

OUP disclaimer: Oxford University Press makes no representation, express or implied, that the drug dosages are correct and that the recommendations are an exclusive or mandatory course of care. All health professionals reading this text have a responsibility to evaluate its appropriateness and take the individual needs of the patient into account.

Local trust guidelines: please refer to your local guidelines as necessary.

Overview

About 30% of men over the age of 65 years experience lower urinary tract symptoms which significantly affect their quality of life. Rarely, lower urinary tract symptoms indicate serious urogenital tract pathology. Assessment aims to identify reversible factors such as infection, to classify symptoms in order to inform management, and to identify cases which warrant specialist input or urgent referral to exclude cancer.

Diagnosis

Differential diagnosis

See Table 97.1.

Table 97.1 Causes of lower urinary tract symptoms in men*

Voiding symptoms predominant	Storage symptoms predominant	Polyuria
Bladder outflow obstruction Benign prostatic enlargement (BPE) Urethral stricture, meatal stenosis, phimosis	**Overactive bladder** Detrusor overactivity	**Endocrine disease** Diabetes mellitus, diabetes insipidus, hypercalcaemia
Detrusor muscle weakness Neurogenic bladder dysfunction, diabetic neuropathy	**Infection** Lower UTI Acute bacterial prostatitis Urethritis	**Renal disease**
Malignancy Bladder cancer Advanced prostate cancer	**Urolithiasis** Bladder, ureteric, or urethral stones	**Heart failure**
Secondary to medication Prescribed: calcium channel blockers, anticholinergics, tricyclic antidepressants, opioids, benzodiazepines Over the counter: antihistamines, decongestants	**Secondary to medication** Prescribed: diuretics, calcium channel blockers, lithium, SSRIs Alcohol Caffeine	
	Neurological Diabetic neuropathy, multiple sclerosis, Parkinson's disease, stroke, spina bifida	**Excessive fluid intake** Including psychogenic polydipsia
	Urethral sphincter disruption Urethral trauma Postoperative (post prostatectomy, other pelvic surgery)	
	Chronic prostatitis/pelvic pain syndrome	
	Malignancy Bladder cancer	

* Categories are in bold, with key examples given in normal text.

History

Characterize symptoms:

- **Voiding:** weak/intermittent stream, straining, terminal dribbling, incomplete emptying
- **Storage:** urgency, frequency, urge incontinence, nocturia
- **Mixed** symptoms.

Assess baseline symptom severity plus functional impact using the **International Prostate Scoring System (IPSS)** (0–7 'mild', 8–19 'moderate', 20–35 'severe' symptoms).

Ask the patient to complete a **urine frequency–volume chart** to distinguish frequency, polyuria, nocturia, and nocturnal polyuria. See Table 97.2.

Table 97.2 Interpretation of urine frequency–volume chart

Frequency	↑ voiding frequency with normal 24-hour urine volume (up to 3L/24 hours)
Polyuria	↑ 24-hour urine volume
Nocturia	Waking at night to urinate
Nocturnal polyuria	Passage of >35% of total 24-hour urine volume at night

Red flag symptoms

New-onset urinary incontinence or impaired awareness of the need to void: THINK could this be cauda equina?

- Lower back pain or nerve root symptoms (e.g. bilateral sciatica)
- Lower limb weakness/sensory loss
- Saddle anaesthesia
- Loss of awareness of bladder fullness/faecal incontinence.

Cauda equina is a spinal emergency. Early diagnosis is imperative to prevent permanent neurological damage. Arrange immediate admission for MRI.

Examination

- **Abdomen:** palpable bladder (retention)
- **External genitalia:** urethral discharge, meatal stenosis, phimosis
- **DRE:** prostate assessment (smooth enlargement suggests BPE; tenderness suggests prostatitis; hard, nodular prostate suggests malignancy)
- **Neurological assessment** where indicated: lower limb motor and sensory function, perineal sensation, anal tone.

Investigations

- **Urinalysis**
- **Urine MC&S:** suspected UTI, prostatitis
- **Sexually transmitted infection screen:** suspected urethritis, consider in suspected prostatitis
- **Bloods: U&E** if suspected renal impairment (recurrent UTI, chronic retention, urolithiasis, nocturnal enuresis). Consider **PSA** if symptoms or examination suggest BPE, or to assess prostate cancer risk in response to clinical suspicion/patient concern. Ideally take PSA level before performing a rectal examination or catheterizing as both may cause a false-positive rise in PSA, see Chapter 111.
- **Other:**
  - Urodynamics
  - Cystoscopy
  - USS/CT kidneys, ureters, and bladder (KUB).

Management

Patient education

Provide information about the suspected diagnosis, further investigation, and management, involving carers where appropriate:

- Bladder and Bowel Foundation: http://www.bladderandbowelfoundation.org
- Prostate Cancer UK: http://www.prostatecanceruk.org (resources on benign prostate disease and prostate cancer).

Lifestyle and simple interventions

Conservative measures alone may be effective for mild symptoms (IPSS ≤7):

- Modify **fluid intake** (total daily intake; ↓ caffeine, artificial sweeteners, carbonated drinks)
- Review **medications**
- **Supervised bladder training** for detrusor overactivity
- Temporary **containment products** (pads, collecting devices) for incontinence.

Catheterization to manage chronic retention or incontinence

- Convene devices (incontinence) and intermittent self-catheterization (retention) are preferable to indwelling catheters
- Indications for indwelling catheter:
  - Chronic retention and renal impairment or hydronephrosis
  - Cannot manage intermittent self-catheterization
  - Skin irritation/ulceration due to urine contamination.

Psychological interventions

CBT may improve pain and quality of life in chronic prostatitis and pelvic pain syndrome.

Pharmacological management

Urinary tract infection, prostatitis, urethritis

Ensure a midstream urine sample is sent prior to starting antibiotics.

Consult local guidelines if available; Table 97.3 summarizes NICE guidance. For urethritis, genitourinary medicine referral is recommended.

Benign prostatic hyperplasia

- **Alpha-blockers** (tamsulosin, alfuzosin, doxazosin, terazosin):
  - Relax prostatic and bladder neck smooth muscle; do not affect symptom progression
  - For moderate–severe symptoms (IPSS score ≥8) or failure of conservative management
  - Side effects: postural ↓ blood pressure ('uroselective' agents ↓ risk—tamsulosin, alfuzosin), erectile dysfunction
  - Review 4–6 weeks after starting and every 6–12 months thereafter
- **5α-reductase inhibitors** (finasteride, dutasteride):
  - Reduce prostatic volume, symptom progression and the risk of acute retention

Table 97.3 NICE-recommended empirical antibiotic treatment for urinary tract infection in men and prostatitis

Indication	First-line antibiotic treatment	Duration
Uncomplicated lower UTI	Trimethoprim 200mg BD	7 days
	Nitrofurantoin modified release 100mg BD	
Pyelonephritis	Cefalexin 500mg BD–TDS	7–10 days
	Ciprofloxacin 500mg BD	7 days
	Co-amoxiclav 625mg TDS*	14 days
	Trimethoprim 200mg BD*	7–10 days
Acute prostatitis	Ciprofloxacin 500mg BD	14 days
	Ofloxacin 200mg BD	

* Select only if in line with urine MC&S sensitivities.

- Alone or in combination with alpha-blockers, if inadequate symptom control with alpha-blockers or high risk of symptom progression (older age, severe symptoms, PSA >1.4ng/mL)
  - Side effects: erectile dysfunction
  - Review 3–6 months after starting and every 6–12 months thereafter
- **PDE-5 inhibitors** (tadalafil):
  - Only tadalafil 5mg OD is licensed for benign prostatic hyperplasia.

Overactive bladder

- **Anticholinergics** (solifenacin, oxybutynin, tolterodine):
  - Reduce detrusor overactivity
  - Side effects: constipation, dry mouth, blurred vision, tachycardia, confusion
  - Review 4–6 weeks after starting and every 6–12 months thereafter
- Consider **alpha-blocker plus anticholinergic** for moderate–severe symptoms (IPSS score ≥8)
- **Mirabegron:**
  - Consider if anticholinergics are ineffective, poorly tolerated, or contraindicated
  - Side effects: tachycardia, rarely severe ↑ blood pressure and associated ischaemic events; avoid in bladder outflow obstruction.

Nocturnal polyuria

- **Loop diuretic** (furosemide 20–40mg taken late afternoon, off-label):
  - Measure baseline U&E. Repeat 1–2 weeks after treatment initiation and dose increases
- **Desmopressin:**
  - Considered if conservative measures and diuretics are ineffective (specialist initiation, sodium monitoring required).

Surgical management

Surgery is more effective than bladder retraining for BPE and should be offered if there is inadequate symptom control with conservative/medical management. For overactive bladder, effectiveness, side effects, and long-term risks of surgical intervention are less well established. See Table 97.4.

Table 97.4 Surgical and interventional procedures for benign prostatic enlargement and detrusor overactivity

Benign prostatic enlargement	Detrusor overactivity
TURP: transurethral resection of the prostate	Bladder wall botulinum toxin injection
TUVP: transurethral vaporization of the prostate	Cystoplasty
HoLEP: holmium laser enucleation of the prostate	Sacral nerve stimulation
TUIP: transurethral incision of the prostate	Urinary diversion
Open prostatectomy	Artificial urethral sphincter implantation

Psychosocial considerations

Explore the emotional, psychosocial, and sexual impact of symptoms, and offer information and support to address these, including self-help resources and support groups, e.g. Bladder and Bowel Foundation.

Specialist referral

Most patients can be managed effectively in primary care. Table 97.5 shows indications for referral to specialist care.

Table 97.5 NICE recommendations for specialist referral for further investigation or management

Referral pathway	Indication
Urology—routine	Recurrent (≥2 episodes in 6 months) or persistent UTI
	Symptoms despite optimal conservative and medical management
	Stress incontinence
	Chronic urinary retention
	Renal impairment with suspected urological cause
Urology—urgent (2 week wait)	**Suspected prostate cancer:** • Abnormal prostate on DRE • Elevated PSA above upper limit of age-specific reference range
	Suspected bladder cancer: • ≥45 years, unexplained visible haematuria after UTI excluded or successfully treated • ≥60 years, unexplained non-visible (dipstick) haematuria and dysuria or leucocytosis
Genitourinary medicine	Suspected urethritis
	Acute prostatitis and confirmed sexually transmitted infection

Complications

- **Urosepsis:** fever, rigors, vomiting, confusion, ↓ blood pressure with lower urinary tract symptoms or abnormal urinalysis (leucocytes, nitrites). Arrange emergency admission
- **Acute urinary retention:** admit for catheterization. Commence an alpha-blocker, wait ≥24–48 hours before attempting a trial without catheter.

Monitoring and follow-up

- Review 4–6-weekly after treatment initiation until symptoms are controlled, then 6–12-monthly. Repeat IPSS at reassessment, comparing follow-up to baseline score.

Special considerations

Renal and hepatic impairment

Many drugs are unsuitable for use or require dose adjustment. Consult the BNF or local formulary.

Elderly

Infection and complications (urosepsis, acute retention) may present atypically. Caution with antimuscarinics (risk of confusion, postural ↓ blood pressure) and alpha-blockers (postural ↓ blood pressure).

Further reading

1. European Association of Urology (2015). Guidelines on the management of non-neurogenic male lower urinary tract symptoms (LUTS), including benign prostatic obstruction (BPO). Available at: https://uroweb.org/wp-content/uploads/EAU-Guidelines-Non-Neurogenic-Male-LUTS-Guidelines-2015-v2.pdf
2. Rees J, Bultitude M, Challacombe B (2014). The management of lower urinary tract symptoms in men. *BMJ*. 348:g3861.
3. Tim Parks (2012). Teach Us to Sit Still: A Skeptic's Search for Health and Healing. Rodale Books.

Chapter 98

Malaria

Guideline:
PHE Advisory Committee on Malaria Prevention in UK Travellers (UK malaria treatment guidelines 2016): https://www.journalofinfection.com/article/S0163-4453(16)00047-5/pdf

OUP disclaimer: Oxford University Press makes no representation, express or implied, that the drug dosages are correct and that the recommendations are an exclusive or mandatory course of care. All health professionals reading this text have a responsibility to evaluate its appropriateness and take the individual needs of the patient into account.

Local trust guidelines: please refer to your local guidelines as necessary.

Overview

Malaria is the most common tropical disease imported into the UK, with approximately 1300–1800 cases each year.

Malaria is a medical emergency and patients with suspected malaria must be evaluated immediately. Malaria is typically divided by species (*Plasmodium falciparum* vs non-*falciparum*) and severity (complicated (otherwise known as severe) vs uncomplicated). The majority of imported cases are caused by the species *P. falciparum*—which can cause serious multiorgan disease and can be life-threatening.

Diagnosis

History

Malaria, a great mimic, can present atypically with a wide range of symptoms:

- **Common symptoms:** fever, headache, and general malaise
- **Other symptoms:** GI disturbance (diarrhoea, vomiting, abdominal pain, and nausea), jaundice, respiratory symptoms, arthralgia, myalgia, somnolence, and lethargy.

Malaria must be considered within the differential diagnosis of any sick or feverish patient who has visited or travelled through a malaria-endemic area. Falciparum malaria most commonly occurs within 6 months of travel, but other species may cause malaria more than a year after travel.

Most missed malaria diagnoses are assumed to be non-specific viral infections, influenza, gastroenteritis, or hepatitis. Other travel-related infections, especially viral haemorrhagic fevers, must also be considered when assessing patients with a fever after they have been travelling outside the UK.

Travel history

As falciparum malaria usually presents within 6 months of travel, a comprehensive travel history is essential (Table 98.1).

Table 98.1 Travel history

Question	Details to ascertain
Where?	Be precise—continent > country > city > town > village, type of accommodation (hotel/hostel/family or friend's home/camping/couch surfing) and remember to ask about 'stopover' countries en route
When?	Find out when symptoms started—is the illness acute (hours to days), subacute (days to weeks), or chronic (weeks to months)
Why?	Find out why they travelled—certain groups of travellers have different risks, particularly those who visit friends and relatives (VFR). They are at higher risk of hospitalization due to less pre-travel advice, underestimation of risk, last-minute/longer trips, and greater exposure to local communities
What?	Ask about potential exposures—**S**exual history, **P**rocedures (medical/tattoos/IV drug use), **A**nimals, **C**ontacts, **E**ating/drinking and **S**wimming (**SPACES**)
Which?	Find out what preparations were made prior to travel—malaria prophylaxis*, vaccinations, and other precautions, e.g. mosquito net, insect repellent, clothing

* Note that the use of malaria prophylaxis does not mean that a diagnosis of malaria is not possible, even if compliance has been good.

Examination

In mild cases, physical examination can be unremarkable. However, it is critical to be able to **quickly identify the clinical features of complicated falciparum malaria**, which requires urgent treatment (Table 98.2).

Table 98.2 Features of complicated falciparum malaria

Generalized features	Renal features	Respiratory features	Neurological features	Haematological features	Biochemical features
Hypotension	Reduced urine output	Acute respiratory distress syndrome	Reduced conscious level	Anaemia (80g/L)	Acidosis (pH <7.3)
Spontaneous bleeding	Haemo-globinuria	Pulmonary oedema	Seizures	Significant parasitaemia (>10%)	Hypo-glycaemia (<2.2mmol/L)
	Renal failure			DIC	

Investigations

Bedside

- CBG
- Urinalysis, urine culture, and stool culture should be considered.

Bloods

Immediately send a malaria blood test:

- **Gold standard = thick and thin blood film**, this will yield information about the species of malaria and degree of parasitaemia, both of which help guide overall management
- There are also **rapid diagnostic tests (RDTs)** available; these are not as sensitive or specific but can be useful out of hours if blood films are not available
- If blood films are negative and clinical suspicion persists, they should be **repeated after 12–24 hours and again at 24 hours**. Three negative blood films, reviewed by **a competent reader**, make a diagnosis of malaria unlikely. Alternative diagnoses should be considered.

Other bloods must also be performed routinely in all patients: FBC, U&E, LFT, and blood glucose.

If the patient is unwell or falciparum malaria is suspected then lactate, coagulation profile, blood cultures, and blood gases must be performed too.

Imaging

- Chest X-ray should be considered to check for pulmonary manifestations of malaria, e.g. acute respiratory distress syndrome, pulmonary oedema.

Other

- If the patient has a seizure and/or a reduced level of consciousness, a LP should also be considered to exclude alternative diagnoses, e.g. meningitis/encephalitis.

Acute management

An ABCDE approach must be adopted to identify features of complicated malaria noted previously.

Supportive treatment must be provided. Empirical malaria treatment is not usually recommended until a positive blood film/RDT is back, unless a patient has features of complicated falciparum malaria (Table 98.2).

The majority of patients with falciparum malaria must be admitted to hospital for at least 24 hours for monitoring due to the risk of sudden deterioration.

Where to turn for help!

Contact the local infectious diseases and/or microbiology team, urgently if falciparum malaria is suspected.

Specialist advice is also available from London (The Hospital for Tropical Diseases, University College London Hospital: http://www.thehtd.org) and Liverpool (Tropical and Infectious Diseases Unit, Royal Liverpool University Hospital: https://www.rlbuht.nhs.uk/). Additionally, the National Travel Health Network and Centre (NaTHNaC) can provide advice on 0845 602 6712.

Treatment must be in consultation with the local infectious diseases/microbiology team and depends on a combination of malaria species and illness severity (Table 98.3).

Table 98.3 Treatment of malaria by severity and species

Falciparum malaria		Non-falciparum malaria	
Complicated	Uncomplicated	Complicated	Uncomplicated
Urgent parenteral antimalarial treatment is essential First line in the UK is IV artesunate; if this is not available, commence IV quinine	Three options: 1. Artemisinin combination therapy (ACT) 2. Oral atovaquone/proguanil 3. Quinine plus doxycycline	Rare, but cases have occurred in patients with *P. vivax*, *P. knowlesi*, and *P. ovale* Seek specialist advice in these circumstances	Chloroquine or ACT (depending on resistance patterns) In cases of *P. vivax* or *P. ovale* check for G6PD deficiency, as concomitant primaquine is required to eliminate parasites hiding in the liver (hypnozoites)

Note: patients with mixed malaria infections (e.g. falciparum plus non-falciparum malaria) must be treated as falciparum malaria.

Patients with severe or complicated malaria should be cared for in a high dependency/intensive care unit as they may require haemodynamic support. They should be monitored for the following:

- Hypoglycaemia
- Acute respiratory distress syndrome
- DIC
- AKI
- Seizures
- Severe intercurrent infection.

Treatment after stabilization

- Consider checking haemoglobin after 2 weeks if IV artesunate is given (causes haemolysis in 10–15%).

Special considerations

- If a patient with malaria is pregnant, they require prompt treatment in hospital and must be managed in collaboration with the obstetric team—there is a higher risk of complicated disease and an association with stillbirths/miscarriages. Pregnancy also complicates diagnosis because parasites in the placenta are not always reflected in blood films
- Malaria is a notifiable disease—Public Health England must be informed (https://www.gov.uk/guidance/notifiable-diseases-and-causative-organisms-how-to-report).

Further reading

1. Fink D, Wani RS, Johnston V (2018). Fever in the returning traveller. *BMJ*. 360:j5773.
2. Travel Health Pro website. Available at: https://travelhealthpro.org.uk/
3. BNF. Malaria, treatment. Available at: https://bnf.nice.org.uk/treatment-summary/malaria-treatment.html

Chapter 99

Venous thromboembolic diseases

Guidelines:
NICE NG158 (Venous thromboembolic diseases: diagnosis, management and thrombophilia testing): https://www.nice.org.uk/guidance/ng158

NICE NG89 (Venous thromboembolism in over 16s: reducing the risk of hospital-acquired deep vein thrombosis or pulmonary embolism): https://www.nice.org.uk/guidance/ng89

ESC (2019 ESC Guidelines for the diagnosis and management of acute pulmonary embolism developed in collaboration with the European Respiratory Society (ERS): The Task Force for the diagnosis and management of acute pulmonary embolism of the European Society of Cardiology (ESC)): https://academic.oup.com/eurheartj/article/41/4/543/5556136

OUP disclaimer: Oxford University Press makes no representation, express or implied, that the drug dosages are correct and that the recommendations are an exclusive or mandatory course of care. All health professionals reading this text have a responsibility to evaluate its appropriateness and take the individual needs of the patient into account.

Local trust guidelines: please refer to your local guidelines as necessary.

Overview

Venous thromboembolic disease includes deep vein thrombosis (DVT) and pulmonary embolism (PE). Virchow's triad describes the three main pathophysiological changes that lead to thromboses (blood stasis, endothelial injury, and hypercoagulability). Thromboses may occur without an identifiable provoking factor or may be provoked by a known risk factor. One example of a provoking factor is malignancy and therefore, a seemingly unprovoked thrombosis may warrant further investigation. This chapter deals with suspected venous thromboembolic disease in non-pregnant adults. For the investigation and management of venous thromboembolic disease in pregnant women, see Chapter 67.

Diagnosis

History

DVT

- Symptoms may include pain, swelling, erythema, tenderness, and oedema of the affected limb
- Risk factors:
  - Hip or knee replacement
  - Hospitalization for AF/atrial flutter or heart failure (within the last 3 months)
  - Lower limb fracture
  - Major trauma
  - Myocardial infarction (within the last 3 months)
  - Previous VTE
  - Spinal cord injury.

PE

- Symptoms may include shortness of breath, pleuritic chest pain, syncope/presyncope, and haemoptysis
- In severe cases (massive PE), patients may be critically unwell due to haemodynamic instability
- Risk factors are the same as for DVT.

Examination

DVT

Examination may reveal distended and hardened superficial veins as well as swelling, pitting oedema, tenderness, and erythema.

PE

Assess using an ABCDE approach. See Table 99.1.

Table 99.1 Possible examination findings in venous thromboembolism

B	Tachypnoea, cyanosis, hypoxia on exertion or at rest
C	Tachycardia, hypotension in massive PE
D	Drowsiness, agitation
E	Signs of DVT, e.g. erythema and swelling of the calf

Investigations

DVT

Use the **DVT Wells score** to direct investigations (Table 99.2).

Table 99.2 Two-level DVT Wells score

Clinical feature	Points
Active cancer (treatment ongoing, within 6 months, or palliative)	1
Paralysis, paresis, or recent plaster immobilization of lower extremities	1
Recently bed-ridden (≥3 days) or major surgery within 12 weeks	1
Localized tenderness along distribution of deep vein	1
Entire leg swollen	1
Calf swelling >3cm versus unaffected side	1
Pitting oedema in symptomatic leg	1
Collateral superficial veins (not varicose)	1
Previous DVT	1
Alternative diagnosis is at least as likely as DVT	−2

If DVT is likely (Wells score ≥2)

- Organize a proximal leg vein USS within 4 hours and if negative send a D-dimer (see Box 99.1)
- If this is not possible, send a D-dimer, anticoagulate, and organize a scan within 24 hours
- Repeat the scan in 6–8 days if D-dimer positive but initial scan negative.

Box 99.1 D-dimer

The specificity of D-dimer results reduces with increasing age and therefore it should be considered whether to use an age-adjusted threshold if age >50 years.

If DVT is unlikely (Wells score ≤1)

- Send a D-dimer so that a result is available within 4 hours. If this is not possible, anticoagulate until the D-dimer result is known
- If the D-dimer is positive, organize an USS as for Wells score ≥2

PE

- Routine observations including temperature, blood pressure, heart rate, respiratory rate, and oxygen saturations
- ECG—possible findings:
  - Sinus tachycardia
  - Right axis deviation and right bundle branch block
  - Right heart strain (T wave inversion in V1–4 and sometimes II, III, and avF)
  - Deep S in lead I, Q wave and inverted T wave in lead III (S1Q3T3)
- Chest X-ray to assess for changes resulting from a PE and also to rule out other causes of dyspnoea
- Consider performing an ABG to assess for respiratory failure as a marker of severity (see Chapter 79).

- If the clinical suspicion of PE is low (felt to be <15% chance), the pulmonary embolism rule-out criteria (PERC) may be used. If the criteria are met, PE may be excluded without the need for further tests.

Use the **PE Wells score** to guide further investigations and management (Table 99.3).

Table 99.3 Two-level PE Wells score

Clinical feature	Points
Clinical signs and symptoms of DVT	3
Alternative diagnosis less likely than PE	3
Heart rate >100bpm	1.5
Immobilization ≥3 days or surgery within 4 weeks	1.5
Previous DVT/PE	1.5
Haemoptysis	1
Malignancy	1

PE is likely (Wells score >4)

- Organize an urgent CTPA.
- If this is not possible, anticoagulate while waiting for a CTPA
- If CTPA is negative but there is still high clinical suspicion, seek senior advice and consider a proximal leg vein USS.

PE is unlikely (Wells score ≤4)

- Send a D-dimer. If positive, perform CTPA as for Wells score>4.

Consider ventilation/perfusion (V/Q, also known as lung scintigraphy) scanning in patients who cannot have a CTPA, i.e. contrast allergy, renal impairment, or high irradiation risk.

Management

Acute management

Thrombolysis

- An UFH infusion and systemic thrombolysis therapy should be considered in patients with PE and haemodynamic instability (Table 99.4).
- Catheter-directed thrombolysis may be offered to patients with an iliofemoral DVT
- Refer to local guidelines and seek senior help immediately.

Table 99.4 Definition of haemodynamic instability, which delineates acute high-risk pulmonary embolism (one of the following clinical manifestations at presentation)

(1) Cardiac arrest	(2) Obstructive shock	(3) Persistent hypotension
Need for cardiopulmonary resuscitation	Systolic BP <90mmHg or vasopressors required to achieve a BP ≥90mmHg despite adequate filling status **AND** End-organ hypoperfusion (altered mental status; cold, clammy skin; oliguria/anuria; increased serum lactate)	Systolic BP <90mmHg or systolic BP drop ≥40mmHg, lasting longer than 15 min and not caused by new-onset arrhythmia, hypovolaemia, or sepsis

BP, blood pressure.

Reprinted from Konstantinides S et al (2020) '2019 ESC Guidelines for the diagnosis and management of acute pulmonary embolism developed in collaboration with the European Respiratory Society (ERS): The Task Force for the diagnosis and management of acute pulmonary embolism of the European Society of Cardiology (ESC)' European Heart Journal 41(4):543–603, with permission from Oxford University Press.

Treatment after stabilization

Anticoagulation

- Anticoagulation should be offered to all patients with confirmed proximal DVT or PE but considering comorbidities, contraindications, and drug costs
- Baseline blood tests should be taken including FBC, U&E, LFT, and coagulation profile. Treatment should not be delayed whilst waiting for the results

Follow local anticoagulation guidelines and remember to adjust for weight and renal function. The patient's bleeding risk should be assessed, either by implicit judgement after evaluating individual risk factors or by the use of a bleeding risk score, at the time of initiation of anticoagulant treatment

- Use the DOAC apixaban or rivaroxaban first line. If unsuitable, LMWH should be provided for 5 days and then the patient should be started on the DOAC dabigatran or edoxaban. Alternatively, a vitamin K antagonist, e.g. warfarin, should be started and LMWH given concurrently for 5 days or until the INR is ≥2 on two consecutive tests
- In renal failure (estimated creatinine clearance <15mL/min) or high bleeding risk, UFH may be appropriate
- Patients with cancer and a confirmed thrombus may be offered a DOAC. If unsuitable, offer LMWH.

> Vena cava filters may be considered acutely in patients with proximal DVT or PE who cannot receive anticoagulation or long-term in patients with recurrent PEs despite pharmacological optimization. Complications with vena cava filters are common and can be serious.

Duration of therapy

- Provide anticoagulation for at least 3 months if provoked (major transient/reversible risk factor) DVT/PE
- Consider providing anticoagulation for >3 months if unprovoked DVT/PE
- Provide anticoagulation to patients with cancer for at least 3–6 months.

Discharge

The Pulmonary Embolism Severity Index (PESI) or Simplified PESI can be used to assess whether early discharge may be safe for the patient. PESI is validated to assess the probability of mortality at 30 and 90 days post PE (Table 99.5).

- If very low or low risk, consider outpatient management
- If intermediate, high, or very high risk, inpatient management may be necessary
- If very high score, seek senior help and consider involving intensive care early.

Table 99.5 PESI score

If yes to any of the following, add on the appropriate number of points:		
Male sex	10 points	
History of heart failure	10 points	
History of chronic lung disease	10 points	
Heart rate ≥110bpm	20 points	
Respiratory rate ≥30/min	20 points	
Temperature <36°C	20 points	
Oxygen saturation <90%	20 points	
Systolic blood pressure <100mmHg	30 points	
History of cancer	30 points	
Altered mental status (reduced GCS score)	60 points	
Subtotal =		
PESI score = subtotal + patient's age =		
Score interpretation		**30-day mortality**
≤65 = very low risk		0.0–1.6%
66–85 = low risk		1.7–3.5%
86–105 = intermediate risk		3.2–7.1%
106–125 = high risk		4.0–11.4%
>125 = very high risk		10–24.5%

Special considerations

Additional testing

A malignancy screen should be considered in patients with unprovoked PE/DVT:

- History and examination
- Blood tests (including FBC, U&E, LFT, and coagulation profile)
- Further testing for malignancy should only be considered if there are relevant signs or symptoms. Consider thrombophilia testing if cessation of anticoagulation is being considered in a patient with an unprovoked PE/DVT and a first-degree relative who had a PE/DVT. Anticoagulation may affect the results of the tests and specialist advice should be sought.

VTE prophylaxis

- All inpatients must be risk assessed for VTE
- Risk of VTE needs to be balanced against risk of bleeding, and both pharmacological and mechanical thromboprophylaxis should be considered. Refer to local guidelines and regularly reassess
- Encourage mobilization and good hydration
- Antiembolism stockings: do not use in those with peripheral arterial disease or grafting, fragile or broken skin, peripheral neuropathy, or severe leg oedema.

Elective surgery

- Advise patients to consider stopping oestrogen-containing oral contraceptives or HRT 4 weeks before elective surgery. Advise on alternative contraception methods.

Antiplatelet agents

- Thromboprophylaxis may be appropriate even if the patient is using antiplatelet agents—discuss with a senior clinician.

Acute coronary syndrome

- Patients receiving anticoagulant drugs as part of their treatment for ACS do not usually need VTE prophylaxis.

Acute stroke

- Consider intermittent pneumatic compression instead of antiembolism stockings.

Elective hip replacement

- LMWH for 10 days then 28 days of aspirin **OR**
- LMWH for 28 days combined with antiembolism stockings with stockings worn until discharge from hospital **OR**
- Rivaroxaban 10mg OD for 2 weeks. Apixaban and dabigatran etexilate could also be considered (refer to local guidelines).

Patient information

When starting anticoagulation, the following topics should be discussed:

- Risks and possible consequence of VTE
- Importance of prophylaxis or treatment

- How to use the treatment correctly (including how to dispose of used needles appropriately if applicable)
- Treatment duration and where this will be reviewed
- Potential side effects and what to do if they occur
- Key interactions with foods, alcohol, and medications, e.g. avoiding grapefruit juice if taking warfarin
- How anticoagulants may affect dental treatment and activities such as sports and travel
- Monitoring requirements if applicable
- Pregnancy and planning pregnancy if relevant
- Use of anticoagulation monitoring booklets if applicable and alert cards
- If using heparins, patients should be aware that some heparins are of animal origin as they may have concerns for religious or ethical reasons
- Lifestyle changes to reduce the risk of VTE, e.g. encouraging mobilization, exercise, and good hydration
- Benefits and correct usage of antiembolism stockings.

Further reading

1. Stein PD, Matta, F, Firth JD (2020). Deep venous thrombosis and pulmonary embolism. In Firth JD, Conlon C, Cox T (eds) *Oxford Textbook of Medicine*, 6th ed (Chapter 16.16.1), Oxford: Oxford University Press. Available at: https://doi.org/10.1093/med/9780198746690.003.0375

Part 15

Cancer guidelines

Chapter 100

Brain and central nervous system cancers

Guideline:
NICE NG12 (Suspected cancer: recognition and referral): https://www.nice.org.uk/guidance/ng12

OUP disclaimer: Oxford University Press makes no representation, express or implied, that the drug dosages are correct and that the recommendations are an exclusive or mandatory course of care. All health professionals reading this text have a responsibility to evaluate its appropriateness and take the individual needs of the patient into account.

Local trust guidelines: please refer to your local guidelines as necessary.

Overview

Brain cancers may be primary or secondary to malignancies elsewhere in the body. Brain cancer can be difficult to detect and there is often a delay in diagnosis. This is because individual symptoms have a low risk of being due to cancer (with the exception of new-onset seizures).[1] Brain and central nervous system cancers in children are covered in Chapter 102.

1 Schmidt-Hansen M, Berendse S, Hamilton W. Symptomatic diagnosis of cancer of the brain and central nervous system in primary care: a systematic review. *Fam Pract*. 2015; 32:618–23.

Diagnosis

See Table 100.1.

Table 100.1 Diagnosis of brain and central nervous system cancers

Symptoms	Examination
New-onset seizures (particularly focal)—occurs in up to 50% of tumours	Full upper and lower limb neurological examination
Progressive motor loss	Cranial nerve exam including ophthalmoscopy looking for papilloedema (↑ intracranial pressure) and cerebellar testing
Progressive visual loss	Cognitive testing
Personality changes	
New-onset cognitive dysfunction	
Dizziness/cerebellar symptoms, e.g. vertigo, ataxia	
Headache with ⚑ features (Box 100.1) (occurs in around 50% of tumours due to ↑ intracranial pressure)	

Box 100.1 Headache red flags

- ⚑ New-onset headache >50 years—think space-occupying lesion/GCA
- ⚑ Progressive or persistent headache that has changed dramatically—think mass/subdural haematoma
- ⚑ Worse on lying down
- ⚑ Triggered by Valsalva manoeuvre, e.g. sneezing, bending, coughing, or exertional activity such as sexual intercourse—think posterior fossa lesion
- ⚑ Immunocompromised, e.g. HIV or on immunosuppressive drugs
- ⚑ Current or past malignancy—common cancers that metastasize to the brain include breast, colon, lung, kidney, and melanoma.

Investigations

Urgent access MRI (CT if MRI contraindicated) within 2 weeks in patients with progressive, subacute loss of central neurological function.

If a LP is being considered as part of the symptoms work-up, it is vital to perform imaging first to ensure it is safe and will not lead to coning.

Acute management

Imaging that shows evidence of a brain cancer should be transferred and discussed with a neurosurgical specialist unit. Consider whether the brain tumour may be secondary and further investigation is required to find a primary source. A biopsy may be considered to provide a tissue diagnosis.

Pharmacological management

- It may be appropriate to prescribe dexamethasone (4–8mg orally) due to cerebral oedema. Consider prescribing gastric protection, e.g. omeprazole 40mg.
- Mannitol may also be suggested following specialist advice for acutely raised intracranial pressure.
- In the absence of a history of seizures, antiseizure prophylaxis is not usually warranted.

Surgical management

- Benign lesions may be resected
- Malignant lesions may be debulked prior to radiotherapy
- A ventriculoperitoneal shunt may be considered for the management of hydrocephalus
- Some tumours are amenable to chemoradiotherapy.

Chapter 101

Breast cancer

Guideline:
NICE NG12 (Suspected cancer: recognition and referral): https://www.nice.org.uk/guidance/ng12

OUP disclaimer: Oxford University Press makes no representation, express or implied, that the drug dosages are correct and that the recommendations are an exclusive or mandatory course of care. All health professionals reading this text have a responsibility to evaluate its appropriateness and take the individual needs of the patient into account.

Local trust guidelines: please refer to your local guidelines as necessary.

Overview

Breast cancer is the most common cancer in women. It is also the second most common cause of death from cancer in the UK, with 55,920 new cases of invasive breast cancer being diagnosed each year.[1]

1 Cancer Research UK. Breast cancer statistics, 2016-2018 average. Available at: https://www.cancerresearchuk.org/health-professional/cancer-statistics/statistics-by-cancer-type/

Diagnosis

History

A breast lump is the commonest symptom. A malignant breast lump may be painful or painless. Other symptoms include bleeding or unusual discharge from the nipple, changes in the shape of the breast, and skin changes including tethering and peau d'orange (Fig. 101.1).

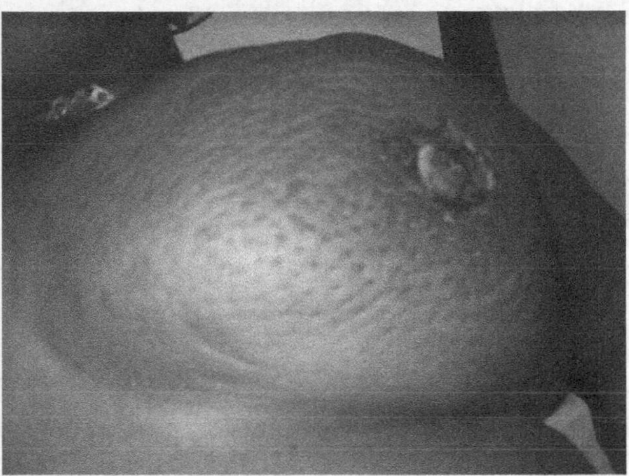

Fig. 101.1 Peau d'orange skin changes which may be seen in breast cancer.

 See colour plate 5.

Risk factors

- Previous history of breast cancer
- Family history of breast cancer in a first-degree relative
- *BRCA1*, *BRCA2*, and *TP53* genetic mutations
- Increasing age
- Childless or birth of first child after the age of 30
- Never having breastfed
- Early menarche and late menopause
- Continuous combined HRT or combined oral contraception
- Previous chest wall radiotherapy
- ↑ BMI after menopause
- ↑ alcohol intake.

Examination

1. Offer a chaperone and gain consent
2. Inspect the patient sat up. While examining, first ask them to place their hands on their thighs, then to press their hands into their hips, then finally to place their hands behind their head and lean forwards
3. Carefully inspect both sides, looking for the following:
   - Changes in breast symmetry
   - Visible lumps
   - Scars
   - Nipple changes, e.g. eczema, inversion, retraction, or discharge
   - Swelling or oedema
   - Skin changes including redness, peau d'orange, tethering or scaling
4. Palpate the breast with a flat hand, with the patient lying at a 45° angle. Using the palmar aspects of the second, third, and fourth fingers held together, move around the breast in discrete circles with light pressure. Ensure that the axillary tail is covered
5. Palpate for lumps as well as asking the patient if they experience any pain or tenderness on palpation
6. If a lump is found, the following characteristics should be described:
   - Location
   - Consistency, e.g. smooth, firm, rubbery
   - Skin changes overlying the mass
   - Size and shape of the mass
   - Mass mobility
   - Mass fluctuance
7. Examine the underarms for enlarged axillary nodes while supporting the weight of the arm with your non-examining hand. It is good practice to also examine the cervical lymph nodes and those around the clavicle and sternum
8. If discharge was mentioned, request that the patient attempt to express some discharge
9. Document your findings accurately to ensure that you can refer according to the pathway shown in Fig. 101.2.

Referrals

See Fig. 101.2.

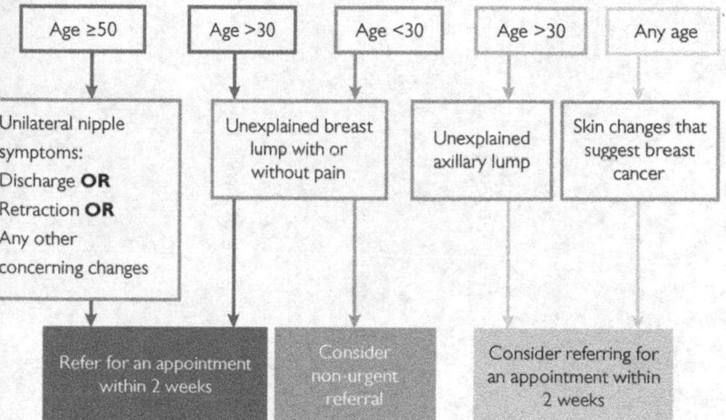

ig. 101.2 Referral pathways for breast cancer.

Investigations

Explain to the patient that they will be seen by a specialist within 2 weeks, ideally in a 'one-stop' clinic where all the investigations can be carried out in 1 day. The process involves a physical examination, followed by either a mammogram or an USS, and potentially a biopsy.

Management

Management options vary according to the grade and stage of the cancer and will be decided by the MDT. Hormone responsiveness also determines whether various treatments will be possible.

Treatments include:

- Chemotherapy
- Radiotherapy—external beam or brachytherapy
- Surgery—wide local excision or mastectomy ± reconstructive surgery
- Hormonal therapy, e.g. tamoxifen if oestrogen receptor positive, letrozole if postmenopausal
- Targeted drugs, e.g. trastuzumab, pertuzumab.

Prognosis

Overall 5-year survival is 90%, although this figure includes cases detected by screening as well as those identified after symptoms have occurred. The five-year survival for stage 4 (metastatic) breast cancer is around 25%.

Further reading

1. Patient UK. Breast lumps and examination. Available at: https://patient.info/doctor/breast-lumps-and-breast-examination
2. GOV.UK. NHS breast screening programme. Available at: https://www.gov.uk/topic/population-screening-programmes/breast

Chapter 102

Childhood cancers

Guideline:
NICE NG12 (Suspected cancer: recognition and referral): https://www.nice.org.uk/guidance/ng12

OUP disclaimer: Oxford University Press makes no representation, express or implied, that the drug dosages are correct and that the recommendations are an exclusive or mandatory course of care. All health professionals reading this text have a responsibility to evaluate its appropriateness and take the individual needs of the patient into account.

Local trust guidelines: please refer to your local guidelines as necessary.

Overview

Childhood cancers are rare, but the majority are curable. They can affect different body systems at any age and present with unexplained symptoms.

In the UK, 1 in 500 children will develop some form of cancer by the age of 14. Prevalence is shown in Table 102.1.[1]

Table 102.1 Incidence of childhood cancers in the UK 2006–2008 (age 0–14 years)

Type of cancer	Incidence (new cases per year)
Leukaemia	468
Brain and central nervous system cancers	412
Lymphoma	167
Soft tissue sarcoma	98
Neuroblastoma	83
Renal cancers (including Wilms' tumour)	82
Bone sarcoma	65
Retinoblastoma	44

1 Cancer Research UK. Children's cancers incidence statistics. Available at: https://www.cancerresearchuk.org/health-professional/cancer-statistics/childrens-cancers/incidence#heading-Three

Diagnosis

Parents/carers have important insight regarding their child, so always take the concern of the parent/carer regarding the child's symptoms seriously, even if the symptoms are very likely to have a benign cause. Referral criteria are shown in Table 102.2.

Table 102.2 Referral criteria for childhood cancers

Type of cancer	Clinical feature	Referral destination and timeline
Brain and central nervous system cancers	Newly abnormal cerebellar or other central neurological function	Specialist appointment within 48 hours
Bone sarcoma	Unexplained bone swelling or pain	X-ray within 48 hours
	X-ray suggesting possible sarcoma	Specialist appointment within 48 hours
Soft tissue sarcoma	Unexplained lump which is increasing in size	USS within 48 hours
	USS findings suggesting possible soft tissue sarcoma **OR** USS findings are ambiguous and there is ongoing clinical concern	Specialist appointment within 48 hours
Neuroblastoma	Palpable abdominal mass **OR** Unexplained enlarged abdominal organ	Specialist appointment within 48 hours
Retinoblastoma	Absent red reflex	Ophthalmological assessment within 2 weeks
Wilms' tumour	Palpable abdominal mass **OR** Unexplained enlarged abdominal organ **OR** Unexplained macroscopic haematuria	Specialist appointment within 48 hours

(Continued)

Table 102.2 *Continued*

Type of cancer	Clinical feature	Referral destination and timeline
Leukaemia	Pallor **OR** Persistent fatigue **OR** Unexplained fever **OR** Unexplained persistent infection **OR** Generalized lymphadenopathy **OR** Persistent or unexplained bone pain **OR** Unexplained bruising or bleeding	FBC within 48 hours
	Unexplained petechiae **OR** Hepatosplenomegaly	Immediate referral for specialist assessment
Hodgkin's and non-Hodgkin's lymphoma	Unexplained lymphadenopathy **OR** Splenomegaly Ask about the following symptoms and include in the referral: • Fever • Night sweats • Pruritis • Shortness of breath • Weight loss	Specialist appointment within 48 hours

Management

Management options are varied and will depend on a number of factors, including the type of cancer, the stage and grade of the cancer, and the age of the child.

Prognosis

See Table 102.3.[2]

Table 102.3 Five-year survival rates for childhood cancers in the UK 2011–2015 (age 0–14 years)

Type of cancer	5-year survival rate (%)
Retinoblastoma	99
Lymphoma	93
Renal cancers (including Wilms' tumour)	88
Leukaemia, myeloproliferative, and myelodysplastic disease	88
Brain and central nervous system cancers	75
Soft tissue sarcoma	74
Bone sarcoma and other malignant bone tumours	71
Neuroblastoma and other peripheral nervous system cancers	71

Further reading

1. Tasker RC, Acerini CL, Holloway E, et al. (eds) (2021). Oncology. In: *Oxford Handbook of Paediatrics*, 3rd ed (pp. 585–620). Oxford: Oxford University Press. Available at: https://doi.org/10.1093/med/9780198789888.003.0015

2 Public Health England. Childhood cancer statistics, England: annual report 2018. 2018. Available at: http://www.ncin.org.uk/view?rid=3715

Chapter 103

Gynaecological cancers

Guideline:
NICE NG12 (Suspected cancer: recognition and referral): https://www.nice.org.uk/guidance/ng12

OUP disclaimer: Oxford University Press makes no representation, express or implied, that the drug dosages are correct and that the recommendations are an exclusive or mandatory course of care. All health professionals reading this text have a responsibility to evaluate its appropriateness and take the individual needs of the patient into account.

Local trust guidelines: please refer to your local guidelines as necessary.

Ovarian cancer

Overview

Ovarian cancer is the leading cause of death from gynaecological malignancy, with 7000 cases diagnosed each year in the UK. Five-year survival is dependent upon the stage at diagnosis. Delays to diagnosis occur as half of women with gynaecological cancers present to a specialty other than gynaecology and 75% present once disease has spread to the abdomen (stage III disease).

History

Aetiology

Aetiology believed to be due to irritation/damage to ovarian epithelium during ovulation.

Risk factors

See Table 103.1.

Table 103.1 Risk factors
(↑ risk if multiple ovulations, ↓ risk if ovulation suppressed)

Increased risk	Decreased risk
Nulliparity	COCP use
Early menarche	Pregnancy
Late menopause	
Family history of gynaecological cancer or cancer syndrome, e.g. BRCA1/2, Lynch syndrome	

Symptoms

Women present with a range of vague and common symptoms which can be misinterpreted as other conditions. Remember: women >50 years rarely present with IBS for the first time.

- Abdominal or pelvic pain
- Abnormal vaginal bleeding
- Loss of weight
- Loss of appetite/early satiety
- Fatigue
- Abdominal distension or bloating
- Change in bowel habit
- ↑ urinary urgency ± frequency.

Examination

Possible findings:

- Ascites
- Abdominal distension
- Abdominal or pelvic mass
- Lymphadenopathy
- Pleural effusion.

Investigations

Carry out tests if the patient (especially if >50 years old) reports persistent or frequent (>12 times/month) abdominal distension, loss of appetite, pelvic pain, or urinary symptoms.

Consider carrying out tests for unexplained weight loss, fatigue, or bowel habit change.

Bloods

- FBC, U&E, LFT (especially albumin)
- Most ovarian cancers lead to a raised cancer antigen (CA) 125.

Imaging

- Transvaginal USS (if CA 125 raised, >35IU/mL or continuing suspicion despite a normal CA 125)
- Definitive diagnosis requires referral to gynaecology.

Two-week wait (2WW) referral

Refer the patient urgently if:

- The USS suggests ovarian cancer
- Examination reveals ascites and/or pelvic or abdominal mass.

Endometrial cancer

Overview

Endometrial cancer is a condition that predominately affects postmenopausal women. About 8000 new cases of endometrial cancer are diagnosed each year in the UK. Five-year survival is almost 80%.

History

Aetiology

- Exposure to unopposed oestrogen.

Risk factors

- Obesity
- Reduced progesterone production:
  - Nulliparity
  - Polycystic ovary syndrome
  - Early menarche/late menopause
- Genetic: Lynch II syndrome
- Exogenous unopposed oestrogen exposure (e.g. tamoxifen, tibolone, oestrogen-only HRT).

Symptoms

The most common symptom is postmenopausal bleeding (PMB). PMB is defined as vaginal bleeding >12 months after menstruation has stopped due to menopause. Other symptoms include:

- Abnormal vaginal bleeding (irregular/heavy) in young women
- Abnormal vaginal discharge/pyometra
- Abdominal pain
- Haematuria.

> Unexplained inter-menstrual bleeding in premenopausal women may also be a symptom of endometrial cancer and warrants investigation.
> Be aware that haematuria, vaginal discharge, and vaginal/rectal bleeding are not always easily differentiated by patients.

Examination

- Abdominal examination
- Bimanual examination: uterine size, adnexal masses
- Speculum examination: rule out other causes of bleeding (vaginal or vulval lesions).

Investigations

Bloods

- FBC, U&E, LFT, glucose.

Imaging

- Consider transvaginal USS
  - Endometrial thickness <4mm indicates a very low risk of endometrial pathology in postmenopausal women.

2WW referrals

- Refer women if aged ≥55 years with PMB
- Consider referring women if <55 years with PMB
- Consider direct access USS to assess for endometrial cancer in women >55 years with:
  - Abnormal vaginal discharge who have thrombocytosis or haematuria
  - Frank haematuria who have anaemia or thrombocytosis or high blood glucose.

Cervical cancer

Overview

Cervical intraepithelial neoplasia is a precursor lesion for cervical cancer and needs persistent infection with human papillomavirus (HPV) to develop. About 3000 new cervical cancers are diagnosed each year in the UK, of which 75% are due to the national screening programme. Five-year survival is approximately 65%.

History

Risk factors

- High-risk HPV infection:
  - Multiple partners ↑ risk of exposure
  - Associated with combined oral contraceptive pill use (believed to be secondary to replacing barrier method)
- Smoking
- Immunocompromise.

Symptoms

- Intermenstrual bleeding
- Postcoital bleeding
- Abnormal vaginal discharge.

Examination

- Abdominal examination
- Bimanual/speculum examination: cervical appearance.

Investigations

Screening

- 3-yearly for women aged 25–50 years; if normal, 5-yearly for women aged 50–64 years.

2WW referrals

- A cervix consistent with the appearance of a cervical cancer should be referred

Vulval cancer

Overview

Vulval cancers are uncommon with around 1000 new cases diagnosed in the UK each year. The majority are squamous cell carcinomas (90%) and the rest are made up of vulval melanomas, Bartholin's gland carcinoma, and sarcomas. Median age at presentation is 74 years.

History

Aetiology

- Patients may have a background of lichen sclerosis or vulval intraepithelial neoplasia.

Symptoms

- Lump, pain, irritation, or bleeding.

Examination

- Inspection of vulva: ulceration (full examination may be too painful!)
- Examine for groin lymphadenopathy.

2WW referrals

- Refer to gynaecology for biopsy if a vulval lump is found on examination or there is ulceration or bleeding.

Vaginal cancer

Overview

Over 250 new vaginal cancers are diagnosed each year in the UK accounting for 1% of all gynaecological cancers. Most lesions found are metastases from other gynaecological malignancies (uterine, cervix, vulva).

History

Risk factors

- Pelvic radiotherapy, long-term inflammation (vaginal pessary, procidentia).

Examination

- Palpable mass or ulceration in the vagina or at the introitus.

2WW referrals

- Refer to gynaecology for biopsy if any suspicion on examination.

Chapter 104

Haematological cancers

Guideline:
NICE NG12 (Suspected cancer: recognition and referral): https://www.nice.org.uk/guidance/ng12

OUP disclaimer: Oxford University Press makes no representation, express or implied, that the drug dosages are correct and that the recommendations are an exclusive or mandatory course of care. All health professionals reading this text have a responsibility to evaluate its appropriateness and take the individual needs of the patient into account.

Local trust guidelines: please refer to your local guidelines as necessary.

Overview

Haematological cancers can present at any age with non-specific symptoms, so vigilance is key. Haematological cancers in children are covered in Chapter 102.

Diagnosis

Differential diagnosis

Haematological cancers include:

- Leukaemia
- Myeloma
- Hodgkin's lymphoma
- Non-Hodgkin's lymphoma.

History and examination

The key features in the history and examination that should raise suspicion of haematological cancer are described in Table 104.1.

Investigations

Bedside

- Pyrexia is common
- Tachycardia (suggests anaemia)
- Hypotension (e.g. due to intercurrent sepsis).

Bloods

- If suspecting leukaemia, a FBC is required within 48 hours (Note in leukaemia, the high number of malignant white cells may give an elevated white cell count. However, these cells are not useful in fighting infection and as such patents may be functionally neutropenic.)
- If suspecting myeloma, perform a FBC, calcium, and plasma viscosity or ESR:
  - If any of these investigations support a diagnosis of myeloma then send an urgent protein electrophoresis and urine Bence Jones protein
  - Serum-free light-chain assay is also being used increasingly to test for myeloma.

Imaging

- A skeletal survey may be requested when working up a patient with suspected myeloma
- CT or ultrasound can be useful to identify lymph nodes for biopsy in suspected lymphoma
- CT staging is required for the MDT to plan treatment in lymphoma.

Other

- Bone marrow aspirate and biopsy is required in most cases of haematological malignancy.

Call for help?

- If the patient presents acutely unwell, escalate early and seek senior advice.

Table 104.1 Clinical features raising suspicion of haematological cancer

	Differential diagnosis			
	Leukaemia	Myeloma	Hodgkin's lymphoma	Non-Hodgkin's lymphoma
Clinical features	• Pallor • Persistent fatigue • Unexplained fever • Unexplained persistent infection • Generalized lymphadenopathy • Unexplained bruising, bleeding, or petechiae • Hepatosplenomegaly	In people aged >60 years: • Persistent bone pain • Persistent back pain • Unexplained fracture	• Unexplained lymphadenopathy Also take into account history of: • Fever • Night sweats • Shortness of breath • Pruritis • Weight loss • Alcohol-induced lymph node pain	• Unexplained lymphadenopathy • Unexplained splenomegaly Also take into account history of: • Fever • Night sweats • Shortness of breath • Pruritis • Weight loss
Initial management	Send FBC within 48 hours	• Send FBC, calcium, and plasma viscosity or ESR • Send electrophoresis and Bence Jones protein within 48 hours if bloods show hypercalcaemia or leucopenia, or if plasma viscosity/ESR is consistent with myeloma		
2WW referral		Refer as a 2WW if electrophoresis or Bence Jones protein is suggestive of myeloma	Consider a 2WW referral for any of the above symptoms	Consider a 2WW referral for any of the above-listed symptoms

Complications

- Sepsis, including neutropenic sepsis (see Chapters 121 and 122)
- Symptomatic anaemia
- Bleeding due to thrombocytopenia (see Chapter 94)
- Thrombosis, including venous sinus thrombosis, due to high plasma viscosity
- Tumour lysis syndrome
- Pericardial effusion in lymphoma
- Cauda equina syndrome due to vertebral fracture in myeloma (see Chapter 53).

All these presentations should be managed as per local/national guidelines and senior help sought early.

Further reading

1. Provan D, Baglin T, Dokal I, et al. (2015). *Oxford Handbook of Clinical Haematology*, 4th ed. Oxford: Oxford University Press. Available at: https://doi.org/10.1093/med/9780199683307.001.0001

Chapter 105

Head and neck cancers

Guideline:
NICE NG12 (Suspected cancer: recognition and referral): https://www.nice.org.uk/guidance/ng12/

OUP disclaimer: Oxford University Press makes no representation, express or implied, that the drug dosages are correct and that the recommendations are an exclusive or mandatory course of care. All health professionals reading this text have a responsibility to evaluate its appropriateness and take the individual needs of the patient into account.

Local trust guidelines: please refer to your local guidelines as necessary.

Overview

Over 11,000 new oral, laryngeal, and thyroid cancers are diagnosed in the UK each year. A significant proportion of these present late.

Unlike many other cancers, the incidence rates of head and neck cancers have been steadily increasing in the UK and have ↑ by a fifth in the last decade.

Diagnosis

Risk factors

See Table 105.1.

Table 105.1 Risk factors for head and neck cancers

Smoking and chewing tobacco	64% of laryngeal cancers and 17% of oral cancers are caused by smoking in the UK[1]
Alcohol	Risk increases with increasing alcohol use and duration of alcohol excess
Age	The most common age group for presentation is 70–74 years
Sex	Laryngeal and oral cancers are more common in men Thyroid cancers are more common in women
Viruses	Some tongue and oropharyngeal cancers are linked to human papillomavirus (HPV) infection Rarely, nasopharyngeal cancers are linked to Epstein–Barr virus (EBV)
Immuno-suppression	↑ risk in patients with prolonged immunosuppression
Diet lacking in fruit and vegetables	Linked with approximately 50% of oral cancer cases[1]
Occupational risk	Prolonged exposure to hardwood dust, leather dust, or formaldehyde

Criteria for two-week wait referrals

Laryngeal cancer

Any patient >45 years with:

- Persistent unexplained hoarseness **OR**
- An unexplained lump in the neck.

Oral cancer

Patient of any age with:

- An unexplained ulcer in the oral cavity lasting >3 weeks
- A persistent and unexplained lump in the neck (*persistent meaning longer than would be expected for a self-limiting condition, e.g. reactive lymphadenopathy*)
- A lump on the lip or in the oral cavity
- A red or red/white patch in the oral cavity consistent with erythroplakia (Box 105.1).

Box 105.1 Erythroplakia

An erythematous area of oral mucous membrane which is not associated with any other oral condition, e.g. a burn. These areas may be smooth or irregular, but tend to be painless and have well-demarcated margins. Areas of erythroplakia commonly contain dysplasia, carcinoma *in situ*, or carcinoma on histological examination.

1 Cancer Research UK. Head and neck cancers statistics. Available at: https://www.cancerresearchuk.org/health-professional/cancer-statistics/statistics-by-cancer-type/head-and-neck-cancers. Accessed October 2022

Thyroid cancer

- Any patient with an unexplained thyroid lump.

Differential diagnosis

See Table 105.2.

Table 105.2 Differential diagnoses of neck lumps and abnormal oral mucosa

Neck lump	**Lymph node:** • Inflammatory (cervical adenitis) in response to local infection • Infective (e.g. TB) • Malignant (metastasis or lymphoma) **Other:** • Benign neoplasm—lipoma, fibroma, neuroma, etc. • Neck abscess • Congenital anomalies—thyroglossal cysts, branchial cysts, fistulae, sinuses • Carotid body aneurysm • Salivary gland—fibrosis or malignancy • Thyroid—goitre, adenoma, cyst, malignancy • Parathyroid—adenoma, cyst, malignancy
Abnormal oral mucosa	• Oral cancer or erythroplakia • Aphthous ulcers • Lichen planus • Pemphigus • Trauma • Infection—candidiasis, deep fungal infection, herpes stomatitis, cytomegalovirus, TB, syphilis (chancre), 'hand, foot, and mouth' infection • Behçet's syndrome • Nutritional deficiency—iron, folate • Drug-related ulcers • Oral hypersensitivity reactions

Investigations

Investigations to confirm diagnosis

- Thyroid or neck lumps: USS or CT
- For oral or throat symptoms/lesions: direct visualization with nasendoscopy, transnasal flexible laryngo-oesophagoscopy, or examination under anaesthetic
- Biopsy: biopsies may be taken using ultrasound guidance or with direct visualization.

Investigations to assess stage

- Imaging may include X-ray, CT, MRI, or CT-PET depending on the type and location of the malignancy.

Management

Management options

See Table 105.3.

Table 105.3 Management options for head and neck cancers

Surgery	Some excisions may be extensive, requiring reconstructive surgery including skin grafts and bone flaps and/or may cause a loss of function, e.g. facial weakness
Radiotherapy	Radiotherapy may be used alone for small cancers, or in combination with surgery, chemotherapy, or biological therapies
Chemotherapy	
Biological therapies	

Further reading

1. NICE Clinical Knowledge Summaries (2021). Head and neck cancers; recognition and referral. Available at: https://cks.nice.org.uk/head-and-neck-cancers-recognition-and-referral#!topic Summary
2. Cancer Research UK. Head and neck cancer statistics. Available at: https://www.cancerresearchuk.org/health-professional/cancer-statistics/statistics-by-cancer-type/head-and-neck-cancers
3. Macmillan. Head and neck cancers. Available at: https://www.macmillan.org.uk/information-and-support/head-and-neck-cancers
4. WHO International Agency for Research on Cancer. A digital manual for the early diagnosis of oral neoplasia: erythroplakia. [For more information on erythroplakia with typical images.] Available at: https://screening.iarc.fr/atlasoral_list.php?cat=A3&lang=1

Chapter 106

Lower gastrointestinal cancers

Guidelines:
NICE NG151 (Colorectal cancer diagnosis and management): https://www.nice.org.uk/guidance/ng151

NICE NG12 (Suspected cancer: recognition and referral): https://www.nice.org.uk/guidance/ng12

OUP disclaimer: Oxford University Press makes no representation, express or implied, that the drug dosages are correct and that the recommendations are an exclusive or mandatory course of care. All health professionals reading this text have a responsibility to evaluate its appropriateness and take the individual needs of the patient into account.

Local trust guidelines: please refer to your local guidelines as necessary.

Overview

Colorectal cancer is the fourth most common cancer in the UK, accounting for 12% of all new cancer cases. It is the second most common cause of death in the UK, accounting for 10% of all cancer deaths. Adenocarcinomas make up the majority of colorectal cancers.

Diagnosis

History

Early stages of colorectal cancer are often asymptomatic and are discovered on routine screening. Symptoms of colorectal cancers are variable and often depend on the tumour site (Table 106.1).

Table 106.1 Symptoms of lower GI cancer

Right-sided/ caecal cancers	Left-sided/sigmoid cancers	Rectal cancer	Metastatic spread
Mass in right iliac fossa	Mass in left iliac fossa	Rectal bleeding	Jaundice
Iron deficiency anaemia	Abdominal pain	Mucus and discharge	Ascites
Weight loss	Rectal bleeding		Pain
Change in bowel habit	Change in bowel habit		Weight loss
	Tenesmus		
	Weight loss		

Specialist referral

Refer to the suspected cancer pathway referral (appointment within 2 weeks) if one of the following is present:

- Rectal/abdominal mass
- Unexplained anal mass or unexplained anal ulceration
- Tests showing positive occult blood
- ≥40 years with unexplained weight loss **AND** abdominal pain
- ≥50 years with unexplained rectal bleeding
- ≥60 years with iron deficiency anaemia **OR** changes in bowel habit.

Consider referring if <50 years old with rectal bleeding **AND** any unexplained abdominal pain/change in bowel habit/weight loss/iron deficiency anaemia

Risk factors

- Old age
- Diet high in red meat, processed meat, and fat
- Alcohol excess
- Family history of bowel cancer or polyps
- Inherited genetic conditions: hereditary non-polyposis colorectal cancer, familial adenomatous polyposis, and Lynch syndrome
- Past medical history of colorectal polyps or pre-existing inflammatory bowel disease.

Examination

- Fresh blood per rectum
- Abdominal/rectal/anal mass
- Anaemia
- Cachexia.

Investigations

Screening

Offer faecal immunochemical test (FIT) (a quantitative faecal occult bloods) if:

- ≥50 years with unexplained abdominal pain **OR** weight loss
- <60 years with changes in bowel habit **OR** iron deficiency anaemia
- ≥60 years with anaemia, even if non-iron deficient.

Bloods

- FBC, haematinics, U&E, calcium, LFT, coagulation profile
- Tumour markers (carcinoembryonic antigen (CEA) and CA 19-9).

Invasive

- Colonoscopy is used as first line and biopsies are often taken for histological diagnosis
- Flexible sigmoidoscopy and barium enema can be used for patients with major comorbidities
- CT colonography can sometimes be used as an alternative investigation. If a suspicious lesion is seen, a colonoscopy and biopsy should then be offered.

Staging

If cancer is confirmed, further imaging is needed for staging:

- CT of the chest, abdomen, and pelvis with contrast to assess for invasion to lymph nodes or metastasis to other organs
- MRI to assess the risk of local recurrence in patients with rectal cancer
- Endorectal ultrasound for patients with rectal cancer if MRI shows disease amenable to local excision or if MRI is contraindicated.

Acute management

All cases of lower GI cancers should be discussed within the MDT.

Pharmacological management

- Short-course preoperative radiotherapy or chemoradiotherapy should be considered for moderate or high-risk operable rectal cancer
- Preoperative chemotherapy should also be considered for T4 colon cancer (where the tumour has breached the outer lining of the bowel)
- Adjuvant chemotherapy is often used after surgery for stage 2 or 3 colon or rectal cancer
- Palliative chemotherapy should be considered for advanced or metastatic disease. This may comprise systemic or oral therapies.

Surgical management

- Local resection if amenable
- Colectomy (total/partial) with colostomy/ileostomy. Laparoscopic resection can also be used if appropriate
- Transanal excision/endoscopic submucosal dissection/total mesorectal excision for rectal cancer
- In metastatic disease, anatomical site-specific multidisciplinary meetings should consider if resection is possible and would be appropriate
- Colonic stents may be used to relieve left-sided bowel obstruction.

Psychosocial considerations

- Offer patients information about the likelihood of having a stoma post surgery. A referral to a stoma nurse for support on how to care for a stoma may be needed
- Inform patients that bowel function may alter after treatment. They may experience symptoms of incontinence, diarrhoea, bloating, mucous discharge, or difficulty emptying bowels. Patients may have to change their eating habits to help reduce symptoms
- Sexual function may be disturbed
- Treatments may result in chronic pain or side effects such as neuropathy
- Treatments may cause cognitive or emotional changes such as anxiety, depression, or chemotherapy-related cognitive impairment.

Complications

- Bowel obstruction
- Metastasis
- Liver failure
- Bleeding
- Colovesical fistula.

Monitoring and follow-up

Following potentially curative surgical treatment for non-metastatic cancer:

- Follow up for the first 3 years
- This should include CT scans of the chest, abdomen, and pelvis, and serum CEA tests.

Further reading

1. Cancer Research UK. Bowel cancer. Available at: https://www.cancerresearchuk.org/about-cancer/bowel-cancer
2. Oxford Medical Education. Colorectal cancer. Available at: http://www.oxfordmedicaleducation.com/oncology/colorectal-cancer/

Chapter 107

Lung cancer

Guideline:
NICE NG12 (Suspected cancer: recognition and referral): https://www.nice.org.uk/guidance/ng12

OUP disclaimer: Oxford University Press makes no representation, express or implied, that the drug dosages are correct and that the recommendations are an exclusive or mandatory course of care. All health professionals reading this text have a responsibility to evaluate its appropriateness and take the individual needs of the patient into account.

Local trust guidelines: please refer to your local guidelines as necessary.

Overview

Lung cancer is the third most common cancer in the UK with approximately 45,000 new cases diagnosed each year.

Non-small cell cancers (85%)

- Adenocarcinoma arising from bronchial mucosal glands (most common)
- Squamous cell carcinoma arising from bronchial respiratory epithelial cells, typically occurring in the centre of the lungs
- Large cell carcinoma
- Undifferentiated.

Small cell cancer ('oat-cell') (15%)

- These arise from endocrine cells. They tend to be aggressive and metastasize early.

Mesothelioma

- A rare cancer that arises from the pleura, or very occasionally from the peritoneum.

Diagnosis

History

Patients are often asymptomatic until the disease is advanced. The symptoms listed in Fig. 107.1 may be suggestive of lung cancer. Smoking is the most important risk factor (see Box 107.1).

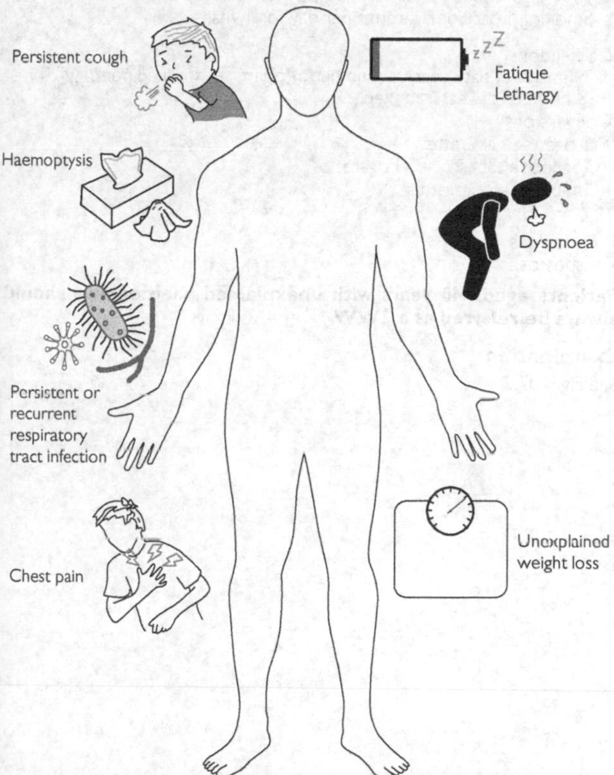

Fig. 107.1 Symptoms of lung cancer.

Ask about occupational exposures as several are known to predispose to the development of lung cancers, e.g.:

- Isocyanates (chemical fumes, especially in the rubber industry)
- Polycyclic hydrocarbons (from burning wood and coal)
- Heavy metals and iron oxides

Box 107.1 Smoking and calculating pack years

Smoking is the most significant risk factor for the development of lung cancer, being responsible for up to 90% of cases. An accurate smoking history should be elicited.

1 pack year can be thought of as:

- 7300 cigarettes smoked, i.e. 20 cigarettes per day **OR**
- Smoking 1 pack of cigarettes per day for 1 year.

Calculation:

Number of pack years = (number of cigarettes smoked per day/20) × number of years smoked

Conversions:

- 1 cigar = 4 cigarettes
- 25g loose tobacco = 50 cigarettes[1]
- 1 pipe = 2.5 cigarettes.

- Radon gas
- Asbestos.

Patients aged >40 years with unexplained haemoptysis should always be referred as a 2WW.

Examination

See Fig. 107.2.

1 Wood DM, Mould MG, Ong SBY, et al. 'Pack year' smoking histories: what about patients who use loose tobacco? *Tob Control*. 2005; 14:141–2.

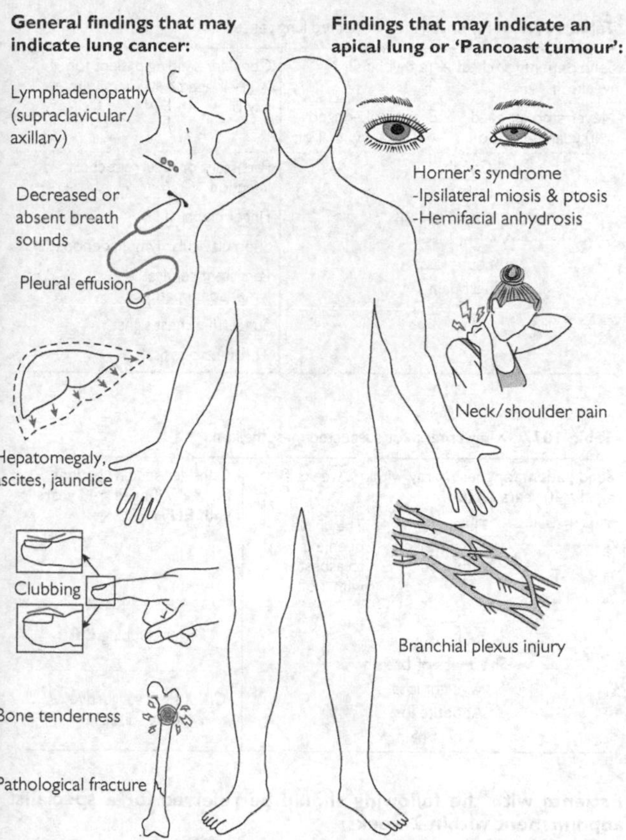

Fig. 107.2 Possible examination findings in lung cancer.

Investigations

Bloods

- FBC may demonstrate anaemia and thrombocytosis.

Imaging

Perform a chest X-ray within 2 weeks if lung cancer is suspected (Table 107.1 and Table 107.2).

Table 107.1 X-ray criteria for suspected lung cancer

Send patient for chest X-ray within 2 weeks if:		Consider sending patient for X-ray if aged >40 years with any of:
Never smoker aged >40 years with 2 of:	Ever smoker aged >40 years with 1 of:	
Cough Fatigue Shortness of breath Weight loss Appetite loss Chest pain		Persistent or recurrent chest infection Finger clubbing Supraclavicular lymphadenopathy Persistent cervical lymphadenopathy Suggestive chest signs Thrombocytosis

Table 107.2 X-ray criteria for suspected mesothelioma

Send patient for chest X-ray within 2 weeks if aged >40 years **AND:**			Consider sending patient for X-ray if aged >40 years with **EITHER:**
They have 2 of:	They have ever smoked with 1 of:	They have been exposed to asbestos with 1 of:	
Cough Fatigue Shortness of breath Weight loss Appetite loss Chest pain			Finger clubbing **OR** Chest signs suggestive of pleural disease

Patients with the following should be referred for a specialist appointment within 2 weeks:

- Chest X-ray findings suggestive of lung cancer **OR**
- Aged >40 years with unexplained haemoptysis.

CT is often required to further assess lesions identified on chest X-ray, and PET is used to radiologically stage the disease.

Other

- Pulmonary function tests and cardiopulmonary exercise testing are used to assess patient suitability for further treatments including radiotherapy and surgical resection
- Tissue biopsy is required to confirm the type of malignancy and allows molecular profiling to determine treatment options and prognosis. Samples may be obtained via thoracoscopy, bronchoscopy, and lymph node biopsy.

Management

Lifestyle and simple interventions

- Ongoing cigarette smoking worsens outcomes after treatment. Offer nicotine replacement therapy and referral to smoking cessation services.

Pharmacological management

- Immunotherapy or targeted therapy may be used with either curative or palliative intent. It may be used as an adjunct to radiotherapy and/or surgery.

Surgical management

- Surgical resection by segmentectomy, lobectomy, or pneumonectomy may be possible.

Psychosocial considerations

Prior to referral, patients should be informed that the purpose of referral is to investigate for suspected cancer, but they can be reassured that in most cases cancer is not found.

If a diagnosis of cancer is made, patients should be offered as much or as little information regarding their prognosis as they want.

A confirmed diagnosis of any cancer is a significant event psychologically and emotionally for patients, their relatives, and carers. Information should be provided in person wherever possible—avoid providing new information in letters or by the phone.

Dedicated cancer care nurses should provide additional support.

Complications

- Hypercalcaemia of malignancy—most commonly occurs in squamous cell carcinoma (see Chapter 16).
- Hypertrophic pulmonary osteoarthropathy—a rare complication of adenocarcinoma characterized by digital clubbing, painful large joint arthritis (often the wrists), and periostitis.
- Effects of local tumour invasion:
  - Nerve injury (brachial plexus, recurrent laryngeal nerve, phrenic nerve)
  - Vascular injury (compression, e.g. superior vena cava syndrome, or erosion leading to bleeding)
  - Airway obstruction.

Prognosis

- Prognosis remains poor; 5-year survival is around 10%.

Special considerations

- Occupational lung diseases, such as mesothelioma, may entitle patients to financial compensation
- All deaths from mesothelioma must be referred to the local Coroner's office.

Further reading

1. Cancer Research UK. Lung cancer. Available at: https://www.cancerresearchuk.org/about-cancer/lung-cancer

Chapter 108

Sarcomas

Guideline:
NICE NG12 (Suspected cancer: recognition and referral): https://www.nice.org.uk/guidance/ng12/

OUP disclaimer: Oxford University Press makes no representation, express or implied, that the drug dosages are correct and that the recommendations are an exclusive or mandatory course of care. All health professionals reading this text have a responsibility to evaluate its appropriateness and take the individual needs of the patient into account.

Local trust guidelines: please refer to your local guidelines as necessary.

Overview

Sarcomas are rare, malignant, connective tissue tumours. They can be divided into sarcomas of the bone and of soft tissues. Sarcomas in children are covered in Chapter 102 on childhood cancers.

Differential diagnosis

See Table 108.1

Table 108.1 Differential diagnosis of sarcoma

Bone sarcoma	Malignant tumours: • Osteosarcoma • Giant cell tumour • Ewing's sarcoma • Chondrosarcoma • Malignant fibrous histiocytoma • Chordoma • Secondary bone tumour Benign tumours: • Osteochondroma • Osteoid osteoma • Chondroma • Fibrous dysplasia of bone
Soft tissue sarcoma	• Lipoma • Lymphoma • Metastatic carcinoma • Neuroma

History and examination

See Table 108.2.

Table 108.2 History and examination findings of sarcoma

Tumour type	Symptoms	Signs
Bone sarcoma	• Bone pain (particularly at night) • Bone swelling • Symptoms of metastases (often to lung or other bones)	• Swelling • Tenderness • Pathological fracture
Soft tissue sarcoma	• Painless lump increasing in size	• Pain/tenderness from muscle or nerve compression • Size of mass >5cm • Mass increasing in size • Located below deep fascia

Red flags

General symptoms of malignancy:

- Weight loss
- Anorexia
- Lethargy
- Night sweats.

Investigations

Bloods

- FBC: check for infection and anaemia
- U&E
- CRP: may be raised in malignancy
- Bone profile: raised calcium may be an indicator of primary disease or metastases
- LFT: may be deranged with metastases.

Imaging

- X-ray if unexplained bone pain or swelling (consider requesting urgently)
- Ultrasound within 2 weeks if unexplained, enlarging soft tissue lump
- Chest X-ray, and CT chest, abdomen, and pelvis may be required for staging after confirmed diagnosis.

Specialist referral

All patients with suspected sarcoma should be referred to a specialist sarcoma MDT.

Referral criteria:

- X-ray findings suggestive of sarcoma
- Ultrasound findings suggestive of sarcoma or inconclusive with ongoing suspicion.

Management

Bone sarcoma

- Complete surgical resection of the tumour (ideally with limb preservation) and chemotherapy is first line. Amputation may be required
- Pre- and postoperative adjuvant chemotherapy and radiotherapy may increase long-term survival
- Radiotherapy may also be used for Ewing's sarcoma and palliation of other incurable bone sarcoma.

Soft tissue sarcoma

- Surgical excision of the tumour with localized wide excision is first line
- Adjuvant chemotherapy ± radiotherapy may be considered for larger tumours to assist surgical removal.

Further reading

1. Sarcoma UK website. Available at: https://sarcoma.org.uk
2. Baldwin A (ed) (2020). *Oxford Handbook of Clinical Specialties*, 11th ed. Oxford: Oxford University Press. Available at: https://doi.org/10.1093/med/9780198827191.001.0001
3. Dangoor A, Seddon B, Gerrand C, et al. (2016). UK guidelines for the management of soft tissue sarcomas. *Clin Sarcoma Res*. 6:20.
4. Gerrand C, Athanasou N, Brennan B, et al. (2016). UK guidelines for the management of bone sarcomas. *Clin Sarcoma Res*. 6:7.
5. NICE (2006). Improving outcomes for people with sarcoma (CSG9). Available at: https://www.nice.org.uk/guidance/csg9

Chapter 109

Skin cancers

Guideline:
NICE NG12 (Suspected cancer: recognition and referral): https://www.nice.org.uk/guidance/ng12/

OUP disclaimer: Oxford University Press makes no representation, express or implied, that the drug dosages are correct and that the recommendations are an exclusive or mandatory course of care. All health professionals reading this text have a responsibility to evaluate its appropriateness and take the individual needs of the patient into account.

Local trust guidelines: please refer to your local guidelines as necessary.

Overview

The UK sees >13,000 diagnoses of malignant melanoma, 25,000 diagnoses of squamous cell carcinoma, and 75,000 diagnoses of basal cell carcinoma per year. Diagnosis can be difficult as skin cancers can appear like many benign conditions, but early diagnosis can be life-saving. Malignant melanoma has a worse prognosis owing to its propensity to metastasize.

Diagnosis

Differential diagnosis

See Table 109.1.

Table 109.1 Differential diagnosis of skin cancer

Skin cancer diagnosis	Possible differential diagnoses
Malignant melanoma	• Benign melanocytic lesions • Non-melanocytic pigmented lesions, e.g. seborrheic keratoses, dermatofibromas, pigmented basal cell carcinomas, lentigines, freckles
Squamous cell carcinoma	• Bowen's disease • Actinic keratoses • Basal cell carcinoma • Malignant melanoma • Keratoacanthoma
Basal cell carcinoma	• Cutaneous squamous cell carcinoma • Keratoacanthoma

History and examination

Malignant melanoma

Pigmented skin lesion demonstrating (Fig. 109.1):

- **A**symmetry
- **B**order irregularity
- **C**olour irregularity
- **D**iameter >7mm
- **E**volution over time
- Inflammation
- Discharge from the lesion
- Change in sensation.

Squamous cell carcinoma

Raised or macular lesion demonstrating (Fig. 109.2):

- Persistent ulceration
- Scale or crust
- Irregular shape
- Bleeding
- Pain.

Basal cell carcinoma

Nodular lesion, often found on sun-exposed areas, e.g. nose, demonstrating (Fig. 109.3 and Fig. 109.4):

- Central induration
- Pearly edge
- Telangiectasia
- Slow growth.

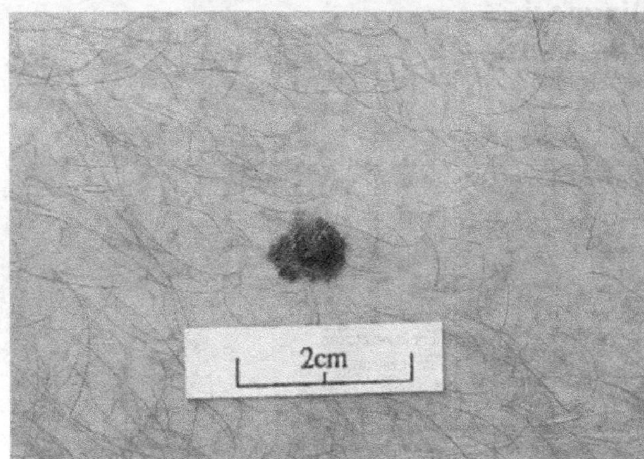

Fig. 109.1 Superficial spreading melanoma.

Reproduced from Firth J, Conlon C, and Cox T (2020) 'Oxford Textbook of Medicine 6th edition' Oxford University Press: Oxford, with permission from Oxford University Press. See colour plate 6.

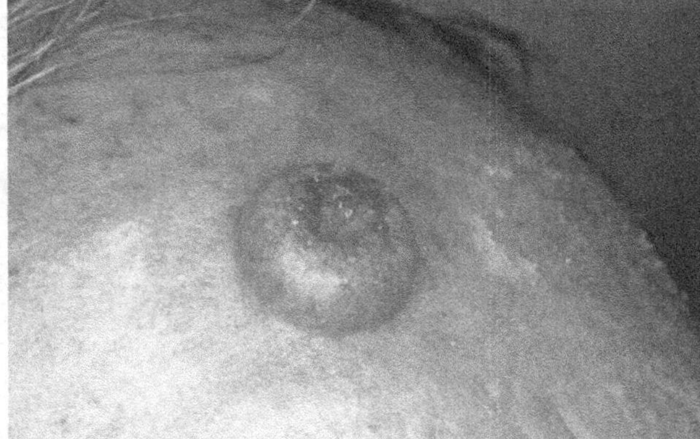

Fig. 109.2 Squamous cell carcinoma presenting as a nodule.

Reproduced from Firth J, Conlon C, and Cox T (2020) 'Oxford Textbook of Medicine 6th edition' Oxford University Press: Oxford, with permission from Oxford University Press. See colour plate 7.

Investigations

Investigations for pigmented skin lesions should be carried out by specialists trained in the diagnosis of skin cancer:

- Dermoscopy: should be conducted for all pigmented or suspicious lesions

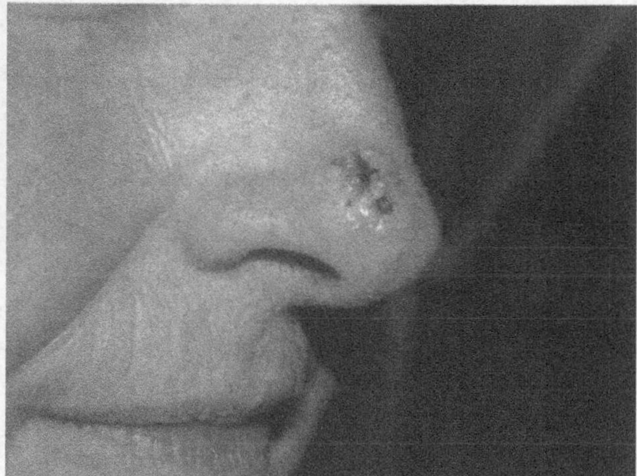

Fig. 109.3 Morphoeic basal cell carcinoma.

Reproduced from Gosney M and Harris T (2009) "Managing Older People in Primary Care: A Practical Guide' Oxford University Press, with permission from Oxford University Press. See colour plate 8.

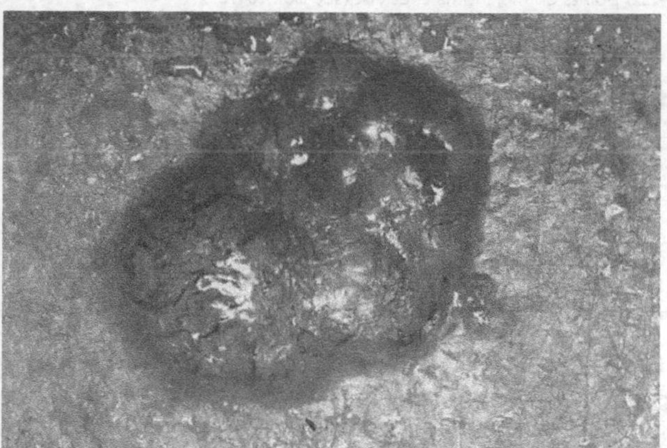

Fig. 109.4 Basal cell carcinoma. See colour plate 9.

- Photography: to be conducted as a baseline for atypical lesions not requiring immediate excision. Lesions can then be followed up at 3 months to determine early changes that would indicate melanoma
- Sentinel lymph node biopsy: to be offered to patients with stage IB–IIC malignant melanoma with a Breslow thickness of >1mm. This acts as a staging procedure to determine if there has been spread to lymph nodes.

Acute management

Referral

Referral must be made to a dermatologist or plastic surgeon with a knowledge and understanding of skin cancer. Information which should be included in the referral is listed in Box 109.1.

Box 109.1 Information about lesion to be included in referral

- Site
- Size
- Shape
- Pigmentation
- Duration of lesion
- Changes (evolution of lesion)
- Symptoms such as bleeding, pustular exudate, and change in sensation
- Palpable lymph nodes
- Patient risk factors for malignancy
- Systemic symptoms.

Malignant melanoma

Appointment within 2 weeks if:

- Dermoscopy indicates melanoma
- ≥3 points on melanoma checklist (see Box 109.2)

Box 109.2 Malignant melanoma referral checklist

Give 2 points for a major feature, and 1 point for a minor feature of the lesion.

Major features:

- Size change
- Irregularity of shape
- Irregularity of pigmentation.

Minor features:

- Largest diameter ≥7mm
- Inflammation
- Oozing
- Altered sensation.

Consider referring if there are suspicious nail changes (any new pigmented line in a nail, or growing under a nail) or any non-resolving skin lesions.

Squamous cell carcinoma

- Appointment within 2 weeks if there is any skin lesion which is suspicious for squamous cell carcinoma.

Basal cell carcinoma

- Appointment within 2 weeks if there is a skin lesion which is suspicious for basal cell carcinoma and that requires urgent management due to factors such as size or location of the lesion, where delay could lead to an adverse impact
- Otherwise, a routine appointment is appropriate.

Chronic management

Patient education

All patients diagnosed with skin cancer should have access to a skin cancer nurse specialist throughout treatment and follow-up in order to aid in the provision of information, psychological support, and palliation if required. They may also be able to advise on local support groups.

Management options

The treatment of skin cancer should be discussed in a MDT which may include a dermatologist, a plastic surgeon, a histopathologist, and a nurse specialist among others. Treatment should be decided upon following discussion with the patient, enabling a full understanding of the options available.

Malignant melanoma

The treatment of malignant melanoma is dependent on stage at diagnosis (Table 109.2).[1]

Table 109.2 Treatment of malignant melanoma

Stage at diagnosis	Potential treatments
0–II (local only)	• Excision • Topical imiquimod
III (nodal spread)	• Excision • Lymph node removal • Chemotherapy • Intralesional treatment • Immunotherapy • Systemic gene-targeted therapy
IV (with metastases)	• Excision • Lymph node removal • Chemotherapy • Intralesional treatment • Immunotherapy • Systemic gene-targeted therapy • Radiotherapy to metastases • Palliative treatment, e.g. palliative surgery

Once diagnosed, it may be helpful to test vitamin D levels as vitamin D deficiency is associated with a worse prognosis.[2] Genetic testing may also be offered if targeted systemic therapy is an option in unresectable or metastatic tumours.

Squamous cell carcinoma

Squamous cell carcinomas are most often managed with surgical excision.

1 Cancer Research UK. Melanoma skin cancer: treatment. 2020. Available at: https://www.cancerresearchuk.org/about-cancer/melanoma/treatment

2 Timerman D, McEnery-Stonelake M, Joyce CJ, et al. Vitamin D deficiency is associated with a worse prognosis in metastatic melanoma. *Oncotarget*. 2016; 8:6873–82.

Basal cell carcinoma

Potential treatments for the management of basal cell carcinoma include:

- Chemotherapy (topical)
- Curettage
- Surgical excision
- Cryotherapy
- Radiotherapy.

Follow-up

Follow-up of skin cancer is dependent on the type and stage of skin cancer and treatment provided. For malignant melanoma, consider whether the patient may have an underlying condition, e.g. atypical mole syndrome, or a family history of a first-degree relative with melanoma which means they require closer follow-up.

Further reading

1. NICE Clinical Knowledge Summaries (2017). Melanoma and pigmented lesions. Available at: https://cks.nice.org.uk/melanoma-and-pigmented-lesions#!topicSummary
2. NICE (2006, updated 2010). Improving outcomes for people with skin tumours including melanoma (CSG8): Available at: https://www.nice.org.uk/guidance/csg8
3. American Joint Committee on Cancer. Cancer staging. Available at: https://cancerstaging.org/references-tools/quickreferences/Pages/default.aspx

Chapter 110

Upper gastrointestinal cancers

Guideline:
NICE NG12 (Suspected cancer: recognition and referral): https://www.nice.org.uk/guidance/ng12

OUP disclaimer: Oxford University Press makes no representation, express or implied, that the drug dosages are correct and that the recommendations are an exclusive or mandatory course of care. All health professionals reading this text have a responsibility to evaluate its appropriateness and take the individual needs of the patient into account.

Local trust guidelines: please refer to your local guidelines as necessary.

Overview

Upper GI cancers frequently have poor prognoses since the presentation is often insidious and non-specific. Early recognition and referral is essential to allow suitable patients to undergo potentially curative surgery.

Oesophageal and stomach cancer

- Incidence: oesophageal, 9100 new cases a year; stomach, 6700 new cases a year (Cancer Research UK)
- Prognosis: oesophageal, 15% 5-year survival; stomach, 20% 5-year survival (all cancer stages, Cancer Research UK).

History

Potential symptoms:
- Dysphagia
- Upper abdominal pain
- Reflux
- Dyspepsia (see Chapter 30)
- Weight loss
- Nausea
- Vomiting.

Examination

- Upper abdominal mass, cachexia
- For stomach cancer, also Virchow's node (large left supraclavicular node) and acanthosis nigricans.

Investigations

Urgent 2WW referral for endoscopy criteria
- Dysphagia **OR**
- Age ≥55 years with weight loss **AND** upper abdominal pain/reflux/dyspepsia.

Routine referral for endoscopy criteria
- Haematemesis **OR**
- Age ≥55 years **AND**:
  - Treatment-resistant dyspepsia **OR**
  - Anaemia with upper abdominal pain **OR**
  - Raised platelet count with nausea/vomiting/weight loss/reflux/dyspepsia/upper abdominal pain **OR**
  - Nausea/vomiting with weight loss/reflux/dyspepsia/upper abdominal pain.

Pancreatic cancer

- Incidence: 10,000 cases a year (Cancer Research UK)
- Prognosis: 5% 5-year survival (all cancer stages, Cancer Research UK).

History

- Painless obstructive jaundice (head of pancreas tumours), epigastric pain radiating to the back (body and tail tumours), anorexia, weight loss, diabetes, pancreatitis.

Examination

- Jaundice and palpable gallbladder (Courvoisier's law), epigastric mass, hepatomegaly, splenomegaly, lymphadenopathy, ascites.

Investigations

Urgent 2WW referral

- Age ≥40 years with jaundice.

Urgent 2WW referral for CT (or ultrasound if CT not available) criteria

- Age ≥60 years **AND** weight loss **AND** any of:
    - Diarrhoea
    - Back pain
    - Abdominal pain
    - Nausea
    - Vomiting
    - Constipation
    - New-onset diabetes.

Gallbladder cancer

- Incidence: 1000 cases a year (Cancer Research UK)
- Prognosis: 15–20% 5-year survival (all cancer stages, Cancer Research UK).

History

- Early disease is often asymptomatic. May present with non-specific symptoms as the disease progresses—e.g. abdominal pain, nausea, vomiting.

Examination

- Upper abdominal mass—Courvoisier's law.

Investigations

Urgent 2WW referral for ultrasound criteria

- Palpable upper abdominal mass consistent with an enlarged gallbladder.

Liver cancer

- Incidence: 5900 cases per year (Cancer Research UK)
- Prognosis: 12% 5-year survival (all cancer stages, Cancer Research UK).

History

- Hepatocellular carcinoma: fatigue, anorexia, right upper quadrant pain, weight loss
- Cholangiocarcinoma: abdominal pain, fever, weight loss, malaise.

Examination

- Hepatomegaly, jaundice, ascites, right upper quadrant tenderness.

Investigations

Urgent 2WW referral for ultrasound criteria

- Palpable upper abdominal mass consistent with an enlarged liver.

Special considerations

Some patients might well fit into more than one of the referral categories previously described. A judgement call may be required as to which is the most appropriate pathway to use initially. More important is to judge the urgency of the referral so that the patient enters the secondary care system promptly.

Further reading

1. Cancer Research UK website. Available at: https://www.cancerresearchuk.org/

Chapter 111

Urological cancers

Guideline:
NICE NG12 (Suspected cancer: recognition and referral): https://www.nice.org.uk/guidance/ng12

OUP disclaimer: Oxford University Press makes no representation, express or implied, that the drug dosages are correct and that the recommendations are an exclusive or mandatory course of care. All health professionals reading this text have a responsibility to evaluate its appropriateness and take the individual needs of the patient into account.

Local trust guidelines: please refer to your local guidelines as necessary.

Overview

This chapter addresses the recognition and referral criteria for suspected prostate, bladder, renal, testicular, and penile cancer (Table 111.1). Prostate cancer is the most common malignancy in men, accounting for one-quarter of male cancer diagnoses (UK lifetime risk: one in six).

Table 111.1 Overview of urological cancers

Site	Histological type	Annual UK incidence	Risk factors	Diagnosis	5-year survival, %
Prostate	Majority adenocarcinoma	>40,000	• Afro-Caribbean ethnicity • BRCA	Image-guided biopsy	80
Bladder	Transitional cell carcinoma (90%) Squamous cell carcinoma	10,000	• Smoking • Aromatic amine exposure (industrial dyes, solvents, etc.) • Schistosomiasis (squamous cell tumours)	Cystoscopy + biopsy	55
Renal	Majority renal cell carcinoma	10,000	• Smoking • Obesity • Hypertension	Ultrasound Image-guided biopsy	55
Testicular	Seminoma Teratoma Yolk sac tumours	2000	• Cryptorchidism • Klinefelter's syndrome	Ultrasound	95
Penile	Squamous cell carcinoma May present as carcinoma *in situ*	500	• Human papillomavirus (HPV)—high risk subtypes, e.g. type 16, 18 • HIV infection	Excision biopsy	75

Diagnosis

History

Table 111.2 outlines common presenting features of urological cancers.

Table 111.2 Presenting features of urological cancers

Site	Presentation
Prostate	• Often asymptomatic • Lower urinary tract symptoms (voiding/storage): weak stream, hesitancy, frequency, urgency, urge incontinence, urinary retention (NB: overlap with BPE, see Chapter 97) • Visible haematuria • Erectile dysfunction • Features of metastatic disease, e.g. bone pain, pathological fractures
Bladder	• Visible haematuria • Lower urinary tract symptoms (storage predominant): dysuria, frequency
Renal	• Visible haematuria • Loin pain • Abdominal/flank mass • Recurrent UTI
Testicular	• Testicular mass/swelling
Penile	• Penile lesion: mass, ulceration • Persistent skin changes affecting the glans/foreskin

Systemic symptoms (anorexia, lethargy, weight loss, cachexia) are non-specific but may be present in locally advanced or disseminated disease.

Examination

- **Abdomen:** palpable bladder; flank mass
- **External genitalia:** testicular mass or scrotal swelling (varicocoele may occur with renal cancer); penile ulceration or mass; abnormal appearance of glans or foreskin (balanoposthitis)
- **DRE:** prostate assessment
- Consider lower limb **neurological assessment** (motor/sensory function, perineal sensation, anal tone) if any features raise suspicion of cauda equina syndrome secondary to metastatic disease (see Chapter 53)
- **Urinalysis:** haematuria (visible/non-visible), leucocytes/nitrites.

Investigations

- **Urine MC&S:** exclude UTI but consider that recurrent UTI may be a sign of bladder or renal cancer
- **Bloods: FBC** (raised white cell count can rarely occur due to a paraneoplastic syndrome in bladder cancer. Also anaemia of chronic disease); consider **PSA** testing in men with any lower urinary tract symptoms, erectile dysfunction, or visible haematuria (prostate cancer).

PSA false positives

Various factors affect PSA level (Table 111.3). Delaying testing is recommended after ejaculation/vigorous exercise (48 hours), DRE (1 week), treatment of UTI (4 weeks) (see 'Further reading').

Table 111.3 Factors affecting PSA levels

Increase PSA level	Reduce PSA level
BPE	5α-reductase inhibitors (finasteride, dutasteride)
Infection: UTI, prostatitis	
Physical factors: ejaculation, DRE, prostate biopsy, vigorous exercise	

- **Sexual health screen:** consider referral to genitourinary medicine or a specialist genital dermatology clinic (penile ulceration/ balanoposthitis)
- **Testicular USS:** consider for evaluation of scrotal mass/swelling. If there is a high index of suspicion for malignancy, do not delay referral.

Screening

- No population screening programme is in place for any urological cancer. Healthy, asymptomatic men >50 years may opt to have a PSA test following an informed discussion in primary care
- Information for patients and GPs to guide decision-making: Prostate Cancer Risk Management Programme (https://www.gov.uk/guidance/prostate-cancer-risk-management-programme-overview); Prostate Cancer UK (http://www.prostatecanceruk.org).

Management

Patient education

Prostate cancer: support shared decision-making about investigation, referral, and treatment. Many prostate cancers progress slowly and never cause symptoms or affect survival, while treatment may cause significant iatrogenic morbidity. Establish patient preference based on symptoms, clinical suspicion, comorbidities, and functional status.

Patients may opt for investigation with PSA testing and referral for further discussion about the advantages and disadvantages of investigation including biopsy, and subsequent treatment.

Specialist referral

Table 111.4 gives indications for urgent and routine referral for suspected urological cancers.

Haematuria may be a presenting symptom of malignancy at different sites (Table 111.2). Referral is typically to a haematuria clinic where dual investigation will take place for urological/renal pathology.

Table 111.4 Indications for urgent and routine referral for suspected urological cancer

Site	Urgent (2WW)	Consider further assessment or routine referral if:
Prostate	• Prostate feels malignant on DRE • Symptoms (see opposite) **AND** PSA level above upper limit of age-specific reference range Age <40 or >79 years: Use clinical judgement Age 40–49 years: >2.5micrograms/litre Age 50–59 years: ≥3.5 micrograms/litre Age 60–69 years: >4.5 micrograms/litre Age 70–79 years: >6.5 micrograms/litre	• Any lower urinary tract symptoms, e.g. nocturia, frequency, hesitancy, urgency, retention • Erectile dysfunction • Visible haematuria
Bladder	• Age ≥45 years **AND** unexplained visible haematuria after UTI excluded, or which persists/recurs after successful treatment of UTI • Age ≥60 years **AND** unexplained non-visible (dipstick) haematuria **AND** dysuria or raised white cell count	• Age ≥60 years **AND** recurrent/persistent unexplained UTI
Renal	• Age ≥45 years **AND** unexplained visible haematuria after UTI excluded, or which persists/recurs after successful treatment of UTI	

Table 111.4 *Continued*

Site	Urgent (2WW)	Consider further assessment or routine referral if:
Testicular	• Painless testicular enlargement or change in shape/texture	• Direct access ultrasound if unexplained or persistent testicular symptoms
Penile	• Unexplained penile mass/ulcerated lesion (following exclusion/ successful treatment of sexually transmitted infection) • Unexplained/persistent symptoms affecting glans or foreskin	

Further reading

1. European Society of Medical Oncology (ESMO). Clinical practice guidelines: genitourinary cancers. Available at: https://www.esmo.org/Guidelines/Genitourinary-Cancers
2. Tchetgen MB, Song JT, Strawderman M, et al. (1996). Ejaculation increases the serum prostate-specific antigen concentration. *Urology*. 47:511–6.
3. Ornstein DK, Rao GS, Smith DS, et al. (1997). Effect of digital rectal examination and needle biopsy on serum total and percentage of free prostate specific antigen levels. *J Urol*. 157:195–8.
4. Zackrisson B, Ulleryd P, Aus G, et al. (2003). Evolution of free, complexed, and total serum prostate-specific antigen and their ratios during 1 year of follow-up of men with febrile urinary tract infection. *Urology*. 62:278–81.

Table 11.4 (Continued)

[illegible]	[illegible]	Consider further assessment or specialist referral if
Testicular	[illegible]	[illegible]
[illegible]	[illegible]	

Further reading

[illegible]

[illegible]

[illegible]

[illegible]

Part 16

Professional guidelines

Chapter 112

Capacity and consent

Guidelines:
General Medical Council (Decision making and consent): https://www.gmc-uk.org/ethical-guidance/ethical-guidance-for-doctors/decision-making-and-consent

General Medical Council (0–18 years: guidance for all doctors): https://www.gmc-uk.org/ethical-guidance/ethical-guidance-for-doctors/0-18-years

OUP disclaimer: Oxford University Press makes no representation, express or implied, that the drug dosages are correct and that the recommendations are an exclusive or mandatory course of care. All health professionals reading this text have a responsibility to evaluate its appropriateness and take the individual needs of the patient into account.

Local trust guidelines: please refer to your local guidelines as necessary.

Overview

Prior to any examination, investigation, or treatment, doctors must be satisfied that they have obtained valid consent (informed, voluntary, and with capacity) from their patient. Consent is also required if doctors wish to involve their patients in teaching or research. Conditions and treatment options should be discussed with patients in a way that they can understand, with their right to make decisions about their care respected. Consent with regard to DNACPR and advanced care planning is covered in Chapter 114.

Ensure that you are following the legal framework for the location in which you are working. This guidance applies to England and may not always be applicable to other parts of the UK.

Capacity

Key principles

Presume capacity

- All adult patients should be presumed to have capacity to make decisions
- Assumptions should not be made based on age, disability, appearance, communication difficulties, beliefs, or behaviours
- Making decisions that are perceived to be 'bad' or irrational does not mean the patient lacks capacity
- Capacity is lacking once it is clear that the patient cannot understand, retain, use, or weigh up the information needed to make the decision, or communicate their wishes, having received all appropriate help and support.

Maximize ability to make decisions

- Patients may have fluctuations in their conditions with associated fluctuations in their capacity and ability to consent; additional time and support should be given to maximize autonomous decision-making
- Reasonable steps should be taken to anticipate foreseeable changes in capacity, e.g. fluctuating delirium. Opportunities should be taken to discuss treatment options during lucid moments when the patient has capacity
- If the patient currently lacks capacity, but they are likely to regain capacity later and the decision can safely be delayed until this time, then the decision should be delayed
- Make enquiries as to what may help the patient meet the requirements for capacity and therefore valid consent. This could include bringing a relative, friend, or carer to consultations, or having written or audio information available, or having discussions in a particular location or at a particular time of day
- For patients who have difficulty retaining information, a written record of your discussions, detailing what decisions were made and why, should be provided
- You should record any decisions that are made, wherever possible, while the patient has capacity to understand and review them. Advance refusals of treatment may need to be recorded, signed, and witnessed.

Capacity assessment

- Capacity is time and decision dependent. A patient's capacity to make a particular decision should be assessed at the time the decision needs to be made. Do not assume that because a patient lacked capacity for a particular decision on a particular occasion that they lack capacity to make any decisions at all
- Requirements for capacity:
  - Understand: understand enough information so that the decision can be considered informed
  - Retain: retain the information for long enough to be able to make the decision
  - Use the information needed to make the decision: i.e. be able to weigh up the pros and cons and come to a decision that is right for them

- Communicate: the patient must be able to communicate their wishes by any means.

If your assessment leaves you in doubt, obtain advice from:

- The mental health team, who are usually the first port of call for support in capacity decisions
- Those close to the patient, nursing staff, or other staff involved in the patient's care, as they may have more knowledge of the patient's usual abilities or particular communication needs
- Specialist colleagues, such as neurologists, or speech and language therapists.

In the event that you remain unsure, legal advice may be necessary.

Making decisions where the patient lacks capacity, in the absence of a power of attorney

- Ensure decisions are made in the patient's best interests
- Treat patients as individuals
- Allow patients to be involved in decisions as much as possible, even if they lack capacity to make a final decision
- Take into account the views of those close to the patient, or the patient's views and beliefs if these are known
- If there is more than one option, choose the option which will be least restrictive to the patient in the future.

> If the patient has a power of attorney (specifically for health and welfare), this only becomes active in the event that the patient lacks capacity. A power of attorney cannot override a decision made by a patient with capacity.

Consent in patients where capacity has been established

Obtaining consent

- Consider who the most appropriate person in the MDT is to deliver the information and obtain consent
- Explain all available options to the patient. When discussing each option, explain the potential benefits and possible risks (including side effects, complications, and failure of treatment if applicable). Try to establish what is important to the patient themselves
- The option of having no examination, investigation, or treatment (including the risks and benefits of this) should always be discussed
- If there is a significant risk of a particular problem occurring during a procedure, patients should be asked in advance what course of action they would like to take should this happen
- Patients **must** be given information about serious adverse outcomes, even if the chances of those outcomes occurring are very small
- Patients should be encouraged to ask questions
- Doctors may recommend the option that they feel is the best in their opinion, but they should not put pressure on the patient to accept their advice
- If the patient requests an investigation or treatment that the doctor does not consider to be in their best interests, the doctor should be prepared to discuss this and explore the reasons behind this. Ultimately, a patient may not demand an investigation or treatment and the doctor is not under any obligation to provide it. The doctor should explain their reasons to the patient, and explain any other options that are available, including the option to seek a second opinion
- Information should be tailored to the individual patient and the amount of information given depends on the complexity of the suggested treatment and the level of associated risk. Patients should be made aware that they can change their mind about a decision at any time
- Information should *not* be shared if this will cause serious harm to the patient (not just causing the patient to become upset, or risking them refusing a treatment). Withholding information from the patient should be documented clearly in the notes with a justification and this is likely to require legal advice
- Patients should be given time to reflect on their options as much as possible before making their decision, and should know who they can contact with questions or requests for further information. However, patients should also be made aware if their decision is time-sensitive, i.e. if there may be an impact from delaying their decision
- Support discussions with written materials and/or visual aids if possible. Ensure that the patient's communication needs are supported, e.g. providing a translator
- Involve the patient's family/friends/carer if this is in line with their wishes
- Keep in mind that pain and anxiety may present barriers to decision-making.

> Before starting a treatment, consent must be checked. This is particularly important if significant time has passed since the decision was originally made, the patient's condition has changed, or new information has become available. Where treatment is ongoing, clear arrangements must be in place to review decisions and, if required, make new ones.

Documentation of obtaining consent

Ensure the following is documented:

- Who was present at the discussion
- Specific information discussed
- Concerns/questions/requests made by the patient
- Additional written/visual/audio information provided
- Details of decisions made.

Consent in an emergency situation

Oral consent can be relied upon in an emergency; however, the patient must still be provided with the required information in order to make an informed decision. Record clearly in the medical records that oral consent was given.

If obtaining consent is not possible, treatment can be given without consent, provided that the treatment is immediately necessary to save their life or to prevent a serious deterioration of their condition. The treatment must be the least restrictive of the patient's future choices. If the patient regains capacity, you should tell them what has been done, and why, as soon as they have recovered enough in order to understand.

Written consent

Consent does not always have to be written; it can also be given orally, or may be implied by virtue of the patient complying with the examination or treatment. This depends on the nature of the decision.

Written consent is required under certain circumstances, including when:

- The proposed treatment is complex or high risk
- The treatment may have a significant impact on the patient's personal life, social life, or employment
- The treatment is part of a research programme or trial.

> When relying on tacit consent for routine procedures, e.g. venepuncture, ensure that you have given a clear explanation of the procedure, that the patient understands that they can refuse or withdraw at any time, and be prepared to stop if the patient withdraws their consent.

Written consent is legally required for certain treatments, such as fertility treatments.

If a patient with capacity refuses to be involved with a consent decision

Where decision-making is deferred by the patient to another person (i.e. the patient asks the doctor to decide for them, or delegates the decision to a friend or relative), the reasons for this should be sought. If the patient refuses to receive even basic information about a procedure or treatment, they must understand that their consent may not be valid as a result. It may be worthwhile getting advice from your medical defence body under these circumstances. This should all be clearly documented.

If a patient with capacity may be making a consent decision under duress

Patients may be put under pressure by third parties such as employers, insurers, or relatives to take a particular course of action. Be mindful of this possibility, particularly if the patient is from a vulnerable background.

Patients admitted under the Mental Health Act

Patients requiring treatment for a psychiatric condition

- Patients admitted under the Mental Health Act may be given treatment for their psychiatric condition without their consent.

Patients requiring treatment for a physical health condition

- Patients admitted under the Mental Health Act for a psychiatric condition are still required to have capacity and give informed consent for treatments aiming to alleviate physical health problems
- Treatments for a physical disorder may only be given without consent if the injury is a direct result of their psychiatric disorder, e.g. treating self-inflicted wounds.

Children and young people

Seek senior advice when considering whether children and young people have capacity to give consent.

Young people aged 16–17 years

- Young people aged ≥16 years usually (but do not always) have capacity to consent
- They should be encouraged to involve their parents in their decision-making, although the young person's decision should be respected.
- If they do not have capacity, the rules differ depending on which country within the UK the young person is based in.

Young people aged <16 years

- Young people aged <16 years may have capacity to consent, and this depends on their maturity and level of understanding
- It is possible to have capacity to consent to a low-risk intervention, e.g. the decision whether to allow a bloods to be taken, but not have capacity for a more complex, higher-risk intervention, e.g. major surgery.

In all cases involving young people aged <18 years

- If the young person does not have capacity, a parent may consent on their behalf. If parents disagree and cannot come to an agreement, legal intervention may be necessary
- If the young person has capacity, it may be helpful to involve an independent advocate or designated doctor for child protection to assist the young person in making a decision
- These team members may also be helpful if a young person with capacity refuses a treatment that has been deemed by the responsible doctor to be in their best interests or if their parent refuses such a treatment. If the issue is not resolved, legal advice should be sought.

Further reading

1. Legislation.gov.uk (2005). Mental Capacity Act 2005. Available at: https://www.legislation.gov.uk/ukpga/2005/9/contents
2. Legislation.gov.uk (2000). Adults with Incapacity (Scotland) Act 2000. Available at: https://www.legislation.gov.uk/asp/2000/4/contents
3. Department of Health (2009). Reference guide to consent for examination or treatment. Available at: https://www.gov.uk/government/publications/reference-guide-to-consent-for-examination-or-treatment-second-edition

Chapter 113

Confidentiality

Guideline:
General Medical Council (Confidentiality: good practice in handling patient information): http://www.gmc-uk.org/guidance/ethical_guidance/confidentiality.asp

OUP disclaimer: Oxford University Press makes no representation, express or implied, that the drug dosages are correct and that the recommendations are an exclusive or mandatory course of care. All health professionals reading this text have a responsibility to evaluate its appropriateness and take the individual needs of the patient into account.

Local trust guidelines: please refer to your local guidelines as necessary.

Overview

Respecting patients' right to confidentiality is one of the duties of a doctor and patients have a right to expect that their information will be held in confidence.

Key principles:
- Use the minimum necessary personal information and anonymize where possible
- Protect against improper access and loss
- Ensure explicit consent is obtained prior to disclosure, unless disclosure is required by law or is justified in the public interest
- Tell patients about disclosures that they would not reasonably expect.

Personal information may be disclosed when:
- The patient gives explicit consent to disclosure
- The patient lacks capacity and disclosure is in their best interests
- Required by law or statutory process
- Justified in the public interest, e.g. for public protection.

In an emergency where consent cannot be obtained, the patient should be informed afterwards if disclosure was in a way that the patient would not reasonably expect.

Consent to disclosure may not be required:
- If doing so would put you or others at risk of serious harm, **OR**
- If doing so would undermine the purpose of the disclosure, e.g. by prejudicing the prosecution of a serious crime, **OR**
- When action must be taken quickly; e.g. in the control of outbreaks of a communicable disease.

You must:
- Keep disclosures to a minimum and keep a written record.

Disclosures to support patient care

Implied consent

You can rely on *implied* consent provided that:

- The disclosure will support the patient's care
- Information is available (leaflets/posters/face to face) explaining how their information will be used and their right to object
- There is no reason to believe the patient has objected
- The recipient understands their duty to respect confidentiality.

Explicit consent

- Explicit consent should be sought if you suspect a patient would be surprised by access to or disclosure of their information; e.g. as part of a shared care record with other agencies or if information is requested by their employment or an insurance company
- Patients should be aware of the potential consequences of not sharing information and how this may impact their care.

If the patient has capacity and refuses disclosure, this should be respected, even if the decision leaves them (but no one else) at risk of death or serious harm.

Sharing information with those close to the patient

- Encourage early discussions about what information the patient wants you to share, with whom, and in what circumstances
- Any explicit wish of the patient *not* to have information disclosed should continue to be respected in the event that they lose capacity or die. You must document their wishes in their records
- In patients who lack capacity, it is reasonable to assume that they would want information to be shared, unless they indicate or have previously indicated otherwise.

Disclosures required by law

- Only disclose what is absolutely necessary
- Wherever possible tell the patient.

You must disclose information if ordered to do so by a court; you should only disclose information that is required by the court, e.g. in the investigation of road accidents.

Disclosures for the protection of patients and others

This includes disclosing information about adults or children who may be at risk of harm or adults who lack capacity.

Disclosing in the public interest

Disclosure may be justified if failure to do so may expose others to a risk of death or serious harm. The benefits to an individual or to society of the disclosure must outweigh both the patient's and the public interest in keeping the information confidential, e.g. when a patient is not fit to drive or has been diagnosed with a serious communicable disease.

If in doubt, seek the advice of an experienced colleague, a Caldicott or data guardian or equivalent, your defence body or professional association, or seek independent legal advice.

Requested disclosures

Requests from employers, insurers, and other third parties; including agencies assessing entitlement to benefits

- The patient must understand the purpose and likely consequences of the disclosure
- Written consent from the patient or authorization to act on their behalf must be sought
- Offer the patient a copy of any report before sending it (unless they do not wish to see it, it could cause serious harm to the patient or someone else, or it could reveal information about another person who does not consent).

Managing and protecting personal information

- You must make sure any personal information about patients is protected at all times
- Do not leave records or notes unattended, either on paper or on screen
- You must not access a patient's personal information unless you have a legitimate reason to view it.

Further reading

1. GMC (2020). Consent: patients and doctors making decisions together. Available at: https://www.gmc-uk.org/ethical-guidance/ethical-guidance-for-doctors/consent
2. GMC (2018). Protecting children and young people: the responsibilities of all doctors. Available at: https://www.gmc-uk.org/ethical-guidance/ethical-guidance-for-doctors/protecting-children-and-young-people

There are six pieces of shorter guidance which explain how to apply the principles of confidentiality to specific situations doctors often encounter or find hard to deal with:

3. GMC (2017). Confidentiality: disclosing information for education and training purposes. Available at: https://www.gmc-uk.org/ethical-guidance/ethical-guidance-for-doctors/confidentiality---disclosing-for-education-and-training-purposes
4. GMC (2017). Confidentiality: disclosing information for employment, insurance and similar purposes. Available at: https://www.gmc-uk.org/ethical-guidance/ethical-guidance-for-doctors/confidentiality---disclosing-information-for-employment-insurance-and-similar-purposes
5. GMC (2017). Confidentiality: disclosing information about serious communicable diseases. Available at: https://www.gmc-uk.org/ethical-guidance/ethical-guidance-for-doctors/confidentiality---disclosing-information-about-serious-communicable-diseases
6. GMC (2017). Confidentiality: patients' fitness to drive and reporting concerns to the DVLA or DVA. Available at: https://www.gmc-uk.org/ethical-guidance/ethical-guidance-for-doctors/confidentiality---patients-fitness-to-drive-and-reporting-concerns-to-the-dvla-or-dva
7. GMC (2017). Confidentiality: reporting gunshot and knife wounds. Available at: https://www.gmc-uk.org/ethical-guidance/ethical-guidance-for-doctors/confidentiality---reporting-gunshot-and-knife-wounds
8. GMC (2017). Confidentiality: responding to criticism in the media. Available at: https://www.gmc-uk.org/ethical-guidance/ethical-guidance-for-doctors/confidentiality---responding-to-criticism-in-the-media

Chapter 114

DNACPR decisions

Guideline:
British Medical Association, Resuscitation Council (UK), Royal College of Nursing (Decisions relating to cardiopulmonary resuscitation): https://www.bma.org.uk/advice-and-support/ethics/end-of-life/decisions-relating-to-cpr-cardiopulmonary-resuscitation

OUP disclaimer: Oxford University Press makes no representation, express or implied, that the drug dosages are correct and that the recommendations are an exclusive or mandatory course of care. All health professionals reading this text have a responsibility to evaluate its appropriateness and take the individual needs of the patient into account.

Local trust guidelines: please refer to your local guidelines as necessary.

Overview

Making timely advance cardiopulmonary resuscitation (CPR) decisions is integral to anticipatory care planning. These decisions are sensitive and effective communication is essential; quality of communication has a lasting impact on the perception of overall care quality for patients and relatives. A DNACPR decision refers to a decision, whether a clinical decision or due to patient choice, not to attempt CPR in the event of a patient suffering a cardiorespiratory arrest.

Background

- **Survival from cardiopulmonary arrest** depends on numerous factors: baseline physiological reserve, cause of arrest, setting (in/out of hospital), time to initiating CPR, and defibrillation
- **Successful resuscitation** (Fig. 114.1) and survival to discharge **is most likely following sudden cardiac arrest with a reversible cause**. CPR will **not** restore long-term cardiopulmonary function following arrest resulting from the progression of advanced, irreversible underlying disease
- **Advance discussion and documentation of CPR decisions** allows communication between patients and healthcare providers about the likely outcome of CPR, enables patients to express their wishes about care at the end of life, and avoids crisis decision-making with limited access to information following acute deterioration
- In an emergency, there must be a **presumption in favour of attempting CPR** if no advance record of a CPR decision is available. Early discussions and clear documentation are important to avoid this situation.

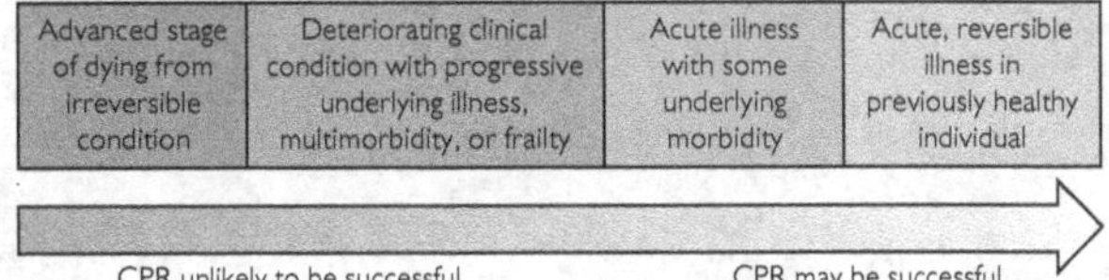

Fig. 114.1 Likelihood of successful outcome of cardiopulmonary resuscitation.

When to consider CPR decisions

- CPR should be discussed with patients at a foreseeable risk of deterioration to cardiopulmonary arrest (e.g. established progressive degenerative disease or multimorbidity)
- Ideally, the discussion should be initiated proactively by experienced professionals well known to the patient and familiar with their care during a period of clinical stability:
  - Typically, the GP or specialist team managing the primary underlying illness
  - Valid CPR decisions made previously should be reviewed following any meaningful change in clinical circumstances, i.e. whenever a patient is acutely admitted to hospital
- In some parts of the UK, the Recommended Summary Plan for Emergency Care and Treatment (ReSPECT) form has been adopted. ReSPECT enables recommendations to be recorded to guide decisions about a person's care and treatment. It highlights what is important to the patient in terms of prolonging life versus providing comfort, and attempting CPR
- **CPR decisions should be discussed with patients** unless to do so would cause material psychological or physical harm, or they express a consistent wish not to discuss CPR. Avoiding discussion in order to avoid distress is not justifiable.

Assessment

- **Establish reason for current presentation/review:** prior anticipatory care/treatment escalation planning discussion/decision? Established CPR decision already in place?
- **Past medical history:** life-limiting or terminal diagnosis? Significant underlying comorbidities, e.g. cardiopulmonary, renal, neurological disease? Consider functional status and estimated survival/ prognosis
- Whether to offer CPR is a **clinical decision**. Consider (Fig. 114.2):
  - Is attempted CPR likely to be successful? Consider the broad context of the patient's condition and treatment plan
  - The patient's expressed wishes
  - Capacity, and if the patient lacks capacity, any applicable advanced statement or appointed attorney/deputy/guardian.

Decisions not to attempt CPR because it will not be successful

- CPR should not be attempted if a person is dying as an inevitable result of progressive underlying disease or a catastrophic acute event, and CPR would not restore cardiopulmonary function for a sustained period
- **Discuss the decision and its rationale** with the patient and those close to them
- Where a DNACPR decision is appropriate on clinical grounds, be clear that consent need not be taken. Patients, relatives, or any appointed attorney/deputy/guardian cannot demand treatment that is clinically inappropriate. A second opinion may be requested where patients or proxy decision-makers disagree with the decision
- Patients should understand that although CPR may restore circulation and breathing, it is almost always heavily invasive, may be traumatic, and that the patient's subsequent quality of life is unlikely to be the same as prior to the cardiac arrest (e.g. due to hypoxic brain injury).

Decision-making where CPR may be successful

- If CPR may be successful, seek to establish the patient's wishes
- Provide information and sufficient time for patients to reach an informed decision.
- Present clinical information relevant to their condition, explore their beliefs and values, and discuss the realistic likelihood of CPR success, potential burdens/harms of attempted CPR, and long-term prognosis
- Capacity assessment should be carried out in accordance with the relevant national legislation (Mental Capacity Act 2005 in England and Wales; Adults with Incapacity (Scotland) Act 2000; Mental Capacity Act (Northern Ireland) 2016)
- **If a patient with capacity refuses CPR**, or a patient who lacks capacity has a valid **advance decision to refuse treatment (ADRT)** detailing refusal of CPR, this must be respected
- **If a patient with capacity declines to discuss CPR**, this should be respected and a clinical decision made in their best interests.
- **Patients who lack capacity:**
  - If a health and welfare attorney is appointed under a Lasting Power of Attorney (LPA) and is authorized to make decisions about life-sustaining treatment, they must be consulted as a proxy decision maker
  - Otherwise, the clinical team must reach a decision in the patient's best interests, establishing their wishes, beliefs, and values by involving relatives or others close to them, or an independent mental capacity advocate (IMCA) where no others can be consulted.

Communication tips

- Recognize that discussions about CPR are sensitive and potentially distressing
- Consider the most appropriate, private setting for discussion. Discuss who the patient would like to be present to support them (relatives or others close to them, members of the MDT)
- Be open and honest
- Use clear, unambiguous language
- Offer as much information as the patient and any others involved in discussion want
- Allow adequate time for discussion, reflection, and review
- Check understanding
- Emphasize that **DNACPR decisions relate to CPR only**, and not to other aspects of monitoring or treatment
- Support verbal information with appropriate written resources (e.g. 'Decisions about Cardiopulmonary Resuscitation (CPR)'[1]).

1 Available at: https://www.resus.org.uk/sites/default/files/2020-06/2016_07_25_CPRdecisions_patientinfo_FINAL.pdf

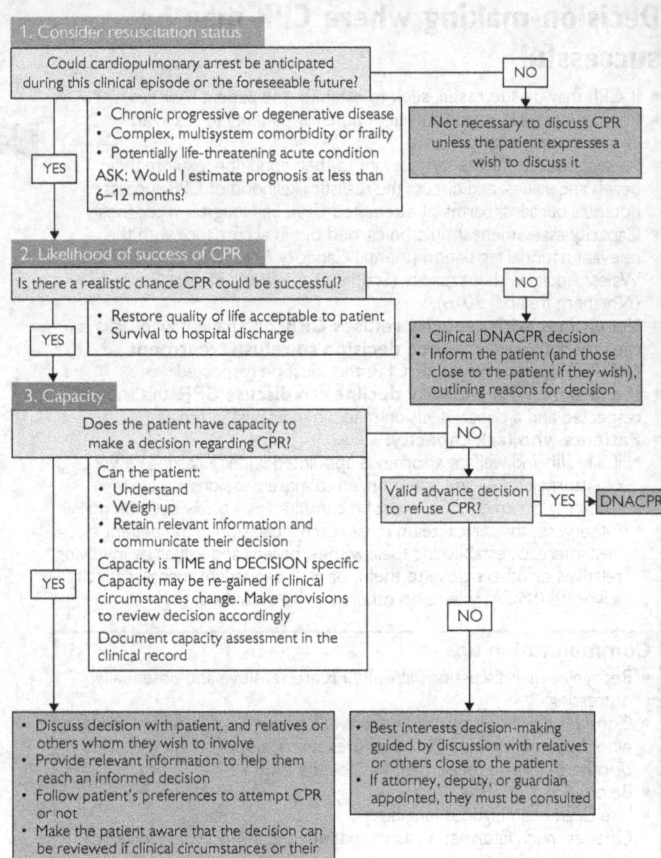

Fig. 114.2 Decision aid to guide decision-making surrounding cardiopulmonary resuscitation.

Record keeping

- Overall responsibility rests with the senior clinician responsible for care (typically the consultant/GP)
- Subject to local policy, junior doctors may complete CPR decision forms; however, the form should be countersigned by the responsible senior clinician as soon as possible
- Document clearly and contemporaneously
- Document DNACPR decisions using standardized forms:
    - Record supplementary detail (e.g. capacity assessment, related treatment planning decisions) separately in the clinical notes
- CPR decision forms are not legally binding documents. They represent an advance clinical assessment used to guide immediate clinical decision-making in an emergency. Final decisions whether to initiate CPR are taken by the clinical team responding at the time of cardiopulmonary arrest.

Information sharing

- The responsible clinician's team should ensure that CPR decisions are communicated to all other relevant professionals/agencies:
    - Clear communication at handover and transfer between wards/departments/care settings
    - Discharge summaries to GP, residential/nursing home staff, and relevant community teams
    - Summary care record information available to out-of-hours/ambulance teams
- Paper DNACPR decision forms should travel with the patient whenever possible. If the form is to be kept at home with the patient, it is essential that the decision has been discussed and the patient understands and accepts the decision.

Special considerations

- **Not the envisaged clinical circumstances:** a DNACPR decision should not override clinical judgement if cardiopulmonary arrest occurs due to a readily reversible cause not matching the circumstances envisaged when the decision was made (e.g. choking, displaced/blocked tracheal or tracheostomy tube)
- **Temporary suspensions:** DNACPR decisions may be suspended during procedures with a high risk of precipitating cardiopulmonary arrest, but where successful resuscitation is likely following prompt treatment (e.g. cardiac catheterization, pacemaker insertion).

Further reading

1. General Medical Council (2010). Treatment and care towards the end of life: good practice in decision making. Available at: https://www.gmc-uk.org/ethical-guidance/ethical-guidance-for-doctors/treatment-and-care-towards-the-end-of-life
2. Pitcher D, Fritz Z, Wang M (2017). Emergency care and resuscitation plans. *BMJ*. 356:j876.
3. ReSPECT (Recommended Summary Plan for Emergency Care and Treatment) process. Available at: https://respectprocess.org.uk/

Chapter 115

Fitness to drive

Guidelines:
DVLA (Assessing fitness to drive: a guide for medical professionals): https://www.gov.uk/government/publications/assessing-fitness-to-drive-a-guide-for-medical-professionals

General Medical Council (Confidentiality: patients' fitness to drive and reporting concerns to the DVLA or DVA): https://www.gmc-uk.org/-/media/documents/gmc-guidance-for-doctors---confidentiality---patients-fitness-to-drive-and-reporting-concer-70063275.pdf

DVLA (Visual disorders: assessing fitness to drive): https://www.gov.uk/guidance/visual-disorders-assessing-fitness-to-drive

OUP disclaimer: Oxford University Press makes no representation, express or implied, that the drug dosages are correct and that the recommendations are an exclusive or mandatory course of care. All health professionals reading this text have a responsibility to evaluate its appropriateness and take the individual needs of the patient into account.

Local trust guidelines: please refer to your local guidelines as necessary.

Overview

Driving is a complex skill, reliant upon multiple physiological processes (Fig. 115.1), and consequently, safe driving (without adaptation) is reliant on the normal functioning of multiple body systems.

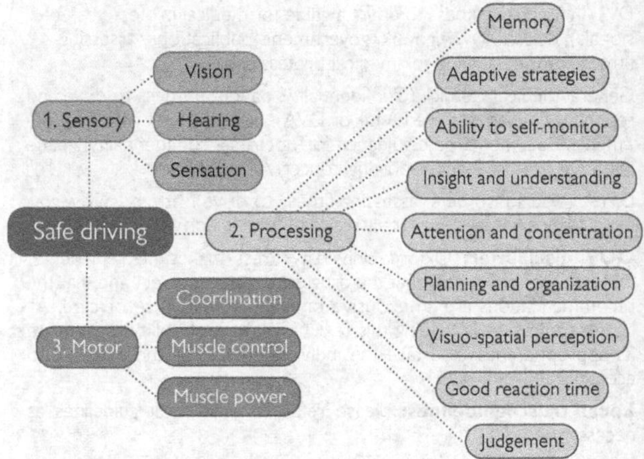

Fig. 115.1 Breakdown of the main physiological processes required for safe driving.

Licence classifications

There are two main groups of drivers which have different rules:

- **Group 1** (cars and motorcycles)
- **Group 2** (lorries and buses).

Common medical conditions (DVLA recommendations)

Neurology

'Collapse query cause' is a common referral to accident and emergency departments. It is essential to get to the bottom of the cause of collapse to make appropriate recommendations for safe driving. See Table 115.1.

Table 115.1 Common neurological conditions requiring safe driving advice

	Group 1 (cars and motorcycles)	Group 2 (lorries and buses)
Fit to drive Do not need to notify the DVLA	• Carotid artery stenosis • Vaso-vagal syncope (which only occurs while standing, or when sitting but due to a specific trigger which will not occur during driving)	
Must not drive while symptomatic May need to notify the DVLA	• Encephalitis (no seizures, full recovery) • Subarachnoid haemorrhage (with treated aneurysm and full recovery)	• Chronic neurological condition, e.g. multiple sclerosis, motor neurone disease (progressing) • Encephalitis (no seizures, full recovery)
Must not drive for a length of time which varies per condition **Need to notify the DVLA**	• Cough syncope • Dizziness (sudden and unprovoked) • Encephalitis (with seizures) • Hypersomnia, e.g. narcolepsy • Seizures • Stroke (with residual neurological weakness after 1 month) • Subarachnoid haemorrhage (untreated) • Subdural haematoma • Vaso-vagal due to unavoidable trigger (while sitting) • Transient ischaemic attack (multiple) • Unexplained syncope	• All syncope • Carotid artery stenosis • Dizziness (sudden and unprovoked) • Encephalitis (with seizures) • Hypersomnia, e.g. narcolepsy • Seizures • Stroke • Subarachnoid haemorrhage • Subdural haematoma • Transient ischaemic attack

Cardiology

See Table 115.2.

Table 115.2 Common cardiology conditions requiring safe driving advice

	Group 1 (cars and motorcycles)	Group 2 (lorries and buses)
Fit to drive Do not need to notify the DVLA	• Aortic aneurysm <6cm in size • Aortic stenosis (asymptomatic) • Heart failure (NYHA I) • Hypertrophic cardiomyopathy • Hypertension (if not malignant hypertension) • Left bundle branch block • Peripheral arterial disease	• Aortic aneurysm ≤5.5cm in size • Aortic stenosis (mild or moderate AND asymptomatic) • Hypertension (if <180/100mmHg and not malignant hypertension)
Fit to drive **Need to notify the DVLA**	• Aortic aneurysm 6–6.4cm in size	• Heart failure (NYHA I) (if ejection fraction ≥40%) • Left bundle branch block* • Peripheral arterial disease
Must not drive while symptomatic Do not need to notify the DVLA	• Angina • Heart failure (NYHA II and III) • Malignant hypertension	
Must not drive while symptomatic **Need to notify the DVLA**		• Angina (if symptoms occur at any time but do not occur regularly) • Heart failure (NYHA II) (if ejection fraction ≥40%) • Long QT syndrome • Malignant hypertension

	Group 1 (cars and motorcycles)	Group 2 (lorries and buses)
Must not drive for a length of time which varies per condition Do not need to notify the DVLA	• ACS** • Arrhythmia that has or is likely to cause incapacity • Catheter ablation • CABG • Elective percutaneous angioplasty • Pacemaker or implantable cardiac defibrillator box change	
Must not drive for a length of time which varies per condition **Need to notify the DVLA**	• Aortic aneurysm >6.5cm in size (until operated on) • Aortic stenosis (symptomatic) • Brugada syndrome • Cardiovascular syncope • Heart failure (NYHA IV) • Implantable cardiac defibrillator insertion • Long QT syndrome • Pacemaker insertion	• ACS • Angina (if symptoms occur regularly) • Aortic aneurysm >5.5cm in size (until operated on) • Aortic stenosis (severe asymptomatic OR symptomatic) • Arrhythmia that has or is likely to cause incapacity • Brugada syndrome • Cardiovascular syncope • Catheter ablation • CABG • Elective percutaneous angioplasty • Heart failure (NYHA III, IV) • Hypertrophic cardiomyopathy • Long QT syndrome • Pacemaker or implantable cardiac defibrillator insertion and box change

* Must have acceptable myocardial perfusion scan or stress echocardiography.

** Recommence driving after 1 week if successful treatment (PCI and no urgent revascularization planned, left ventricular ejection fraction >40% and no other disqualifying conditions).

Diabetes

Most of the guidance is determined by the risk of severe hypoglycaemia (defined as 'an episode of hypoglycaemia requiring the assistance of a third party'). There are strict requirements for patients on insulin, including regular monitoring of blood sugars before and during driving. See Table 115.3.

Table 115.3 Safe driving advice for patients with diabetes

	Group 1 (cars and motorcycles)	Group 2 (lorries and buses)
Fit to drive Do not need to notify the DVLA	• Diet-controlled diabetes or orally treated (excluding sulphonylureas and glinides) with no end-organ damage	• Diet-controlled diabetes with no end-organ damage
Must not drive while symptomatic Do not need to notify the DVLA	• Sulphonylurea and glinide treated diabetes (if the last severe hypoglycaemic episode was >3 months ago and there has been no more than one severe episode in the last 12 months)	
Must not drive while symptomatic **Need to notify the DVLA**	• Insulin-controlled diabetes	• Sulphonylurea, glinide and insulin treated diabetes (if full awareness of hypoglycaemia and there has been no more than one severe episode in the last 12 months)
Must not drive for a length of time which varies per condition **Need to notify the DVLA**	• Impaired awareness of hypoglycaemia	• Impaired awareness of hypoglycaemia

Drug or alcohol misuse

All patients who have alcohol or drug misuse or dependence must not drive while symptomatic and need to notify the DVLA. See Table 115.4.

Table 115.4 Length of driving licence suspension in drug or alcohol misuse

Medical condition	Group 1 (cars and motorcycles)	Group 2 (lorries and buses)
Alcohol dependence	Must not drive until 1 year free of alcohol problems (medical reports and DVLA independent medical examination and bloods). Abstinence is a requirement	Must not drive until 3 years free of alcohol problems (medical reports and DVLA independent medical examination and bloods). Abstinence is a requirement
Persistent alcohol misuse	Must not drive until 6 months of controlled alcohol intake or abstinence and normalization of bloods	Must not drive until 1 year of controlled alcohol intake or abstinence and normalization of bloods
Drug misuse or dependence (cannabis, amphetamines, ecstasy, ketamine, other psychoactive substances)	Must not drive for at least 6 months—during which they must not use these drugs. Additional rules and an independent assessment including urine screen may be arranged for ketamine users	Must not drive for at least 1 year—during which they must not use these drugs. An independent medical assessment is usually required prior to re-licencing
Drug misuse or dependence (heroin, morphine, methadone, cocaine, methamphetamine, benzodiazepines)	Must not drive for at least 1 year—during which they must not use these drugs	Must not drive for at least 3 years—during which they must not use these drugs. An independent medical assessment is usually required prior to re-licencing

Mental health

Mild to moderate anxiety and depression episodes, which are short-lived and do not result in significant impairment, do not need to be notified to the DVLA. However, severe, recurrent anxiety, depression, or psychotic episodes resulting in significant impairment require DVLA notification and for the individual to immediately stop driving. Any mental health condition in which there is a risk of suicide at the wheel is notifiable to the DVLA.

A formal diagnosis of dementia should be notified to the DVLA. Those that are not fit to drive typically include those with poor short-term memory, disorientation and lack of insight and judgement. Patients with a group 1 licence may be able to drive following assessment and patients with a group 2 licence are not allowed to drive.

Visual disorders

All drivers

For it to be legally permissible to drive, drivers must:

- Be able to read a numberplate correctly during daylight from 20 metres away (20.5 metres on some larger numberplates).

Group 1 drivers

Must have:

- A minimum visual acuity of Snellen 6/12 with both eyes, or one eye if monocular
- A visual field of at least 120° horizontally and 50° extension left and right
- No visual field defect that encroaches within 20° of the fixation point.

Group 2 drivers

Must have:

- A minimum visual acuity of Snellen 6/7.5 in the better eye and 6/60 in the poorer eye
- A visual field of at least 160° horizontally and 70° extension left and right and at least 30° above and below the horizontal plane
- No visual field defect that encroaches within 30° of the fixation point
- No other impairment, e.g. glare sensitivity.

DVLA notification—who is responsible?

Patient's responsibilities

It is the patient's responsibility to notify the DVLA of any health condition that impacts on their ability to drive safely. They are also required to respond fully and accurately to information requests from the DVLA and healthcare professionals and to comply with any routine medical reviews required by the DVLA.

Doctor's responsibilities

1. **To advise** the patient of the health impact on driving and their legal obligation to notify the DVLA
2. **To monitor** the patient's ongoing fitness to drive
3. **To notify** the DVLA if a patient cannot or will not notify the DVLA themselves. The patient should ideally be informed prior to contacting the DVLA and should be informed in writing after doing so.

Confidentiality and consent

Consent should be obtained from the patient before their information is shared with the DVLA. However, if it is not possible or appropriate to request consent and/or if the risk to the public is deemed to outweigh the benefit of respecting confidentiality, it may be appropriate to share information with the DVLA without the patient's consent. See also Chapter 112 and Chapter 113.

Part 17

Resuscitation

Chapter 116

Advanced life support

Guidelines:
Resuscitation Council UK (Adult advanced life support guidelines): https://www.resus.org.uk/library/2021-resuscitation-guidelines/adult-advanced-life-support-guidelines

Resuscitation Council UK (The ABCDE approach): https://www.resus.org.uk/library/abcde-approach

OUP disclaimer: Oxford University Press makes no representation, express or implied, that the drug dosages are correct and that the recommendations are an exclusive or mandatory course of care. All health professionals reading this text have a responsibility to evaluate its appropriateness and take the individual needs of the patient into account.

Local trust guidelines: please refer to your local guidelines as necessary.

Overview

Advanced life support (ALS) refers to the management of the deteriorating patient and of cardiac arrest. In a deteriorating patient, the ABCDE approach allows life-threatening issues to be addressed in a systematic order. This chapter covers the diagnosis and management of a deteriorating adult patient and the adult patient in cardiac arrest. This chapter does not cover paediatric life support; however, at the end of this chapter links are given to relevant sections in this book covering some of the underlying conditions which can lead to paediatric cardiac arrest.

Diagnosis

History

History may be limited and history taking should be succinct, using all available resources, and is often conducted alongside initial management steps. If possible, establish the specific complaint (such as chest pain, palpitations, or shortness of breath), past medical history, and drug history (including allergies) that may help guide management.

Examination and investigations

Initial approach

- Ensure it is safe to approach the patient
- Call for help!
- Assess if the patient is conscious (communicating or responsive to stimulus) and breathing. **If unresponsive, or not breathing properly, switch to the ALS algorithm** (Fig. 116.1).

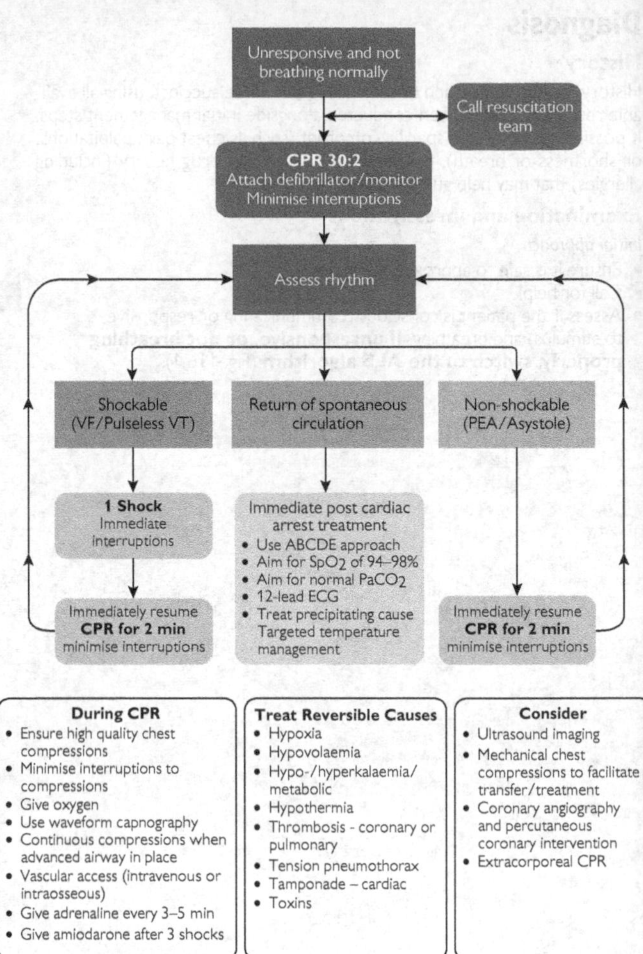

Fig. 116.1 Adult ALS algorithm.

If the patient is conscious but critically unwell

- Examination should follow an ABCDE approach (Table 116.1)
- **If the patient becomes unconscious and is not breathing properly, switch to the ALS algorithm** (Fig. 116.1)
- The patient should be frequently reassessed, particularly after any intervention.

Table 116.1 ABCDE assessment of the critically unwell patient

A	• Look/listen for obvious airway obstruction (absent sounds suggest complete airway obstruction, while noisy breathing suggests partial obstruction) • If there are any concerns about airway obstruction, attempt airway manoeuvres, apply high-flow oxygen, and call for help immediately • Look for central cyanosis (late sign of airway obstruction)
B	• Look for signs of respiratory distress such as tachypnoea and accessory muscle use • Measure the respiratory rate and note the saturations • Palpate the trachea • Percuss and auscultate the lungs • The above may point towards a diagnosis such as pneumothorax, chest sepsis (see Chapter 83), or heart failure (see Chapter 2) • Saturations >94% are not normal if the patient is requiring oxygen to maintain them!
C	• Feel the hands, assess the pulse, and measure capillary refill time • Measure the blood pressure and record the heart rate • Examine for other signs of poor cardiac output, e.g. urine output, and look for possible causes, e.g. haemorrhage • Auscultate for cardiac murmurs (including 'muffled' sounds of cardiac tamponade) • Attach the patient to a cardiac monitor and/or defibrillator pads • Insert two wide-bore cannulae (and withdraw blood for testing—see Box 116.1) • In shock, treat the patient for hypovolaemia (see Chapter 96) until an alternative cause is found • A low diastolic blood pressure (<70mmHg) is indicative of arterial vasodilation (commonly due to sepsis; see Chapter 122), while a narrow pulse pressure (systolic–diastolic: normal value = 35–45mmHg) is often due to arterial vasoconstriction (commonly due to cardiogenic shock or hypovolaemia)
D	• Assess pupils, establish GCS score, and try to elicit any lateralizing neurological signs • Check temperature • Check CBG, as hypoglycaemia (see Chapter 21) is a common and easily reversible cause of deterioration
E	• Expose the patient and perform a top-to-toe examination. This may elicit clues as to the cause of their deterioration, such as rashes or abdominal tenderness, or evidence of injury • Review the drug chart and consider any causative agents, e.g. sedatives or opiates • Examine the upper arms and back for topical medications, e.g. transdermal opiate patches or for evidence of needle track marks

Box 116.1 Bloods

Blood is often taken at the same time as cannulation and the following tests should be sent (this should not delay management and therefore should ideally be processed by a second person):

- FBC
- U&E
- LFT
- Troponin
- Calcium, magnesium, and phosphate
- Coagulation profile
- Group and save
- Blood culture (if infection suspected).

Cardiac arrest

Examination will be limited and should only be performed if it does not interrupt life-saving management .

Investigations should focus on identifying reversible causes. These can be categorized into four 'Hs and Ts':

- **H**ypoxia: pre-arrest oxygen saturations
- **H**ypothermia: temperature
- **H**yperkalaemia (see Chapter 48)/hypokalaemia: VBG
- **H**ypovolaemia (see Chapter 96): pre-arrest blood pressure and heart rate and review of recent fluid balance/history of fluid or blood loss, e.g. burns, diarrhoea, vomiting
- **T**ension pneumothorax: clinical examination (including deviated trachea) and history (e.g. recent chest trauma)
- **T**amponade: bedside echocardiogram
- **T**oxins: history, VBG, and specific bloods (consider paracetamol and salicylate levels)
- **T**hrombus: history, e.g. recent DVT or PE (see Chapter 99).

Management

Acute management

If the patient is conscious but critically unwell

- Monitor and support the airway with oxygen and adjuncts if required
- If hypotensive, give a bolus of 500mL crystalloid stat
- Monitor the heart rate and blood pressure
- Repeat the fluid bolus if there is no improvement and monitor for fluid overload
- Other examples of causes of acute deterioration are listed in Table 116.2.

Table 116.2 Examples of acute management following an ABCDE approach

System	Problem identified on examination	Immediate management
Airway	Anaphylaxis (see Chapter 117)	IM adrenaline, steroids, high-flow oxygen, IV fluids
Breathing	Pneumothorax	Chest decompression either with a needle or drain
	Asthma (see Chapter 80)	Oxygen, nebulized bronchodilator therapy
Circulation	Septic shock (see Chapter 122)	IV fluids, antibiotics, consider need for vasopressors and higher-level care
	Myocardial infarction (see Chapter 1)	Dual antiplatelet therapy and consider PCI
Disability	Hypoglycaemia (see Chapter 21)	PO or IV glucose/dextrose, IM glucagon
Exposure	Opiate overdose	IV or IM naloxone

Cardiac arrest

- If a patient is found or becomes unconscious, they should be managed in line with the ALS algorithm, see Fig. 116.1
- Place defibrillator pads, routinely underneath the right clavicle (second intercostal space) and in the left mid-axillary line (fifth/sixth intercostal space). Alternative placement may be needed if the patient has a pacemaker, if the patient is prone, or has chest trauma
- Obtain a secure airway and give high-flow oxygen
- Get urgent IV access or intraosseous if IV is unsuccessful or not possible
- Consider the 4Hs and 4Ts as quickly as possible
- When the patient is intubated, waveform capnography may be used to confirm tube placement, monitor cardiopulmonary resuscitation (CPR) quality, and help to identify return of spontaneous circulation.

Non-shockable rhythms (pulseless electrical activity or asystole)

- Immediate 1mg IV/IO adrenaline repeated every 3–5 minutes (every alternate cycle).

Shockable rhythms (pulseless ventricular tachycardia or ventricular fibrillation)

- Open circuit oxygen should be moved at least 1m away before a shock is given

- After a shock is given (120–360J), compressions should be restarted as quickly as possible (<5 second delay)
- Patients sometimes develop asystole following a shock and this may last for >2 minutes before there is return of spontaneous circulation
- Give adrenaline 1mg IV/IO after the third shock and further doses after alternate shocks (i.e. approximately every 3–5 minutes)
- Give amiodarone 300mg IV/IO after the third shock and a further 150mg dose after the fifth shock.

> After the first rhythm check, CPR will be recommenced for 2 minutes. This is a good time to consider the reversible causes of cardiac arrest and ensure appropriate treatment is given (Table 116.3). Point-of-care ultrasound (POCUS) may be useful for diagnosis but disruptions to chest compressions must be minimized.

Table 116.3 Management of reversible causes of cardiac arrest

Cause	Immediate management
Hypoxia (see Chapter 79)	• High-flow oxygen via non-rebreathe mask/supraglottic airway device/ endotracheal intubation
Hypovolaemia (see Chapter 96)	• Crystalloid fluids • Check for haemorrhage as this is the most common cause of hypovolaemic cardiac arrest, and obtain control of any bleeding
Hyperkalaemia (see Chapter 48), hypocalcaemia (see Chapter 20), or calcium channel blocker overdose	• 10mL of 10% IV calcium chloride over 5–10 minutes
Hypothermia	• Continued CPR with temperature monitoring • Consider using a warming blanket • Consider other methods of active warming, e.g. forced air warming, warm inspired air, warm IV fluids, and cardiopulmonary bypass
Tension pneumothorax	• Needle decompression in second intercostal rib space, followed by an urgent chest drain
Tamponade	• Resuscitative thoracotomy
Thrombus	• If PE (see Chapter 99), give a fibrinolytic drug and consider performing CPR for 60–90 minutes after the drug has been given • If cardiac thrombus (see Chapter 1) is suspected, consider performing angiography and PCI
Toxins	• Specific antidote, e.g. naloxone for opiate overdose

Treatment after stabilization

- Once return of spontaneous circulation is achieved, it is important to reassess using the ABCDE approach. Furthermore, it is imperative to maintain normal temperature, glucose, oxygen, and carbon dioxide levels
- Reassess using the ABCDE approach
- Consider whether a satisfactory cause has been identified and if not, consider further investigations. Make plans for definitive treatment (such as PCI) or admit to intensive care
- Update the next of kin as soon as possible.

Paediatric conditions that if untreated can lead to cardiac arrest

The most common underlying causes of cardiac arrest in children are respiratory or circulatory failure. Some common causes and pre-arrest management of the acutely unwell child are covered in the following chapters:

- Chapter 70. Fever in under 5s
- Chapter 71. Neonatal infections
- Chapter 72. Paediatric asthma
- Chapter 73. Paediatric meningitis
- Chapter 74. Paediatric bronchiolitis
- Chapter 76. Paediatric gastroenteritis
- Chapter 77. Paediatric type 1 diabetes
- Chapter 117. Anaphylaxis and drug allergy
- Chapter 119. Choking.

Further reading

1. European Resuscitation Council (2021). ERC guidelines. Available at: https://cprguidelines.eu
2. Resuscitation Council UK (2021). Paediatric basic life support. Available at: https://www.resus.org.uk/library/2021-resuscitation-guidelines/paediatric-basic-life-support-guidelines
3. Resuscitation Council UK (2021). Paediatric advanced life support. Available at: https://www.resus.org.uk/library/2021-resuscitation-guidelines/paediatric-advanced-life-support-guidelines

Chapter 117

Anaphylaxis and drug allergy

Guidelines:
NICE CG134 (Anaphylaxis: assessment and referral after emergency treatment): https://www.nice.org.uk/guidance/cg134

NICE CG183 (Drug allergy: diagnosis and management): https://www.nice.org.uk/guidance/cg183

Resuscitation Council UK (Emergency treatment of anaphylaxis): https://www.resus.org.uk/media/337/download

Local trust guidelines: please refer to your local guidelines as necessary.

Overview

Anaphylaxis is a life-threatening hypersensitivity reaction and is characterized by the rapid development of airway and/or breathing and/or circulatory compromise, often accompanied by skin and mucosal changes. Precipitants include drugs, foods, and insect bites/venom. Refractory anaphylaxis refers to anaphylaxis that has not responded to two doses of IM adrenaline. The management in this chapter relates to adult management except for the paediatric management section at the end of the chapter.

Drug allergies are a common cause of anaphylaxis; however, drugs may precipitate a variety of other reactions as well. There are three categories of drug allergy:

- Immediate reactions (within 1 hour):
  - Anaphylaxis
  - Urticaria or angioedema without systemic features
  - Acute bronchospasm, or exacerbation of asthma (e.g. with NSAIDs)
- Non-immediate reactions without systemic involvement (within 3–10 days):
  - Widespread red macules or papules
  - Fixed drug eruption
- Non-immediate reactions with systemic involvement (within 3 days–6 weeks):
  - Drug hypersensitivity syndrome
  - Stevens–Johnson syndrome or toxic epidermal necrolysis
  - Acute generalized exanthematous pustulosis.

Diagnosis

See Box 117.1.

Box 117.1 Anaphylaxis criteria

If all three of the following are present, anaphylaxis is likely:

1. Sudden onset, rapidly progressing symptoms
2. Life-threatening airway and/or breathing and/or circulation problems
3. Skin and/or mucosal changes.

If anaphylaxis is present, move immediately to acute management (see later in the chapter).

History

- Taking a history must not delay emergency treatment
- When possible, a thorough medication history should be taken, including over-the-counter products. Other precipitants include insect bites and certain foods, including shellfish and peanuts.

Examination

Systemically examine the patient using an ABCDE approach (Table 117.1).

Investigations

- **ECG:** anaphylaxis can cause ischaemic changes even with normal coronary vasculature
- **Bloods:** FBC, U&E, LFT, ABG, serum mast cell tryptase if the diagnosis is uncertain (see Box 117.2)
- **Chest X-ray:** to exclude other causes of breathlessness/hypoxia.

Table 117.1 Examination findings in allergy and anaphylaxis

A	Throat, tongue, and lip swelling Hoarseness Stridor Difficulty swallowing
B	Tachypnoea Hypoxia Wheeze (bronchospasm) Cyanosis (late feature) Exhaustion Respiratory arrest
C	Tachycardia Hypotension Cool peripheries Pallor Clammy Dizziness/collapse Bradycardia (late feature) Cardiac arrest
D	Confusion Agitation Reduced GCS score Sense of impending doom Fever
E	Skin erythema and/or mucosal changes Urticaria Angioedema Vomiting/nausea Abdominal pain Incontinence Lymphadenopathy

Box 117.2 Serum mast cell tryptase levels

Serum mast cell tryptase levels are taken in suspected anaphylaxis. Take an initial sample immediately after emergency treatment has started. A second sample should be taken within 1–2 hours of symptom onset, and a third sample after 24 hours/during follow-up.

Management

Acute management

Assess and manage the patient using an ABCDE approach (see Table 117.1).

Anaphylaxis

- Call for help
- **Stop the drug or remove the trigger**
- **In cardiac arrest, commence ALS (see Chapter 116)**
- Lie the patient flat, or sit them up if this makes their breathing easier. Pregnant women should lie on their left side instead
- Give IM adrenaline 500 micrograms of 1:1000 (0.5mL) into the anterolateral aspect of the middle third of the thigh. Repeat after 5 minutes if no improvement
- Establish airway and administer high-flow oxygen
- Give IV fluid bolus 500–1000mL of crystalloid if poor response to initial dose of adrenaline, hypotension, or shock
- If refractory, get critical care support early as the patient will require a low-dose IV adrenaline infusion. If this is not possible, IM adrenaline should be given every 5 minutes for as long as the patient has life-threatening symptoms
- Steroids are not routinely given but may be useful for refractory reactions, ongoing asthma, or shock
- Use continuous pulse oximetry, ECG, and blood pressure monitoring.

Biphasic reactions

Biphasic anaphylactic reactions can occur in around 5% of cases. Patients with anaphylaxis must be admitted to hospital for a minimum of 6–12 hours of observation from symptom onset and reviewed by a senior clinician before discharge.

Non-anaphylaxis reaction

- Stop the drug or trigger
- Treat symptomatically, e.g. cetirizine 10mg.

Treatment after stabilization

Pharmacological treatments

- Non-sedating oral antihistamines, e.g. cetirizine 10–20mg OD, may be used to treat skin symptoms
- Bronchodilators may be helpful for patients with asthmatic symptoms
- Patients with suspected anaphylaxis must be given an adrenaline injector (e.g. EpiPen® or Jext®) on discharge and be taught how to use it. Ideally, close family, friends, and carers should also be taught
- If the patient had an anaphylactic reaction, consider discharging them with a 3-day supply of antihistamines and oral steroids.

Referral

- Patients with anaphylaxis or severe non-immediate cutaneous reactions must be referred to a specialist allergy service.

Patient education

- Patients must be counselled regarding their allergy, including how to avoid triggers and what to do should their reaction recur
- The patient should be informed of the importance of alerting health professionals to their allergy at all appointments, and they should be clear on what may be included in their allergy, e.g. Tazocin® contains a penicillin
- Advise patients to consider wearing a bracelet or other allergy identifier.

Documentation

- Document clearly the events leading up to the reaction, the time of onset of symptoms, and possible triggers
- Ensure any possible triggering medications have been stopped. Patient allergy details must be updated on all computer systems and the patient's GP must be informed.

Paediatric differences in the management of anaphylaxis

The following doses should be used in children:

Adrenaline

As per the adult guidelines, doses should be repeated after 5 minutes if no improvement:

- *Child >12 years:* IM adrenaline 500 micrograms of 1:1000 (0.5mL)
- *Child 6–12 years:* IM adrenaline 300 micrograms of 1:1000 (0.3mL)
- *Child 6 months–6 years:* IM adrenaline 150 micrograms of 1:1000 (0.15mL)
- *Child <6 months:* IM adrenaline 100–150 micrograms of 1:1000 (0.1–0.15mL).

IV fluids

- Give IV fluid bolus 10mL/kg of crystalloid.

Cetirizine

- *Child ≥12 years:* PO cetirizine 10–20mg OD
- *Child 6–11 years:* PO cetirizine 5–10mg OD
- *Child 2–6 years:* PO cetirizine 2.5–5mg OD
- *Child <2 years:* PO cetirizine 250 micrograms/kg OD.

Further reading

1. Ramrakha P, Moore K, Amir S (2019). Anaphylaxis. In: *Oxford Handbook of Acute Medicine*, 4th ed (pp. 342–3). Oxford: Oxford University Press. Available at: https://doi.org/10.1093/med/9780198797425.003.0005
2. Tasker RC, Acerini CL, Holloway E, et al. (eds) (2021). Anaphylaxis. In: *Oxford Handbook of Paediatrics*, 3rd ed (p. 52). Oxford: Oxford University Press. Available at: https://doi.org/10.1093/med/9780198789888.003.0003
3. Anaphylaxis Campaign website. Available at: https://www.anaphylaxis.org.uk/

Chapter 118

Bradycardia

Guideline:
Resuscitation Council UK (Bradycardia): https://www.resus.org.uk/library/2021-resuscitation-guidelines/adult-advanced-life-support-guidelines

OUP disclaimer: Oxford University Press makes no representation, express or implied, that the drug dosages are correct and that the recommendations are an exclusive or mandatory course of care. All health professionals reading this text have a responsibility to evaluate its appropriateness and take the individual needs of the patient into account.

Local trust guidelines: please refer to your local guidelines as necessary.

Overview

Bradycardia is defined as a heart rate <60bpm. This may be physiological or due to a range of pathological causes (Table 118.1). Initially, the most important distinction to make is between symptomatic patients, where treatment is urgently required, and asymptomatic patients.

Table 118.1 Causes of bradycardia

Physiological	Sleep Athletes
Cardiac	Atrioventricular (AV) nodal block First degree: ↑ PR interval Second degree: Mobitz I and II and 2:1 block Third degree: complete AV dissociation Sinus node block Sick sinus syndrome (tachy-brady syndrome) *The above-listed causes may result from acute myocardial infarction or ischaemia, myocarditis, or myocardial fibrosis*
Medications	Beta-blockers Calcium channel blockers Diltiazem Digoxin Amiodarone Verapamil Clonidine
Other	Vasovagal syncope Hypothyroidism Hypothermia Hyperkalaemia Cushing's reflex—↑ intracranial pressure causing hypertension and bradycardia

Diagnosis

History

The patient may be asymptomatic or may present with any of the following features:

- Dizziness
- Collapse
- Fatigue
- Chest pain
- Shortness of breath.

Important points to elicit in the history include:

- Previous episodes of bradycardia
- Previous cardiac arrest resulting from bradycardia
- Past medical history with an emphasis on conditions that may lead to bradycardia (Table 118.1)
- Medication history with an emphasis on drugs that may lead to bradycardia (Table 118.1).

Examination

During the examination, it is important to elicit any adverse features (Box 118.1) and identify precipitating causes of bradycardia.

Box 118.1 Adverse features of bradycardia

The presence of these features signify that the patient is unstable and at high risk of sudden deterioration and death.

- Heart failure:
  - Pulmonary oedema, raised JVP
- Ischaemia:
  - Ongoing chest pain and/or features of ischaemia on ECG
- Shock:
  - Systolic blood pressure <90mmHg, cold or clammy peripheries, confusion or impaired consciousness, diaphoresis, pallor
- Syncope:
  - Loss of consciousness due to reduced cardiac output leading to impaired cerebral perfusion.

Table 118.2 Bradycardia examination findings using an ABCDE approach

A	Partial or complete airway obstruction due to ↓ conscious level
B	Cyanosis Bilateral coarse crepitations on auscultation ↓ oxygen saturations
C	Heart rate <60bpm Hypotension Hypertension in Cushing's reflex with ↑ intracranial pressure Cool extremities Capillary refill time >2 seconds Elevation of JVP (cannon waves in complete heart block)

(Continued)

Table 118.2 *Continued*

D	GCS score—confusion or reduced level of consciousness
E	Hypothermia Hypoglycaemia

Investigations

Bedside

- Continuous monitoring of vital signs
- A 12-lead ECG looking particularly for features suggesting a risk of asystole (Box 118.2).

Bloods

- FBC, U&E including magnesium and calcium, glucose, troponin, TFT, and toxicology including a digoxin level if appropriate.

Imaging

- Chest X-ray to look for features of heart failure.

Box 118.2 Factors which increase the risk of asystole

- Recent asystole
- Mobitz II AV block
- Complete heart block with widened QRS
- Ventricular pause >3 seconds.

Management

Acute management

- Use an ABCDE approach: intervene as problems arise and regularly reassess
- Ensure continuous cardiac monitoring
- Gain IV access early
- Correct electrolytes and glucose, warm hypothermic patients, and treat any other reversible causes
- Treat according to the presence of adverse features as per Table 118.3.

Table 118.3 Acute management of bradycardia

Situation	Management
If adverse features present (Box 118.1)	500mcg atropine IV
If inadequate response to atropine or risk of asystole (Box 118.2)	Interim measures: • 500mcg atropine IV to be repeated every 3–5 minutes (not to exceed 3mg) (caution if acute myocardial infarction or ischaemia as mentioned in 'Special considerations') **OR** • Transcutaneous pacing (with analgesia or sedation)/fist pacing (Box 118.3) **OR** • Isoprenaline 5mcg per minute IV • Adrenaline 2–10 mcg per minute IV • Alternative medications (Box 118.4)
If requiring interim measures	**INVOLVE CARDIOLOGY TEAM**: transvenous pacing required

Box 118.3 Fist pacing

If atropine has been given but there has not been a good response and transcutaneous pacing has not yet commenced, fist pacing may be considered. This should **only** be performed in life-threatening bradycardia (significant haemodynamic instability) and may be performed until transcutaneous pacing is possible. A closed fist can be thumped over the left lower sternum at a rate of 50–70bpm.

Box 118.4 Alternative medications

- Aminophylline
- Dopamine (requires central venous access)
- Glucagon (in beta-blocker- or calcium channel blocker-induced bradycardia)
- Glycopyrrolate (alternative to atropine).

Treatment after stabilization

- Treatment of the underlying cause of bradycardia
- Medication review by a senior clinician with possible cessation of contributing medications
- Referral to the cardiology team and consideration of permanent pacemaker insertion.

Special considerations

Acute myocardial infarction or ischaemia

An increase in heart rate due to atropine use, and the subsequent increase in cardiac oxygen demand, may extend the area of infarction or ischaemia.

Cardiac transplants

- Do **NOT** give atropine. Transplanted hearts do not have the same nerve supply as native hearts and therefore will not respond to the mechanism of action of atropine (vagus nerve block)
- Atropine may instead result in sinus node block, Mobitz type II or complete AV block
- IV theophylline may be used for bradycardia in the presence of inferior wall myocardial infarction, spinal cord injury, or a cardiac transplant. This should be done under senior and/or specialist advice.

Further reading

1. Ramrakha P, Hill J (eds) (2012). Arrhythmias. In: *Oxford Handbook of Cardiology*, 2nd ed (pp. 477–540). Oxford: Oxford University Press. Available at: https://doi.org/10.1093/med/9780199643219.003.0010

Chapter 119

Choking

Guidelines:
Resuscitation Council UK (Choking: adult basic life support and automated external defibrillation): https://www.resus.org.uk/resuscitation-guidelines/adult-basic-life-support-and-automated-external-defibrillation/#foreign

Resuscitation Council UK (Choking: paediatric basic life support): https://www.resus.org.uk/resuscitation-guidelines/paediatric-basic-life-support/#choking

OUP disclaimer: Oxford University Press makes no representation, express or implied, that the drug dosages are correct and that the recommendations are an exclusive or mandatory course of care. All health professionals reading this text have a responsibility to evaluate its appropriateness and take the individual needs of the patient into account.

Local trust guidelines: please refer to your local guidelines as necessary.

Overview

Choking is caused by airway obstruction due to a foreign body, usually a food bolus, and is life-threatening unless managed promptly. The management described in this chapter relates to adult management. Special considerations in paediatric patients are covered at the end of the chapter.

Diagnosis

History

- Commonest when eating/drinking
- Risk factors:
  - Reduced GCS score
  - Intoxication
  - Impaired airway reflexes
  - Respiratory disease
  - Dementia
  - Poor dentition
  - Child or elderly.

Examination

Ask the patient 'Are you choking?':

- **Mild airway obstruction**: the patient can speak and cough
- **Severe airway obstruction:** the patient has a weak or absent cough and struggles to breathe or speak.

Management

Acute management

Mild airway obstruction

- If the foreign body is easy to visualize and accessible in the mouth, remove it (do not perform blind finger sweeps of the mouth)
- Avoid aggressive treatment of mild obstruction as this could worsen the obstruction
- Patients should be encouraged to cough and be monitored until they improve
- Mild airway obstruction may progress to severe obstruction.

Severe airway obstruction

If unconscious, start CPR (see Chapter 116).

If conscious, successful relief of the obstruction is made more likely by alternating between five back blows and five abdominal thrusts:

Back blows

- Stand to the side and support the chest
- Lean the victim forward
- Give five sharp blows between the shoulder blades with the heel of your hand (Fig. 119.1).

Abdominal thrusts

- To be used if back blows are ineffective
- Stand behind the victim, put both arms around the upper abdomen
- Lean the victim forward
- Clench one fist and place below the ribcage
- Grasp your fist with the other hand and pull sharply inwards and upwards (Fig. 119.1).

Treatment after stabilization

- There is a risk of foreign material persisting in the airway
- This may lead to a persistent cough, difficulty swallowing, or the sensation of a foreign body
- Anyone receiving abdominal thrusts/chest compressions should be examined afterwards for injury
- Patients on anticoagulants/antiplatelets are at ↑ risk of intra-abdominal haemorrhage, so have a low threshold for senior review or thoracoabdominal CT
- Discuss with a senior whether further investigations such as X-rays/CT of the neck/chest or bronchoscopy are required to investigate the possibility of a retained aspirated foreign body causing ongoing partial obstruction.

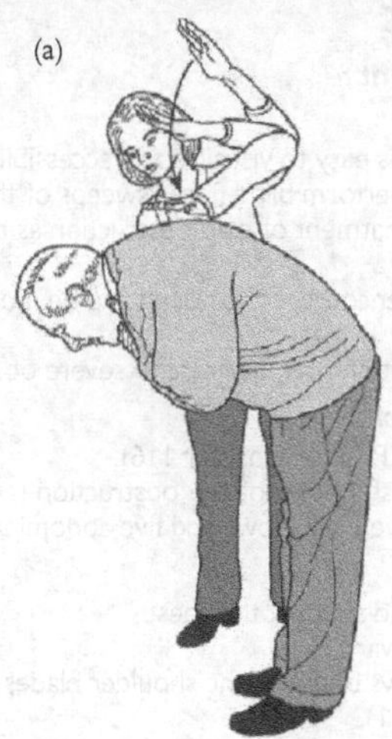

• If the back blows fail, carry out abdominal thrusts:

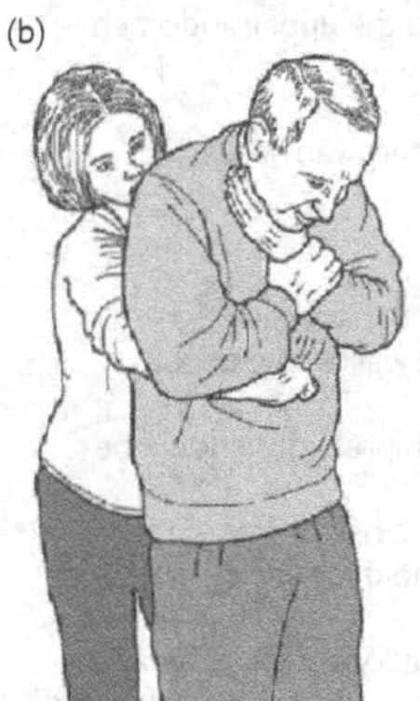

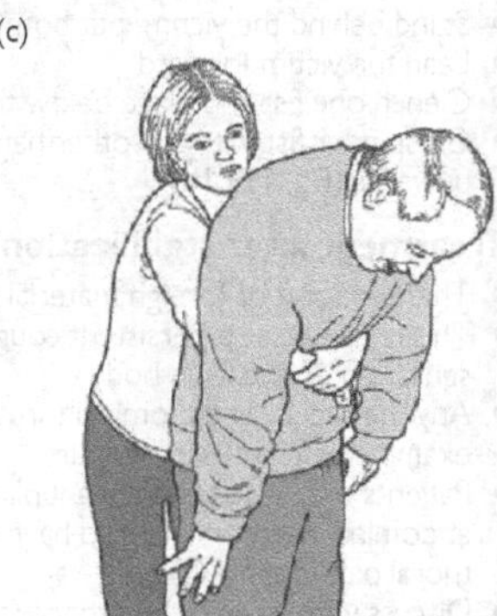

• Stand behind the patient and put both your arms around the upper part of the abdomen.

• Clench your fist and grasp it with your other hand.
• Pull sharply inwards and upwards with the aim of producing sudden expulsion of air, together with the foreign body, from the airway.

Fig. 119.1 Back blows and abdominal thrusts.

Reproduced with kind permission from Basic Adult Life Support Manual, Chapter: 10 Conflict resolution 10: Choking © (2015) Resuscitation Council UK.

Special considerations in paediatric patients

Airway obstruction due to a foreign body (often food, but virtually any small object could be inhaled by children) is an important differential diagnosis for sudden-onset respiratory distress, particularly if associated with gagging, stridor, or coughing. The diagnosis may not be clear-cut, especially in non-verbal or preschool children.

For children aged >1 year, management is very similar to adults as described previously:

- If effective cough (mild obstruction): support and continuously reassess
- If ineffective cough (severe obstruction): use back blows and abdominal thrusts to attempt to relieve airway obstruction
- If the child is unconscious: follow paediatric cardiac arrest algorithm.

For infants aged <1 year, different techniques are required as abdominal thrusts may cause intra-abdominal injury in infants. Use the following procedures to attempt to relieve airway obstruction.

Back blows

- Support the infant in a head-down **prone** position, i.e. across the lap
- Support the head by gently holding the jaw—avoid the soft tissues as this will worsen obstruction
- Deliver five sharp back blows with the heel of the hand between the shoulder blades (Fig. 119.2).

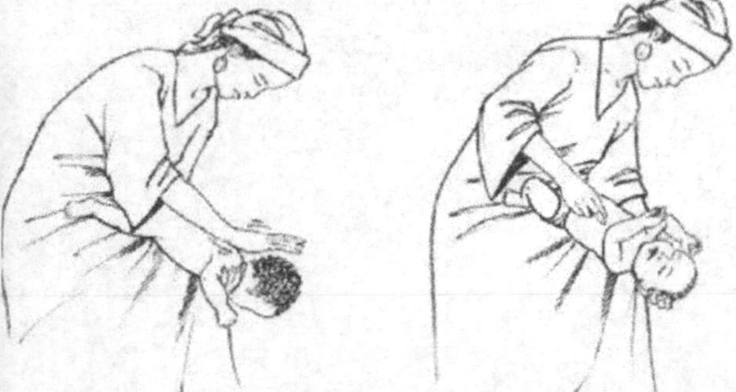

Fig. 119.2 Back blows (left) and chest thrusts (right) to relieve airway obstruction in a choking infant.

Reproduced from World Health Organization, Pocket Book of Hospital Care for Children 2005: 6–7, with permission of WHO.

Chest thrusts

- Support the infant in a head-down **supine** position
- Place them on your arm or lap with your hand holding the occiput
- Deliver up to five chest thrusts, a fingers breadth above the xiphisternum

- These are similar to infant chest compressions, i.e. using two fingers to a depth of 1/3 of the chest
- Chest thrusts are sharper and at a slower rate (Fig. 119.2).

The same principles of treatment after stabilization apply to children as those described previously for adults.

Chapter 120

Major trauma

Guidelines:

NICE NG39 (Major trauma: assessment and initial management): https://www.nice.org.uk/guidance/ng39

NICE CG176 (Head injury: assessment and early management): https://www.nice.org.uk/guidance/cg176

NICE NG41 (Spinal injury: assessment and initial management): https://www.nice.org.uk/guidance/ng41

OUP disclaimer: Oxford University Press makes no representation, express or implied, that the drug dosages are correct and that the recommendations are an exclusive or mandatory course of care. All health professionals reading this text have a responsibility to evaluate its appropriateness and take the individual needs of the patient into account.

Local trust guidelines: please refer to your local guidelines as necessary.

Overview

Major trauma is the leading cause of death in people aged <45 years. It encompasses any limb- or life-threatening injury that may lead to death or prolonged disability. Initial assessment involves a primary survey to identify and treat injuries that may cause imminent morbidity or mortality. This should be followed by prompt transfer to a major trauma centre for definitive management. This chapter covers the basic principles of assessment and management of major trauma in adult patients aged >16 years.

Diagnosis

History

May be collateral depending on the level of consciousness, confusion, or amnesia. The following information should be recorded if possible:

Patient demographics and incident description

- Age and sex of patient
- Time of incident
- Mechanism of injury (see Box 120.1), e.g. driver in small car versus motorcyclist approximately 20mph; seatbelt on, airbag deployed, car written off
- Extrication, e.g. did they stand and walk unaided after the incident, was fire service input required?

Box 120.1 Examples of dangerous mechanisms of injury

- Pedestrian or cyclist hit by a vehicle
- Car accident of sufficient force to eject the patient from the vehicle
- Fall from height of >1m or >5 stairs
- Accident where the car has rolled
- High-speed collision
- Diving or horse-riding accidents.

Patient condition

- Injuries suspected
- Vital signs and GCS score (including E/V/M breakdown)
- Head trauma:
  - Current GCS score and whether this has changed since the injury
  - Behavioural change
  - Focal neurological deficit
  - Seizures
  - Headache
  - Amnesia
  - Vomiting
- Evidence of alcohol or drug use
- Interventions or treatments given prior to arrival in hospital
- Location of pain (distracting injuries) and timing of onset (e.g. immediate or delayed neck pain)
- Time of last meal (in case anaesthesia is required).

Past medical history

- General past medical, drug, and allergy history, specifically including:
  - Bleeding or coagulation profile disorders, or anticoagulation use
  - Previous spinal problems or surgeries that may predispose to spinal instability
  - Previous brain surgery.

Examination

Examination should take place according to the CABCDE structure, similar to the traditional ABCDE structure but modified for major trauma to include haemorrhage control and C-spine immobilization. See Table 120.1.

Table 120.1 Potential examination findings in a primary survey of a major trauma patient

C (catastrophic haemorrhage)	Exsanguination
A (with in-line spinal immobilization)	Orofacial or neck trauma Blood/vomit/foreign body occluding the airway
B	Hypoxia and tachypnoea Reduced chest expansion and absent breath sounds Flail chest (due to fracture of ≥3 ribs)
C	Hypotension and tachycardia Evidence of bleeding Prolonged capillary refill time
D	Reduced or decreasing GCS score (if <8 involve anaesthetist urgently for airway protection) Unequal or fixed unreactive pupils
E	Patient complaining of spinal pain, altered sensation, or weakness Priapism (due to spinal cord injury) Hypothermia Neurovascular status of obviously deformed/ fractured limbs

Following any life- or limb-saving interventions, initiation of resuscitation, and transfer to appropriate facilities, a secondary survey should be conducted. This should be a thorough head-to-toe assessment including a full neurological examination, 30° tilt, palpation of the length of the spine, and rectal examination.

Re-examination is essential: injuries in a major trauma can become apparent as distracting injuries are managed or may become increasingly evident after arrival in hospital.

Investigations

General trauma

Bloods

- Group and save or cross-match (activate the major haemorrhage protocol in patients with significant haemorrhage)
- ABG/VBG, FBC, U&E, LFT, troponin (if cardiac muscle damage is suspected), creatinine kinase (for patients with crush injuries or long lie), amylase, and coagulation profile.

Imaging

- A whole-body CT or 'pan scan' (head, neck, thorax, abdomen, and pelvis) should be considered if multiple injuries are suspected or there is a high-risk mechanism of injury (see Box 120.1). The patient should be haemodynamically stable and their bleeding should be controlled before transfer to CT.

Suspected head injury

- In those with a suspected head injury, CT head should be performed urgently within 1 hour if any of the following apply:
    - GCS score <13 on initial assessment
    - GCS score <15 at 2 hours after the injury
    - Suspected skull fracture or any sign of basal skull fracture (haemotympanum, 'panda' eyes, CSF rhinorrhoea or otorrhoea, Battle's sign)
    - Post-traumatic seizure
    - Focal neurological deficit
    - >1 episode of vomiting
- In patients with any of the following, who have had either amnesia or loss of consciousness since their head injury, a CT head should be performed within 8 hours of the injury:
    - Age >65 years
    - History of bleeding or coagulation profile disorders
    - Dangerous mechanism of injury (see Box 120.1)
    - >30 minutes' retrograde amnesia of events leading up to the injury
- Patients on anticoagulants but with no other risk factors should have a CT head within 8 hours of the injury
- Patients with any of the following also require CT C-spine within 1 hour:
    - GCS score <13 on initial assessment
    - Intubated patient
    - Plain X-ray was inadequate for diagnosis, or is suspicious or clearly abnormal
    - A definitive diagnosis is needed urgently, e.g. prior to surgery
    - The patient is being scanned for head injury or multi-region trauma
    - The patient is alert, stable, and at least one of the following apply:
        - Is aged >65 years
        - Had a dangerous mechanism of injury (see Box 120.1)
        - Has a peripheral focal neurological defect
        - Has limb paraesthesia.

Suspected spinal trauma

- Thoracolumbar radiograph is the first line for those with suspected spinal column injury **without** neurological signs (T1–L3) followed by CT if abnormalities are identified
- If a spinal column fracture is identified, the rest of the spine should be imaged
- The Canadian C-spine rule (Fig. 120.1) has a high sensitivity for cervical spine injury and can aid the clinician in deciding if imaging is necessary
- Carry out full in-line spinal immobilization and request a CT if:
    - High risk on Canadian C-spine rule

 - Low risk on Canadian C-spine rule and the patient is unable to rotate their neck 45° to left/right
 - Suspected thoracic or lumbosacral spinal injury and:
   - Age >65 years with spinal pain
   - Dangerous mechanism of injury (see Box 120.1)
   - Pre-existing spinal pathology
   - Current or risk of osteoporosis
   - Suspected fracture in another part of the spine
   - Focal neurology
   - New spinal deformity or midline tenderness
   - Pain or neurological symptoms on mobilization
- This should be done by fitting an appropriately sized semi-rigid collar (unless airway compromise or spinal deformity prevents this), securing the patient on a scoop stretcher, and securing the patient with head blocks and tape
- Three-view cervical spine X-rays may be appropriate if the patient does not have the above-listed risk factors but it is not safe to assess the movement in their neck, or if they clearly have a reduced range of movement
- MRI is the gold standard for identifying ligamentous, soft tissue, or spinal cord injury.

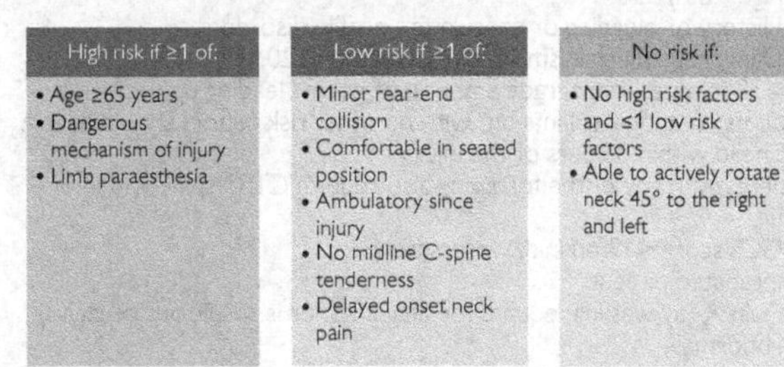

High risk if ≥1 of:
• Age ≥65 years
• Dangerous mechanism of injury
• Limb paraesthesia
Low risk if ≥1 of:
• Minor rear-end collision
• Comfortable in seated position
• Ambulatory since injury
• No midline C-spine tenderness
• Delayed onset neck pain
No risk if:
• No high risk factors and ≤1 low risk factors
• Able to actively rotate neck 45° to the right and left

Fig. 120.1 Canadian C-spine injury rules.

Management

Acute management

Catastrophic haemorrhage

- Apply direct pressure to external bleeding, or apply a tourniquet if external pressure is not sufficient
- Insert two large-bore IV cannulae while awaiting central access. Consider intraosseous access early if peripheral cannulation is difficult
- Transfuse blood as soon as it is available. Give crystalloids, e.g. 500mL boluses, as necessary to maintain blood pressure if blood components are not available
- 1 unit of plasma should be given with every 1 unit of red blood cells
- Administer IV tranexamic acid (1g over 10 minutes) within 8 hours of trauma, followed by 1g every 8 hours
- Reverse anticoagulation:
  - Prothrombin complex concentrate to reverse a vitamin K antagonist
  - Urgent haematology advice for any other anticoagulants
- Consider 'damage control' or definitive surgery or interventional radiology for uncontrolled bleeding.

Airway management

- If the airway is blocked because of liquid, use suction to remove, e.g. blood, saliva, vomit
- If the airway is obstructed, use manoeuvres to relieve the blockage including head tilt, chin lift, or jaw thrust (if there is suspected spinal trauma, **do not** excessively tilt the head and try to maintain the head and neck in a neutral position)
- Consider using airway adjuncts, particularly if the patient has reduced consciousness. This includes oropharyngeal and nasopharyngeal airways
- Get anaesthetic help early, particularly if there has been trauma to the face or neck.

Head injury

- Attempt full cervical spinal immobilization if any of the following:
  - GCS score <15 on initial assessment
  - Neck pain/tenderness
  - Focal neurology
  - Paraesthesia in the extremities
- Perform rapid sequence induction and intubation, led by an anaesthetist if:
  - GCS score <8
  - Unable to maintain airway (loss of protective laryngeal reflexes, unstable facial fractures, significant bleeding within the mouth, seizures)
  - Inadequate ventilation (PaO_2 <13kPa on oxygen, $PaCO_2$ >6kPa, spontaneous hyperventilation causing $PaCO_2$ <4kPa, irregular breathing)
- If rapid sequence induction is unsuccessful, use basic airway manoeuvres and adjuncts until a surgical airway can be procured.

Pneumothorax

- Needle decompression followed by chest drain insertion if a tension pneumothorax is suspected and there is haemodynamic instability or severe respiratory compromise

- Cover an open pneumothorax with an occlusive dressing and monitor for a tension pneumothorax.

Analgesia and patient comfort

- Titrate IV morphine to pain. Second-line agents include intranasal diamorphine and ketamine
- Keep the patient warm
- Catheterization is usually appropriate as a full bladder can cause distress to the patient
- Splint fractures early.

Treatment after stabilization

- Re-evaluate the patient and carry out a complete secondary survey (head-to-toe assessment to identify any further injuries, including relevant investigations and imaging)
- Discuss any intracranial bleed or spinal column/cord injury with appropriate specialists for consideration of surgery and transfer
- Update the patient (if conscious), and family members. Try to:
  - Manage expectations
  - Avoid being overly optimistic or pessimistic
  - Avoid speculation and answer questions within the limits of your knowledge
- Patients with a head injury may need to be admitted for a period of observation
- Observations should be half hourly until GCS score is 15 and should include:
  - GCS score
  - Pupil size and reactivity
  - Limb movements
  - Respiratory rate, heart rate, blood pressure, temperature, and oxygen saturations
- Once the GCS score is 15, assess: half hourly for 2 hours, 1-hourly for 4 hours, then 2-hourly
- The supervising doctor should reassess urgently, and consider a CT if:
  - The patient becomes agitated or displays abnormal behaviour
  - There is a drop in GCS score
  - The patient complains of severe or worsening headache
  - The patient vomits persistently
  - The patient displays new or evolving neurological symptoms, e.g. unequal pupils
- Once the GCS score is 15, patients should be discharged only if there is someone appropriate to supervise them at home.

Further reading

1. Henry S (2018). ATLS 10th edition offers new insights into managing trauma patients. Bulletin of the American College of Surgeons. Available at: http://bulletin.facs.org/2018/06/atls-10th-edition-offers-new-insights-into-managing-trauma-patients/
2. RCEM Learning (2017). Cervical spine injury. Available at: https://www.rcemlearning.co.uk/references/cervical-spine-injury/
3. Michaleff ZA, Maher CG, Verhagen AP, et al. (2012). Accuracy of the Canadian C-spine rule and NEXUS to screen for clinically important cervical spine injury in patients following blunt trauma: a systematic review. Available at: https://www.ncbi.nlm.nih.gov/books/NBK110125/

Chapter 121

Neutropenic sepsis

Guideline:
NICE CG151 (Neutropenic sepsis: prevention and management in people with cancer): https://www.nice.org.uk/guidance/cg151

OUP disclaimer: Oxford University Press makes no representation, express or implied, that the drug dosages are correct and that the recommendations are an exclusive or mandatory course of care. All health professionals reading this text have a responsibility to evaluate its appropriateness and take the individual needs of the patient into account.

Local trust guidelines: please refer to your local guidelines as necessary.

Overview

Neutropenic sepsis is a medical emergency and a potentially serious complication of anticancer therapies. Systemic therapies to treat cancer such as chemotherapy, and in some cases radiotherapy, lower the body's natural immune system via bone marrow suppression. This results in increased susceptibility to, and poorer defence against, bacterial and viral infections which can lead to sepsis. Mortality from neutropenic sepsis can be as high as 21%, but this figure can be significantly reduced with rapid recognition and management.

Although many of the following principles apply, the management of acutely ill children with cancer is highly specialist and senior help should be sought if neutropenic sepsis is suspected in a child.

Diagnosis

History/diagnostic criteria

Neutropenic sepsis is defined as neutropenia (a low neutrophil count) ≤0.5 × 10^9/L, in conjunction with a temperature >38°C, or other symptoms consistent with sepsis.

> **All unwell patients on anticancer treatment should be considered as having neutropenic sepsis until proven otherwise.**

When neutropenic sepsis is suspected or patients are at risk of neutropenic sepsis, take a history to include the following:

- Fevers, rigors, hypothermia
- Symptoms suggesting a focus of infection: productive cough, shortness of breath, dysuria, diarrhoea
- Dehydration, reduced urine output
- Cognitive changes
- Risk factors for infection: central venous access, recent surgery or hospital admission, fungal infections
- Cancer treatment: type of chemotherapy, timing and duration of last dose, number of cycles
- Recent treatments: antibiotic therapy, granulocyte colony-stimulating factor (G-CSF) or corticosteroids
- Previous episodes of neutropenic sepsis
- Recent travel, contact with infectious diseases, animal exposure.

Examination

Use an ABCDE approach for examination (Table 121.1). Patients who are immunocompromised often do not present with an obvious source of infection.

Table 121.1 Examination findings in neutropenic sepsis

B	Signs suggestive of a respiratory source: productive cough, wheeze, crepitations Reduced oxygen saturations (may indicate poor peripheral perfusion) Tachypnoea
C	Tachycardia Hypotension Prolonged capillary refill time Mottled or cyanosed skin Cold peripheries ↓ urine output
D	Fever or hypothermia ↓ level of consciousness
E	Abdominal tenderness, particularly suprapubic (UTI) Rash: non-blanching (may indicate meningococcal disease), viral exanthem Breaks in skin integrity (ulcers, cellulitis, cuts, burns, skin infections) Ports, lines, and other central venous access devices

Investigations

Bedside

Urinalysis and MC&S: if urinary source of infection is suspected.

Bloods

- Blood gas: a VBG or ABG to include glucose and lactate can provide a rapid indication of the severity of illness
- FBC: demonstrates the extent of neutropenia and thrombocytopenia
- CRP: typically raised in infection and inflammation
- U&E: will highlight AKI or dehydration
- LFT: including albumin
- Coagulation profile
- Blood cultures: ideally taken before antibiotic treatment is commenced, providing that treatment is not delayed. Cultures should also be taken from any ports or lines the patient has.

Imaging

Chest X-ray if clinically indicated. It can be used to identify respiratory foci of infection. More sophisticated imaging such as CT or MRI may be indicated to further investigate in prolonged cases of neutropenic sepsis.

Management

All management should take place in liaison with the patient's named oncologist.

Acute management

- Neutropenic sepsis is a form of sepsis, therefore the usual sepsis protocols (see Chapter 122) should be followed. However, there are specific guidelines for the use of antimicrobial treatments in neutropenic sepsis (as follows)
- It is usual to isolate the patient in a side room if possible, as they are immunocompromised
- Central venous access devices should not be removed empirically
- Involve critical care early if the patient responds poorly to initial antibiotic and fluid therapy, as inotropic and vasopressor support may be required.

Antimicrobials

- **Do not** delay antibiotic treatment to await confirmation of neutropenia
- Empirical monotherapy with an IV beta lactam agent such as piperacillin with tazobactam (Tazocin®) should be given, unless the patient is penicillin allergic or local guidelines advise otherwise
- Do not switch the empirical antibiotics only because patients have a persistent fever. The antibiotics should be changed only if they deteriorate clinically or if there are microbiology results to prove that the empirical choice would be ineffective
- Consider switching IV to oral therapy after 48 hours in patients at low risk of complications
- Additional agents may be considered in the presence of persistent pyrexia or ongoing deterioration, suggesting a fungal or atypical source of infection
- Outpatient therapy may be appropriate for patients at low risk of developing complications, but appropriate safety net advice should be given to return to hospital in the event of deterioration
- Stop therapy when the patient has responded to treatment clinically, irrespective of their neutrophil count.

Special considerations

Patient education is imperative in aiding the rapid diagnosis of neutropenic sepsis. Teaching patients to seek medical attention early when they have worrying symptoms could drastically reduce their mortality.

Consider giving patients at risk of neutropenic sepsis the following advice in verbal and written form:

- Explain what neutropenia is and the signs of infection and sepsis
- Ensure that the patient has access to a thermometer
- Infection prevention: good oral hygiene, handwashing, cooking foods thoroughly, wearing hand protection for household cleaning or gardening
- How to obtain specialist oncology advice 24/7 and when to attend the emergency department
- Certain patients may be eligible for prophylaxis with fluoroquinolone antibiotics when they are expected to become neutropenic.

Further reading

1. Baid H, Creed F, Hargreaves J (eds) (2016). Sepsis. In: *Oxford Handbook of Critical Care Nursing*, 2nd ed (pp. 327–41). Oxford: Oxford University Press. Available at: https://doi.org/10.1093/med/9780198701071.003.0011
2. Watson M, Ward S, Vallath N, et al. (eds) (2019). Sepsis in the neutropenic patient. In: *Oxford Handbook of Palliative Care*, 3rd ed (pp. 785–8). Oxford: Oxford University Press. Available at: https://doi.org/10.1093/med/9780198745655.003.0029

Chapter 122

Sepsis

Guideline:
NICE NG51 (Sepsis: recognition, diagnosis, and early management): https://www.nice.org.uk/guidance/ng51

OUP disclaimer: Oxford University Press makes no representation, express or implied, that the drug dosages are correct and that the recommendations are an exclusive or mandatory course of care. All health professionals reading this text have a responsibility to evaluate its appropriateness and take the individual needs of the patient into account.

Local trust guidelines: please refer to your local guidelines as necessary.

Overview

Sepsis is a potentially life-threatening systemic response to an infection. It can be difficult to recognize, presenting in a myriad of ways, and it may mimic other conditions such as influenza or gastroenteritis. There is no single test or scoring system that accurately identifies sepsis; diagnosis relies on having a high index of suspicion. Sepsis carries a high morbidity and mortality, with the best outcomes resulting from early recognition and management. For pregnant patients, refer to Chapter 66. For neutropenic patients, refer to Chapter 121.

Diagnosis

History/diagnostic criteria

Patients may present with symptoms of a specific infection or in a vague, non-specific manner:

- Weakness/lethargy
- Altered behaviour/reduced consciousness
- Fevers, chills, rigors, sweats
- Myalgia/arthralgia
- Diarrhoea, vomiting
- Reduced fluid intake and reduced urine output.

Risk factors

- Aged >75 years or frail
- Immunosuppression (recent chemotherapy (see Chapter 121), taking steroids or other immunosuppressive drugs, diabetes mellitus, HIV infection, splenectomy, sickle cell disease)
- Recently postpartum or post miscarriage/termination of pregnancy (see Chapter 66)
- Recent trauma, surgery, or invasive procedure
- IV drug users
- Indwelling line/catheter
- Burns, skin infections, or other breach of skin integrity.

Examination

Take a full set of observations, then use an ABCDE approach to examine. Be systematic and thorough, especially in patients who are more difficult to assess (e.g. learning disabled, language barrier, etc.). For findings see Table 122.1.

Common examination pitfalls

- Temperature:
  - Patients who are elderly, very frail, receiving cancer treatments, or very unwell may not develop a raised temperature in sepsis
- Heart rate:
  - Elderly patients may develop an arrhythmia with sepsis rather than tachycardia
  - Patients may be on medications such as beta-blockers giving the false impression that their heart rate is normal
- Oxygen saturations:
  - Very low or unreadable oxygen saturations may be suggestive of poor peripheral circulation, which may or may not be due to shock.

Investigations

No test can 'prove' sepsis. Investigations help to identify potential sources of infection and assess the degree of organ dysfunction, e.g. AKI (see Chapter 46).

Table 122.1 Clinical findings in sepsis

	High risk findings	Moderate risk findings
B	• Respiratory rate ≥25 per minute • New need for supplemental oxygen (>40%) to maintain target saturations >92% • Cyanosis of lips, skin, or tongue	• Respiratory rate 21–24 per minute
C	• Systolic blood pressure <90mmHg **OR** >40mmHg drop from baseline • Heart rate >130bpm • Not passed urine in 18 hours **OR** <0.5mL/kg/hour urine output in catheterized patients • Mottled, ashen skin • Delayed capillary refill >3 seconds	• Systolic blood pressure 91–100mmHg • Heart rate 90–130bpm **OR** new arrhythmia • Not passed urine in 12–18 hours **OR** 0.5–1mL/kg/hr urine output in catheterized patients
D	• Objective evidence of altered mental state	• History from patient, friend, or relative of altered behaviour, mental state, or reduced functional ability • Temperature <36°C
E	• Non-blanching rash of skin	• Redness, swelling, or discharge at surgical site or breakdown of wound

Bedside
- ECG to assess potential new dysrhythmia
- Urine MC&S
- Sputum MC&S
- Blood glucose.

Bloods
- FBC
- U&E
- LFT
- Coagulation profile
- CRP
- VBG to include lactate and glucose
- Blood cultures.

Imaging
- Chest X-ray
- Abdominal USS/CT in suspected intra-abdominal sepsis.

Other
- Joint fluid aspiration in suspected septic arthritis (see Chapter 86)
- Ascitic fluid aspiration in suspected spontaneous bacterial peritonitis
- Skin swabs if suspected skin infection, e.g. diabetic ulcers
- Lumbar puncture if suspected meningitis (see Chapter 52) or encephalitis (see Chapter 49).

Management

Acute management

If in the community, transfer a patient meeting any of the high risk criteria in Table 122.1 to hospital urgently. Otherwise, clinical judgement should be used to decide if they can be treated safely in the community.

If meningitis is suspected, IM benzylpenicillin should be given prior to (but should not delay) hospital transfer (see Chapter 52). See Table 122.2 for management of the septic patient.

Discussion with a senior clinician

All patients diagnosed with suspected sepsis should be discussed with a senior clinician.

Patients who deteriorate despite appropriate treatment should be discussed with the critical care team as they may require multiorgan support, which might include:

- Invasive ventilation
- Vasopressor/inotropic support to maintain blood pressure and organ perfusion
- Renal replacement therapy to correct acidaemia and/or electrolyte imbalances.

Table 122.2 Management based on clinical findings

Clinical findings		Management
≥1 high risk criteria **OR** ≥2 moderate risk criteria **PLUS EITHER** lactate >2mmol/L **OR** has evidence of AKI	→	• Check bloods (see 'Investigations') • Give maximum dose broad-spectrum antibiotics with 1 hour, e.g. Tazocin® 4.5g • Immediate senior review and discuss with consultant
Any high risk criteria **PLUS EITHER** lactate >4mmol/L **OR** systolic blood pressure <90mmHg	→	• Give IV fluid bolus urgently (see Chapter 96) • Refer to critical care
Any high risk criteria **AND** lactate of 2–4mmol/litre	→	• Give IV fluid bolus urgently
Any high risk criteria **BUT** lactate <2mmol	→	• Consider giving IV fluid bolus
≥2 moderate risk criteria **OR** Systolic blood pressure of 90–100mmHg	→	• Check bloods as above • Review within 1 hour

In all of the above scenarios:

- Monitor continuously or at least every 30 minutes
- Request consultant review if failure to respond to antibiotics/fluids within 1 hour:
  - Systolic blood pressure persistently <90mmHg
  - Reduced GCS score despite resuscitation
  - Respiratory rate >25/minute or new need for mechanical ventilation
  - Lactate not reduced by >20%

Sepsis Six

The 'Sepsis Six' is a commonly used mnemonic to remember the steps which should be implemented within an hour of identifying sepsis:

- Take blood cultures
- Take bloods for lactate
- 'Take' urine, i.e. catheterize and monitor urine output
- Give oxygen if appropriate
- Give IV antibiotics
- Give a fluid challenge.

Treatment after stabilization

Monitoring

Initially patients should be observed at least hourly. Consider admitting to a monitored or high-dependency bed.

Antibiotics

Antibiotic therapy should be 'targeted' as soon as possible; continuing broad-spectrum antibiotics unnecessarily carries a risk of diarrhoea, *Clostridium difficile* infection, and antibiotic resistance. Once a source of infection has been identified, local guidelines should be followed to convert to narrow-spectrum therapy guided by microbiology results and sensitivities. Discuss with the duty microbiologist if unsure about the type and/or duration of antibiotic therapy needed.

Regular medications

Consider which should be withheld or stopped; these might include nephrotoxic agents, agents that may interact with antibiotics, or agents that may lower blood pressure. Review the patient's drug chart carefully and if unsure speak to a senior clinician or pharmacist.

Treatment of underlying source

Some infections causing sepsis will require surgical intervention for definitive treatment, e.g. abscesses/collections, appendicitis, perforated abdominal viscus, retained products of conception. Adequate resuscitation is critical as unstable, under-resuscitated septic patients are extremely high risk when undergoing general anaesthesia. If a septic patient requires emergency surgery, an early anaesthetic review is vital.

Special considerations

Pregnancy

Some antibiotics (e.g. tetracyclines) are contraindicated and others may require dose adjustment—consult the BNF and/or a pharmacist if unsure.

Radiation risk to fetus and maternal breast tissue must be weighed against the diagnostic benefits of X-ray and CT. Discussion may be required between senior clinicians and radiologists.

Renal and hepatic impairment

Some antibiotics require dose adjustment—consult the BNF and/or a pharmacist if unsure.

Further reading

1. The UK Sepsis Trust website. Available at: www.sepsistrust.org
2. qSOFA. What is qSOFA? Available at: https://qsofa.org/what.php

Chapter 123

Tachycardia

Guideline:
Resuscitation Council UK (Tachycardias): https://www.resus.org.uk/library/2021-resuscitation-guidelines/adult-advanced-life-support-guidelines

OUP disclaimer: Oxford University Press makes no representation, express or implied, that the drug dosages are correct and that the recommendations are an exclusive or mandatory course of care. All health professionals reading this text have a responsibility to evaluate its appropriateness and take the individual needs of the patient into account.

Local trust guidelines: please refer to your local guidelines as necessary.

Overview

Tachycardia is defined as a heart rate >100bpm. Tachycardia encompasses a number of different arrhythmias, some of which are unstable and require urgent treatment to avoid the patient deteriorating to the point of cardiac arrest.

Diagnosis

Risk factors

- Cardiac:
  - Underlying cardiac disease, e.g. AF, cardiomyopathy
  - Ischaemia
- Respiratory:
  - PE
- Endocrine:
  - Hyperthyroidism
  - Phaeochromocytoma
  - Acromegaly
- Metabolic:
  - Alcohol
  - Caffeine
  - Hypoglycaemia
  - Hyperkalaemia
  - Illicit drugs, e.g. cocaine
  - Iatrogenic, e.g. atropine
- Neurological:
  - Anxiety
  - Pain
- Systemic:
  - Exercise
  - Hypovolaemia
  - Anaemia
  - Infection/sepsis
  - Severe fatigue
  - Pregnancy.

History

If the patient is stable, a brief history should include:

- Symptoms of tachycardia (syncope/presyncope, chest pain, dyspnoea)
- Duration of tachycardia symptoms and whether symptoms are exercise related
- Past medical history and cardiovascular risk factors
- Medication history including alcohol and drug use
- Presence of family history of sudden cardiac death.

Examination

Use an ABCDE approach (Table 123.1), paying particular attention to adverse features (Box 123.1).

Table 123.1 ABCDE approach to examination and initial investigations in a tachycardic patient

B	• Respiratory rate • Oxygen saturations—check for hypoxia • Auscultate—bibasal crepitations might indicate heart failure (Box 123.1)
C	• Palpate central pulse—if absent proceed to cardiac arrest algorithm (see Chapter 116) • Blood pressure—may be low due to shock (Box 123.1) • Heart rate—determine if pulse is regular or irregular • Auscultate for murmurs • Assess JVP (if raised might indicate heart failure) (Box 123.1) • Peripheral perfusion—peripheries might be cool and clammy with prolonged capillary refill time • Insert a wide-bore cannula and send bloods
D	• Assess for new confusion or altered GCS score (Box 123.1) • Measure blood glucose
E	• Examine for peripheral oedema • Examine for pacemaker or implantable cardiac defibrillator

Box 123.1 Adverse features of tachycardia

The presence of these features signify that the patient is unstable and at high risk of sudden deterioration and death.

- Heart failure:
  - Pulmonary oedema, raised JVP
- Ischaemia:
  - Ongoing chest pain and/or features of ischaemia on ECG
- Shock:
  - Systolic blood pressure <90mmHg, cold or clammy peripheries, confusion or impaired consciousness, diaphoresis, pallor
- Syncope:
  - Loss of consciousness due to reduced cardiac output leading to impaired cerebral perfusion.

Investigations

Bedside

- ECG (Table 123.2):
  - Determine the heart rate, QRS duration, if the RR interval is regular or irregular, QTc interval
  - Look for features of ischaemia: ST-segment and T wave changes, pathological Q waves.

Table 123.2 Classification of tachycardias

QRS duration	Regular RR interval	Irregular RR interval
>120ms (broad)	• Ventricular tachycardia (VT) • Supraventricular tachycardia with bundle branch block	• Ventricular fibrillation (VF) • AF with pre-excitation • AF with bundle branch block • Polymorphic VT (torsades de pointes)
<120ms (narrow)	• Sinus tachycardia • AV node re-entry tachycardia (AVNRT) • AV re-entry tachycardia (AVRT) • Atrial flutter with regular AV conduction block	• AF • Atrial flutter with variable AV conduction block

Bloods

- FBC—anaemia may exacerbate symptoms
- U&E, including phosphate, calcium, and magnesium—deranged renal function may lead to electrolyte disturbances, and derangement of electrolytes affects myocardial stability and thus predisposes to arrhythmias
- Cardiac troponins—interpret with caution as cardiac troponins can be raised by tachycardia without underlying myocardial infarction
- TFT—hyperthyroidism can cause tachycardia.

Imaging

- Chest X-ray:
  - Pulmonary oedema, cardiomegaly
- Echocardiogram:
  - Interpretation is difficult during tachycardia
  - Once heart rate is controlled, echocardiography can give aetiological information (regional wall motion abnormalities due to infarction, structural and valvular abnormalities, and heart failure).

Management

Acute management

Unstable patient with adverse features

Confirm the presence of a pulse and then proceed with an ABCDE approach. Seek senior help.

A. Ensure airway is patent, secure, and protected
B. Give oxygen if hypoxic
C. Obtain IV access. Perform emergency synchronized DC cardioversion (with anaesthetic support for sedation):
  - Broad complex tachycardia and AF: start with 120–150J. Gradually increase the energy with each shock if this fails
  - Atrial flutter and regular narrow complex tachycardia: start with 70–120J. Gradually increase the energy with each shock if this fails
  - After three unsuccessful attempts, give 300mg amiodarone IV over 10–20 minutes before the next shock
D. Treat any underlying reversible causes (electrolyte abnormalities, ischaemia, sepsis, hypovolaemia).

Stable patient with no adverse features

The management depends on the type of the tachycardia (Table 123.2). Definitive treatment may not be required in some cases although it may be necessary to treat the underlying cause. Assess with an ABCDE approach before starting specific treatments.

A. Ensure airway is patent, secure, and protected
B. Give oxygen if hypoxic
C. Record a 12-lead ECG, consider continuous cardiac monitoring, obtain adequate IV access.
D. Identify and treat any underlying causes (electrolyte abnormalities, ischaemia, sepsis, hypovolaemia, pain, anxiety, etc.).

Regular narrow complex tachycardia

- Sinus tachycardia:
  - This is not an arrhythmia
  - Treat underlying causes, e.g. anaemia, infection
- Supraventricular tachycardia:
  - Start with vagal manoeuvres, e.g. Valsalva manoeuvres
  - If vagal manoeuvres fail, give adenosine IV (do not administer if the patient has asthma). Ensure ongoing cardiac monitoring and recording of rhythm strip. Use a large cannula in a large vein so it can be given as a rapid bolus, and warn the patient that they will feel very unwell while the medication is being administered:
    - Start with 6mg
    - If this fails, give 12mg
    - If this fails, give a further 12mg
    - If adenosine is contraindicated, consider verapamil 2.5–5mg IV over 2 minutes
  - If adenosine fails, seek expert advice:
    - Failure of vagal manoeuvres and adenosine suggests underlying atrial flutter with regular AV block. This may respond to rate control with beta-blockers or diltiazem.

Irregular narrow complex tachycardia

- AF (see Chapter 4) or atrial flutter with variable AV block:
  - Rate control:
    - Beta-blockers are first line, e.g. bisoprolol 2.5mg
    - Diltiazem or verapamil can be used if beta-blockers are contraindicated or not tolerated
    - In heart failure, consider digoxin or amiodarone
  - Rhythm control with chemical or electrical cardioversion:
    - Chemical cardioversion with amiodarone, flecainide, or propafenone may be done under senior supervision if duration of AF <48 hours
    - Electrical cardioversion is also an option if duration of AF <48 hours
  - Assess the risk of thromboembolism and the need for anticoagulation—if the patient has been in AF for >48 hours, cardioversion should not be attempted until they have been anticoagulated for 3 weeks.

Regular broad complex tachycardia

- Monomorphic VT:
  - 300mg amiodarone IV over 20–60 minutes, followed by an amiodarone infusion (900mg over 24 hours)
- Tachycardia with bundle branch block:
  - Treat as for regular narrow complex tachycardia
  - **NOTE:** if there is any doubt about this diagnosis, then treat as monomorphic VT.

Irregular broad complex tachycardia

- VF:
  - VF is not compatible with life
  - Initiate cardiac arrest algorithm (see Chapter 116)
- AF with pre-excitation (includes Wolff–Parkinson–White syndrome):
  - There is high risk of deterioration to VF
  - Synchronized DC cardioversion is advised
- Polymorphic VT (torsades de pointes):
  - 2g IV magnesium (8mmol or 4mL of 50% magnesium sulphate) over 10 minutes
  - Stop all drugs that prolong QTc
  - Correct electrolyte abnormalities
- AF with bundle branch block:
  - Treat as irregular narrow complex arrhythmia
  - **NOTE:** if there is any doubt about this diagnosis, then treat as AF with pre-excitation.

Treatment after stabilization

- Repeat ABCDE assessment
- Repeat 12-lead ECG to confirm termination of the tachycardia and identify any aetiological factors (ischaemia, long QTc, etc.)
- Repeat bloods: electrolytes to ensure adequate correction, cardiac troponin to assess the trend of change
- Consider echocardiography
- Discuss with cardiology for advice on further investigations, management, and outpatient follow-up.

Further reading

1. Life in the Fastlane. ECG differentiation of VT versus SVT with bundle branch block. Available at: https://litfl.com/vt-versus-svt-ecg-library/
2. Life in the Fastlane. Example ECGs. Available at: https://litfl.com/ecg-differential-diagnosis-ecg-library/

Index

For the benefit of digital users, indexed terms that span two pages (e.g., 52–53) may, on occasion, appear on only one of those pages.

Notes
Tables, figures, and boxes are indicated by *t*, *f*, and *b* following the page number

J

K

L

T